DISEASE CONTROL PRIORITIES • THIRD EDITION

Essential Surgery

DISEASE CONTROL PRIORITIES • THIRD EDITION

Series Editors

Dean T. Jamison

Rachel Nugent

Hellen Gelband

Susan Horton

Prabhat Jha

Ramanan Laxminarayan

Volumes in the Series

Essential Surgery

Reproductive, Maternal, Newborn, and Child Health

Cancer

Mental, Neurological, and Substance Use Disorders

Cardiovascular, Respiratory, Renal, and Endocrine Disorders

HIV/AIDS, STIs, Tuberculosis, and Malaria

Injury Prevention and Environmental Health

Child and Adolescent Development

Disease Control Priorities: Improving Health and Reducing Poverty

DISEASE CONTROL PRIORITIES

Budgets constrain choices. Policy analysis helps decision makers achieve the greatest value from limited available resources. In 1993, the World Bank published *Disease Control Priorities in Developing Countries* (DCP1), an attempt to systematically assess the cost-effectiveness (value for money) of interventions that would address the major sources of disease burden in low- and middle-income countries. The World Bank's 1993 *World Development Report* on health drew heavily on *DCP1*'s findings to conclude that specific interventions against noncommunicable diseases were cost-effective, even in environments in which substantial burdens of infection and undernutrition persisted.

DCP2, published in 2006, updated and extended *DCP1* in several aspects, including explicit consideration of the implications for health systems of expanded intervention coverage. One way that health systems expand intervention coverage is through selected platforms that deliver interventions that require similar logistics but deliver interventions from different packages of conceptually related interventions, for example, against cardiovascular disease. Platforms often provide a more natural unit for investment than do individual interventions. Analysis of the costs of packages and platforms—and of the health improvements they can generate in given epidemiological environments—can help to guide health system investments and development.

The third edition of *DCP* is being completed. *DCP3* differs importantly from *DCP1* and *DCP2* by extending and consolidating the concepts of platforms and packages and by offering explicit consideration of the financial risk protection objective of health systems. In populations lacking access to health insurance or prepaid care, medical expenses that are high relative to income can be impoverishing. Where incomes are low, seemingly inexpensive medical procedures can have catastrophic financial effects. *DCP3* offers an approach to explicitly include financial protection as well as the distribution across income groups of financial and health outcomes resulting from policies (for example, public finance) to increase intervention uptake. The task in all of the *DCP* volumes has been to combine the available science about interventions implemented in very specific locales and under very specific conditions with informed judgment to reach reasonable conclusions about the impact of intervention mixes in diverse environments. *DCP3*'s broad aim is to delineate essential intervention packages and their related delivery platforms to assist decision makers in allocating often tightly constrained budgets so that health system objectives are maximally achieved.

DCP3's nine volumes are being published in 2015 and 2016 in an environment in which serious discussion continues about quantifying the sustainable development goal (SDG) for health. *DCP3*'s analyses are well-placed to assist in choosing the means to attain the health SDG and assessing the related costs. Only when these volumes, and the analytic efforts on which they are based, are completed will we be able to explore SDG-related and other broad policy conclusions and generalizations. The final *DCP3* volume will report those conclusions. Each individual volume will provide valuable specific policy analyses on the full range of interventions, packages, and policies relevant to its health topic.

More than 500 individuals and multiple institutions have contributed to *DCP3*. We convey our acknowledgments elsewhere in this volume. Here we express our particular gratitude to the Bill & Melinda Gates Foundation for its sustained financial support, to the InterAcademy Medical Panel (and its U.S. affiliate, the Institute of Medicine of the National Academy of Sciences), and to the External and Corporate Relations Publishing and Knowledge division of the World Bank. Each played a critical role in this effort.

Dean T. Jamison
Rachel Nugent
Hellen Gelband
Susan Horton
Prabhat Jha
Ramanan Laxminarayan

VOLUME **1**

DISEASE CONTROL PRIORITIES • THIRD EDITION

Essential Surgery

EDITORS

Haile T. Debas
Peter Donkor
Atul Gawande
Dean T. Jamison
Margaret E. Kruk
Charles N. Mock

WORLD BANK GROUP

ISBN (paper): 978-1-4648-0346-8
ISBN (electronic): 978-1-4648-0367-3
DOI: 10.1596/978-1-4648-0346-8

Cover photo: The 16 Makara hospital in Cambodia's remote Preah Vihear province is equipped with modern equipment. The maintenance of 16 Makara is supported by the World Bank and other international donors through the Health Sector Support Program and the Cambodia Second Health Sector Support Program. Photo: © Chhor Sokunthea/World Bank. Further permission required for reuse.

Cover and interior design: Debra Naylor, Naylor Design, Washington, DC

Library of Congress Cataloging-in-Publication Data
Essential surgery / volume editors, Haile T. Debas, Peter Donkor, Atul Gawande, Dean T. Jamison, Margaret E. Kruk, Charles N. Mock.
 p ; cm. — (Disease control priorities ; v. 1)
 Previously published in: Disease control priorities in developing countries, 2nd ed. c2006.
 ISBN 978-1-4648-0346-8 (v. 1 : pb) — ISBN 978-1-4648-0097-9 (v. 1 : hc)
 I. Debas, Haile T., editor. II. Disease control priorities in developing countries. III. Series: Disease control priorities ; v. 1.
 [DNLM: 1. General Surgery—economics. 2. Developing Countries.   WA 395]
 RD27.42
 362.197—dc23
                                        2014037594

Contents

Foreword

The past few decades have seen enormous changes in the global burden of disease. Although many people, especially those living in (or near) poverty and other privations, are familiar with heavy burdens and much disease, the term "global burden of disease" emerged in public health and in health economics only in recent decades. It was coined to describe what ails people, when, and where, and just as reliable quantification is difficult, so too is agreeing on units of analysis. Does this term truly describe the burden of disease of the globe? Of a nation? A city?

We have also learned a thing or two about how to assess this global burden, and how to reveal its sharp local variation and transformation with changing conditions ranging from urbanization to a global rise in obesity (Murray, Lopez, and Jamison 1994; Murray and Lopez 1997; Lopez and others 2006; Mathers, Fat, and Boerma 2008; Jamison and others 2013; Lozano and others 2013). Measuring illness has never been easy, nor has attributing a death—whether premature or at the end of fourscore years—to a specific cause (Yarushalmy and Palmer 1959; Rothman 1976; Byass 2010; Byass and others 2013). Even countries with sound vital registries generate data of varying quality, given that cause of death is rarely confirmed by autopsy (Mathers and others 2005; Mahapatra and others 2007). When nonlethal or slowly debilitating illness is added to considerations of burden of disease, the challenge of both measurement and etiologic claims can appear overwhelming (Kleinman 1995; Arnesen and Nord 1999; Salomon and others 2012; Voigt and King 2014).

The challenges of measuring the burden of disease only get more complex when attempting to use the category of surgical disease. For starters, even experts do not agree on definitions of ostensibly simple terms such as "surgical disease" (Debas and others 2006; Duba and Hill 2007;

Ozgediz and others 2009; Bickler and others 2010). Some illnesses rarely considered to be surgical problems pose threats to health if neglected long enough. Some trends are clear, however. Take the examples offered by Haiti and Rwanda, where different types of trauma (intentional or the result of crush injuries) account for a majority of young-adult deaths. How many of these deaths are classified as attributable to surgical disease? If someone dies of acute abdomen—and if his or her death is recorded at all—was it attributed to appendicitis or to enteric fever? Are these infectious complications of surgical disease or surgical complications of infectious disease? If a child with untreated epilepsy falls into a fire and succumbs from burns, how is this death reported, if it is registered at all? Clinicians who work in settings far from any pathology laboratory have seen infected tumors (misdiagnosed as primary infection) as often as they have discovered that a suspected breast cancer was a long-untreated canalicular abscess. Brain tumors are revealed to be tuberculomas and vice versa.

A sound grasp of the burden of disease is essential to those seeking data-driven methods to design and evaluate policies aimed at decreasing premature death and suffering (Nordberg, Holmberg, and Kiugu 1995; Taira, McQueen, and Burkle 2009; Poenaru, Ozgediz, and Gosselin 2014). But surgical disease was not often on the agenda. The immensity and complexity of the task of quantifying the surgical burden of disease has led many to avoid that task, leading to an analytic vacuum with adverse consequences. For too long, the global health movement has failed to count surgery as an integral part of public health. Prevailing wisdom dictated that the surgical disease burden was too low, surgical expenses too high, and delivery of care too complicated. The predecessor to this volume, the second edition of *Disease Control Priorities in Developing Countries*

(*DCP2*; Jamison and others 2006), changed this paradigm. Published in 2006, it included, for the first time in a major global health platform, sustained attention to surgery. The editors sought to marshal the experience of its contributors to help quantify and classify the burden of surgical disease. Admittedly, this most widely cited estimate of surgical need—11 percent of the global burden of disease was surgical—was based on the best educated guesses of a convenience sample of 18 surgeons on an online survey. Nonetheless, this figure was later validated by the common experience of providers and patients alike from the poorest reaches of the world: the burden of surgical disease was never trivial.

DCP3 builds upon this foundation and substantially improves it. It enhances our understanding of *DCP2*'s pioneering work with more robust methodology. Over the years, researchers—led by the editors of and many of the contributors to this volume—have devoted attention to cancers, orthopedic injuries, disfigurements after burns, congenital defects such as cleft lip and palate, blindness from cataracts, and the many causes of death from acute surgical needs. This volume collates the knowledge gained through the increased attention to global surgery since 2006.

This new volume of *DCP* underlines the central importance of surgical care because, by these measures, surgical disease is thought to account for a significant portion of the global disease burden. The *Essential Surgery* volume of *DCP3* helps definitively dispel many of the myths about surgery's role in global health, in part by showing the very large health burden from conditions that are primarily or extensively treatable by surgery. It dispels the myth that surgery is too expensive by showing that many essential surgical services rank among the most cost-effective of all heath interventions. This volume begins to dispel the myth that surgery is not feasible in settings of poverty by documenting many successful programs that have improved capacity, increased access, and enhanced quality of surgical care in countries across the globe.

As argued many times in the past—and worth repeating to clinical colleagues, students, trainees, and diverse interlocutors—global surgery is one of the most exciting frontiers in the quest for global health equity. Patients and providers, along with those who set and evaluate policies, will want (or need) to join this quest if we are to avert unnecessary suffering. We all have cause to be grateful for the many individuals whose time and energy have been invested in producing the wealth of knowledge presented in the *Essential Surgery* volume of *DCP3*.

Paul Farmer
Harvard Medical School
Brigham and Women's Hospital
Partners in Health

REFERENCES

Arnesen, T., and E. Nord. 1999. "The Value of DALY Life: Problems with Ethics and Validity of Disability Adjusted Life Years." *BMJ* 319 (7222): 423–25.

Bickler, S., D. Ozgediz, R. Gosselin, T. Weiser, D. Speigel, and others. 2010. "Key Concepts for Estimating the Burden of Surgical Conditions and the Unmet Need for Surgical Care." *World Journal of Surgery* 34 (3): 374–80.

Byass, P. 2010. "The Imperfect World of Global Health Estimates." *PLOS Medicine* 7: e1001006.

———, M. de Courten, W. J. Graham, L. Laflamme, A. McCaw-Binns, and others. 2013. "Reflections on the Global Burden of Disease 2010 Estimates." *PLOS Medicine* 10: e1001477.

Debas, H. T., R. Gosselin, C. McCord, and A. Thind. 2006. "Surgery." In *Disease Control Priorities in Developing Countries*, 2nd edition, edited by D. T. Jamison, J. G. Breman, A. R. Measham, G. Alleyene, M. Claeson, D. B. Evans, P. Jha, A. Mills, and P. Musgrove, 1245–59. Washington, DC: World Bank and Oxford University Press.

Duba, R. B., and A. G. Hill. 2007. "Surgery in Developing Countries: Should Surgery Have a Role in Population-Based Health Care?" *Bulletin of the American College of Surgeons* 92 (5): 12–18.

Jamison, D. T., J. G. Breman, A. R. Measham, G. Alleyne, M. Claeson, D. B. Evans, P. Jha, A. Mills, and P. Musgrove, eds. 2006. *Disease Control Priorities in Developing Countries*, 2nd edition. Washington, DC: World Bank and Oxford University Press.

Jamison, D. T., L. H. Summers, G. Alleyne, K. J. Arrow, S. Berkley, and others. 2013. "Global Health 2035: A World Converging within a Generation." *The Lancet* 382 (9908): 1898–955.

Kleinman, A. 1995. "A Critique of Objectivity in International Health." In *Writing at the Margin: Discourse between Anthropology and Medicine*, edited by A. Kleinman. Berkeley, CA: University of California Press.

Lopez, A. D., C. D. Mathers, M. Ezzati, D. T. Jamison, and C. J. L. Murray. 2006. "Global and Regional Burden of Disease and Risk Factors, 2001: Systematic Analysis of Population Health Data." *The Lancet* 367 (9524): 1747–57.

Lozano, R., M. Naghavi, K. Foreman, S. Lim, K. Shibuya, and others. 2013. "Global and Regional Mortality from 235 Causes of Death for 20 Age Groups in 1990 and 2010: A Systematic Analysis for the Global Burden of Disease Study 2010." *The Lancet* 380 (9859): 2095–128.

Mahapatra, P., K. Shibuya, A. D. Lopez, F. Coullare, F. C. Notzon, and others. 2007. "Civil Registration Systems and Vital Statistics: Successes and Missed Opportunities." *The Lancet* 370 (9599): 1653–63.

Mathers, C., D. M. Fat, and J. T. Boerma. 2008. *The Global Burden of Disease: 2004 Update*. Geneva, Switzerland: World Health Organization.

Mathers, C. D., M. A. Fat, M. Inoue, C. Rao, and A. D. Lopez. 2005. "Counting the Dead and What They Died From: An Assessment of the Global Status of Cause of Death Data." *Bulletin of the World Health Organization* 83 (3): 161–240.

Murray, C. J. L., and A. D. Lopez. 1997. "Global Mortality, Disability, and the Contribution of Risk Factors: Global Burden of Disease Study." *The Lancet* 349 (9063): 1436–42.

———, and D. T. Jamison. 1994. "The Global Burden of Disease in 1990: Summary Results, Sensitivity Analysis and Future Directions." *Bulletin of the World Health Organization* 72 (3): 495–509.

Nordberg, E., S. Holmberg, and S. Kiugu. 1995. "Output of Major Surgery in Developing Countries: Towards a Quantitative Evaluation and Planning Tool." *Tropical and Geographical Medicine* 47 (5): 206–11.

Ozgediz, D., R. Hsia, T. Weiser, R. Gosselin, D. Spiegel, and others. 2009. "Population Health Metrics for Surgery: Effective Coverage of Surgical Services in Low-Income and Middle-Income Countries." *World Journal of Surgery* 33 (1): 1–5.

Poenaru, D., D. Ozgediz, and R. A. Gosselin. 2014. "Burden, Need, or Backlog: A Call for Improved Metrics for the Global Burden of Surgical Disease." *International Journal of Surgery* 12 (5): 483–86.

Rothman, K. J. 1976. "Causes." *American Journal of Epidemiology* 104 (6): 587–92.

Salomon, J. A., T. Vos, D. R. Hogan, M. Gagnon, M. Naghavi, and others. 2012. "Common Values in Assessing Health Outcomes from Disease and Injury: Disability Weights Measurement Study for the Global Burden of Disease Study 2010." *The Lancet* 380 (9859): 2129–43.

Taira, B. R., K. McQueen, and F. M. Burkle. 2009. "Burden of Surgical Disease: Does the Literature Reflect the Scope of the International Crisis?" *World Journal of Surgery* 33 (5): 893–98.

Voigt, K., and N. B. King. 2014. "Disability Weights in the Global Burden of Disease 2010 Study: Two Steps Forward, One Step Back?" *Bulletin of the World Health Organization* 92 (3): 226–28.

Yerushalmy, J., and C. E. Palmer. 1959. "On the Methodology of Investigations of Etiologic Factors in Chronic Diseases." *Journal of Chronic Disease* 10 (1): 27–40.

Preface

Conditions that are treated primarily or frequently by surgery constitute a significant portion of the global burden of disease. In 2012, injuries killed nearly 5 million people, and about 270,000 women died from complications of pregnancy. Many of these deaths, as well as deaths from abdominal emergencies, congenital anomalies, and other causes, could be prevented by improved access to quality surgical care. However, surgical care itself has barely been addressed within the field of global health. A growing number of people from diverse backgrounds are attempting to change this, and to increase access to appropriate, safe, surgical care in low- and middle-income countries. The *Essential Surgery* volume of *Disease Control Priorities*, third edition (*DCP3*), contributes to these efforts by (1) better defining the health burden from conditions requiring surgery, (2) identifying those surgical procedures that are the most cost-effective and cost-beneficial, and (3) describing the health care policies and platforms that can universally deliver these procedures safely and effectively.

Essential Surgery identifies and studies a group of "essential" surgical conditions and the procedures needed to treat them. These surgical conditions can be defined as those that (1) are primarily or extensively treated by surgery, (2) have a large health burden, and (3) can be successfully treated by surgical procedures that are cost-effective and feasible to promote globally. To address these conditions, the authors derive a set of 44 essential surgical procedures. These include procedures to treat injuries, obstetric complications, abdominal emergencies, cataracts, and congenital anomalies, among others. We estimate that universal access to this package of essential procedures would prevent about 1.5 million deaths per year or 6 to 7 percent of all preventable deaths in low- and middle-income countries. These procedures rank among the most

cost-effective of all health interventions. They are eminently feasible to promote globally, and many could be delivered at first-level hospitals.

The large burden of surgical conditions, cost-effectiveness of essential surgical procedures, and strong public demand for those procedures suggest that universal coverage of essential surgery should be implemented early on the path to universal health coverage. Implementation would include measures such as using public funds to ensure access to essential procedures and including them in the packages covered by national health insurance programs. Such measures would also offer financial risk protection against medical impoverishment from the costs of surgical care. Surgery should be considered an indispensable component of a properly functioning health system and can be a means for strengthening the entire system, thus increasing the return on investment.

Not covered in this volume are procedures to treat other surgical conditions, such as transplantation, or surgery for cancer and vascular disease. Improving access to these procedures will also have benefits. But for prioritization of the sequencing and use of public funds, efforts to ensure greater access to the essential surgical services should be undertaken first, relative to increased investment in those conditions that are more expensive to treat or that have smaller health impacts.

The editors and authors of *Essential Surgery* hope that this volume will increase efforts to improve access to and quality of essential surgical care in low- and middle-income countries. We especially hope to stimulate increased attention to addressing essential surgery on the part of two very different communities: the global health community and the surgical community. With the exception of obstetric care, the global health community has largely failed to address the unmet need for surgery. The surgical community, in turn, has not tackled broader requirements for incorporating surgery into resource-constrained health systems (with the important exceptions of exploring task-sharing and improving safety of care). We hope that this volume invigorates the global health community to advocate for inclusion of essential surgery as part of universal health coverage and as an integral part of a well-functioning health system. Likewise, we hope that this volume motivates the surgical community to advocate for increased investment in surgical capabilities in first-level hospitals and for greater access to the basic essential procedures. Ensuring that essential surgical services are available to everyone who needs them when they need them is in part about improving training in safe surgical care and techniques, and in part about improving the functioning of health systems, including better monitoring and evaluation and developing appropriate financing mechanisms. It is also about promoting equity, social justice, and human rights.

We thank the following individuals who provided valuable comments and assistance on this effort: Brianne Adderley, Elizabeth Brouwer, Kristen Danforth, Anna Dare, Mary Fisk, Nancy Lammers, Rachel Nugent, Devlan O'Connor, Zach Olson, Rumit Pancholi, Carlos Rossel, Nopadol Wora-Urai, and *The Lancet* Commission on Global Surgery, especially John Meara, Sarah Greenberg, Andrew Leather, and Gavin Yamey. The authors also thank the reviewers organized by the Institute of Medicine and the InterAcademy Medical Panel (listed separately in this volume) and the following additional reviewers for their insightful comments: Wame Baravilala, Michael Cotton, Raul Garcia, John S. Greenspan, Caris Grimes, Russell Gruen, Jaymie Henry, Robert Lane, Jenny Löfgren, Jane Maraka, Pär Nordin, Ebenezer Anno Nyako, Akinyinka O. Omigbodun, Norgrove Penny, Dan Poenaru, Teri Reynolds, Nitin Verma, Lee Wallis, Benjamin C. Warf, David Watters, and Andreas Wladis. We also thank the following professional societies that helped to identify reviewers: the African Federation for Emergency Medicine; the American College of Surgeons; the College of Surgeons of East, Central and Southern Africa; the International Collaboration for Essential Surgery; the International Society of Surgery; the Panamerican Trauma Society; and the West African College of Surgeons. We especially thank Rachel Cox for her hard work keeping this large endeavor well organized.

Haile T. Debas
Peter Donkor
Atul Gawande
Dean T. Jamison
Margaret E. Kruk
Charles N. Mock

Abbreviations

ADLA	adenolymphangitis
AIDS	acquired immune deficiency syndrome
ALS	advanced life support
AMO	assistant medical officer
ANAC	African Network of Associate Clinicians
ARM	anorectal malformation
ASA	American Society of Anesthesiologists
BC	benefit-cost
BCA	benefit-cost analysis
BCVA	best-corrected visual acuity
BCR	benefit-cost ratio
BLD	banana leaf dressing
BLS	basic life support
bpm	beats per minute
BPOC	Basic Package of Oral Care
CC	Copenhagen Consensus
CEA	cost-effectiveness analysis
CFR	case fatality rate
CLP	cleft lip and palate
CYP	couple-year of protection
DALY	disability-adjusted life year
DCP	Disease Control Priorities
DCP2	*Disease Control Priorities in Developing Countries*, second edition
DCP3	*Disease Control Priorities*, third edition
D&C	dilation and curettage
ECCE	extracapsular cataract extraction
ECG	electrocardiogram
EESC	Emergency and Essential Surgical Care
EHCP	Essential Health Care Program
EMLA	eutectic mixture of local anesthetics
EMRI	Emergency Management and Research Institute
EMS	emergency medical service
ETV	endoscopic third ventriculostomy
EVA	electric vacuum aspiration
FI	fascial interposition
FIGO	International Federation of Gynecology and Obstetrics

GBD	Global Burden of Disease study
GCCCC	Guwahati Comprehensive Cleft Care Center
GCS	Glasgow Coma Score
GDP	gross domestic product
GHE	Global Health Estimates
GHS	Ghana Hernia Society
GIEESC	Global Initiative for Emergency and Essential Surgery Care
GNI	gross national income
GPELF	Global Programme to Eliminate Lymphatic Filariasis
HD	Hirschsprung's disease
HDI	Human Development Index
HIC	high-income country
HIV	human immunodeficiency virus
HPV	human papilloma virus
IA	inflammatory arthropathies
ICD-9	International Classification of Diseases, Ninth Revision
ICER	incremental cost-effectiveness ratio
IMEESC	Integrated Management of Emergency and Essential Surgical Care
ISO	International Organization for Standardization
ISOFS	International Society of Obstetric Fistula Surgeons
IOL	intraocular lens
IUD	intrauterine device
IVD	intra vas device
LBP	low back pain
LE	life expectancy
LF	lymphatic filariasis
LIC	low-income country
LMICs	low- and middle-income countries
LYS	life-year saved
M&M	Morbidity and Mortality Conference
MBBHS	
M&E Matrix	*Monitoring the Building Blocks of Health Systems* Monitoring and Evaluation Matrix
MDA	mass drug administration
MDG	Millennium Development Goals
MEBO	moist exposed burn ointment
MIC	middle-income country
MLP	midlevel provider
MMR	maternal mortality ratio
mm	millimeter
MSICS	manual small-incision cataract surgery
MSK	musculoskeletal system
MVA	manual vacuum aspiration
NGO	nongovernmental organization
NHANES	National Health and Nutrition Examination Survey (U.S.)
NHS	National Health Service (U.K.)
NIS	Nationwide Inpatient Sample
NPC	nonphysician clinician
NSAID	nonsteroidal anti-inflammatory drug
OA	osteoarthritis
PE	phacoemulsification
PCO	posterior capsule opacification
PCR	posterior capsular rupture
PMMA	polymethylmethacrylate

POMR	perioperative mortality rate
PPP	purchasing power parity
QALY	quality-adjusted life year
QI	quality improvement
QOL	quality of life
RA	rheumatoid arthritis
RTI	road traffic injury
RVF	recto-vaginal fistula
SIA	surgically induced astigmatism
TBA	traditional birth attendant
TBSA	total body surface area
TBI	traumatic brain injury
TC	*técnicos de cirurgia* (Mozambique)
TJR	total joint replacement
TTO	time tradeoff
UCVA	uncorrected visual acuity
UMIC	upper-middle-income country
UNFPA	United Nations Population Fund
VA	vacuum aspiration
VSL	value of a statistical life
VSLY	value of a statistical life year
VVF	vesico-vaginal fistula
WFSA	World Federation of Societies of Anaesthesiologists
WHA	World Health Assembly
WHO	World Health Organization
WTP	willingness to pay
YLD	years lived with disability
YLL	years of life lost
YLS	years of life saved

Income Classifications

World Bank Income Classifications as of July 2014 are as follows, based on estimates of annual gross national income (GNI) per capita for 2013:

- Low-income countries (LICs) = US$1,045 or less
- Middle-income countries (MICs) are subdivided:
  a) lower-middle-income = US$1,046 to US$4,125
  b) upper-middle-income (UMICs) = US$4,126 to US$12,745
- High-income countries (HICs) = US$12,746 or more.

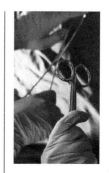

Chapter 1

Essential Surgery: Key Messages of This Volume

Charles N. Mock, Peter Donkor, Atul Gawande,
Dean T. Jamison, Margaret E. Kruk, and Haile T. Debas

VOLUME SUMMARY

Essential Surgery reflects an increased emphasis on health systems relative to previous editions of *Disease Control Priorities*. This volume identifies 44 surgical procedures as essential on the basis that they address substantial needs, are cost-effective, and can feasibly be implemented. This chapter summarizes and critically assesses the volume's key findings:

- Provision of essential surgical procedures would avert an estimated 1.5 million deaths a year, or 6 percent to 7 percent of all avertable deaths in low- and middle-income countries (LMICs).
- Essential surgical procedures rank among the most cost-effective of all health interventions. The surgical platform of first-level hospitals delivers 28 of the 44 essential procedures, making investment in this platform also highly cost-effective.
- Measures to expand access to surgery, such as task-sharing, have been shown to be safe and effective while countries make long-term investments in building surgical and anesthesia workforces. Because emergency procedures constitute 23 of the 28 procedures provided at first-level hospitals, such facilities must be widely geographically available.
- Substantial disparities remain in the safety of surgical care, driven by high perioperative mortality rates

and anesthesia-related deaths in LMICs. Feasible measures, such as the World Health Organization's (WHO's) Surgical Safety Checklist (WHO 2008a), have led to improvements in safety and quality.
- The large burden of surgical conditions, the cost-effectiveness of essential surgery, and the strong public demand for surgical services suggest that universal coverage of essential surgery (UCES) should be financed early on the path to universal health coverage. We point to estimates that full coverage of the component of UCES applicable to first-level hospitals would require slightly more than $3 billion annually of additional spending and yield a benefit:cost ratio of better than 10:1. It would efficiently and equitably provide health benefits and financial protection, and it would contribute to stronger health systems.

INTRODUCTION

Conditions that are treated primarily or frequently by surgery constitute a significant portion of the global burden of disease. In 2011, injuries killed nearly 5 million people; 270,000 women died from complications of pregnancy (WHO 2014). Many of these injury- and obstetric-related deaths, as well as deaths from other causes such as abdominal emergencies and congenital anomalies, could be prevented by improved access to surgical care.

Despite this substantial burden, surgical services are not being delivered to many of those who need them most. An estimated 2 billion people lack access to even the most basic surgical care (Funk and others 2010). This need has not been widely acknowledged, and priorities for investing in health systems' surgical capacities have only recently been investigated. Indeed, until the 1990s, health policy in resource-constrained settings focused sharply on infectious diseases and undernutrition, especially in children. Surgical capacity was developing in urban areas but was often viewed as a secondary priority that principally served those who were better off.

In the 1990s, a number of studies began to question the perception that surgery was costly and low in effectiveness. Economic evaluations of cataract surgery found the procedure to be cost-effective, even under resource-constrained circumstances; Javitt pioneered cost-effectiveness analysis (CEA) for surgery, including his chapter on cataract in *Disease Control Priorities*, first edition (*DCP1*) in 1993 (Javitt 1993). In 2003, McCord and Chowdhury enriched the approach to economic evaluation in surgery in a paper looking at the overall cost-effectiveness of a surgical platform in Bangladesh (McCord and Chowdhury 2003). By design, *DCP2*, published in 2006, placed much more emphasis on surgery than had previous health policy documents. *DCP2* included a dedicated chapter on surgery that amplified the approach of McCord and Chowdhury and provided an initial estimate of the amount of disease burden that could be addressed by surgical intervention in LMICs (Debas and others 2006). *DCP3* places still greater emphasis on surgery by dedicating this entire volume (out of a total of nine volumes) to the topic. There is also a growing academic literature on surgery's importance in health system development; for example, Paul Farmer and Jim Kim's paper observes that "surgery may be thought of as the neglected stepchild of global public health" (Farmer and Kim 2008, 533). The WHO is paying increasing attention to surgical care through such vehicles as its Global Initiative for Emergency and Essential Surgical Care. Finally, the creation of *The Lancet* Commission on Global Surgery, now well into its work, points to a major change in the perceived importance of surgery.

The chapter seeks to do the following:

- Better define the health burden of conditions requiring surgery
- Identify those surgical procedures that are the most cost-effective and cost-beneficial
- Describe the health care policies and platforms that can universally deliver these procedures at high quality. In particular, *Essential Surgery* seeks

to define and study a package of essential surgical procedures that would lead to significant improvements in health if they were universally delivered. This chapter and the volume focus on the situation of low-income countries (LICs) and lower-middle-income countries.

Box 1.1 describes the history, objectives, and contents of DCP3 (Jamison 2015).

DEFINITIONS

Health conditions cannot be neatly split between conditions that require surgery and those that do not. Different diagnoses range widely in the proportion of patients requiring some type of surgical procedure. At the upper end are admissions for musculoskeletal conditions; 84 percent of these patients underwent some type of surgical procedure in an operating room in the United States in 2010. At the lower end are admissions for mental health conditions (0.4 percent) (Rose and others 2014).

The surgical capabilities required are not only those related to performing operations. Surgical care also involves preoperative assessment, including the decision to operate; provision of safe anesthesia; and postoperative care. Even when patients do not need surgical procedures, surgical providers often provide care, such as management of severe head injuries and resuscitation for airway compromise and shock in patients with trauma. Such care occurs in contexts in which clinicians must be prepared to intervene operatively as complications arise or conditions deteriorate.

Within the limitations inherent in defining surgical conditions, *DCP3* has outlined, by consensus, a group of essential surgical conditions and the procedures and other surgical care needed to treat them. Essential surgical conditions can be defined as those that meet the following criteria:

- Are primarily or extensively treated by surgical procedures and other surgical care
- Have a large health burden
- Can be successfully treated by a surgical procedure and other surgical care that is cost-effective and feasible to promote globally (Bellagio Essential Surgery Group 2014; Luboga and others 2009; Mock and others 2010).

In most situations, procedures to treat these conditions, for example, cesarean section, can be done at first-level hospital—those that have 50–200 beds, serve 50,000–200,000 people, and have basic surgical capabilities.

Box 1.1

From the Series Editors of *Disease Control Priorities*, Third Edition

Budgets constrain choices. Policy analysis helps decision makers achieve the greatest value from limited available resources. In 1993, the World Bank published *Disease Control Priorities in Developing Countries (DCP1)*, an attempt to systematically assess the cost-effectiveness (value for money) of interventions that would address the major sources of disease burden in low- and middle-income countries (Jamison and others 1993). The World Bank's 1993 *World Development Report* on health drew heavily on *DCP1*'s findings to conclude that specific interventions against noncommunicable diseases were cost-effective, even in environments in which substantial burdens of infection and undernutrition persisted.

DCP2, published in 2006, updated and extended *DCP1* in several respects, including explicit consideration of the implications for health systems of expanded intervention coverage (Jamison and others 2006). One way that health systems expand intervention coverage is through selected platforms that deliver interventions that require similar logistics but address heterogeneous health problems. Platforms often provide a more natural unit for investment than do individual interventions, and conventional health economics has offered little understanding of how to make choices across platforms. Analysis of the costs of packages and platforms—and of the health improvements they can generate in given epidemiological environments—can help guide health system investments and development.

The third edition of *DCP* is being completed. *DCP3* differs substantively from *DCP1* and *DCP2* by extending and consolidating the concepts of platforms and packages and by offering explicit consideration of the financial risk protection objective of health systems. In populations lacking access to health insurance or prepaid care, medical expenses that are high relative to income can be impoverishing. Where incomes are low, seemingly inexpensive

medical procedures can have catastrophic financial effects. *DCP3* offers an approach that explicitly includes financial protection as well as the distribution across income groups of financial and health outcomes resulting from policies (for example, public finance) to increase intervention uptake (Verguet, Laxminarayan, and Jamison 2015). The task in all the volumes has been to combine the available science about interventions implemented in very specific locales and under very specific conditions with informed judgment to reach reasonable conclusions about the impact of intervention mixes in diverse environments. *DCP3*'s broad aim is to delineate essential intervention packages—such as the essential surgery package in this volume—and their related delivery platforms. This information will assist decision makers in allocating often tightly constrained budgets so that health system objectives are maximally achieved.

DCP3's nine volumes are being published in 2015 and 2016 in an environment in which serious discussion continues about quantifying the sustainable development goal (SDG) for health (United Nations 2015). *DCP3*'s analyses are well-placed to assist in choosing the means to attain the health SDG and assessing the related costs. Only when these volumes, and the analytic efforts on which they are based, are completed will we be able to explore SDG-related and other broad policy conclusions and generalizations. The final *DCP3* volume will report those conclusions. Each individual volume will provide valuable specific policy analyses on the full range of interventions, packages, and policies relevant to its health topic.

Dean T. Jamison
Rachel Nugent
Hellen Gelband
Susan Horton
Prabhat Jha
Ramanan Laxminarayan

However, treatments for some conditions, for example, cataract extraction, are primarily provided at higher level or specialized facilities. Table 1.1 lists the procedures that we define to be essential; this chapter addresses those conditions listed. We acknowledge that the list is not exhaustive, and other procedures might be considered as essential. For many countries, though, table 1.1 will provide a reasonable starting point for an essential surgical package, although there will be country-specific variations. Safe anesthesia and perioperative care are necessary components of all of these procedures.

KEY MESSAGES

This chapter synthesizes the main results of the individual chapters of *Essential Surgery* to provide broad directions for policy. The key messages deriving from our analysis are summarized and explained in the following sections and concern five categories of results: the surgically avertable disease burden, cost-effectiveness and economics, improving access, improving quality, and essential surgery in the context of universal health coverage (UHC).

Table 1.1 The Essential Surgery Package: Procedures and Platforms[a,b]

| Type of procedure | Platform for delivery of procedure[c] | | |
	Community facility and primary health center	First-level hospital	Second- and third-level hospitals
Dental procedures	1. Extraction 2. Drainage of dental abscess 3. Treatment for caries[d]		
Obstetric, gynecologic, and family planning	4. Normal delivery	1. Cesarean birth 2. Vacuum extraction/forceps delivery 3. Ectopic pregnancy 4. Manual vacuum aspiration and dilation and curettage 5. Tubal ligation 6. Vasectomy 7. Hysterectomy for uterine rupture or intractable postpartum hemorrhage 8. Visual inspection with acetic acid and cryotherapy for precancerous cervical lesions	1. Repair obstetric fistula
General surgical	5. Drainage of superficial abscess 6. Male circumcision	9. Repair of perforations: for example, perforated peptic ulcer, typhoid ileal perforation 10. Appendectomy 11. Bowel obstruction 12. Colostomy 13. Gallbladder disease, including emergency surgery 14. Hernia, including incarceration 15. Hydrocelectomy 16. Relief of urinary obstruction: catheterization or suprapubic cystostomy	

table continues next page

Table 1.1 The Essential Surgery Package: Procedures and Platforms[a,b] (continued)

| Type of procedure | Platform for delivery of procedure[c] | | |
	Community facility and primary health center	First-level hospital	Second- and third-level hospitals
Injury[e]	7. Resuscitation with basic life support measures	17. Resuscitation with advanced life support measures, including surgical airway	
	8. Suturing laceration	18. Tube thoracostomy (chest drain)	
	9. Management of non-displaced fractures	19. Trauma laparotomy[f]	
		20. Fracture reduction	
		21. Irrigation and debridement of open fractures	
		22. Placement of external fixator; use of traction	
		23. Escharotomy/fasciotomy (cutting of constricting tissue to relieve pressure from swelling)	
		24. Trauma-related amputations	
		25. Skin grafting	
		26. Burr hole	
Congenital			2. Repair of cleft lip and palate
			3. Repair of club foot
			4. Shunt for hydrocephalus
			5. Repair of anorectal malformations and Hirschsprung's Disease
Visual impairment			6. Cataract extraction and insertion of intraocular lens
			7. Eyelid surgery for trachoma
Nontrauma orthopedic		27. Drainage of septic arthritis	
		28. Debridement of osteomyelitis	

Sources: This list of essential surgical procedures is based on the authors' judgment in light of the burden, implementation feasibility, and cost-effectiveness information contained in *DCP3* volume 1, *Essential Surgery*. Earlier assessments of essential surgical interventions also provide useful information (WHO 2015b; Luboga and others 2009; Mock and others 2004, 2010).

a. Red type implies emergency procedure or condition.

b. All procedures listed in this table are discussed in *DCP3*, volume 1, *Essential Surgery*, with three exceptions, which will be covered in other *DCP3* volumes: male circumcision, visual inspection and treatment of precancerous cervical lesions, and eyelid surgery for ocular trachoma.

c. All of the procedures listed under community health and primary health centers are also frequently provided at first-level and second-level hospitals. All of the procedures under first-level hospitals are also frequently provided at second-level hospitals. The column in which a procedure is listed is the lowest level of the health system in which it would usually be provided. Not included in the table are prehospital interventions, such as first aid, basic life support procedures, or advanced life support procedures done in the prehospital setting. Health systems in different countries are structured differently, and what might be suitable at the various levels of facilities will differ. In this table, *community facility* implies primarily outpatient capabilities (as would be used to provide the elective procedures such as dental care), whereas *primary health center* implies a facility with overnight beds and 24-hour staff (as would be needed for procedures such as normal delivery). *First-level hospitals* imply fairly well-developed surgical capabilities with doctors with surgical expertise; otherwise, many of the procedures would need to be carried out at higher-level facilities. *Referral and specialized hospitals* (which could also be considered as second- and third-level hospitals) imply facilities that have advanced or subspecialized expertise for treatment of one or more surgical conditions, not usually found at lower-level facilities.

d. Treatment for caries can include one or more of the following, depending on local capabilities: silver diamine fluoride application, atraumatic restoration, or fillings.

e. Trauma care includes a wide variety of procedures. Not included in the list of essential procedures would be procedures that are more applicable at higher-level facilities: repair of vascular injury, open reduction and internal fixation, drainage of intracranial hematoma other than through burr hole, or exploration of neck or chest.

f. Trauma laparotomy applicable at first-level hospitals: exploratory laparotomy for hemoperitoneum, pneumoperitoneum, or bowel injury; specific procedures include splenectomy, splenic repair, packing of hepatic injury, and repair of bowel perforation.

Disease Burden Avertable by Essential Surgery

The conditions treated at least in part by the procedures in table 1.1 account for 4.7 million deaths (nearly 10 percent of all deaths) in LMICs (table 1.2). This figure is likely to be an underestimate; the burden of several common surgical conditions listed in table 1.1, for example, bowel obstruction or gallbladder disease, are not estimated as distinct entities in the WHO Global Health Estimates and hence not included in table 1.2. With UCES in LMICs, 1.5 million deaths per year could be averted (table 1.3), representing 6.5 percent of all avertable deaths in LMICs.

In comparison, *DCP2* estimated that 11 percent of the total global burden of death and disability was from conditions that were very likely to require surgery (Debas and others 2006; Laxminarayan and others 2006). The current estimates are based on a more rigorous estimation method and a more narrowly defined subset of essential surgical conditions (figure 1.1) that excludes other highly prevalent conditions often treated by surgery, such as cancer and vascular disease.

Obtaining more accurate estimates of the avertable burden from surgically treatable conditions will require broad agreement on a definition of the concept of avertable burden and the methods for its measurement. The steps taken in *Essential Surgery* should be regarded as preliminary. Better estimates of the avertable burden will require more systematic data gathering from hospitals and population-based surveys on the significant proportion of the world's people who lack access to surgical care. Such a survey recently conducted in Sierra Leone indicated that 25 percent of deaths might have been prevented with timely surgical care (Groen and others 2012). Similar studies need to be repeated more widely. In addition to individual research studies, the international community could contribute to developing and promoting metrics for ongoing monitoring of the burden of essential surgical conditions, as is currently done for maternal mortality.

Table 1.2 Total Burden of Conditions Addressed by Essential Surgery, Low- and-Middle-Income Countries, 2011

Category	Deaths (thousands)	DALYS (thousands)
Category 1. Communicable, maternal, perinatal, and nutritional		
Maternal conditions	280	19,000
Birth asphyxia and birth trauma	780	78,000
Category 2. Noncommunicable diseases		
Cataracts	< 1	7,000
Peptic ulcer disease	230	7,000
Appendicitis	38	2,000
Skin diseases[a]	90	16,000
Cleft lip and palate	5	< 1,000
Oral conditions[b]	< 1	13,000
Category 3. Injuries[c]		
Road traffic crash	1,160	72,000
Other unintentional injuries	1,550	96,000
Intentional injuries	540	34,000
Burden from these conditions	4,700	340,000
Total burden from all causes	45,000	2,400,000
Share of burden due to conditions addressable by essential surgery (percent)	10.4	14.2

Source: Data are from WHO 2014.
Note: DALYs = disability-adjusted life years.
a. Skin diseases include abscess and cellulitis.
b. Oral conditions include caries, periodontal disease, and edentulism.
c. Other unintentional injury includes falls, fires (and heat and hot substances), and exposure to forces of nature; it excludes drowning and poisoning. Intentional injury includes violence and collective violence or legal intervention; it excludes self-harm.

Table 1.3 Disease Burden Avertable by Essential Surgery, Low- and Middle-Income Countries, 2011

	Deaths (thousands)	DALYs (thousands)
1. Total burden[a]	45,000	2,400,000
2. Total avertable burden[b]	23,000	1,300,000
3. Burden from conditions addressable by essential surgery[c]	4,700	340,000
4. Burden avertable by essential surgery[d]	1,500	87,000
5. Burden avertable by essential surgery as a % of total burden [(4) ÷ (1)]	3.3%	3.6%
6. Burden avertable by essential surgery as a % of avertable burden [(4) ÷ (2)]	6.5%	6.6%

Note: DALYs = disability-adjusted life years.
a. Total disease burden from all causes in low- and middle-income countries (WHO 2014).
b. Total avertable burden: number of deaths and DALYs that would be averted if all-cause, age-adjusted rates of death and disability in high-income countries pertained in low- and middle-income countries (WHO 2014).
c. From table 1.2.
d. From Bickler and others 2015. The burden avertable from essential conditions reported in this table is adjusted downward from what is estimated in the chapter; this chapter does not categorize as essential the surgery to address congenital cardiac disease or neural tube defects, while the burden from those conditions is included in the chapter estimates. Furthermore, the total and avertable burden estimates in rows 1 and 2 of this table are slightly higher than those underlying the data in the chapter. This leads to the percentages reported in rows 5 and 6 being very slight underestimates.

Economic Evaluation of Essential Surgery

Surgical Procedures. At the time of *DCP2*, a small number of cost-effectiveness analyses had found specific surgical procedures to be very cost-effective. Since then, the literature has expanded and consistently documented that many of the essential surgical services identified in this chapter rank among health care's most cost-effective interventions (figure 1.2). A few examples, all context-specific, include cleft lip repair (US$10–US$110 per disability adjusted life year [DALY] averted), inguinal hernia repair (US$10–US$100 per DALY averted), cataract surgery (US$50 per DALY averted), and emergency cesarean section (US$15–US$380 per DALY averted). Many of the widely disseminated public health measures are of similar cost-effectiveness or are not as cost-effective: of vitamin A supplementation (US$10 per DALY averted), oral rehydration solution (more than US$1,000 per DALY averted), and antiretroviral therapy for HIV/AIDS (US$900 per DALY averted) (Chao and others 2014; Grimes and others 2014).

Benefit-cost analyses have shown similar findings. An analysis of the benefits from cleft lip repair looked at the costs needed to run a specialized cleft clinic in India and the resulting health benefits, to which a monetary benefit was ascribed. Cleft surgery had a cost of approximately US$300 per DALY averted and a benefit-cost ratio (BCR) of 12 (Alkire, Vincent, and Meara 2015). These findings put cleft repair within the BCR range for the key investment priorities for disease control established by the Copenhagen Consensus, an organization that asks experts to rank global health and development interventions (Jamison, Jha, and

Figure 1.1 Deaths, Avertable Deaths, and Surgically Avertable Deaths in Low- and Middle-Income Countries, 2011

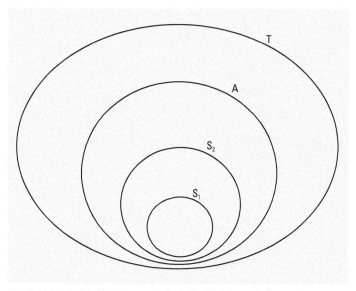

Note: T= total deaths (45 million); A = avertable deaths (23 million); S$_2$ = surgically avertable deaths (estimate not available); S$_1$ = deaths avertable by essential surgery (1.5 million).
Definitions
1. S$_1$ = 2011 deaths in low- and middle-income countries (LMICs) that would have been averted by the universal coverage of essential surgery (UCES).
2. (S$_1$ / T) × 100 = percentage of total deaths in 2011 in LMICs that would have been averted by UCES.
3. (S$_1$ / A) × 100 = percentage of avertable deaths in 2011 in LMICs that would have been averted by UCES.

others 2013). The BCR for cleft surgery is also very high in the range of BCRs across different development sectors. Box 1.2 provides an overview of approaches to economic evaluation of surgical procedures and an overview of findings.

Figure 1.2 Cost-Effectiveness of Surgical Interventions

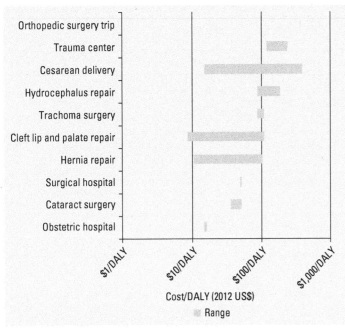

Source: Data from Prinja and others 2015.
Note: DALY = disability-adjusted life year. This figure summarizes the cost-effectiveness of surgical interventions in low- and middle-income countries according to available literature.

Surgical Platforms. The cost-effectiveness of certain platforms or facility types for providing surgical care also needs to be considered. *Essential Surgery* includes a chapter on CEA (Prinja and others 2015). Basic essential procedures are likely to be cost-effective when delivered at any level of the health care system. However, the first-level hospital has been found to be especially cost-effective as a surgical delivery platform, with costs of US$10–US$220 per DALY averted for all surgical care delivered, across a wide range of LMICs (Gosselin and Heitto 2008; Gosselin, Maldonado, and Elder 2010; Gosselin, Thind, and Bellardinelli 2006; McCord and Chowdhury 2003). Most surgery in first-level hospitals is emergency surgery. Therefore, health systems need to disperse surgical facilities widely in the population, and surgical teams working in first-level hospital should have a broad array of basic emergency skills rather than a narrow range of specialized skills.

Our analysis also considered a range of other surgical platforms. Short-term surgical missions by outside surgeons appear beneficial only if no other option is available; otherwise, suboptimal outcomes, unfavorable cost-effectiveness, and lack of sustainability limit their usefulness. Self-contained mobile platforms, such as hospital ships, appear to offer good outcomes for people who can reach them, but there are no data on their cost-effectiveness and obvious limitations for scale-up

and national ownership. Specialized hospitals, including those providing surgery for cataract and obstetric fistula, appear to be among the most cost-effective of the competing options for specialized platforms (Shrime, Sleemi, and Ravilla 2015). Such specialized hospitals would be most sustainable if they develop strong links with local practitioners living and working in that country to promote training and to ensure appropriate postsurgical care, and if they eventually evolve to be led by these local professionals. Since most essential procedures undertaken in specialized hospitals are elective rather than urgent, patients can be scheduled to achieve high volumes, contain costs, and improve technical quality.

Many people with surgical conditions, especially trauma, die in prehospital settings. For example, one study found that 81 percent of trauma deaths were in prehospital settings in Kumasi, Ghana (Mock and others 1998). Most prehospital deaths occur in areas of LMICs where formal emergency medical services are rudimentary or absent. Improving the first aid skills of lay first responders can cost less than US$10 per year of life gained, making it one of the most cost-effective of all health interventions. Similarly, basic ambulance services can cost less than US$300 per year of life gained, which is still highly cost-effective (Thind and others 2015).

Cost of Universal Access. Jamison and colleagues estimate that it would cost approximately US$3 billion annually to scale up delivery of the component of the essential surgery package shown in table 1.1 that is applicable to first-level hospitals, so that this package would be available universally (Jamison, Jha, and others 2013). This expenditure would have a BCR of 10:1, which is broadly consistent with the BCR of other surgical procedures as described by Alkire, Vincent, and Meara (2015).

Improving Access

Challenges. The significant avertable burden from surgical conditions is directly related to the low capacity for surgical care in many LMICs, as reflected in the numbers of surgical procedures performed globally (map 1.1). Most operations (60 percent) take place in wealthier countries where 15 percent of the world's people live. Only 3.5 percent of operations take place in the poorer countries where 35 percent of the world's people live (Weiser and others 2008).

Across 23 LMICs, the ratio of general surgeons per population ranges from 0.13 to 1.57 per 100,000; the ratio of anesthesiologists per population ranges from 0 to 4.9 per 100,000 (Hoyler and others 2014). In contrast, the United States has 9 general surgeons and 11.4 anesthesiologists

Economic Evaluation of Investments in Surgery

Economic evaluations aim to inform decision making by quantifying the tradeoffs between resource inputs required for alternative investments and resulting outcomes. Four approaches to economic evaluation in health are particularly salient:

- *Assessing how much of a specific health outcome,* for example, HIV infections averted, can be attained for a given level of resource input.
- *Assessing how much of an aggregate measure of health*—such as deaths or disability or quality adjusted life years (DALYs or QALYs)—can be attained from a given level of resource inputs applied to alternative interventions. This cost-effectiveness analysis (CEA) approach enables the attractiveness of interventions addressing many different health outcomes to be compared, for example, tuberculosis treatment versus cesarean section.
- *Assessing how much health and financial risk protection* can be attained for a given level of public sector finance of a given intervention. This approach, extended cost-effectiveness analysis (ECEA), enables the assessment not only of efficiency in improving the health of a population but also of efficiency in achieving the other major goal of a health system, that is, protecting the population from financial risk.
- *Assessing the economic benefits,* measured in monetary terms, from investment in a health intervention, and weighing that benefit against its

cost (benefit-cost analysis or BCA). BCA enables health investments to be compared with investments in other sectors.

CEAs predominate among economic evaluations in surgery and for health interventions more generally. Three recent overviews of CEA findings for surgery (one in chapter 18 of this volume) underpin this chapter's conclusion that many essential surgical procedures are highly cost-effective even in resource-constrained environments (Grimes and others 2014; Chao and others 2014; Prinja and others 2015). This volume's chapter 18 looks as well at the cost-effectiveness of the first-level hospital surgical platform.

The Lancet Commission on Investing in Health applied BCA to broad investments in health and found B:C ratios often in excess of 10 (Jamison, Summers, and others 2013). This volume contains BCA evaluations of selected surgical procedures reporting similarly high BCAs (Alkire, Vincent, and Meara 2015). Earlier, the Copenhagen Consensus for 2012 used BCA to rank "strengthening surgical capacity" as number 8 in a list of 30 attractive priorities for investment in development across all sectors (Jamison, Jha, and others 2013; Kydland and others 2013).

ECEAs remain a relatively new evaluation approach. This volume's chapter 19 applies ECEA to surgical intervention in Ethiopia and finds substantial financial protection benefits (Shrime and others 2015).

---

per 100,000 (Stewart and others 2014). Striking differences also exist in the ratio of operating theaters per population across countries at different economic levels: 25 per 100,000 in Eastern Europe, 14–15 in North America and Western Europe, 4–14 in Latin America and the Caribbean, 4.7 in East Asia, but only 1.3 in South Asia, and 1–1.2 in Sub-Saharan Africa (Funk and others 2010).

Two related WHO efforts have defined optimal infrastructure needs for first-level hospitals for surgical care in general (the Programme for Emergency and Essential Surgical Care [WHO 2015a]), and for trauma care at all levels of the health care system (the Essential Trauma Care Project [WHO 2015b]). Surveys conducted using

these WHO guidelines and tools have shown the consistent absence of many low-cost pieces of equipment and supplies, such as chest tubes, oxygen, and equipment for airway management and anesthesia, in many locations, but especially in LICs and at first-level hospitals. In some cases, items are physically present but nonfunctional, such as equipment awaiting repairs. Often, equipment is functional, but it is only available to those who can pay, sometimes in advance; many of those who need the services are unable to access them (Belle and others 2010; Kushner and others 2010; Mock and others 2004, 2006; Ologunde and others 2014; Vo and others 2012; WHO 2003; WHO 2015a; WHO 2015b).

Map 1.1 Number of Surgical Procedures per 100,000 Population, 2004

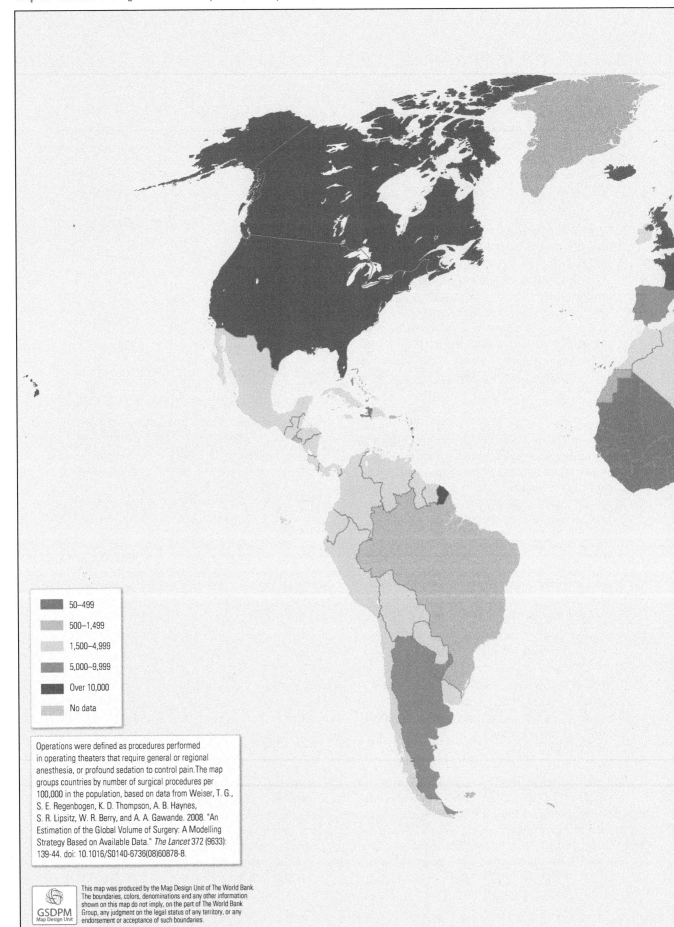

50–499

500–1,499

1,500–4,999

5,000–9,999

Over 10,000

No data

Operations were defined as procedures performed
in operating theaters that require general or regional
anesthesia, or profound sedation to control pain. The map
groups countries by number of surgical procedures per
100,000 in the population, based on data from Weiser, T. G.,
S. E. Regenbogen, K. D. Thompson, A. B. Haynes,
S. R. Lipsitz, W. R. Berry, and A. A. Gawande. 2008. "An
Estimation of the Global Volume of Surgery: A Modelling
Strategy Based on Available Data." *The Lancet* 372 (9633):
139-44. doi: 10.1016/S0140-6736(08)60878-8.

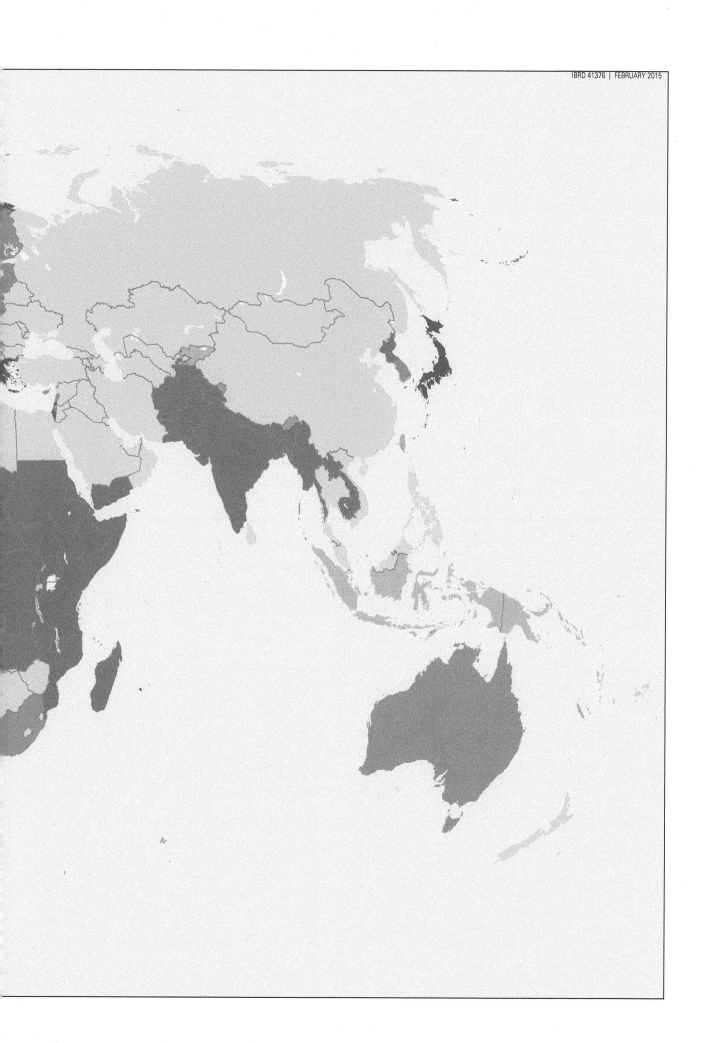

Approaches to Improve Access. Some institutions and health systems have successfully overcome these barriers. For example, the Hanoi Health Department steadily improved its physical resources for trauma care in its network of clinics and hospitals. Such improvements have been stimulated in part by research defining substantial gaps in availability of low-cost items recommended in the WHO's *Guidelines for Essential Trauma Care* and by advocacy to remedy those gaps (Nguyen and Mock 2006). There have also been improvements in the availability of human resources for surgical care. For example, the establishment of the Ghana College of Physicians and Surgeons in 2003 created the first in-country credentialing process for surgeons and led to an expansion of the workforce of fully trained general surgeons and obstetricians. As of June 2014, 284 specialist surgeons and obstetrician-gynecologists had graduated from the college and been posted to first- and second-level hospitals throughout the country to serve as both providers and trainers.

It will likely be impossible to expand access to essential surgical services in rural areas of LMICs in the foreseeable future by depending only on fully certified surgeons and anesthesiologists. Innovative solutions to the surgical workforce crisis are imperative. Evidence shows that mid-level operators can safely perform a number of essential surgical procedures, provided they are properly trained and supervised and perform the operations frequently (McCord and others 2009; Pereira and others 2011). In some locations, these operators are general practitioners. In other cases, they are nonphysician clinicians (NPCs), such as *técnicos de cirurgia* (TCs) in Mozambique or assistant medical officers (AMOs) in Tanzania.

Outcomes such as maternal and neonatal mortality rates after cesarean section and other emergency obstetric procedures were similar for AMOs, compared with doctors in Tanzania (McCord and others 2009; Pereira and others 2011). Although cost studies are few, preliminary evidence shows the cost-effectiveness of task-sharing. For example, in Mozambique, it was three times more cost-effective to train and deploy TCs than to train and deploy physicians to provide obstetric surgery; the 30-year cost per major operation was US$40 for TCs and US$140 for physicians (Kruk and others 2007). Similarly, emergency obstetric care provided by general practitioners was found to be more cost-effective than that provided by fully trained obstetricians in Burkina Faso (Hounton and others 2009).

NPCs are more likely than physicians to stay in underserved rural areas, and they are less likely to emigrate, so their deployment significantly increases the availability of surgical services in underserved rural areas.

In Mozambique and Tanzania, NPCs perform about 90 percent of major emergency obstetric surgery in rural areas where most of the population live (Bergström and others 2015). Challenges continue for many countries, including physicians' acceptance of NPCs, as well as of standardizing their training, supervision, regulatory mechanisms, continuing skills improvement, and remuneration and nonfinancial incentives. The long-range goal is expanding the number of fully trained surgeons. However, general practitioners and NPCs, with appropriate support from surgeons, can be an important intermediate solution to the problem of access to basic surgery.

Many essential physical resources, such as equipment and supplies, are low cost and could be better supplied through improved planning and logistics. The availability of some of the more expensive items, such as x-ray machines and ventilators, would be improved by research on product development. Such research should address improved durability, lower cost of both purchasing and operating, and increased ease of operation. Similarly, the availability of many items could be improved by increased capabilities for local manufacture (WHO 2012). However, international assistance for provision of basic essential equipment and supplies will be needed for the immediate future for the poorest countries. An often overlooked ingredient is the need to ensure local capacity to maintain and repair equipment.

Population, policy, and implementation research (PPIR) could contribute by identifying more efficient and lower-cost delivery methods. The WHO has made significant contributions by establishing norms for human and physical resources for surgical and trauma care and by documenting success stories of individual countries (Mock and others 2004; WHO 2010; WHO 2015b); this is a role for the WHO and other stakeholders that should be expanded.

Surgical training has traditionally emphasized decision making and operative technique for individual patient care; this is appropriate, given the clinical role that most surgeons play. However, those surgeons who wish to address the systems-level barriers to achieving UCES will need additional skills in management and supervision of health care systems, quality improvement (QI), and public health.

A considerable additional barrier to access to surgical care is financial, especially in situations in which user fees are high or where out-of-pocket payments are required. The cost of surgical care is also a significant contributor to medical impoverishment (Schecter and Adhikari 2015). Including UCES within universal public finance would remove financial barriers to access to essential surgical care and would offer financial risk protection, as discussed in the conclusions of this chapter.

Improving the Safety and Quality of Anesthesia and Surgery

Surgical care in all settings is fraught with hazards, including risks from the diseases themselves, the operation, and the anesthesia. These hazards translate into dramatically different risks of death and other complications in different settings. For example, compared with Sweden's rate of 0.04 deaths per 1,000 cesarean sections, mortality is at least 2–4 times higher in Latin America and the Caribbean, 6–10 times higher in South Asia, and 100 times higher in Sub-Saharan Africa (Hogberg 1989; Weiser and Gawande 2015).

A large component of the differences in postoperative mortality is due to differences in anesthesia-related mortality. Major advances have occurred in anesthesia safety in high-income countries (HICs), primarily due to improved monitoring and increased standardization and professionalization. In wealthier countries (those with higher scores on the human development index), mortality per million anesthetics has decreased from 357 deaths per million anesthetics before 1970 to 25 deaths per million anesthetics in the 1990s–2000s, but high rates of anesthetic deaths remain prevalent in most LMICs. Deaths solely attributable to anesthesia are estimated to occur at a rate of 141 deaths per million anesthetics in poorer countries, that is, those with lower score on the human development index, in comparison with the noted 25 deaths per million anesthetics in wealthier countries (Bainbridge and others 2012).

Many of the deaths and complications from surgery in LMICs are potentially preventable with three specific affordable and sustainable improvements:

- Use of a surgical safety checklist
- Improved monitoring and related safety practices during anesthesia
- Improved systems-wide monitoring and evaluation of surgical care overall.

The use of the simple, 19-item WHO Surgical Safety Checklist across eight countries was found to double adherence to basic perioperative safety standards (Haynes and others 2009; WHO 2008a), such as confirmation of the procedure and operative site, objective airway assessment, and completion of instrument and sponge counts at the end of the procedure. Use of the checklist reduced deaths by 47 percent (the postoperative death rate fell from 1.5 percent before introduction of the checklist to 0.8 percent afterward) and

inpatient complications by 35 percent, from 11 percent to 7 percent. The checklist improved outcomes in HICs and upper-middle-income countries (UMICs), LMICs, LICs, and in elective and emergency cases.

The safety of anesthesia in HICs has been achieved by adopting standards of care, such as the continuous presence of a trained anesthesia provider and uninterrupted monitoring of oxygenation, ventilation, and perfusion (Eichhorn and others 1986). Anesthesia delivery systems have been better standardized, with safety features engineered into the machines. One critical technology is pulse oximetry, an essential standard in HICs, which allows ongoing monitoring of oxygenation status so that problems can be corrected early, before they lead to serious or lethal consequences. In one study in Moldova, the introduction of a surgical safety checklist and pulse oximetry led to a significant drop in the number of hypoxic episodes and in the complication rate (Kwok and others 2013). A barrier to pulse oximetry availability has been its cost, although a concerted global effort is underway to lower these costs and increase its availability in LMICs. With lower-cost options now available, the cost-effectiveness of introducing pulse oximetry appears very favorable (Burn and others 2014).

Improved monitoring and evaluation of surgical care across institutions, such as through QI programs, help to better inform administration and management. QI programs range from very simple outcome assessments, such as morbidity and mortality conferences, to more complex monitoring, such as surveillance of complications and use of risk-adjusted mortality. Many hospitals in LMICs have some type of basic QI activities. The effectiveness of these activities could be increased by simple measures, such as more systematic recording of proceedings, more purposeful enactment of corrective action, and monitoring of the outcome of corrective action. A WHO review of QI programs for trauma care shows that most programs led to improvements in patient outcomes, including mortality, or process of care; many also reported cost savings (Juillard and others 2009). Although most of the programs were in HICs, two were in Thailand, an upper-middle-income country, where a model QI program led to sustained improvements in both process of care and mortality rates. Despite their effectiveness, simplicity, and affordability, QI programs are at a rudimentary level of development and implementation in most LMICs (Juillard and others 2009; Mock and others 2006).

An important role for the international community is to support PPIR that (1) addresses affordable and sustainable methods to improve quality of care and (2) documents and disseminates specific case studies of sustaining good practices. The WHO has already made significant contributions by establishing norms, such as the Surgical Safety Checklist (WHO 2008a). This role of governments, the WHO, and other stakeholders needs to be expanded, by establishing and promoting standards for safer, lower-cost anesthesia machines, and norms for monitoring and evaluation procedures for surgical care. Definition and tracking of a variety of quality indicators, such as the perioperative mortality rate needs to be better globally (McQueen 2013; Weiser and others 2009).

Surgery: A Core Component of Universal Health Coverage

Our results point to the potential for essential surgery to cost-effectively address a large burden of disease. Moreover, there are several viable short- and longer-term options for improving access to and safety and quality of surgical care. Figure 1.3 illustrates alternative uses for incremental resources in light of these findings. A country's situation today could be portrayed as a point in the cube: its position on dimension Q depicts the current average quality of care. Its position on dimension A reflects the proportion of the population with access to care, and its position on dimension R reflects the range of services available. Investment choice requires assessment of whether to put incremental money into improving access, improving average quality, or increasing the range of services to be offered. *Our interpretation of the results presented is that it will generally prove both equitable and efficient to achieve full access to essential surgery at high quality before committing public resources to expanding the range of services for a smaller percentage of the population.* The shading in figure 1.3 depicts this situation, which we have termed UCES. UCES should appear early on the pathway to UHC (Jamison, Summers, and others 2013).

Other surgical conditions and procedures merit consideration, such as those for cancer; vascular disease; and conditions requiring more advanced treatments, such as transplantation. Improving access to these procedures will also provide benefits. With regard to sequencing and use of public funds, efforts to ensure greater access to the essential services should be undertaken first, relative to increased investment in those conditions that are more expensive to treat or that have smaller health impacts.

CONCLUSIONS

There is a high burden of avertable death and disability from conditions that can be successfully treated by surgery. Many of the surgical procedures and capabilities needed to treat these conditions are among the most cost-effective of all health interventions and most in demand from the population. These include procedures to treat injuries, obstetric complications, abdominal emergencies, cataracts, obstetric fistula, and congenital anomalies. Many of the most needed procedures are affordable and feasible to deliver, but improving their coverage and quality will require a focused effort to strengthen the health system, particularly at first-level hospitals.

With the exception of obstetric care, the global health community has largely failed to address the unmet need for surgery. The surgical community, in turn, has not tackled the broader requirements for incorporating surgery into resource-constrained health systems—with the important exceptions of exploring task-sharing and improving quality of care.

Ensuring access to essential surgical services for everyone who needs them, when they need them, is in part about improving training in safe surgical care and technique, and in part about improving the functioning of health systems, including better monitoring and evaluation, developing appropriate financing mechanisms, and promoting equity, social justice, and human rights. The global system can play an important role in these efforts through informed leadership and advocacy, support for PPIR, and financial transfers to LICs to assist in attaining UCES.

Improved access to essential surgery should be implemented early in the path to UHC as part of the overall essential benefit package advocated by the Commission on Investing in Health (Jamison, Summers, and others 2013). Implementation would include measures such as using public funds to ensure access to essential surgery and including essential surgery in the packages covered

Figure 1.3 Dimensions of Universal Coverage of Essential Surgery

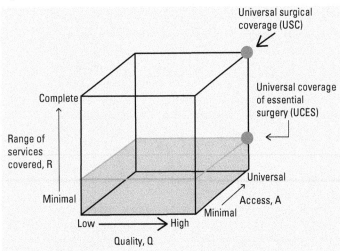

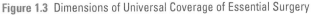

Note: Access is defined as the extent to which services are available to the population—geographically, socially, and financially, for example, with low or zero out-of-pocket payment at the point of service.

by national health insurance schemes. Such measures would also offer financial risk protection against medical impoverishment from the costs of surgical care. Surgery should be considered an indispensable component of a properly functioning health system and can indeed be a means for strengthening the entire system, thereby increasing the return on investment (Jamison, Summers, and others 2013; WHO 2008b). Investments to provide and maintain equipment and to ensure a steady flow of supplies required for a functioning surgical service can strengthen the supply chain for an entire facility.

The nascent literature in this area also suggests positive spillovers between surgical investments and the functioning of and demand for health care. For example, upgrading facilities to provide surgery improved the confidence of providers in their facility and in their own clinical skills in Uganda (Kruk, Rabkin, and others 2014). Several studies show that availability of surgical services increased demand for health care in potentially high-risk conditions, such as labor and delivery or emergency care (Kruk, Hermosilla, and others 2014; Yaffee and others 2012).

Commitments by national governments and the international community to UCES would substantially reduce the mortality and suffering from treatable surgical conditions. Such commitments would also protect populations from financial risk and contribute to the development of the broader health system.

ACKNOWLEDGMENTS

The Bill & Melinda Gates Foundation provides financial support for the Disease Control Priorities Network project, of which this volume is a part. The following individuals provided valuable comments and assistance on this chapter: Elizabeth Brouwer, Rachel Cox, Anna Dare, Sarah Greenberg, Andrew Leather, Rachel Nugent, Zachary Olson, and Gavin Yamey.

Members of the *DCP3* Essential Surgery Author Group wrote the chapters on which this initial chapter draws. The Group includes Richard M. K. Adanu, Sweta Adhikari, Asa Ahimbisibwe, Blake C. Alkire, Joseph B. Babigumira, Jan J. Barendregt, Jessica H. Beard, Staffan Bergström, Stephen W. Bickler, David Chang, Anthony Charles, Meena Cherian, Thomas Coonan, Dawit Desalegn, Catherine R. deVries, Delanyo Dovlo, Richard P. Dutton, Mike English, Diana Farmer, Magda Feres, Zipporah Gathuya, Richard A. Gosselin, Hideki Higashi, Susan Horton, Renee Hsia, Kjell Arne Johansson, Clark T. Johnson, Timothy R. B. Johnson, Manjul Joshipura, Nicholas J. Kassebaum, Ramanan Laxminarayan, Carol Levin, Katrine Lofberg, Svjetlana Lozo, Jackie Mabweijano, Colin McCord, Barbara McPake, Kelly McQueen, John G. Meara, Nyengo Mkandawire, Mark A. Morgan, Mulu Muleta Bedane, Arindam Nandi, Richard Niederman, Emilia V. Noormahomed, Florian R. Nuevo, Eyitope Ogunbodede, Michael Ohene-Yeboah, Andrew Ottaway, Doruk Ozgediz, Caetano Pereira, Mary Lake Polan, N. Venkatesh Prajna, Raymond R. Price, Shankar Prinja, Thulasiraj D. Ravilla, Eduardo Romero Hicks, Sarah Russell, William P. Schecter, Nicole Sitkin, Ambereen Sleemi, David Spiegel, Mark G. Shrime, Sathish Srinivasan, Andy Stergachis, Amardeep Thind, Stéphane Verguet, Jeffrey R. Vincent, Michael Vlassoff, Johan von Schreeb, Theo Vos, Thomas G. Weiser, Iain H. Wilson, and Ahmed Zakariah.

NOTE

World Bank Income Classifications as of July 2014 are as follows, based on estimates of gross national income (GNI) per capita for 2013:

- Low-income countries (LICs) = US$1,045 or less
- Middle-income countries (MICs) are subdivided:
  - lower-middle-income = US$1,046 to US$4,125
  - upper-middle-income (UMICs) = US$4,126 to US$12,745
- High-income countries (HICs) = US$12,746 or more.

REFERENCES

Alkire, Blake, Jeffrey Vincent, and John Meara. 2015. "Benefit-Cost Analysis for Selected Surgical Interventions in Low and Middle Income Countries." In *Disease Control Priorities* (third edition): Volume 1, *Essential Surgery*, edited by H. T. Debas, P. Donkor, A. Gawande, D. T. Jamison, M. E. Kruk, and C. N. Mock. Washington, DC: World Bank.

Bainbridge, D., J. Martin, M. Arango, D. Cheng, and Evidence-based Peri-operative Clinical Outcomes Research (EPiCOR) Group. 2012. "Perioperative and Anaesthetic-Related Mortality in Developed and Developing Countries: A Systematic Review and Meta-Analysis." *The Lancet* 380 (9847): 1075–81.

Bellagio Essential Surgery Group. 2014. http://essentialsurgery.org/bellagio/.

Belle, J., H. Cohen, N. Shindo, M. Lim, A. Velazquez-Berumen, and others. 2010. "Influenza Preparedness in Low-Resource Settings: A Look at Oxygen Delivery in 12 African Countries." *Journal of Infection in Developing Countries* 4: 419–24.

Bergström, S., B. McPake, C. Pereira, and D. Dovlo. 2015. "Workforce Innovations to Expand the Capacity for Surgical Services." In *Disease Control Priorities* (third edition): Volume 1, *Essential Surgery*, edited by H. T. Debas, P. Donkor, A. Gawande, D. T. Jamison, M. E. Kruk, and C. N. Mock. Washington, DC: World Bank.

Bickler, S., T. Weiser, N. Kassebaum, H. Higashi, D. Chang, and others. 2015. "Global Burden of Surgical Conditions." In *Disease Control Priorities* (third edition): Volume 1,

Essential Surgery, edited by H. T. Debas, P. Donkor, A. Gawande, D. T. Jamison, M. E. Kruk, and C. N. Mock. Washington, DC: World Bank.

Burn, S., P. Chilton, A. Gawande, and R. Lilford. 2014. "Peri-Operative Pulse Oximetry in Low-Income Countries: A Cost–Effectiveness Analysis." *Bulletin of the World Health Organization* 14: 137315.

Chao, T. E., K. Sharma, M. Mandigo, L. Hagander, S. C. Resch, and others. 2014. "Cost-Effectiveness of Surgery and Its Policy Implications for Global Health: A Systematic Review and Analysis." *The Lancet Global Health* 2: e334–45.

Debas, H. T., R. Gosselin, C. McCord, and A. Thind. 2006. "Surgery." In *Disease Control Priorities in Developing Countries*, (second edition): edited by D. T. Jamison, J. Breman, A. Measham, G. Alleyne, M. Claeson, D. B. Evans, P. Jha, A. Mills, and P. Musgrove, 1245–60. Washington, DC: Oxford University Press and World Bank.

Eichhorn, J. H., J. B. Cooper, D. J. Cullen, W. R. Maier, J. H. Philip, and others. 1986. "Standards for Patient Monitoring During Anesthesia at Harvard Medical School." *Journal of the American Medical Association* 256: 1017–20.

Farmer, P. E., and J. Y. Kim. 2008. "Surgery and Global Health: A View from Beyond the OR." *World Journal of Surgery* 32 (4): 533–36.

Funk, L. M., T. G. Weiser, W. R. Berry, S. R. Lipsitz, A. F. Merry, and others. 2010. "Global Operating Theatre Distribution and Pulse Oximetry Supply: An Estimation from Reported Data." *The Lancet* 376: 1055–61.

Gosselin, R., and M. Heitto. 2008. "Cost-Effectiveness of a District Trauma Hospital in Battambang, Cambodia." *World Journal of Surgery* 32: 2450–53.

Gosselin, R., A. Maldonado, and G. Elder. 2010. "Comparative Cost-Effectiveness Analysis of Two MSF Surgical Trauma Centers." *World Journal of Surgery* 34: 415–19.

Gosselin, R., A. Thind, and A. Bellardinelli. 2006. "Cost/DALY Averted in a Small Hospital in Sierra Leone: What Is the Relative Contribution of Different Services?" *World Journal of Surgery* 30: 505–11.

Grimes, C. E., J. A. Henry, J. Maraka, N. C. Mkandawire, and M. Cotton. 2014. "Cost-Effectiveness of Surgery in Low- and Middle-Income Countries: A Systematic Review." *World Journal of Surgery* 38: 252–63.

Groen, R. S., M. Samai, K. A. Stewart, L. D. Cassidy, T. B. Kamara, and others. 2012. "Untreated Surgical Conditions in Sierra Leone: A Cluster Randomised, Cross-Sectional, Countrywide Survey." *The Lancet* 380 (9847): 1082–87.

Haynes, A. B., T. G. Weiser, W. R. Berry, S. R. Lipsitz, A. H. Breizat, and others. 2009. "A Surgical Safety Checklist to Reduce Morbidity and Mortality in a Global Population." *New England Journal of Medicine* 360: 491–99.

Hogberg, U. 1989. "Maternal Deaths Related to Cesarean Section in Sweden, 1951–1980." *Acta Obstetricia et Gynecologica Scandinavica* 68: 351–57.

Hounton, H., D. Newlands, N. Meda, and V. Brouwere. 2009. "A Cost-Effectiveness Study of Caesarean-Section Deliveries by Clinical Officers, General Practitioners and Obstetricians in Burkina Faso." *Human Resources for Health* 7: 34.

Hoyler, M., S. R. Finlayson, C. D. McClain, J. G. Meara, and L. Hagander. 2014. "Shortage of Doctors, Shortage of Data: A Review of the Global Surgery, Obstetrics, and Anesthesia Workforce Literature." *World Journal of Surgery* 38: 269–80.

Jamison, D. T. 2015. "Disease Control Priorities, 3rd edition: Improving Health and Reducing Poverty." *The Lancet*. February 5. http://dx.doi.org/10.1016/S0140-6736(15)60097-6.

Jamison, D. T., J. G. Breman, A. R. Measham, G. Alleyne, M. Claeson, and others. 2006. *Disease Control Priorities In Developing Countries,* second edition. Washington, DC: Oxford University Press and World Bank.

Jamison, D. T., P. Jha, R. Laxminarayan, and T. Ord. 2013. "Infectious Disease, Injury, and Reproductive Health." In *Global Problems, Smart Solutions: Costs and Benefits*, edited by Bjørn Lomborg. Cambridge, UK: Cambridge University Press for Copenhagen Consensus Center.

Jamison, D. T., W. Mosley, A. R. Measham, and J. Bobadilla. 1993. *Disease Control Priorities in Developing Countries.* 1st ed. New York: Oxford University Press.

Jamison, D. T., L. H. Summers, G. Alleyne, K. J. Arrow, S. Berkley, and others. 2013. "Global Health 2035: A World Converging within a Generation." *The Lancet* 382 (9908): 1898–955.

Javitt, J. C. 1993. "The Cost-Effectiveness of Restoring Sight." *Archives of Ophthalmology* 111 (12): 1615.

Juillard, C., C. Mock, J. Goosen, M. Joshipura, and I. Civil. 2009. "Establishing the Evidence Base for Trauma Quality Improvement Programs: A Collaborative WHO-IATSIC Review." *World Journal of Surgery* 33: 1075–86.

Kruk, M. E., S. Hermosilla, E. Larson, and G. M. Mbaruku. 2014. "Bypassing Primary Clinics for Childbirth: A Cross-Sectional Study in the Pwani Region, United Republic of Tanzania." *Bulletin of the World Health Organization* 92: 246–53.

Kruk, M. E., C. Pereira, F. Vaz, S. Bergstrom, and S. Galea. 2007. "Economic Evaluation of Surgically Trained Assistant Medical Officers in Performing Major Obstetric Surgery in Mozambique." *BJOG* 114: 1253–60.

Kruk, M. E., M. Rabkin, K. A. Grépin, K. Austin-Evelyn, D. Greeson, and others. 2014. "'Big Push' to Reduce Maternal Mortality in Uganda and Zambia Enhanced Health Systems but Lacked a Sustainability Plan." *Health Affairs (Millwood)* 33: 1058–66.

Kushner, A., M. N. Cherian, L. Noel, D. A. Spiegel, S. Groth, and others. 2010. "Addressing the Millennium Development Goals from a Surgical Perspective: Essential Surgery and Anesthesia in 8 Low- and Middle-Income Countries." *Archives of Surgery* 145: 154–59.

Kwok, A. C., L. M. Funk, R. Baltaga, S. R. Lipsitz, A. F. Merry, and others. 2013. "Implementation of the World Health Organization Surgical Safety Checklist, Including Introduction of Pulse Oximetry, in a Resource-Limited Setting." *Annals of Surgery* 257: 633–39.

Kydland, F. E., R. Mundell, T. Schelling, V. Smith, and N. Stokey. 2013. "Expert Panel Ranking." In *Global Problems, Smart Solutions: Costs and Benefits*, edited by B. Lomborg, 701–16. Cambridge, UK: Cambridge University Press.

Laxminarayan, R., A. J. Mills, J. G. Breman, A. R. Measham, G. Alleyne, and others. 2006. "Advancement of Global Health: Key Messages from the Disease Control Priorities Project." *The Lancet* 367 (9517): 1193–208.

Luboga, S., S. B. Macfarlane, J. von Schreeb, M. E. Kruk, M. N. Cherian, and others. 2009. "Increasing Access to Surgical Services in Sub-Saharan Africa: Priorities for National and International Agencies Recommended by the Bellagio Essential Surgery Group." *PLoS Med* 6 (12): e1000200.

McCord, C., and Q. Chowdhury. 2003. "A Cost Effective Small Hospital in Bangladesh: What It Can Mean for Emergency Obstetric Care." *International Journal of Gynecology and Obstetrics* 81: 83–92.

McCord, C., G. Mbaruku, C. Pereira, C. Nzabuhakwa, and S. Bergstrom. 2009. "The Quality of Emergency Obstetrical Surgery by Assistant Medical Officers in Tanzanian District Hospitals." *Health Affairs (Millwood)* 28: w876–85.

McQueen, K. A. 2013. "Editorial Perspective: Global Surgery: Measuring the Impact." *World Journal of Surgery* 37: 2505–06.

Mock, C. N., M. Cherian, C. Juillard, P. Donkor, S. Bickler, and others. 2010. "Developing Priorities for Addressing Surgical Conditions Globally: Furthering the Link between Surgery and Public Health Policy." *World Journal of Surgery* 34: 381–85.

Mock, C. N., G. J. Jurkovich, D. nii-Amon-Kotei, C. Arreola-Risa, and R. V. Maier. 1998. "Trauma Mortality Patterns in Three Nations at Different Economic Levels: Implications for Global Trauma System Development." *Journal of Trauma* 44: 804–12.

Mock, C. N., J. D. Lormand, J. Goosen, M. Joshipura, and M. Peden. 2004. *Guidelines for Essential Trauma Care.* Geneva: WHO.

Mock, C. N., S. Nguyen, R. Quansah, C. Arreola-Risa, R. Viradia, and M. Joshipura. 2006. "Evaluation of Trauma Care Capabilities in Four Countries using the WHO-IATSIC Guidelines for Essential Trauma Care." *World Journal of Surgery* 30: 946–56.

Nguyen, S., and C. N. Mock. 2006. "Improvements in Trauma Care Capabilities in Vietnam through Use of the WHO-IATSIC Guidelines for Essential Trauma Care." *Injury Control and Safety Promotion* 13 (2): 125–72.

Ologunde, R., J. P. Vogel, M. N. Cherian, M. Sbaiti, M. Merialdi, and others. 2014. "Assessment of Cesarean Delivery Availability in 26 Low- and Middle-Income Countries: A Cross-Sectional Study." *American Journal of Obstetrics and Gynecology* 211 (5): 504. ajog.2014.05.022. Electronic publication ahead of print.

Pereira, C., G. Mbaruku, C. Nzabuhakwa, S. Bergstrom, and C. McCord. 2011. "Emergency Obstetric Surgery by Non-Physician Clinicians in Tanzania." *International Journal of Gynecology and Obstetrics* 114: 180–83.

Prinja, S., A. Nandi, S. Horton, C. Levin, and R. Laxminarayan. 2015. "Costs, Effectiveness, and Cost-Effectiveness of Selected Surgical Procedures and Platforms: A Summary." In *Disease Control Priorities* (third edition): Volume 1, *Essential Surgery*, edited by H. T. Debas, P. Donkor,

A. Gawande, D. T. Jamison, M. E. Kruk, and C. N. Mock. Washington, DC: World Bank.

Rose, J., D. Chang, T. Weiser, N. Kassebaum, and S. Bickler. 2014. "The Role of Surgery in Global Health: Analysis of United States Inpatient Procedure Frequency by Condition Using the Global Burden of Disease 2010 Framework." *PLoS One* 9 (2): e89693. doi:10.1371/journal.pone.0089693.

Schecter, W. P., and S. Adhikari. 2015. "Global Surgery and Poverty." In *Disease Control Priorities* (third edition): Volume 1, *Essential Surgery*, edited by H. T. Debas, P. Donkor, A. Gawande, D. T. Jamison, M. E. Kruk, and C. N. Mock. Washington, DC: World Bank.

Shrime, M., A. Sleemi, and T. Ravilla. 2015. "Specialized Surgical Platforms." In *Disease Control Priorities* (third edition): Volume 1, *Essential Surgery*, edited by H. T. Debas, P. Donkkor, A. Gawande, D. T. Jamison, M. E. Kruk, and C. N. Mock. Washington, DC: World Bank.

Shrime, M., S. Verguet, K. A. Johansson, D. Desalegne, D. T. Jamison, and others. 2015. "Task-Sharing or Public Finance for the Expansion of Surgical Access in Rural Ethiopia: An Extended Cost-Effectiveness Analysis." In *Disease Control Priorities* (third edition): Volume 1, *Essential Surgery*, edited by H. A. Debas, P. Donkor, A. Gawande, D. T. Jamison, M. E. Kruk, and C. N. Mock. Washington, DC: World Bank.

Stewart, B., P. Khanduri, C. McCord, M. Ohene-Yeboah, S. Uranues, and others. 2014. "Global Disease Burden of Conditions Requiring Emergency Surgery." *British Journal of Surgery* 101 (1): e9–22.

Thind, A., R. Hsia, J. Mabweijano, E. Romero Hicks, A. Zakariah, and C. N. Mock. 2015. "Prehospital and Emergency Care." In *Disease Control Priorities* (third edition), Volume 1, *Essential Surgery*, edited by H. T. Debas, P. Donkor, A. Gawande, D. T. Jamison, M. E. Kruk, and C. N. Mock. Washington, DC: World Bank.

United Nations. 2015. "Sustainable Development Goals." http://sustainabledevelopment.un.org/?menu=1300.

Verguet, S., R. Laxminarayan, and D. T. Jamison. 2015. "Universal Public Finance of Tuberculosis Treatment In India: An Extended Cost-Effectiveness Analysis." *Health Economics* 24 (3): 318–32.

Vo, D., M. Cherian, S. Bianchi, L. Noel, G. Lundeg, and others. 2012. "Anesthesia Capacity in 22 Low- and Middle-Income Countries." *Journal of Anesthesia and Clinical Research* 3: 207. doi:10.4172/2155-6148.1000207. http://omicsonline.org/2155-6148/2155-6148-3-207.pdf.

Weiser, T., and A. Gawande. 2015. "Excess Surgical Mortality: Strategies for Improving Quality of Care." In *Disease Control Priorities* (third edition): Volume 1, *Essential Surgery*, edited by H. T. Debas, A. Gawande, D. T. Jamison, M. E. Kruk, and C. N. Mock. Washington, DC: World Bank.

Weiser, T. G., M. A. Makary, A. B. Haynes, G. Dziekan, W. R. Berry, and others, for the Safe Surgery Saves Lives Measurement and Study Groups. 2009. "Standardised Metrics for Global Surgical Surveillance." *The Lancet* 374: 1113–17.

Weiser, T. G., S. E. Regenbogen, K. D. Thompson, A. B. Haynes, S. R. Lipsitz, and others. 2008. "An Estimation of the

Global Volume of Surgery: A Modelling Strategy Based on Available Data." *The Lancet* 372 (9633): 139–44.

WHO (World Health Organization). 2003. *Surgical Care at the District Hospital.* Geneva: WHO. http://www.int/surgery/publications/scdh_manual/en.

———. 2008a. *Surgical Safety Checklist and Implementation Manual* [Internet]. Geneva: WHO. http://www.who.int/patientsafety/safesurgery/tools_resources/SSSL_Checklist_finalJun08.pdf?ua=1.

———. 2008b. *World Health Report 2008: Primary Health Care: Now More Than Ever.* Geneva: WHO.

———. 2010. *Strengthening Care for the Injured: Success Stories and Lessons Learned from around the World.* Geneva: WHO.

———. 2012. *Local Production and Technology Transfer to Increase Access to Medical Devices.* Geneva: WHO. http://www.int/medical_devices/1240EHT_final.pdf.

———. 2014. "Global Health Estimates (2011)." http://www.who.int/healthinfo/global_burden_disease/en/.

———. 2015a. Essential Trauma Care Project, www.who.int//violence_injury_prevention/services/traumacare/en/.

———. 2015b. Global Initiative for Emergency and Essential Surgical Care, http://www.who.int/surgery/en/.

Yaffee, A. Q., L. Whiteside, R. A. Oteng, P. M. Carter, P. Donkor, and others. 2012. "Bypassing Proximal Health Care Facilities for Acute Care: A Survey of Patients in a Ghanaian Accident and Emergency Centre." *Tropical Medicine & International & International Health* 17: 775–81.

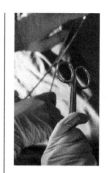

Chapter 2

Global Burden of Surgical Conditions

Stephen W. Bickler, Thomas G. Weiser, Nicholas Kassebaum,
Hideki Higashi, David C. Chang, Jan J. Barendregt,
Emilia V. Noormahomed, and Theo Vos

INTRODUCTION

Approximately 2 billion people lack access to emergency and essential surgical care (Funk and others 2010). Most of the need is in rural and marginalized populations living in low- and middle-income countries (LMICs), where the poorest one-third of the world's population receives only 3.5 percent of all surgical procedures (Weiser and others 2008). The lack of surgical care takes a serious human and economic toll and can lead to acute, life-threatening complications. In other instances, poor-quality care results in chronic disabilities that make productive employment impossible and impose a burden on family members and society.

The failure to appreciate the role of surgery in addressing important public health problems is the main cause of disparities in surgical care worldwide. Yet, surgically treatable conditions—such as obstructed labor (Alkire and others 2012; Ndour and others 2013); injuries (Abdur-Rahman, van As, and Rode 2012; Mock and others 2012); intra-abdominal emergencies (Stewart and others 2014); correctable congenital anomalies, such as clubfoot and cleft lip or palate (Mossey and Modell 2012; Wu, Poenaru, and Poley 2013); symptomatic hernias (Beard and others 2013); cataracts (Rao, Khanna, and Payal 2011); osteomyelitis (Bickler and Rode 2002; Stanley and others 2010); and otitis media (Monasta and others 2012)—contribute to premature deaths or ill health of populations.

In this chapter, we explore surgery's multifaceted contribution to global public health. We begin by providing an overview of the public health dimensions of surgical care in LMICs and examine the current challenges of making a comprehensive assessment of the global burden of surgical diseases. Next, we estimate the public health impact in LMICs if basic and selected subspecialty surgical care could be scaled up to meet standards that currently exist in high-income countries (HICs). Finally, we attempt to define where surgical care fits among other global health priorities and discuss areas toward which future research should be focused. Our analysis uses the 21 epidemiology regions from the Global Burden of Diseases, Injuries, and Risk Factors Study 2010.

ROLE OF SURGERY IN GLOBAL HEALTH

Public Health Dimensions

In the second edition of *Disease Control Priorities in Developing Countries*, Debas, McCord, and Thind (2006) describe four types of surgical interventions that have a public health dimension:

- The provision of competent, initial surgical care to injury victims to reduce preventable deaths, as well as to decrease the number of survivable injuries that result in disability

Corresponding author: Stephen W. Bickler, Rady Children's Hospital and University of California, San Diego, MD, DTM&H, FACS, sbickler@ucsd.edu

- The handling of obstetrical complications, such as obstructed labor and hemorrhage
- The timely and competent surgical management of a variety of abdominal and extra-abdominal emergency and life-threatening conditions
- The elective care of simple surgical conditions, such as hernia, clubfoot, cataract, hydroceles, and otitis media

Based on expert opinion, Debas, McCord, and Thind (2006) estimate that 11 percent of the global burden of disease measured in disability-adjusted life years (DALYs) could be treated with surgery. Their estimates range from 7 percent for Sub-Saharan Africa to as high as 15 percent for Europe. Although based on incomplete information and a limited number of surgical procedures, the 11 percent estimate is one of the most widely quoted figures in global surgery.

Why surgically treatable conditions are not more widely appreciated as a critical public health problem is an important question. Although the answer is complex, it is in part related to the misconception that surgical care is too costly. Surgical care can, in fact, be remarkably cost-effective, even in comparison with nonsurgical interventions that are commonly implemented as public health measures. For example, the cost of emergency obstetric care at a rural hospital in Bangladesh was estimated to be US$11 per DALY averted (McCord and Chowdhury 2003). The same measurement for all surgical care services provided by a hospital in Sierra Leone was just US$33 per DALY averted (Gosselin, Thind, and Bellardinelli 2006). These costs compare favorably with many other primary interventions, such as vitamin A distribution (US$9 per DALY averted), acute lower respiratory infection detection and home treatment (US$20 per DALY averted), or measles immunization (US$30 per DALY averted) (Grimes and others 2014; Ozgediz and Riviello 2008).

Importance of Preventive and Curative Services

During the past several decades, public health professionals have come to understand that successful health care depends on both prevention and curative intervention. Because prevention is rarely 100 percent effective, clinical services will always be needed. This principle applies to a broad spectrum of health care problems in LMICs. Examples include malaria control programs, through which bed nets can reduce but not eliminate the need to treat symptomatic cases, as well as maternal health programs, in which cesarean section must be an available treatment option for cases of obstructed labor. With respect to the latter, approximately 10 percent

to 15 percent of pregnancies will require emergency obstetrical care (Gibbons and others 2010). The experience with controlling HIV infection in LMICs is particularly germane because programs are most successful when screening and prevention strategies are combined with treatment. Striking a balance between prevention and clinical programs has proved to be especially challenging in LMICs, where there is fierce competition for limited resources. Nevertheless, clinical services must be available if the health needs of a population are to be appropriately met.

CHALLENGES ESTIMATING A GLOBAL BURDEN OF SURGICAL DISEASE

The Global Burden of Diseases, Injuries, and Risk Factors Study 2010 (known as GBD 2010) (Murray, Vos, and others 2012) reinforces use of the DALY as the preferred metric for determining the relative contribution of disease categories to the overall burden of disease. The DALY is a summary measure of population health that sums up fatal burden and nonfatal burden into a single index: years of life lost (YLLs) and years lived with disability (YLDs). Because the GBD framework is increasingly used as a factor to inform resource allocation in LMICs, it is extremely important that the impact of surgical care be estimated using the DALY metric, if possible. Nevertheless, in the process of trying to estimate a global burden of surgical disease, we encountered several challenges when analyzing surgical care using this metric.

Challenge 1: Defining Surgical Care

Confusion persists about what constitutes surgical care and the role surgery should have in settings of limited resources. Surgery is often defined as it relates to specific procedures, but this definition fails to recognize the larger role that surgical care has in clinical practice. Our preferred surgical definitions are shown in box 2.1. In addition to the technical execution of an operation, surgical care encompasses the preoperative assessment of patients, including deciding whether to operate; intraoperative anesthetic management; and postoperative care—all of which are major determinants of surgical outcomes.

More important and frequently ignored is that surgeons often provide nonoperative care to their patients. Examples include the airway management of injured patients; the use of traction in extremity fractures; the care of most head injuries; and the nonoperative management of the majority of blunt abdominal injuries, for example, a spleen injury in a child. Although surgical care has an important role in the diagnosis and treatment of many diseases, it can also have a role in prevention, as in the use of circumcision to prevent HIV infection.

Challenge 2: Distinguishing between Surgical and Nonsurgical Conditions in the GBD 2010 Study

Efforts to estimate a global burden of surgical disease have been predicated on the idea that GBD causes must be classified as either surgical or nonsurgical. To test this assertion, and to gain better insight into the role of surgery in a high-functioning health system, we queried the U. S. National Inpatient Sample (NIS)[1] to determine operative rates for each of the GBD 2010 disease and injury categories (Rose and others 2014). This database is the largest all-payer inpatient care database in the United States, containing data on more than 7 million hospital stays each year. This database cannot be expected to represent what occurs globally, but it can provide insight into operative rates in a well-resourced health system.

We compiled all International Classification of Diseases, Version 9 (ICD-9) codes from the NIS from 2010 and grouped the NIS primary diagnosis codes into GBD 2010 disease categories. The ICD-9 codes used in the GBD 2010 were extracted from table 4 of the Supplement material of the GBD 10 (annex 2A to this chapter; Lozano and others 2012). We determined the fraction of admitted patients in each GBD cause category who underwent an operation. *Operation* was defined as a surgical procedure performed in an operating room on inpatients. This definition and corresponding ICD-9 procedure codes are standardized and publicly available through the Agency for Healthcare Research and Quality (AHRQ 2008). The details of our analysis, along with the AHRQ list of surgical procedures, can be found in annexes 2B and 2C.

In 2010, 10 million inpatient operations were performed in the United States and were associated with 28.6 percent of all admissions. Operations were performed in every GBD 2010 cause subcategory (frequency prevalence ranged from 0.2 percent to 84.0 percent). The highest frequencies were in the subcategories of musculoskeletal (84.0 percent); neoplasm (61.4 percent); and diabetes, urological, blood, and endocrine disease (33.3 percent) (figure 2.1). The GBD 2010 framework captured 80.1 percent of inpatient operations; 19.9 percent of operations were performed on patients with a primary diagnosis not included in the GBD 2010 framework. The two most common missed ICD-9 codes were single live birth, both with and without cesarean section. With childbirth being a precarious process in many settings, it illustrates that this important process is not captured in the GBD framework.

Surgical care thus cuts across the entire spectrum of GBD 2010 cause categories, calling into question dichotomous traditional classifications of *surgical* versus *nonsurgical* disease. There was no disease subcategory that required an operation 100 percent of the time, nor was there any that never required an operation. The neoplasm subcategory is an excellent example. In our study, 61.4 percent of patients admitted for treatment of a neoplasm diagnosis underwent a surgical procedure. Certainly there is disagreement about whether to classify all patients with a neoplasm as surgical patients. Yet surgical care plays an important role in the diagnosis (biopsy), treatment (resection), and supportive care (chronic intravenous access) of patients with tumors. Although operative rates vary by country, and our study could not evaluate specific indications or outcomes of procedures, the findings illustrate the integrative nature of surgical care within a health system.

Figure 2.1 Chance of a Patient Admitted to the Hospital in a Well-Resourced Health System Requiring a Surgical Procedure in the Operating Room

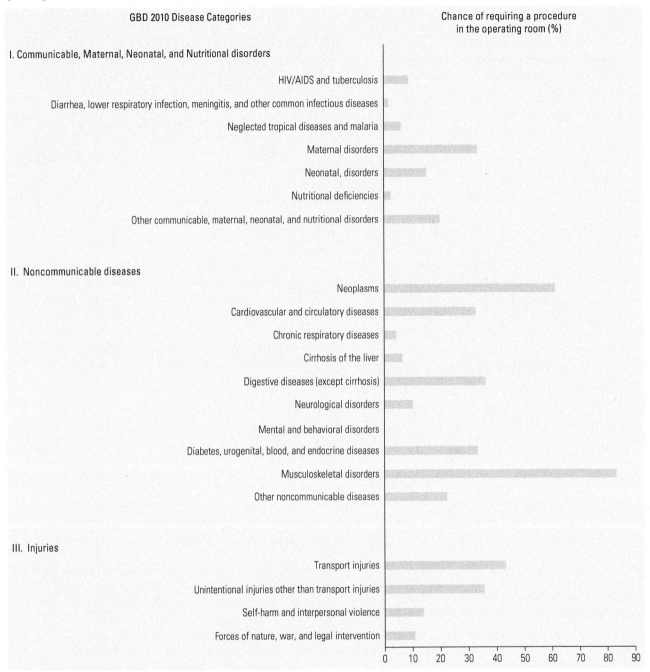

Source: Rose and others 2014, based on the National (Nationwide) Inpatient Sample (NIS), 2010, Healthcare Cost and Utilization Project, Agency for Healthcare Research and Quality, Rockville, MD, http://www.hcup-us.ahrq.gov/db/nation/nis/nisdbdocumentation.jsp.

Challenge 3: Assigning DALYs Averted Values to Large Numbers of Surgical Procedures

Modern surgical care has an impressive armamentarium of surgical procedures—everything from the drainage of a simple abscess to the repair of complex congenital heart anomalies. The AHRQ list used in the database analysis includes ICD-9 procedure codes for more than 2,500 major operations (annex 2C). To accurately calculate DALYs averted by a given surgical procedure, one must know the disability weight associated with a particular condition, the effectiveness of the operation in reducing incidence and mortality, and its ability to affect duration or severity of the condition. The effectiveness of an operation varies by the type of operation; resources available to conduct the operation; operative skills of the surgeon; capability and resources of anesthesia personnel; and patient factors, such as nutritional status and other comorbidities. The large number of surgical procedures and the variability in operative outcomes make a comprehensive calculation difficult, if not impossible.

Strategy for Assessing the Public Health Impact of Surgical Care in LICs and MICs

Given the complexities and inherent challenges of estimating an accurate global burden of surgical disease, we adopted an alternative strategy for assessing the public health impact of surgical care in LMICs. Instead of trying to make a comprehensive assessment of all surgical care, we focused our efforts on estimating the public health impact of scaling up basic surgical care deliverable at first-level hospitals and selected subspecialty care. Our goal was to capture the most important surgical procedures that have the highest impact on improving public health.

BURDEN AVERTED BY SCALING UP BASIC SURGICAL CARE[2]

Rationale

During the past decade, interest in building surgical capacity at first-level hospitals in LMICs has increased. The rationale for this strategy is that a large percentage of the world's population receives emergency care at first-level facilities. Moreover, many surgical conditions—particularly obstetric emergencies, intra-abdominal catastrophes, and life-threatening injuries—require that appropriate care be immediately available if lives are to be saved.

In response to this challenge, the World Health Organization (WHO) launched two complementary initiatives: the Emergency and Essential Surgical Care (EESC) program in 2004 and the Global Initiative for Emergency and Essential Surgical Care (GIEESC) in 2005 (Abdullah, Troedsson, and Cherian 2011; Bickler and Spiegel 2010; Spiegel and others 2013). The goal of the EESC project was the development and implementation of training materials to improve care for surgical conditions at first-level facilities in LMICs; the objective of the GIEESC project was to stimulate collaboration among governments, organizations, agencies, and institutions involved in reducing death and disability from surgically treatable conditions. The 2012 Copenhagen Consensus reaffirmed the need to strengthen surgical capacity in the developing world, emphasizing that very low-cost investments could be highly effective (Copenhagen Consensus Center 2012).

As funders and national policy makers consider the expansion of health systems in LMICs, it is imperative that they understand the potential impact that scaling up basic surgical care deliverable at first-level hospitals could have on population health.

Methodology

Our analysis assumes a basic surgical package with various therapeutic interventions that could be provided at first-level hospitals. These conditions were selected based on recommendations and guidelines in the literature (Mock and others 2010; WHO 2003); consultation with experts in global surgery; practicality in quantifying health outcomes, for example, the existence of clear health outcomes corresponding to specific surgical procedures; and a corresponding cause in GBD 2010. We examined the following:

- *Four digestive diseases:* Appendicitis, paralytic ileus[3] and intestinal obstruction, inguinal and femoral hernia, and gallbladder and bile duct disease
- *Four maternal-neonatal conditions:* Maternal hemorrhage, obstructed labor, abortion, and neonatal encephalopathy
- *Injuries that could be treated with basic interventions:* Resuscitation, surgical airway, peripheral venous access, suturing, laceration and wound management, chest tube or needle decompression, fracture reduction, escharotomy, fasciotomy, skin grafting, trauma-related amputation, and trauma-related laparotomy

To investigate which surgical procedures would be required to treat this group of surgical conditions, we searched Surgical Care for the District Hospital (WHO 2003) for procedures that corresponded to the GBD causes. Our review showed that almost 50 surgical procedures are required to treat these GBD causes, illustrating that a broad spectrum of procedures are required to treat even a limited list of surgical conditions (annex 2D).

Our burden estimates were based on data from the GBD 2010 (Murray, Vos, and others 2012). Parameters included population, standard life expectancy, cause-specific mortality, incidence, prevalence, and disability weights (Lozano and others 2012; Salomon and others 2012; Vos and others 2012). The parameters were specific by cause, age, gender, region, and year. The GBD 2010 groups countries into 21 epidemiological regions (17 of which contain LMICs) and seven superregions (six of which contain LMICs) (table 2.1). Our analysis was conducted at the superregion level by aggregating regional-level parameters.

Our approach recognized that some conditions, such as maternal hemorrhage and neonatal encephalopathy, are not fully amenable to surgical care and required adjustments to limit the effect of surgery. Other GBD causes (such as drowning, poisoning, self-harm, venomous animal contact, and injuries not classified elsewhere) were assumed to be not amenable to surgery. When questions on the proportions of conditions that could be managed by surgical care arose, we referred to the literature and adjusted the avertable burden accordingly. Additional details on the adjustments to account for the burden not amenable to surgical care can be found in annex 2E.

The overall concept of the approach was to split the reported DALYs of surgical conditions in 2010 into

surgically avertable burden and surgically nonavertable burden. The avertable burden was calculated as follows:

$$\text{Avertable burden} = DALY^{Current} - DALYcf, \quad (2.1)$$

in which $DALY^{Current}$ denotes the DALYs reported in GBD 2010, and $DALYcf$ the estimated DALYs if the delivery of surgical care had existed in a counterfactual state in which the entire population had access to appropriate and safe surgical care appropriate for delivery at the first-level hospital. The counterfactual level equates to the outcome that is achievable across all segments of the health care system in HICs.

To determine the $DALYcf$ quantity, we estimated $YLLcf$ and $YLDcf$ for the counterfactual state in separate steps. Such separation in estimating fatal and nonfatal burden is consistent with the approach used in generating the GBD 2010 estimates.

We first estimated the number of deaths for the counterfactual state in LMIC superregions with the following equation:

$$DEATHcf^{superregion}_{age,\,gender} = Incidence^{superregion}_{age,\,gender} \times CFRcf_{age,\,gender}, \quad (2.2)$$

in which $DEATHcf^{superregion}_{age,\,gender}$ is the age- and gender-specific number of deaths for the counterfactual state in each superregion, $Incidence^{superregion}_{age,\,gender}$ the age- and gender-specific number of incident cases from GBD 2010 in each superregion, and $CFRcf_{age,\,gender}$ the age- and gender-specific case fatality rates for the counterfactual state.

$CFRcf_{age,gender}$ values would ideally be informed by complete data on coverage, access, quality, and effectiveness of surgical care in each region. Although such data exist for some LMICs and a subset of causes in our analysis, it is very sparse (Choo and others 2010; Galukande and others 2010; Kushner and others 2010).

We therefore assigned the lowest fatality rates among the 21 epidemiological regions for each age and gender to be representative of $CFRcf_{age,gender}$. In addition to being consistent across conditions, we believe this value best reflects the situation of the counterfactual state in which diagnosis is reasonably prompt, treatment is available, and there is access to appropriate and safe surgical care. Not surprisingly, the majority of lowest CFRs were from one of the HICs: high-income Asia Pacific, Western Europe, Australasia, and high-income North America.

After calculating $DEATHcf^{superregion}_{age,\,gender}$, we multiplied this quantity by the age-specific standard life expectancy used in GBD 2010 to estimate the fatal burden for the

Table 2.1 GBD 2010 Epidemiological Regions and Groupings into LMIC Superregions

GBD 2010 epidemiological regions		LMIC superregions
High-income countries	1. High-income Asia Pacific	
	2. Western Europe	
	3. Australasia	
	4. High-income North America	
Low- and middle-income countries	5. Central Europe	Eastern Europe and Central Asia
	6. Eastern Europe	
	7. Central Asia	
	8. Southern Sub-Saharan Africa	Sub-Saharan Africa
	9. Eastern Sub-Saharan Africa	
	10. Central Sub-Saharan Africa	
	11. Western Sub-Saharan Africa	
	12. North Africa and Middle East	Middle East and North Africa
	13. South Asia	South Asia
	14. Southeast Asia	
	15. East Asia	East Asia and Pacific
	16. Oceania	
	17. Southern Latin America	Latin America and the Caribbean
	18. Tropical Latin America	
	19. Central Latin America	
	20. Andean Latin America	
	21. Caribbean	

counterfactual state (Lozano and others 2012; Murray, Ezzati, and others 2012) using the following formula:

$$YLLcf_{age,\ gender}^{superregion} = Deathcf_{age,\ gender}^{superregion}$$
$$\times Standard\ life\ expectancy_{age,\ gender}. \quad (2.3)$$

The next step was to estimate the nonfatal burden (*YLDcf*) for the counterfactual state. Although scaling up surgical coverage would reduce fatal burden (YLL), the averted deaths would still contribute to the nonfatal burden for a shorter—or sometimes longer—duration, as estimated by YLDs. YLDs in GBD 2010 were calculated by multiplying the prevalent cases by disability weights that are unique to each health state. However, we did not know the direct impact of reduced CFRs on prevalence. For diseases that had a short duration, defined as less than one year, we calculated the YLDs for the counterfactual state as follows:

$$YLDcf_{age,\ gender}^{superregion} = \left(Incidence_{age,\ gender}^{superregion} - Deathcf_{age,\ gender}^{superregion} \right)$$
$$\times Duration \times DW, \quad (2.4)$$

in which $YLDcf_{age,\ gender}^{superregion}$ is the nonfatal burden in the counterfactual state, *Duration* is the duration of disease calculated by dividing the prevalence by incidence, and *DW* the disability weight attached to each condition from the GBD 2010 study. For injury conditions with long-term sequelae that exceeded a year, we used a slightly different equation:

$$YLDcf_{age,\ gender}^{superregion} = Incidence_{age,\ gender}^{superregion}$$
$$\times YLD\ per\ incident\ case_{age,\ gender}^{lowest\ from\ all\ regions}. \quad (2.5)$$

The final step was to calculate the avertable burden, which was accomplished by summing the *YLDcf* and *YLLcf* for each region and then subtracting the total from the total DALYs estimate from GBD 2010, and aggregating the results to the superregion level. Additional details on how burden calculations were performed can be found in the four manuscripts included in annex 2F.

Results were expressed as the number of deaths and burden (DALYs) that would be averted per year by scaling up care for a group of surgically treatable conditions in LMICs. This care would be appropriate for first-level hospitals and would include treatment for four digestive diseases, four maternal-fetal conditions, and injuries that could be treated with basic interventions. Our estimates are based on the assumption that surgical care could be

scaled up to match the accessibility and quality of care provided in HICs—the counterfactual rate—either at first-level hospitals or at higher levels of care.

Because surgical care can never completely prevent or reverse disability, we have also included an estimate of the nonavertable burden. The nonavertable burden refers to the fraction of the burden that is currently not preventable or reversible with surgical care. Perhaps the best examples of nonavertable burden occur in injured patients for whom death and disability often occur even when the best possible surgical care is available. Two examples are an amputation for a severely mangled extremity and a fatality from a severe head injury before the patient arrives at the hospital. The outcomes are unavoidable and thus nonavertable with surgical care.

Some may question the value of including data on the nonavertable burden given that we have focused our efforts on trying to define the role of surgery in reducing death and disability. Nevertheless, we have included these data for two important reasons. First, nonavertable does not necessarily imply a problem that cannot be addressed: nonavertable burden can be reduced through nonsurgical means, for example, injury prevention, improved delivery of care, or innovation. Second, without a complete accounting of total burden—the avertable and nonavertable burden—it is impossible to appreciate the magnitude of the problem and the limitations of surgical care.

Impact on Population Health

Scaling up basic surgical care across all sectors of the health care system in LMICs could prevent 1.4 million deaths and 77.2 million DALYs per year. The details of these preventable deaths and avertable DALYs, by superregion, are shown in tables 2.2 and 2.3. Overall, scaling up surgical care to treat four gastrointestinal diseases, four maternal-neonatal conditions, and injuries treated with simple interventions could prevent 3.2 and 3.5 percent of all deaths and DALYs, respectively, that occur each year in LMICs.

The majority of the preventable deaths were due to injuries (77 percent), followed by maternal-neonatal conditions (14 percent) and digestive diseases (9 percent). Road injury (292,000 deaths per year) and falls (184,000 deaths per year) were the two most common causes of preventable death. In the maternal-neonatal category, neonatal encephalopathy was the leading cause of preventable death (166,000 deaths per year). The South Asia and Sub-Saharan Africa superregions have the largest number of preventable deaths per year, 485,000 and 327,000 deaths, respectively.

Table 2.2 Estimated Number of Deaths per Year That Could Be Prevented If Basic Surgical Care Could Be Provided in LMICs

Surgical condition		Eastern Europe and Central Asia	Sub-Saharan Africa	Middle East and North Africa	South Asia	East Asia and Pacific	Latin America and the Caribbean	LMIC total	Major category totals (percent)
Digestive diseases	Appendicitis	1,773	14,248	1,035	1,712	3,905	3,614	26,286	145,292 (9.0)
	Gall bladder and bile duct disease	3,672	9,123	1,950	2,087	21,605	9,477	47,914	
	Hernia	3,810	816	0	4,459	1,279	3,700	14,065	
	Paralytic ileus and bowel obstruction	938	17,637	4,622	23,360	4,525	5,945	57,027	
Maternal-neonatal	Maternal hemorrhage	63	10,228	703	6,147	2,424	478	20,042	233,658 (14.4)
	Obstructed labor	8	2,248	59	8,284	255	28	10,882	
	Abortion	333	16,756	364	15,179	3,440	862	36,935	
	Neonatal encephalopathy	1,475	62,271	2,477	91,286	5,871	2,420	165,800	
Injuries	Road injury	14,342	59,218	19,832	86,610	76,976	34,894	291,872	1,042,292 (76.6)
	Other transport injury	405	3,618	633	3,325	2,220	715	10,916	
	Falls	18,731	15,823	3,224	35,239	95,405	15,148	183,570	
	Drowning	0	0	0	0	0	0	0	
	Fire, heat, and hot substances	6,772	44,754	5,016	104,373	7,583	3,922	172,421	
	Poisoning	0	0	0	0	0	0	0	
	Exposure to mechanical forces	24,602	25,333	12,094	40,270	24,560	8,370	135,229	
	Adverse effects of medical treatment	2,305	11,774	1,048	12,789	8,707	6,563	43,186	
	Animal contact (venomous)	0	0	0	0	0	0	0	
	Animal contact (nonvenomous)	491	1,508	216	802	1,335	424	4,777	
	Unintentional injuries not classified elsewhere	13,342	10,054	1,898	32,828	22,081	11,335	91,537	
	Self-harm	0	0	0	0	0	0	0	
	Interpersonal violence	9,905	21,997	3,261	16,723	12,557	44,342	108,784	
	Exposure to forces of nature	0	0	0	0	0	0	0	
	Collective violence and legal intervention	0	0	0	0	0	0	0	
Preventable deaths in LMICs		102,966	327,405	58,432	485,472	294,730	152,238	1,421,242	
Total deaths in LMICs		4,861,515	8,291,833	2,109,258	12,537,748	12,649,687	3,623,093	44,073,134	
Fraction of LMIC deaths (percent)		2.1	3.9	2.8	3.9	2.3	4.2	3.2	

Note: LMIC = low- and middle-income countries. The basic surgical care would treat four gastrointestinal diseases, four maternal-fetal conditions, and injuries that require simple interventions. Estimates are based on the assumption that surgical care could be scaled up to match the accessibility and standard of care in high-income countries across all sectors of the health care system.

Table 2.3 Estimated Number of DALYs per Year That Could Be Averted If Basic Surgical Care Could Be Provided in LMICs

Surgical condition		Eastern Europe and Central Asia	Sub-Saharan Africa	Middle East and North Africa	South Asia	East Asia and Pacific	Latin America and the Caribbean	LMIC total	Major category totals (percent)
Digestive diseases	Appendicitis	52,513	715,487	43,104	91,989	140,253	110,468	1,153,814	4,848,078 (6.3)
	Gall bladder and bile duct disease	74,813	327,655	48,675	104,648	447,519	188,670	1,191,981	
	Hernia	68,822	37,015	0	119,929	24,260	75,281	325,308	
	Paralytic ileus and bowel obstruction	50,726	663,486	164,888	975,976	175,431	146,468	2,176,975	
Maternal-neonatal	Maternal haemorrhage	3,485	577,146	39,034	346,842	132,128	26,409	1,125,044	20,024,726 (25.9)
	Obstructed labor	439	125,618	3,230	462,367	13,636	1,543	606,833	
	Abortion	18,411	953,725	20,397	863,443	189,761	48,443	2,094,180	
	Neonatal encephalopathy	168,036	5,956,409	292,750	8,744,616	749,316	287,542	16,198,669	
Injuries	Road injury	779,308	3,507,638	1,093,122	4,692,999	4,336,877	1,691,314	16,101,257	52,316,946 (67.8)
	Other transport injury	47,120	270,686	66,709	340,760	309,928	59,125	1,094,328	
	Falls	772,809	934,208	346,824	2,031,692	3,902,220	524,038	8,511,792	
	Drowning	0	0	0	0	0	0	0	
	Fire, heat, and hot substances	270,469	3,010,660	291,629	5,559,069	403,174	173,684	9,708,685	
	Poisoning	0	0	0	0	0	0	0	
	Exposure to mechanical forces	371,523	721,882	285,019	1,422,803	394,083	147,054	3,342,364	
	Adverse effects of medical treatment	97,135	689,029	80,351	688,719	395,255	221,024	2,171,513	
	Animal contact (venomous)	0	0	0	0	0	0	0	
	Animal contact (nonvenomous)	15,857	99,707	12,394	49,961	59,451	15,136	252,507	
	Unintentional injuries not classified elsewhere	557,481	740,551	164,376	1,616,624	1,262,528	560,301	4,901,861	
	Self-harm	0	0	0	0	0	0	0	
	Interpersonal violence	461,613	1,378,702	206,024	1,043,360	761,912	2,381,028	6,232,639	
	Exposure to forces of nature	0	0	0	0	0	0	0	
	Collective violence and legal intervention	0	0	0	0	0	0	0	
Avertable DALYs		3,810,561	20,709,604	3,158,526	29,155,798	13,697,732	6,657,528	77,189,749	
Total DALYs in LMICs		160,209,494	574,216,660	122,217,565	679,620,290	525,029,717	169,976,643	2,231,270,369	
Fraction of LMIC DALYs (percent)		2.4	3.6	2.6	4.3	2.6	3.9	3.5	

Note: DALY = disability-adjusted life year; LMIC = low- and middle-income country. The basic surgical care would treat four gastrointestinal diseases, four maternal-fetal conditions, and injuries that require simple interventions. Estimates are based on the assumption that surgical care for these conditions could be scaled up to match the accessibility and standard of care in high-income countries across all sectors of the health care system.

Figure 2.2 Distribution of Burden Avertable by Scaling Up Basic Surgical Care Deliverable at First-Level Hospitals in Low- and Middle-Income Countries
Percent

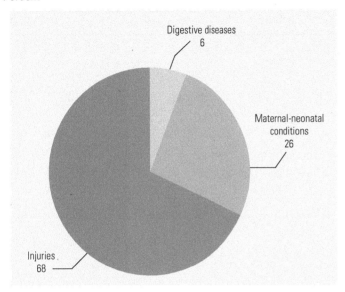

Source: Data in table 2.3.
Note: Percentages are based on a surgical package that could treat four gastrointestinal diseases, four maternal-neonatal conditions, and injuries that could be managed with simple interventions.

Injuries also accounted for the largest fraction of avertable DALYs (figure 2.2). Road injury is the leading cause of injury-related avertable DALYs in LMICs (16.1 million DALYs per year) followed by fire, heat, and hot substances (9.7 million DALYs per year) (table 2.3). Of the total injury burden in LMICs, 21 percent is potentially avertable by providing basic trauma care at first-level hospitals and higher levels of care. Sub-Saharan Africa has the largest proportion of potentially avertable DALYs related to injuries (25 percent); South Asia the highest absolute number of avertable DALYs (17.4 million per year).

Of the burden associated with the maternal-neonatal conditions that we analyzed, 36 percent is potentially avertable by full coverage of quality obstetric surgery in LMICs (20.0 million DALYs). The South Asia superregion has the highest total number of avertable maternal-neonatal DALYs (10.4 million). Neonatal encephalopathy comprises the largest portion of avertable burden among the five conditions analyzed, followed by abortion (16.2 and 2.1 million DALYs, respectively).

Of the burden related to the four digestive diseases (4.8 million DALYs per year), 65 percent is potentially avertable with first-level surgical care in LMICs. Sub-Saharan Africa has the largest avertable burden in absolute DALYs (1.7 million per year) and in avertable proportion (83 percent). Paralytic ileus and intestinal obstruction accounted for the largest portion of avertable burden among the four digestive diseases (2.2 million DALYs per year; 64 percent avertable).

The majority of the burden associated with the four gastrointestinal diseases, four maternal-neonatal conditions, and injuries analyzed cannot be averted by surgical care (table 2.4). The nonavertable burden from the group (238.5 million DALYs per year; 10.7 percent of the GBD in LMICs) was 2.5 times greater than the burden averted by the basic surgical package. The majority (84 percent) of the total nonavertable burden was due to injuries (200.4 million DALYs per year), followed by maternal-neonatal conditions (34.5 million DALYs per year). Figure 2.3 shows the nonavertable burden by LMIC superregion and its relationship to the avertable burden. South Asia had the largest number of nonavertable DALYs (75.6 million DALYs per year), while the Latin American and the Caribbean superregion had the highest fraction of the total regional GBD (17.9 percent). The latter reflects the devastating earthquake in Haiti in January 2010.

BURDEN AVERTED BY SCALING UP SELECTED SUBSPECIALTY SURGICAL CARE

Rationale

Subspecialty surgical care refers to highly specialized procedures that require advanced technical skills and training. Although some third-level referral hospitals in LMICs may provide surgical care for these conditions, the advanced skills required for these procedures have prevented them being incorporated into the general health care system. Consequently, these conditions have often been managed by establishing vertical, single-procedure-based programs in LMICs, frequently supported by international funding and surgical missions. Nevertheless, because these procedures are relatively common, life changing, and often involve children, they offer a potentially large source of avertable DALYs.

Methodology

We examined five conditions: cataract, clefts (both lip and palate), congenital heart anomalies, neural tube defects, and obstetric fistula. We selected these conditions from the GBD 2010 cause list for which clearly corresponding and well-established surgical programs exist. Similar to the analysis of surgical burden at first-level hospitals, we obtained demographic and epidemiological parameters from the GBD 2010.

Table 2.4 Nonavertable Burden (DALYs) Associated with a Group of Conditions That Can Be Treated with Basic Surgical Care in LMICs

Surgical condition		Eastern Europe and Central Asia	Sub-Saharan Africa	Middle East and North Africa	South Asia	East Asia and Pacific	Latin America and the Caribbean	LMIC total	Major category totals (percent)
Digestive diseases	Appendicitis	19,536	40,564	21,724	60,541	91,505	30,921	264,791	2,569,667 (1.1)
	Gall bladder and bile duct disease	84,517	86,298	46,506	171,374	228,275	96,787	713,756	
	Hernia	24,234	50,564	27,799	101,544	136,906	37,116	378,163	
	Paralytic ileus and bowel obstruction	178,522	178,767	88,595	384,235	302,702	80,136	1,212,957	
Maternal-neonatal	Maternal hemorrhage	9,551	1,049,909	76,887	701,056	263,167	49,947	2,150,516	35,484,201 (14.9)
	Obstructed labor	100	7,962	1,700	23,261	2,495	1,106	36,624	
	Abortion	4,769	3,068	3,528	5,153	13,647	3,354	33,520	
	Neonatal encephalopathy	1,439,805	9,159,407	1,345,063	12,856,954	6,364,307	2,098,006	33,263,541	
Injuries	Road injury	3,595,438	10,438,956	3,705,845	13,102,811	18,456,805	4,236,206	53,536,062	200,495,053 (84.0)
	Other transport injury	506,046	863,473	391,651	993,914	1,253,312	334,767	4,343,163	
	Falls	2,100,073	3,087,910	1,247,749	6,769,471	5,823,690	1,345,565	20,374,457	
	Drowning	1,280,302	3,241,397	699,575	7,152,853	5,518,534	1,234,016	19,126,677	
	Fire, heat, and hot substances	499,174	2,811,538	358,772	3,928,508	907,600	303,034	8,808,626	
	Poisoning	817,934	1,502,573	345,178	3,437,583	2,009,199	150,428	8,262,895	
	Exposure to mechanical forces	1,184,059	1,496,743	544,190	2,377,539	1,620,976	339,263	7,562,770	
	Adverse effects of medical treatment	169,265	232,522	135,416	201,614	349,494	280,437	1,368,748	
	Animal contact (venomous)	41,796	923,985	55,456	1,403,954	179,762	103,217	2,708,170	
	Animal contact (nonvenomous)	17,706	363,505	15,345	165,198	77,752	16,669	656,174	
	Unintentional injuries not classified elsewhere	1,332,066	2,079,247	649,305	3,462,963	3,581,777	942,741	12,048,099	
	Self-harm	3,792,899	2,175,157	735,231	14,721,081	8,472,490	1,775,160	31,672,018	
	Interpersonal violence	1,578,109	3,950,824	683,929	3,034,727	2,980,006	5,590,425	17,818,020	
	Exposure to forces of nature	0	5,519	0	0	0	11,373,271	11,378,790	
	Collective violence and legal intervention	6,228	179,868	61,659	582,628	0	0	830,383	
Nonavertable DALYs		18,682,128	43,929,755	11,241,103	75,638,960	58,634,402	30,422,573	238,548,921	
Total DALYs in LMICs		160,209,494	574,216,660	122,217,565	679,620,290	525,029,717	169,976,643	2,231,270,369	
Fraction of LMIC DALYs (percent)		11.7	7.7	9.2	11.1	11.2	17.9	10.7	

Note: DALY = disability-adjusted life year; LMIC = low- and middle-income countries. The group includes four digestive diseases, four maternal-fetal conditions, and injuries that can be treated with simple interventions. The nonavertable burden refers to the burden associated with a particular condition that is not preventable or reversible with surgical care.

Figure 2.3 Burden Associated with a Group of Conditions That Can Be Treated with Basic Surgical Care in Low- and Middle-Income Countries

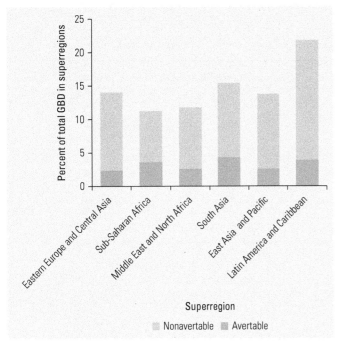

Source: Data from tables 2.3 and 2.4.

Note: GBD = global burden of disease. The group includes four gastrointestinal diseases, four maternal-neonatal conditions, and injuries that can be managed with simple interventions. Results are expressed as the percentage of the total superregion global burden of disease.

The burden of obstetric fistula and cataract in the GBD 2010 comprised YLDs only. We estimated the burden of fistula in the counterfactual state by adjusting the successful closure rate of surgical repair with the risk of residual urinary incontinence that may take over:

$$YLDcf_{age,\,gender}^{superregion} = Prevalence_{age,\,gender}^{superregion} \times (1 - SuccessRate)$$
$$\times DW^{fistula} + SuccessRate \times UIRate \times DW^{urinary\ incontinence},$$
$$(2.6)$$

in which *SuccessRate* is the successful closure rate and *UIRate* the risk of urinary incontinence after surgery.

The burden of cataract in its counterfactual state was calculated by assuming that the lowest age- and sex-specific YLD rates per capita reflect the counterfactual situation:

$$Pop'n_{age,\,gender}^{superregion} \times YLDRate_{age,\,gender}^{lowest\ from\ all\ regions},\qquad (2.7)$$

where *Pop'n* is the population in each superregion, and *YLDRate* the per capita YLD of cataract in each region.

For congenital anomalies, we first estimated the nonfatal burden if the counterfactual surgical coverage could be provided in LMICs. This estimation was made by assuming that the difference in prevalence between a particular age group and the age group immediately following that in the high-income superregion reflects the excess mortality for the counterfactual surgical coverage. Beginning with the birth prevalence that varies between LMIC regions, we applied this assumption to age one year and above to follow the prevalence. The resulting prevalence for each gender and age was then multiplied by the disability weights of each condition to derive the YLDs. Next, we estimated the fatal burden attributable to congenital anomalies in the counterfactual situation. We then estimated the YLLs and DALYs for the counterfactual state in the same manner as we did in our analysis of basic surgical care in the previous section. Finally, the avertable burden was calculated using equation (2.1).

Because it is well known that persons with congenital anomalies, especially those without access to treatment, are at risk for any number of other fatal complications, such as malnutrition or pneumonia, we performed an additional analysis to more accurately quantify the avertable burden of cleft lip and palate, congenital heart anomalies, and neural tube defects. This step was necessary because deaths and YLLs for congenital anomalies reported in the GBD 2010 are limited to only those deaths for which the underlying cause is coded as being due to congenital conditions. Furthermore, natural history modeling of the GBD 2010 data shows a sharp decline in the prevalence of non-operated cases compared with those who received operations. The excess number of deaths compared with the number predicted by the cause-code deaths and YLLs clearly illustrate this excess mortality phenomenon. Accordingly, to avoid underestimating the potential impact of surgical care in treating congenital anomalies, we based our avertable DALY estimates on the excess mortality related to all causes, not only the DALYs reported for a particular congenital anomaly in the GBD study. Additional details on how these burden calculations were performed can be found in manuscript B listed in annex 2F.

Impact on Population Health

Scaling up selected subspecialty surgical care in LMICs could prevent 388,000 deaths and avert 38.9 million DALYs per year. The details of these preventable deaths and avertable DALYs, by superregion, are shown in table 2.5. This impact, although smaller than the total burden averted by scaling up basic surgical care, is still substantial and could increase the number of surgically preventable deaths and DALYs by 27.3 and 50.4 percent, respectively. Overall, scaling up surgical care to treat cataract, cleft lip and palate, congenital heart anomalies,

Table 2.5 Estimated Number of Preventable Deaths and Avertable, and Nonavertable DALYs Associated with Scaling Up Selected Subspecialty Surgical Care

Surgical condition		Eastern Europe and Central Asia	Sub-Saharan Africa	Middle East and North Africa	South Asia	East Asia and Pacific	Latin America and the Caribbean	LMIC total	Fraction of total (percent)
Preventable deaths	Cataract	n.a.	n.a.	n.a.	n.a.	n.a.	n.a.	n.a.	n.a.
	Cleft lip and palate	1,915	16,863	8,330	21,905	13,631	3,004	65,648	16.9
	Congenital heart anomalies	4,844	89,231	21,742	99,414	32,905	8,045	256,180	66.0
	Neural tube defects	500	18,162	5,395	39,934	1,736	619	66,346	17.1
	Obstetric fistula	n.a.	n.a.	n.a.	n.a.	n.a.	n.a.	n.a.	n.a.
	Total preventable deaths	7,259	124,256	35,467	161,253	48,273	11,668	388,174	
	Total deaths in LMICs	4,861,515	8,291,833	2,109,258	12,537,748	12,649,687	3,623,093	44,073,134	
	Fraction of LMIC deaths (percent)	0.2	1.5	1.7	1.3	0.4	0.3	0.9	
Avertable DALYs	Cataract	306,592	306,441	288,451	2,043,146	988,834	274,295	4,207,758	10.8
	Cleft lip and palate	147,661	1,447,813	601,006	1,705,359	965,032	209,701	5,076,572	13.0
	Congenital heart anomalies	442,648	7,726,243	1,898,098	8,938,691	2,893,186	697,631	22,596,497	58.1
	Neural tube defects	46,399	1,602,477	495,807	3,669,764	175,503	57,880	6,047,830	15.5
	Obstetric fistula	1,525	415,241	50,472	225,218	298,628	5,471	996,553	2.6
	Total avertable DALYs	944,823	11,498,214	3,333,834	16,582,177	5,321,183	1,244,978	38,925,209	
	Total DALYs in LMICs	160,209,494	574,216,660	122,217,565	679,620,290	525,029,717	169,976,643	2,231,270,369	
	Fraction of LMIC DALYs (percent)	0.6	2.0	2.7	2.4	1.0	0.7	1.7	
Nonavertable DALYs	Cataract	69,600	41,459	31,647	115,320	222,271	49,772	530,068	1.1
	Cleft lip and palate	54,930	250,262	75,040	311,746	232,878	54,035	978,889	2.1
	Congenital heart anomalies	1,116,728	14,502,230	3,046,252	15,196,430	5,229,279	1,903,422	40,994,342	88.1
	Neural tube defects	66,776	1,073,060	295,829	1,763,196	611,067	110,549	3,920,477	8.4
	Obstetric fistula	191	51,998	6,320	28,202	37,395	685	124,791	0.3
	Total nonavertable DALYs	1,308,225	15,919,009	3,455,087	17,414,894	6,332,890	2,118,463	46,548,568	
	Total DALYs in LMICs	160,209,494	574,216,660	122,217,565	679,620,290	525,029,717	169,976,643	2,231,270,369	
	Fraction of LMIC DALYs (percent)	0.8	2.8	2.8	2.6	1.2	1.2	2.1	

Note: DALY = disability-adjusted life year; LMIC = low- and middle-income countries. Estimates are based on the assumption that care for cataract, cleft lip and palate, congenital heart anomalies, neural tube defects, and obstetric fistula could be scaled up to match the accessibility and standard of care in high-income countries. Estimates for cleft lip and palate, congenital heart anomalies, and neural tube defects account for the excess mortality due to any cause. n.a. = not applicable.

neural tube defects, and obstetric fistula could prevent 0.9 and 1.7 percent of all deaths and DALYs, respectively, that occur each year in LMICs.

The largest number of preventable deaths occurred in the congenital heart anomalies category (66 percent), followed by neural tube defects (17 percent). This finding may underestimate the actual mortality because not all deaths are necessarily coded to these causes. Figure 2.4 shows the distribution of the burden that could be averted by scaling up advanced surgical treatment of cataract, cleft lip and palate, congenital heart anomalies, neural tube defects, and obstetric fistula. These avertable DALY estimates, which include the correction for the excess mortality due to other causes, shows that the majority of avertable burden would result from scaling up surgical care to treat congenital heart anomalies (58 percent) and neural tube defects (15 percent). The South Asia and Sub-Saharan Africa superregions have the highest total number of avertable DALYs per year, 16.6 million and 11.5 million, respectively; the Eastern Europe and Central Asia superregion has the least (945,000 DALYs per year).

The subspecialty surgical care we analyzed is better at addressing burden compared with basic surgical care provided at first-level hospitals. Of the burden associated with cataract, cleft lip and palate, congenital heart anomalies, neural tube defects, and obstetric fistula, 46 percent is avertable with surgical care, compared with 24.1 percent of the burden related to the gastrointestinal diseases, maternal-neonatal conditions, and injuries we analyzed. An advantage of subspecialty surgical care is that it can be planned, is usually reproducible, and can be done on an elective basis.

LIMITATIONS OF CURRENT ANALYSIS

Our methodology relied on the assumption that the lowest fatality and disability estimates for persons with surgically treatable conditions from the 21 epidemiological regions reflect the case of full surgical coverage. The estimates of impact of full coverage on disease burden were from high-income regions, and whether these figures are applicable to other settings is not clear.

Even if geographic and financial barriers to surgical care are removed, health-seeking behavior may vary substantially among contexts. The nontrivial variations of fatality rates among HICs suggest that none of the health systems truly reflect the counterfactual state, although differences in coding practices and data-gathering mechanisms may contribute to the variations.

In addition to full population coverage, the quality of surgery and anesthesia is a critical precondition of this analysis that, if compromised, could separately add to excess mortality.

We may also be overestimating the burden that could be averted with first-level surgical care because our analysis is based on the lowest rates of case fatality and disability in HICs. In HICs, the sickest patients are often transferred to higher levels of care where they benefit from advanced care provided in intensive care units—this higher level of care is often not available in LICs, resulting in higher fatality rates.

Furthermore, the parameters for our analysis are primarily from the GBD 2010. This is a major advantage in that our results are thus directly comparable with those from the GBD 2010, but it also implies that our analysis is fully prone to the GBD 2010's limitations.

Finally, we did not attempt to make any estimates of uncertainty. Uncertainty estimates are reported in the GBD 2010, but to propagate these estimates through to our analysis did not seem practical given that we needed to make numerous assumptions to arrive at our results.

WHERE SURGICAL CARE FITS AMONG GLOBAL HEALTH PRIORITIES

LMICs are increasingly using burden-of-disease data to allocate limited resources and to prioritize funding for research and treatment programs at the global level.

Figure 2.4 Distribution of Burden That Could Be Averted by Scaling Up Selected Subspecialty Surgical Care in Low- and Middle-Income Countries
Percent

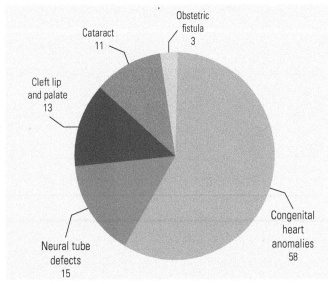

Source: Data from table 2.5.
Note: Percentages are based on surgical care that would treat cataracts, cleft lip and palate, congenital heart anomalies, neural tube defects, and obstetric fistula.

Table 2.6 Public Health Impact of Scaling Up Surgical Care in Low- and Middle-Income Countries

| | | Burden | | | |
| | | Avertable | | Nonavertable | |
Type of surgical care	Preventable deaths (millions)	DALYs per year (millions)	Fraction of LMIC total GBD (percent)	DALYs per year (millions)	Fraction of LMIC total GBD (percent)
Basic surgical care[a]	1.4	77.2	3.5	238.5	10.7
Subspecialty surgical care[b]	0.4	38.9	1.7	46.5	2.1
Totals	1.8	116.1	5.2	285.0	12.8

Note: DALY = disability-adjusted life year; GBD = global burden of disease; LMIC = low- and middle-income countries.
a. Designed to treat four gastrointestinal diseases, four maternal-fetal conditions, and injuries that can be managed with simple interventions. Basic surgical care refers to emergency and essential surgical care that is deliverable with the resources available at first-level hospitals.
b. Surgical care for cataract, cleft lip and palate, congenital heart anomalies, neural tube defects, and obstetrical fistula.

It is important that our burden estimates be properly represented and interpreted. Table 2.6 summarizes the potential impact on public health in LMICs if surgical care could be scaled up to meet the standard of care and accessibility that exists in HICs. Included in the table are our estimates of the number of preventable deaths and surgically avertable and nonavertable DALYs and their respective fraction of the total GBD in LMICs. Overall, our analysis suggests that scaling up basic and selected subspecialty surgical care could avert 5.2 percent of the total burden of disease in LMICs.

Care should be exercised in interpreting this 5.2 percent figure because it does not represent the global surgical burden or the total burden that could be averted by surgical care in LMICs. To estimate a global surgical burden, it would be necessary to extend our analysis to include surgical care provided in HICs. It would also be necessary to account for the almost 20 percent of patients in our NIS database analysis whose primary diagnoses were not captured by the GBD 2010 cause list. A more complete assessment of the burden that could be averted by surgical care in LMICs would need to include the following:

- Care for other common surgical conditions that could be or is already being, done at first-level hospitals, for example, treatment of surgical infections such as incision and drainage of abscesses, tube thoracostomy for empyema, irrigation of septic joints, and sequestrectomy for chronic osteomyelitis
- Surgical care provided at second- and third-level hospitals, for example, complex gastrointestinal surgery, resection of tumors, and major pediatric surgical procedures

Given what seems like the ability to prevent only a small fraction of total GBD in LMICs, how then does surgical care fit among other global health priorities? To address this question, we compared our surgical burden estimates to the global burden of tuberculosis, HIV/AIDS, malaria, and ischemic heart disease. These four conditions were selected because they are currently recognized as some of our most important global health problems. Ischemic heart disease (129.8 million DALYs) ranks first on the GBD 2010 cause list (Murray, Vos, and others 2012). The other three have been the targets of the Global Fund to Fight AIDS, Tuberculosis and Malaria since 2002. Because patients with tuberculosis, HIV/AIDS, and ischemic heart disease may sometimes require surgical care, it is important to not interpret this simply as a comparison between surgical and nonsurgical conditions; rather, it is intended to illustrate the magnitude of the disease burden amenable to a select number of surgical interventions.

Figure 2.5 illustrates the burden of high-priority global health problems and compares them with our surgical burden estimates. The avertable burden from scaling up basic surgical care at first-level hospitals and advanced care in specialized clinics in LMICs (116.1 million DALYs per year) exceeds the unaddressed global burdens of HIV/AIDS (81.6 million DALYs), tuberculosis (49.4 million DALYs), or malaria (82.7 million DALYs) individually, but it is less than the unaddressed burden associated with ischemic heart disease (130.0 million DALYs per year). Perhaps a better comparison would be between the burden that could be addressed with surgical care and the burden that could be averted by treatment of the other conditions—for example, the burden averted by antiretroviral medication to treat HIV—but these data do not exist.

Figure 2.5 Burden of Important Global Health Problems

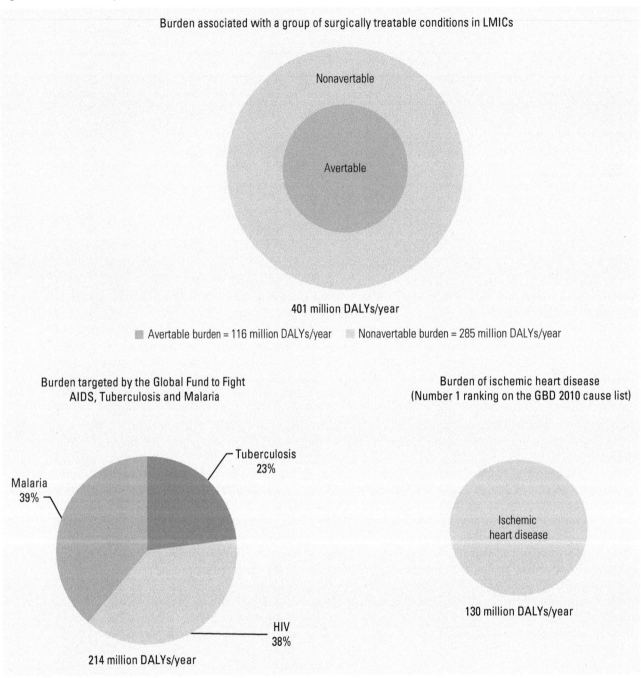

Burden associated with a group of surgically treatable conditions in LMICs

Nonavertable

Avertable

401 million DALYs/year

Avertable burden = 116 million DALYs/year   Nonavertable burden = 285 million DALYs/year

Burden targeted by the Global Fund to Fight
AIDS, Tuberculosis and Malaria

Tuberculosis
23%

Malaria
39%

HIV
38%

214 million DALYs/year

Burden of ischemic heart disease
(Number 1 ranking on the GBD 2010 cause list)

Ischemic
heart disease

130 million DALYs/year

Note: DALY = disability-adjusted life year; GBD 2010 = Global Burden of Disease 2010. Area of circles represents the relative number of DALYs per year. The "avertable burden" area depicts the burden that could be averted by scaling up surgical care in low- and middle-income countries (basic surgical care that can be delivered at first-level hospitals and selected subspecialty surgical care). The burden averted from scaling up surgical care (116.1 million DALYs per year) exceeds the global burden of HIV/AIDS (81.6 million DALYs per year) and malaria (82.7 million DALYs per year). The total burden associated with the surgical conditions analyzed is almost twice the burden targeted by the Global Fund to Fight AIDS, Tuberculosis and Malaria.

Just as not all of the HIV (or other disease burden) can be addressed with currently available treatments, the magnitude of the nonavertable surgical burden should be interpreted as providing crucial direction for development of strategies to prevent and more effectively treat these conditions. To place the nonavertable surgical burden (285 million DALYs per year) in perspective, that number is more than twice that associated with ischemic heart disease; it is more than 1.3 times larger than the total burden targeted by the Global Fund to Fight AIDS, Tuberculosis and Malaria. Given that the largest portion of this nonavertable burden is related to injuries (200.5 million DALYs per year; 70.3 percent of the nonavertable burden), development of injury prevention programs and improvement of prehospital care for injured patients in LMICs are critical. To provide the best possible care for our patients, we must advocate for a comprehensive strategy that includes both surgical and nonsurgical interventions.

In conclusion, surgically treatable conditions are an important public health problem in LMICs; the magnitude of avertable burden exceeds the burden of some of the most widely recognized global health problems.

FUTURE DIRECTIONS

Health Systems and Performance of Surgical Services

Global health initiatives have often struggled to implement changes at scale. It is reasonable to expect that scaling up surgical care in LMICs will face similar problems unless the understanding of the factors that determine the performance of surgical services is improved. Performance refers to the ability of the surgical service to deliver safe, effective, accessible, and cost-efficient care—and ultimately whether that surgical service meets the needs of the population. A health system encompasses the individuals, organizations, and processes—from the national government to the private sector to community-based organizations—that focus primarily on ensuring health outcomes (WHO 2007). Surgery performance can vary markedly in different health systems, even at similar levels of health care expenditure.

The recent focus on strengthening health systems in LMICs (Mills, Rasheed, and Tollman 2006; Palen and others 2012), and, in particular, the role of primary health care, means that this is an opportune time to develop strategies for examining the performance of surgical services. An evolving theme is that surgical care is an essential component of primary health care (WHO 2008). In the new conceptual model, primary health care is viewed as a hub of coordination within the health system, with the first-level hospital serving as one of many components (figure 2.6). The challenge for surgery is to integrate the organizational structure of surgical care into the larger health system and to concurrently develop methods for measuring its performance. Meeting this challenge will require moving beyond the reductionist view that surgical care is simply a collection of components that includes infrastructure, human resources, financing, and supplies. A more comprehensive view is needed, one that recognizes that surgical care is part of a larger health system in which performance is determined by critical interrelationships.

Research and Development Goals

The literature on surgical care in LMICs is growing rapidly. Nevertheless, major knowledge gaps remain, especially related to optimal strategies for delivering surgical care at first-level hospitals and measuring its impact. Based on the work done in preparing this chapter, the following are some of the areas that require investments in research and development.

- *Improved methodology for assessing the public health impact of surgical care.* As noted by Gosselin, Ozgediz, and Poenaru (2013) and further illustrated by the challenges we encountered in trying to estimate a global burden of surgical disease, DALY-based approaches may not be the best metric for global surgery or for measuring the impact of surgical interventions. The ideal metric would be simple to measure, oriented toward quantifying outcomes of interventions, and easy for policy makers and health planners to interpret. Alternatives include measurement of disease prevalence, backlogs in treatment, disability incurred by delays in care, and value of a statistical life (Gosselin, Ozgediz, and Poenaru 2013). The value of a statistical life is of particular interest because it widens the spectrum of tools available to estimate the cost-effectiveness of surgical care (Corlew 2010). Research is needed to explore these and other alternatives and to determine their utility in HICs as well as LMICs.
- *Better estimates of the avertable and nonavertable burden of surgically treatable conditions in LMICs.* Although population-based countrywide surgical surveys in LMICs have been undertaken (Groen and others 2013; Petroze and others 2013), these data are not of sufficient detail to be used in GBD calculations. Data collection needs to be standardized so that data generated in community-based surveys can be used in future GBD studies.

Figure 2.6 Primary Care as a Hub of Coordination: Networking within the Community Served and Outside Partners

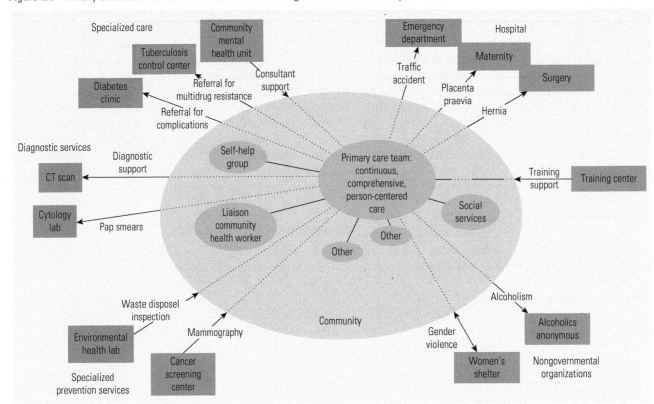

Source: WHO 2008.

Note: CT = computed tomography. The emergency, maternity, and surgery departments are included as essential components.

Moreover, these data could be used to support the case for expanding the purview of future GBD studies. Because our analysis was based heavily on methodological assumptions, our estimates need to be validated. Validation could perhaps be undertaken in prospective pilot studies from a sample of hospitals or populations, or by comparing appropriately matched hospitals in high- and low-income settings.

- *Identified strategies to address the nonavertable surgical burden.* One of the most important findings in our study was that the majority of the surgical burden is currently nonavertable. Nonavertable does not necessarily imply a problem that cannot be addressed; the nonavertable burden can be reduced through nonsurgical means, such as injury prevention, improved delivery of care, or innovation. Research priorities include a more detailed analysis of the nonavertable burden, ways in which injury prevention strategies can best be implemented in settings of limited resources, and identification of areas in which surgical innovation might have the greatest impact in LMICs.

- *Tools to assess surgical care within primary health care systems.* Although the development of indicators for monitoring and evaluating project and system performance is commonplace within health and economic development programs, this process has not been applied in a systematic way to the field of essential and emergency surgery in LMICs. One approach might be to adapt the WHO's *Monitoring the Building Blocks of Health Systems* Monitoring and Evaluation Matrix (MBBHS M&E Matrix) (WHO 2010) or similar tool for surgical care. Within the MBBHS M&E Matrix are health system building blocks that represent discrete areas of policy making, inputs into the health system, and direct outputs. Improvements in the health system are measured in four domains: improved health, responsiveness, social and financial risk protection, and improved efficiency. The MBBHS M&E strategy seeks to create government accountability for progress and performance toward health goals, to facilitate results-based financing of health programs, to measure the impact of interventions and inputs, and to create sustainable measurement strategies (WHO 2010). The matrix provides a comprehensive strategy for assessing the function of primary health care systems, but it has not been adapted to monitor and evaluate surgical care. Adapting the MBBSHS M&E Matrix or a similar framework for assessing surgical care in LMICs could help facilitate surgery's integration into health systems and simultaneously provide a mechanism for measuring its performance.

- *Models of how surgical care can best be implemented in LMICs.* Perhaps the most pressing research need in global surgery is to determine how emergency and essential surgical services can best be implemented in countries where the needs are greatest and where health systems are least developed. At present, far too few examples of well-functioning surgical services in LMICs can be found, and little research on what factors make them successful has been conducted. Scaling up surgical care in LMICs requires much more than theater personnel, equipment, and infrastructure; it also requires education and training, functioning methods and processes, data systems, and an enabling environment (Akenroye, Adebona, and Akenroye 2013). Research priorities include the design of a basic surgical package that is flexible enough to be adapted to local needs, benchmarks to assess what is required for health systems to deliver emergency and essential surgical care at first-level hospitals, strategies for measuring the impact of the improvements, and most important, cost estimates.

- *Research to better understand the surgical workforce needs in LMICs.* One of the greatest challenges of scaling up surgical care worldwide lies in deficiencies in the supply, training, and distribution of human resources. Training surgeons takes time and is expensive; once qualified, they are reluctant to serve in rural first-level hospitals where the needs are greatest. Nonetheless, various countries have successfully trained doctors to perform surgical care in rural areas (Sani and others 2009); in other cases, countries have introduced nonphysician cadres specializing in surgery. Mozambique, for example, began training nonphysician surgeons (*técnicos de cirurgia*) in 1984, a program involving a three-year degree (Cumbi and others 2007; Pereira and others 2007; Vaz and others 1999). Important questions remain regarding how surgical providers in LMICs should be trained, their scope of practice, and how best to assess their surgical skills.

- *Studies to define how quality of surgical care affects the entire health service.* Assessment of surgical care in settings of limited resources has typically focused on physical and human resources and has neglected the process and outcomes components. However, understanding how the physical and human resources affect processes and outcomes is necessary to gain a proper understanding of the factors that determine quality of care. The link between quality of surgical care and the public's perception of the health system needs further study.

- *Initiatives to better align surgical care with other global health movements.* Surgery has an important role in meeting the 2015 United Nations Millennium Development Goals (PLoS Medicine Editors 2008). Scaling up surgical care in LMICs will be required if infectious, child, and maternal mortality rates are to be brought down to universally low rates by 2035 (Jamison and others 2013). No detailed studies have been made of the role surgical care has in meeting the Millennium Development Goals and Global Health 2035 targets. Because both initiatives link health improvement to economic growth, integrating surgical care into these important movements could be an important strategy for encouraging investment in surgical care in LMICs.

ANNEXES

The annexes to this chapter are as follows. They are available at http://www.dcp-3.org/surgery:
- Annex 2A. ICD-9 Codes Included in the GBD 2010 Study
- Annex 2B. The Role of Surgery in Global Health: Analysis of United States Inpatient Procedure Frequency by Condition Using the Global Burden of Disease 2010 Framework
- Annex 2C. AHRQ ICD-9 Procedure Codes
- Annex 2D. Surgical Procedures Required to Treat the GBD 2010 Causes Included in the Basic Surgical Care Scale-Up Model
- Annex 2E. Adjustments to Account For The Burden Not Amenable to Surgical Care
- Annex 2F. Additional Details on How Burden Calculations Were Performed

1. Higashi, H., J. J. Barendregt, N. J. Kassebaum, T. G. Weiser, S. W. Bickler, and others. 2014. "Burden of Injuries Avertable by a Basic Surgical Package in Low- and Middle-Income Regions: A Systematic Analysis from the Global Burden of Disease 2010 Study." *World Journal of Surgery* 39 (1):1–9. doi:10.1007/s00268-014-2685-x.

2. Higashi, H., J. J. Barendregt, N. J. Kassebaum, T. G. Weiser, S. W. Bickler, and others. 2014. "The Burden of Selected Congenital Anomalies Amenable to Surgery in Low and Middle-Income Regions: Cleft Lip and Palate, Congenital Heart Anomalies and Neural Tube Defects." *Archives of Disease in Childhood.* September 26. Electronic publication ahead of print.

3. Higashi, H., J. J. Barendregt, N. J. Kassebaum, T. G. Weiser, S. W. Bickler, and others. 2014. "Surgically-Avertable Burden of Digestive Diseases at First-Level Hospitals in Low and Middle-Income Regions." *Surgery.* October 22. Electronic publication ahead of print.

4. Higashi, H., J. J. Barendregt, N. J. Kassebaum, T. G. Weiser, S. W. Bickler, and T. Vos. 2015. "Surgically-Avertable Burden of Obstetric Conditions in Low and Middle-Income Regions: A Modelled Analysis." *BJOG* 122 (2): 228–36.

• Annex 2G. WHO Monitoring the Building Blocks of Health Systems

NOTES

This research was supported by grant number R24TW008910 from the Fogarty International Center (Stephen Bickler, David Chang, and Emilia Noormahomed) and the Bill and Melinda Gates Foundation (Hideki Higashi, Jan Barendregt, and Theo Vos) under the Disease Control Priorities Network Project. The content is solely the responsibility of the authors and does not necessarily represent the official views of the Fogarty International Center, the National Institutes of Health (NIH), and the Bill and Melinda Gates Foundation. The NIH Common Fund supports the first award.

The World Bank classifies countries according to four income groupings. Income is measured using gross national income (GNI) per capita, in U.S. dollars, converted from local currency using the *World Bank Atlas* method. Classifications as of July 2014 are as follows:

• Low-income countries (LICs) = US$1,045 or less in 2013
• Middle-income countries (MICs) are subdivided:
  • Lower-middle-income = US$1,046 to US$4,125
  • Upper-middle-income (UMICs) = US$4,126 to US$12,745
• High-income countries (HICs) = US$12,746 or more

1. The National (Nationwide) Inpatient Sample (NIS), 2010, Healthcare Cost and Utilization Project, Agency for Healthcare Research and Quality, Rockville, MD, http://www.hcup-us.ahrq.gov/db/nation/nis/nisdbdocumentation.jsp.
2. *Basic surgical care* refers to emergency and essential surgical care that can be provided with the resources available at first-level hospitals. Because emergency and essential surgical care is often provided at higher levels of care—secondary and tertiary hospitals—our estimates are based on the effects of scaling up basic surgical care across all sectors of the health care system.
3. Paralytic ileus is grouped with intestinal obstruction in GBD 2010.

REFERENCES

Abdullah, F., H. Troedsson, and M. Cherian. 2011. "The World Health Organization Program for Emergency Surgical, Obstetric, and Anesthetic Care: From Mongolia to the Future." *Archives of Surgery* 146 (5): 620–23.

Abdur-Rahman, L. O., A. B. van As, and H. Rode. 2012. "Pediatric Trauma Care in Africa: The Evolution and Challenges." *Seminars in Pediatric Surgery* 21 (2): 111–15.

AHRQ (Agency for Healthcare Research and Quality). 2008. "Appendix A." In *Patient Safety Indicators: Technical Specifications*, Version 3.2., A-1—A-20. http://www.qualityindicators.ahrq.gov/downloads/modules/psi/v32/psi_technical_specs_v32.pdf.

Alkire, B. C., J. R. Vincent, C. T. Burns, I. S. Metzler, P. E. Farmer, and J. G. Meara. 2012. "Obstructed Labor and Caesarean Delivery: The Cost and Benefit of Surgical Intervention." *PLoS One* 7 (4): e34595.

Akenroye, O. O., O. T. Adebona, and A. T. Akenroye. 2013. "Surgical Care in the Developing World—Strategies and Framework for Improvement." *Journal of Public Health in Africa* 4: e20.

Beard, J. H., L. B. Oresanya, M. Ohene-Yeboah, R. A. Dicker, and H. W. Harris. 2013. "Characterizing the Global Burden of Surgical Disease: A Method to Estimate Inguinal Hernia Epidemiology in Ghana." *World Journal of Surgery* 37 (3): 498–503.

Bickler, S., D. Ozgediz, R. Gosselin, T. Weiser, D. Spiegel, and others. 2010. "Key Concepts for Estimating the Burden of Surgical Conditions and the Unmet Need for Surgical Care." *World Journal of Surgery* 34 (3): 374–80.

Bickler, S. W., and H. Rode. 2002. "Surgical Services for Children in Developing Countries." *Bulletin of the World Health Organization* 80 (10): 829–35.

Bickler, S. W., and D. Spiegel. 2010. "Improving Surgical Care in Low- and Middle-Income Countries: A Pivotal Role for the World Health Organization." *World Journal of Surgery* 34 (3): 386–90.

Choo, S., H. Perry, A. A. Hesse, F. Abantanga, E. Sory, and others. 2010. "Assessment of Capacity for Surgery, Obstetrics and Anaesthesia in 17 Ghanaian Hospitals Using a WHO Assessment Tool." *Tropical Medicine and International Health* 15 (9): 1109–15.

Copenhagen Consensus Center. 2012. "Copenhagen Consensus." http://www.copenhagenconsensus.Com/sites/default/files/Outcome_Document_Updated_1105.pdf.

Corlew, D. S. 2010. "Estimation of Impact of Surgical Disease through Economic Modeling of Cleft Lip and Palate Care." *World Journal of Surgery* 34 (3): 391–96.

Cumbi, A., C. Pereira, R. Malalane, F. Vaz, C. McCord, and others. 2007. "Major Surgery Delegation to Mid-level Health Practitioners in Mozambique: Health Professionals' Perceptions." *Human Resources for Health* 5: 27.

Debas, H. T., C. McCord, and A. Thind. 2006. "Surgery." In *Disease Control Priorities in Developing Countries*, 2nd ed., edited by D. T. Jamison, J. G. Breman, A. R. Measham, G. Alleyene, M. Claeson, D. B. Evans, P. Jha, A. Mills, and P. Musgrove, 1245–59. Washington, DC: Oxford University Press and World Bank.

Funk, L. M., T. G. Weiser, W. R. Berry, S. R. Lipsitz, A. F. Merry, and others. 2010. "Global Operating Theatre Distribution and Pulse Oximetry Supply: An Estimation from Reported Data." *The Lancet* 376 (9746): 1055–61.

Galukande, M., J. von Schreeb, A. Wladis, N. Mbembati, H. de Miranda, and others. 2010. "Essential Surgery at the District Hospital: A Retrospective Descriptive Analysis in Three African Countries." *PLoS Med* 7 (3): e1000243.

Gibbons, L., J. M. Belizán, J. A. Lauer, A. P. Betrán, M. Merialdi, and F. Althabe. 2010. "The Global Numbers and Costs of Additionally Needed and Unnecessary Caesarean Sections Performed per Year: Overuse as a Barrier to Universal Coverage." World Health Report Background Paper 30. http://www.who.int/healthsystems/topics/financing/healthreport/30C-sectioncosts.pdf.

Gosselin R., D. Ozgediz, and D. Poenaru. 2013. "A Square Peg in a Round Hole? Challenges with DALY-Based 'Burden of Disease' Calculations in Surgery and a Call for Alternative Metrics." World Journal of Surgery 37 (11): 2507–11.

Gosselin, R. A., A. Thind, and A. Bellardinelli. 2006. "Cost/DALY Averted in a Small Hospital in Sierra Leone: What Is the Relative Contribution of Different Services?" World Journal of Surgery 30 (4): 505–11.

Grimes, C. E., J. A. Henry, J. Maraka, N. C. Mkandawire, and M. Cotton. 2014. "Cost-Effectiveness of Surgery in Low- and Middle-Income Countries: A Systematic Review." World Journal of Surgery 38 (1): 252–63. doi: 10.1007/s00268-013-2243-y.

Groen, R. S., M. Samai, R. T. Petroze, T. B. Kamara, L. D. Cassidy, and others. 2013. "Household Survey in Sierra Leone Reveals High Prevalence of Surgical Conditions in Children." World Journal of Surgery 37 (6): 1220–26.

Jamison, D. T., L. H. Summers, G. Alleyne, K. J. Arrow, S. Berkley, and others. 2013. "Global Health 2035: A World Converging within a Generation." The Lancet 382 (9908): 1898–955.

Kushner, A. L., M. N. Cherian, L. Noel, D. A. Spiegel, S. Groth, and C. Etienne. 2010. "Addressing the Millennium Development Goals from a Surgical Perspective: Essential Surgery and Anesthesia in 8 Low- and Middle-Income Countries." Archives of Surgery 145 (2): 154–59.

Lozano, R., M. Naghavi, K. Foreman, S. Lim, K. Shibuya, and others. 2012. "Global and Regional Mortality from 235 Causes of Death for 20 Age Groups in 1990 and 2010: A Systematic Analysis for the Global Burden of Disease Study 2010." The Lancet 380 (9859): 2095–128.

McCord, C., and Q. Chowdhury. 2003. "A Cost Effective Small Hospital in Bangladesh: What It Can Mean for Emergency Obstetric Care." International Journal of Gynecology and Obstetrics 81 (1): 83–92.

Mills, A., F. Rasheed, and S. Tollman. 2006. "Strengthening Health Systems." In Disease Control Priorities in Developing Countries, 2nd ed., edited by D. T. Jamison, J. G. Breman, A. R. Measham, G. Alleyne, M. Claeson, D. B. Evans, P. Jha, A. Mills, and P. Musgrove, 87–102. Washington, DC: World Bank and Oxford University Press.

Mock, C., M. Cherian, C. Juillard, P. Donkor, S. Bickler, and others. 2010. "Developing Priorities for Addressing Surgical Conditions Globally: Furthering the Link between Surgery and Public Health Policy." World Journal of Surgery 34 (3): 381–85.

Mock, C., M. Joshipura, C. Arreola-Risa, and R. Quansah. 2012. "An Estimate of the Number of Lives That Could Be Saved through Improvements in Trauma Care Globally." World Journal of Surgery 36 (5): 959–63.

Monasta, L., L. Ronfani, F. Marchetti, M. Montico, L. Vecchi Brumatti, and others. 2012. "Burden of Disease Caused by Otitis Media: Systematic Review and Global Estimates." PLoS One 7 (4): e36226.

Mossey, P. A., and M. B. Modell. 2012 "Epidemiology of Oral Clefts 2012: An International Perspective." Frontiers of Oral Biology 16: 1–18.

Murray, C. J., M. Ezzati, A. D. Flaxman, S. Lim, R. Lozano, and others. 2012. "GBD 2010: Design, Definitions, and Metrics." The Lancet 380 (9859): 2063–66.

Murray, C. J., T. Vos, R. Lozano, M. Naghavi, A. D. Flaxman, and others. 2012. "Disability-Adjusted Life Years (DALYs) for 291 Diseases and Injuries in 21 Regions, 1990–2010: A Systematic Analysis for the Global Burden of Disease Study 2010." The Lancet 380 (9859): 2197–23.

Ndour, C., S. Dossou Gbété, N. Bru, M. Abrahamowicz, A. Fauconnier, and others. 2013. "Predicting In-Hospital Maternal Mortality in Senegal and Mali." PLoS One 8(5): e64157.

Ozgediz, D., and R. Riviello. 2008. "The 'Other' Neglected Diseases in Global Public Health: Surgical Conditions in Sub-Saharan Africa." PLoS Med 5 (6): e121.

Palen, J., W. El-Sadr, A. Phoya, R. Imtiaz, R. Einterz, and others. 2012. "PEPFAR, Health System Strengthening, and Promoting Sustainability and Country Ownership." Journal of Acquired Immune Deficiency Syndrome 60 (Suppl. 3): S113–19.

Pereira, C., A. Cumbi, R. Malalane, F. Vaz, C. McCord, and others. 2007. "Meeting the Need for Emergency Obstetric Care in Mozambique: Work Performance and Histories of Medical Doctors and Assistant Medical Officers Trained for Surgery." BJOG 114 (12): 1530–33.

Petroze, R. T., R. S. Groen, F. Niyonkuru, M. Mallory, E. Ntaganda, and others. 2013. "Estimating Operative Disease Prevalence in a Low-Income Country: Results of a Nationwide Population Survey in Rwanda." Surgery 153 (4): 457–64.

PLoS Medicine Editors. 2008. "A Crucial Role for Surgery in Reaching the UN Millennium Development Goals." PLoS Medicine 5 (8): e182.

Rao, G. N., R. Khanna, and A. Payal. 2011. "The Global Burden of Cataract." Current Opinion in Ophthalmology 22 (1): 4–9.

Rose, J., D. C. Chang, T. G. Weiser, N. J. Kassebaum, and S. W. Bickler. 2014. "The Role of Surgery in Global Health: Analysis of United States Inpatient Procedure Frequency by Condition Using the Global Burden of Disease 2010 Framework." PLoS One 9 (2) e89693.

Salomon, J. A., T. Vos, D. R. Hogan, M. Gagnon, M. Naghavi, and others. 2012. "Common Values in Assessing Health Outcomes from Disease and Injury: Disability Weights Measurement Study for the Global Burden of Disease Study 2010." The Lancet 380 (9859): 2129–43.

Sani, R., B. Nameoua, A. Yahaya, I. Hassane, R. Adamou, and others. 2009. "The Impact of Launching Surgery at the District Level in Niger." World Journal of Surgery 33 (10): 2063–68.

Spiegel, D. A., F. Abdullah, R. R. Price, R. A. Gosselin and S. W. Bickler. 2013. "World Health Organization Global Initiative for Emergency and Essential Surgical Care: 2011 and Beyond." World Journal of Surgery 37 (7): 1462–69.

Stanley, C. M., G. W. Rutherford, S. Morshed, R. R. Coughlin, and T. Beyeza. 2010. "Estimating the Healthcare Burden of Osteomyelitis in Uganda." *Transactions of the Royal Society of Tropical Medicine and Hygiene* 104 (2): 139–42.

Stewart, B., P. Khanduri, C. McCord, M. Ohene-Yeboah, S. Uranues, and others. 2014. "Global Disease Burden of Conditions Requiring Emergency Surgery." *British Journal of Surgery* 101 (1): e9–22.

Vaz, F., S. Bergstrom, L. Vaz Mda, J. Langa, and A. Bugalho. 1999. "Training Medical Assistants for Surgery." *Bulletin of the World Health Organization* 77 (8): 688–91.

Vos, T., A. D. Flaxman, M. Naghavi, R. Lozano, C. Michaud, and others. 2012. "Years Lived with Disability (YLDs) for 1160 Sequelae of 289 Diseases and Injuries 1990–2010: A Systematic Analysis for the Global Burden of Disease Study 2010." *The Lancet* 380 (9859): 2163–96.

Weiser, T. G., S. E. Regenbogen, K. D. Thompson, A. B. Haynes, S. R. Lipsitz, and others. 2008. "An Estimation of the Global Volume of Surgery: A Modelling Strategy Based on Available Data." *The Lancet* 372 (9633): 139–44.

Wu, V. K., D. Poenaru, and M. J. Poley. 2013. "Burden of Surgical Congenital Anomalies in Kenya: A Population-Based Study." *Journal of Tropical Pediatrics* 59 (3): 195–202.

WHO (World Health Organization). 2003. *Surgical Care at the District Hospital.* Geneva: WHO. http://www.who.int/surgery/publications/scdh_manual/en/.

———. 2007. *Everybody's Business: Strengthening Health Systems to Improve Health Outcomes: WHO's Framework for Action.* Geneva: WHO. http://www.who.int/healthsystems/strategy/everybodys_business.pdf.

———. 2008. *World Health Report 2008: Primary Health Care—Now More Than Ever.* Geneva: WHO.

———. 2010. *Monitoring the Building Blocks of Health Systems: A Handbook of Indicators and Their Measurement Strategies.* Geneva: WHO.

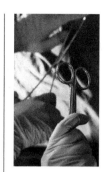

Chapter 3

Surgery and Trauma Care

Richard A. Gosselin, Anthony Charles,
Manjul Joshipura, Nyengo Mkandawire,
Charles N. Mock, Raymond R. Price, and David Spiegel

INTRODUCTION

The burden of death and disability attributable to lack of access to surgical care for traumatic injuries, as well as of nontraumatic chronic conditions and soft tissue and bone infections, falls most heavily on people in low- and middle-income countries (LMICs) (Ozgediz and others 2008; Spiegel and others 2008). Human and technical capacities are insufficient to address the existing burden of injuries in these countries. Selected surgical interventions for trauma have proven cost-effective in these settings, and innovative low-cost programs and interventions have improved trauma care outcomes at individual hospitals. It is critical that LMICs create or strengthen existing trauma systems to improve outcomes. Identifying effective and cost-effective interventions and strategies to inform the future direction of these resource-challenged countries is an essential step in this process.

The chapter on surgery in the *Disease Control Priorities in Developing Countries*, second edition (*DCP2*) (Jamison and others 2006) exposed the scarcity of relevant evidence on outcomes, effectiveness, and cost-effectiveness in the literature from the developing world; unfortunately, this situation has improved only mildly. Although some interventions and strategies have been identified (Tollefson and Larrabee 2012), deficiencies in both the quantity and the quality of data remain glaring (Vos 2009).

This chapter addresses the surgical aspects of care for these conditions. It presents available epidemiological data, as well as data on systematic approaches to trauma and interventions in specific anatomic areas.

International and National Advocacy for Improved Trauma Care

International and national organizations have begun to recognize and implement strategies for addressing the worldwide trauma pandemic. The World Health Organization (WHO) has developed guidelines with an internationally applicable metric for countries to use to evaluate and monitor resources for trauma care in their health care facilities and system-wide parameters. The creation of the WHO Global Alliance for Care of the Injured provides a common platform for greater political advocacy for increased attention and resource allocation to trauma care. World Health Assembly (WHA) Resolution 60.22 on trauma and emergency care services provides a high-level global political endorsement for improvements in trauma care. The Ministry of Health in Uganda targeted trauma care and injury prevention as one of the nation's top 10 health care priorities, following the review of data collected from a WHO-supported hospital-based injury surveillance system that demonstrated the significant burden of disease arising from injuries.

Corresponding author: Richard A. Gosselin, MD, MPH, MSc, FRCS(C), University of California, San Francisco, froggydoc@gmail.com

GLOBAL BURDEN OF TRAUMA

One of the findings of the 2013 Global Health Estimates (GHE) study is that the ongoing epidemiological transition is shifting the global disease burden away from premature deaths (years of life lost, YLLs) and toward years lived with disability (YLDs) (WHO 2013b). Worldwide, the percentage of deaths due to injury has fallen from 9.4 percent to 9.1 percent.

During the same period, deaths due to musculoskeletal disorders have increased 34 percent (WHO 2013b), as summarized in table 3.1. The WHO report on road safety estimates that 1.25 million people died from road traffic injuries (RTIs) in 2010 (WHO 2013c). More than 75 percent of those were young males in their productive years. More than 50 percent of all deaths in LMICs were pedestrians and cyclists. For every death, it is estimated that 20 people are injured; of these injured, one will experience some form of permanent disability. The burden of RTIs is already disproportionally shouldered by LMICs (Ameratunga, Hijar, and Norton 2006), and most of the projected increase of this burden will occur in countries with rapid economic growth, in particular, China and India (Mathew and Hanson 2009; WHO 2013c).

Epidemiological Burden of Preventable Trauma Deaths

Decreasing the heavy burden imposed on individuals and society is the overarching mission of trauma systems and

Figure 3.1 Case Fatality Rates for Severely Injured People, 1998

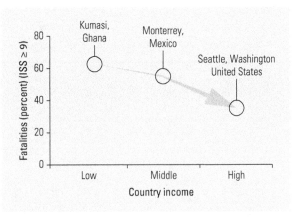

Source: Data based on Mock and others (1998). Illustration courtesy of Intermountain Healthcare.
Note: ISS = Injury Severity Score. Income classifications are based on status at the time of the study. Ghana is now a lower-middle-income country, and Mexico is an upper-middle-income country.

one of the main challenges for public health in this century (ACS 2006; Mock and others 2004). People in LMICs have as yet been unable to benefit as significantly from trauma system development as those in high-income countries (HICs) have. Case fatality rates for seriously injured patients (Injury Severity Score [ISS] ≥ 9) were significantly lower in an HIC (the United States), compared with a middle-income country (MIC) (Mexico), or a low-income country (LIC) (Ghana), as shown in figure 3.1 (Mock and others 1998).

Between 1.7 and 1.9 million lives, or 34–38 percent of all injury deaths in LMICs, could be saved if trauma care initiatives could be designed and implemented to reduce the case fatality rates among seriously injured patients to equal those in HICs (Mock and others 2012).

Systematic Approach to Trauma Care

Although this chapter concentrates on the effectiveness of individual interventions, such as operations, the overall organizational context within which these interventions are provided needs to be considered as an integral part of the health care system. Trauma care necessitates the rapid availability of trained personnel and readily available and sufficient equipment and supplies. Improving the availability of these human and physical resources and monitoring the care-provision process can significantly improve the outcomes. Better system-wide organization and planning for trauma care can help achieve these goals.

A trauma system encompasses the entire spectrum of services that a country or region has in place: prehospital care, initial emergency care, definitive hospital care

Table 3.1 Worldwide Rankings of Injuries and Musculoskeletal Conditions for Deaths, YLDs, and DALYs, 2000–11

		Ranking		Change in rates per 100,000 population (percent)
		2000	2011	
All injuries	Deaths	n.a.	n.a.	−8.7
	YLDs	n.a.	n.a.	8.7
	DALYs	n.a.	n.a.	−15.3
Road traffic injuries	Deaths	11	9	8.9
	YLDs	16	15	−2.4
	DALYs	10	8	+0.9
Falls	Deaths	n.a.	n.a.	13.7
	YLDs	8	8	12.0
	DALYs	n.a.	17	4.0
Musculoskeletal disorders	Deaths	n.a.	n.a.	+34.0
	YLDs	n.a.	n.a.	+7.2
	DALYs	n.a.	n.a.	+8.3

Source: Data based on Global Health Estimates (WHO 2013b).
Note: DALYs = disability-adjusted life years; YLDs = years lived with disability; n.a. = not available.

(care provided after initial resuscitation to definitively treat injuries), and long-term rehabilitation of injured survivors. It also encompasses the information systems needed to monitor and ensure quality of care along this spectrum. In HICs, a variety of elements commonly constitute a formal and well-organized trauma system (table 3.2).

These elements are facilitated by enabling legislation and oversight by appropriately empowered governmental agencies to achieve the basic goals for trauma systems (box 3.1).

Table 3.2 Elements of Trauma Care Systems that Coordinate with the Public Health System

Prevention
Prehospital Care
Standards for training for paramedics and for equipment on ambulances
Triage protocols for prehospital care
Definitive Hospital Care
Network of facilities with increasing trauma care capabilities
External verification of hospitals and trauma centers with different levels of capability for trauma care
Transfer guidelines and interfacility protocols
Rehabilitation
Process Improvement and Patient Safety Initiatives
Research
Trauma registries

Source: Authors.

Box 3.1

Trauma Care System Goals

- Decrease the incidence and severity of trauma
- Ensure optimal, equitable, accessible care for all trauma patients
- Prevent unnecessary deaths and disabilities from trauma
- Contain costs and enhance efficiency
- Implement quality- and performance-improvement processes
- Identify appropriate resources and ensure their availability

Source: Adapted from U.S. DHHS (2006).

EFFECTIVENESS OF TRAUMA CARE SYSTEMS

Geographic areas that implement better-organized trauma systems that include the elements listed in table 3.2 are able to decrease trauma mortality. Better-organized trauma systems have been consistently shown to decrease mortality by 15–20 percent among treated patients. The effect is even more pronounced in lowering medically preventable deaths, that is, deaths from causes that should be able to be treated well in most locations, such as deaths from airway obstruction or splenic lacerations. Such medically preventable deaths are typically decreased by 50 percent in better-organized trauma systems. These findings are fairly consistent across multiple states in the United States and provinces in Canada, as well as several other HICs, including Australia, Israel, the Netherlands, and the United Kingdom (Siman-Tov, Radomislensky, and Peleg 2012; Tallon and others 2012). Better-organized trauma systems have also demonstrated improved functional outcomes among survivors of severe injuries (Gabbe and others 2012).

Improvements in the organization of trauma systems have generally been very low cost in comparison with the overall cost of trauma care. For example, strengthening the trauma care system in Quebec Province, Canada, led to a notable decrease in mortality of all severely injured persons province-wide from 50 percent in the early 1990s to 10 percent in the early 2000s. The costs of this reduction were low and sustainable. An initial expenditure of Can$2 million (US$1.5 million) was invested to elevate the four major trauma centers in the province to minimum criteria, especially with respect to infrastructure. This expenditure amounted to far less than 1 percent of the provincial health budget for that year. Subsequently, the only ongoing cost has been for the monitoring, evaluation, and regulatory oversight provided by the accreditation committee. These costs have been minimal because the work was mostly done by volunteer academics and trauma care clinicians (WHO 2010) (box 3.2).

The ability to demonstrate systemwide improvements in trauma mortality rates requires regionwide trauma registries or other health information systems to monitor mortality rates among injured persons. Such information systems are rudimentary or nonexistent in most LMICs. There have been almost no reports of effectiveness of systemwide improvements in these countries. Many lack designated national lead agencies to oversee trauma-related issues, including policy making, finance, establishment of trauma systems, training of personnel, and accreditation or licensing of trauma care providers (Zong and others 2011).

Story of a Successful System-Wide Improvement: The Quebec Trauma System

The Problem

In 1989, trauma-related mortality was higher in Quebec than in the rest of Canada and the United States because of the following deficiencies:

- No prehospital triage system
- No communication system among centers to facilitate the arrival, referral, and transport of patients
- No prehospital treatment guidelines
- No province-wide, uniform hospital management standards
- No mechanism for quality control.

The Solution

The implementation of a province-wide trauma registry that included all trauma admissions allowed evidence-based policy decisions to be made and led to the phased implementation of a comprehensive trauma system:

- **Phase 1** (1993–94): Accreditation of trauma centers and initiation of a trauma care network, following American College of Surgeons guidelines
- **Phase 2** (1994–97): Creation of prehospital triage and interhospital transfer protocols. The registry

had allowed the identification of a subset of patients with severe injuries, and these patients were now brought directly to first-level trauma centers.

- **Phase 3** (1997–present): Review, evaluation, and consolidation of the system. New second-level and third-level centers were accredited, and some older centers lost their accreditation. Protocols were reviewed and updated, as necessary; areas of subspecialty care were made operational.

The Results

- Overall mortality fell from 20 percent to 10 percent after accreditation of first-level trauma centers.
- Mean prehospital time declined from 62 to 44 minutes.
- Proportion of patients with Injury Severity Score > 25 treated at first-level centers went from 36 percent to 84 percent.
- Mortality for the subset of severely injured patients fell from 52 percent to 10 percent.
- The overall costs were very low (Can$2 million to start the program) and have remained sustainable.

Source: WHO 2010.

Nevertheless, several countries have made progress in implementing systemwide improvements. Sri Lanka has put in place a national trauma secretariat that is implementing some of the trauma system elements used in HICs, including a National Injury Surveillance System to monitor trauma care nationwide. Similarly, the Hanoi Health Department has documented progressive, sustainable improvements in the capabilities of its network of hospitals through better organization and planning, with no additional budget allocation to trauma care.

Although data to monitor patient outcomes systemwide are sparse in most LMICs, documented improvements in outcome have been made in some components of the trauma system, such as in prehospital settings. For example, improvements in prehospital care capabilities, especially through the provision of widespread first aid training for lay first responders, were found to be among the most cost-effective of all surgical

interventions studied by *DCP3*, discussed in more detail in chapter 14.

Definitive Hospital Care

Poor infrastructure, limited human resources, unavailability of acute interventions, and lack of life-saving equipment and essential supplies for resuscitation plague health care facilities in LMICs trying to provide trauma care for their injured people (Choo and others 2010; Kushner and others 2010). The WHO and the International Association for Trauma Surgery and Intensive Care developed guidelines for essential trauma care services, including the following (Mock and others 2004):

- Standards for the care of the injured person
- Set of essential trauma care services

- Suggested resources necessary to offer these services
- Guidance to promote national efforts to deliver resources and services

The Essential Trauma Care Project established a set of 11 essential trauma care services that should be made available to all injured patients in any setting worldwide. This list can help hospitals, health care providers, ministries of health, and other stakeholders develop appropriate trauma care improvement initiatives (Mock and others 2006) (box 3.3).

In addition, the Essential Trauma Care Project, recognizing that every facility cannot have all the resources and skills of third-level care facilities, categorized resources and skills (essential, desired, irrelevant, or possibly required) to match the capabilities of different levels of facilities (first level, general practice, specialist, or third level) in an attempt to encourage appropriate improvements across the entire spectrum of fixed facilities in the system.

Box 3.3

Essential Trauma Care Services

Airway: Appropriately managed

Breathing: Supported until able to breathe independently

Pneumothorax/hemothorax: Diagnosed and treated expeditiously

Bleeding: Stopped, whether external or internal

Shock: Recognized and treated; intravenous fluids available

Brain injuries: Space-occupying lesions decompressed in a timely manner

Abdominal injuries: Promptly identified and treated appropriately

Extremity injuries: Corrected

Unstable spinal cord injuries: Recognized and managed with appropriate immobilization

Rehabilitation services: Provided to minimize long-term impairment

Medications: Made available for these services and for pain control.

Source: Mock and others 2004.

Although a network of facilities with increasing resources and capabilities may provide the best use of limited resources in LMICs, a variety of systems provide definitive care in different countries and regions of the world.

In China, 400,000 people die from trauma-related deaths each year (Zong and others 2011); trauma is the leading cause of death in males ages 18–40 years in China. Although no national guidelines or protocols guide trauma care, China has developed various types of regionalized trauma systems that have resulted in improved patient outcomes. Despite these regional improvements, only 1 percent of 19,712 hospitals in the country have established trauma departments.

Several LMICs have improved trauma care in the rural areas through education and simple infrastructure development (Henry and others 2012; Mock and others 2005). A trauma continuing education course taught in rural Ghana showed improvements in the initial management of trauma patients with torso and orthopedic injuries, in plastic surgical care, and in radiologic interpretation one year following training. Basic airway maneuvers (93 percent) and proper chest tube insertion (67 percent) increased significantly, while advanced airway utilization remained low (20 percent). Areas with less improvement appeared to be those requiring more advanced training, such as open fractures (33 percent), closed fractures (20 percent), and diagnosis of intra-abdominal injuries (20 percent) (Mock and others 2005).

Mongolia, using the Global Initiative for Emergency and Essential Surgical Care program, increased the percentage of rural health facilities with actual emergency rooms from 25 percent to 83 percent; the emergency room supplies availability increased from 5 percent to 65 percent over a two-year period (Henry and others 2012). Basic skills in wound debridement (15 percent to 55 percent), resuscitation (5 percent to 15 percent), fracture management (9 percent to 14 percent), and penetrating injuries (5 percent to 15 percent) all improved.

Interventions to improve prehospital trauma care have proven effective, but this area remains a significant challenge for poorer countries (Jayaraman and others 2009; Nielsen and others 2012). The quality of hospital care varies considerably according to available human and material resources (Mock 2011). Facilities that are integrated into a broader trauma system generally have better outcomes (Gruen and others 2012; O'Reilly and others 2013). McCord and Chowdhury (2003) were the first to report the cost-effectiveness analysis of a first-level hospital in rural Bangladesh that handled a heavy caseload of obstetrics but also general trauma: US$11 per disability-adjusted life year (DALY) averted.

A subsequent study in a pure trauma first-level hospital in Cambodia found a cost-effectiveness of US$78 per DALY averted (Gosselin and Heitto 2008). Another study comparing two Médecins Sans Frontières trauma hospitals in Haiti and Nigeria found a cost-effectiveness ratio of US$223 and US$172 per DALY averted, respectively, with almost all the difference attributable to pay scales and employee-benefit schemes (Gosselin, Maldonado, and Elder 2010).

Transfer Guidelines and Capabilities

The guidelines that have been refined over the past 30 years in HICs for transferring more severely injured patients to facilities with increased capabilities rely on physiologic, anatomic, and mechanistic indicators of severe injury (MacKenzie and others 2006). However, in many LMICs, formal referral systems do not exist or function poorly. In Cambodia, informal systems are used in which patients are transferred by taxi, accompanied by community volunteers (Nakahara and others 2010). Referral distances are often long and cost prohibitive for many families. Coordinated transfer of more critically injured patients to regional facilities with adequate human and physical resources could be an important method for more effectively using the limited resources in LMICs.

Rehabilitation

As injury-related disabilities increase, rehabilitation that assists with the reintegration of injured patients into functional society has broad implications. Physiotherapy and occupational therapy linked with vocational skills training programs are needed in LMICs to address the 1 billion people who are experiencing disabilities by providing the tools needed to help patients attain physical and socioeconomic independence and remain productive members of their communities (WHO 2013a).

LMICs are home to 80 percent of people with disabilities, and they are typically among the very poorest. In Haiti, the poorest country in the Western Hemisphere, Healing Hands for Haiti, a nonprofit nongovernmental organization working closely with the local health care community, provides rehabilitation education and training, clinical treatment, disability prevention, and public awareness of disability and rehabilitation.[1]

Land mines, which are prevalent in many LMICs, are responsible for approximately 26,000 new amputees per year; worldwide, there are more than 250,000 such amputees. Estimates range as high as 10 million to 25 million amputees worldwide when the effects of untreated chronic diseases, such as diabetes or vascular disease, are included. The Jaipur prosthesis, named for the town where it was designed, is a culturally appropriate, socially acceptable, low-cost but high-quality prosthetic foot that was developed in India through a partnership between an orthopedic surgeon (P. D. Sethi) and a local craftsman (Ram Chandra Sharma). Using local production methods, the Jaipur foot has been used in more than 22 countries, helping more than 900,000 amputees in developing and landmine-affected countries (Price 2013).

At its 66th assembly in 2013, the WHA adopted a resolution that calls for the WHO and member states to ensure equal access to health services for people with disabilities. This resolution, supported by 98 countries, serves as a clarion call for improved rehabilitation services in LMICs (WHO 2013a).

Research, Quality Improvement, and Patient Safety Initiatives

Trauma registries are integral for trauma research that can help monitor and improve trauma care, yet relatively few trauma registries exist in developing countries (O'Reilly and others 2013). A literature review of trauma registries in LMICs identified 84 articles; of these, 76 were sourced from 47 registries. Most were from China, the Islamic Republic of Iran, Jamaica, South Africa, and Uganda (O'Reilly and others 2013). There were large variations in processes and variables collected—some collecting less than 20 variables. A variety of ISSs were used, most commonly the standard ISS. Using information obtained from the Injury Control Center in Uganda, the Ministry of Health included injury as one of the top 10 health priorities facing the Ugandan people.[2]

Quality improvement (QI) programs have been shown to be valuable and inexpensive tools for strengthening the care of severely injured patients. The Royal Australasian College of Surgeons convened a meeting in Melbourne, Australia, in 2012 to explore experiences with trauma QI activities in LMICs in the East Asia and Pacific region (Stelfox and others 2012). Only 56 percent of the respondents reported having morbidity and mortality conferences, 31 percent monitored complications, 25 percent conducted preventable-death studies, and 6 percent used statistical methods for analyzing morbidity and mortality rates. The barriers for instituting QI programs included limited engagement and support from leaders, organizational diversity, heavy clinical workloads, and medico-legal concerns. One QI program implemented successfully at the facility level in Thailand is described in box 3.4.

Success Story: A Quality Improvement Program at Khon Kaen Hospital, Thailand

The Problem

Clinicians at Khon Kaen Hospital in northern Thailand knew that they were seeing increasing trauma cases but lacked ways to document the increase to inform their recommendations for better prevention and improved trauma care.

The Solution

The hospital initiated a quality improvement (QI) program based on a trauma registry.

- **Phase 1:** Data retrieval, collection, and storage using participatory action research, peer review, and medical audits.
- **Phase 2:** Data generation to allow the identification of general problems involving diagnosis, early management, resuscitation, and monitoring, as well as specific problems involving rapid recognition and management of limb- and life-threatening injuries.
- **Phase 3:** Development of key performance indicators for the overall management of trauma patients, from prehospital care to rehabilitation after discharge upon recognition of potential pitfalls, such as delays, errors, and systemic inadequacies.

Examples include the following:

- Penetrating injuries are explored within one hour of arrival.
- Long-bone fractures are fixed within 48 hours of arrival.
- All patients with Glasgow Coma Scale <13 receive a head computed tomography scan.
- All patients are seen within four hours of arrival.

This QI program has been regularly evaluated and updated, as necessary.

The Results

Direct improvements: Mortality rates decreased 50 percent, delays in diagnosis decreased 70 percent, and diagnostic or therapeutic errors decreased 50 percent.

Indirect improvements: Improvements were made in the trauma referral plan, as well as in prehospital care and survival.

Source: WHO 2010.

Their recommendations on trauma QI and better data were included in the 2007 WHA resolution on trauma and emergency care (Mock 2007).

TRAUMA CARE OF SPECIFIC BODY REGIONS

Head, Neck, Face, and Spine

Traumatic injury epidemiology in LICs and LMICs remains a relatively neglected subject (Sitsapesan and others 2013). However, identifying the most commonly injured body regions is important in the design of the most appropriate and cost-effective treatment strategies (Stewart and others 2013). Health care providers trained in neurosurgery, otolaryngology, ophthalmology, plastic surgery, or dentistry would be better able to treat face, head, and neck injuries. Orthopedic and reconstructive surgical training might be more critical for addressing fractures.

Head injury is the leading cause of injury death in many countries (Qureshi and others 2013). An estimated 10 million people suffer traumatic brain injuries (TBIs) annually, making TBI an important public health problem. TBIs pose especially difficult problems in LICs and LMICs, where TBI rates are higher than in HICs, but existing health systems are inadequate to address the resulting disabilities (Hyder 2013). Authors in HICs, where resources are much greater, have published most of the guidelines for the management of severe brain injuries.

In Uganda, minor head injury (12 percent) was the third most common cause for trauma admission in one hospital; more severe injuries, such as intracranial hemorrhage (1.9 percent) and skull fracture (1.5 percent), were much less common (Hulme 2010). In Sierra Leone, a population survey identified injuries to the face, head, and neck combined as the second most common cause of injuries reported (16 percent), following extremity injuries (55 percent) (Stewart and others 2013).

Access to dedicated neurosurgical care is limited in LICs and LMICs (Alexander and others 2009). General surgeons or even medical officers with limited training care for the vast majority of head injury patients. Dedicated neurosurgical units are uncommon. Although TBI is a frequent problem in South Africa (25 percent of hospital admissions are due to TBI), only a small subset of patients actually require specialized neurosurgical care.

In resource-constrained settings, basic clinical evaluation tools such as the Glasgow Coma Score (GCS) and heart rate can effectively triage head injury patients and identify those most critically ill. In Malawi, a multivariate logistic regression model revealed that GCS and heart rate changes correlated closely with mortality: a drop in heart rate below 60 beats per minute (bpm) or an increase in heart rate above 100 bpm increased the odds of dying by 10.9 and 11.6 times, respectively (Qureshi and others 2013). Based on the GCS, the odds of mortality for moderate and severe head injury increases by 4- and 88-fold, respectively, compared with mild head injury. The presence of multiple injuries exacerbated head trauma; all deaths in the moderate head injury group were associated with multiple trauma.

Accordingly, simple methods to improve care for head injuries in LMICs could include the following:

- Immediate measurement should be made of GCS and vital signs.
- Triage guidelines should be based on GCS and neurologic examination.
- Health care personnel treating patients should consider whether injured patients with GCS 3 should take up limited beds and resources in intensive care units.
- Patients with multiple trauma injuries should receive higher triage priority and appropriate and accurate resuscitation to limit mortality and morbidity.

Survival rates among the most critical neurotrauma patients depend on the development of the trauma system, including access to emergency and neurointensive care units and neurosurgeons. Low compensation for trauma care and fear of being sued may serve as disincentives to the few neurosurgeons in these areas from participating fully in integrated neurotrauma care (Rubiano and others 2013).

Spinal cord injuries usually result from road traffic accidents, falls, or sports. In Nigeria, cervical spine injuries represent 46.2 percent of all spinal injuries; the two most common causes of cervical spine injuries are RTIs (67 percent) and falls (23 percent) (Solagberu 2002). Back injuries represent 12 percent of traumatic injuries in Sierra Leone (Stewart and others 2013). In austere environments where specialized rehabilitation resources are lacking, conservative management of spine injuries with complete paralysis almost inevitably leads to sores, infections, and sepsis (Gosselin and Coppotelli 2005). Those patients with no or incomplete spinal cord injuries generally fare better than those patients with complete paralysis, but the recovery time and amount of residual disability are worse than if they had received surgical treatment.

A study from Pakistan compares costs of operative and nonoperative management of spinal injuries with complete neurological deficits. The authors find that outcomes are worse for the patients who had received surgery, as evidenced by longer length of stay, longer rehabilitation time, and higher infection rates. The mean cost of treatment is higher in the operative group (US$6,500) as compared with the nonoperative group (US$1,490). The researchers conclude that, in their setting, patients with complete spinal cord injuries should be managed nonoperatively, with surgery only if rehabilitation is impeded as the result of pain or deformity (Shamim, Ali, and Enam 2011).

Thorax and Abdomen

Patients with injuries to the thorax and abdomen may present with higher ISS scores. Information on injuries to these areas is extremely limited in LMICs and may be underdiagnosed because of patient deaths in the field, the unavailability of diagnostic capability with computed tomography scanning, and the scarcity of comprehensive registries.

Qureshi and others (2013) suggest that patients with moderate head trauma and multiple trauma may have died because of the inability to diagnose and treat abdominal injuries. Perforation of abdominal viscera was only reported in 0.5 percent of trauma cases in a Ugandan hospital, while no chest injuries were reported (Hulme 2010). Twenty-three cases of isolated small bowel perforation from blunt abdominal trauma were identified over a four-year period in a hospital in Cameroon (Chichom Mefire and others 2014). Timely diagnosis was difficult because of lack of awareness of this injury by clinicians and poor diagnostic capability. Improved education and clinical awareness, serial exams, and repeated upright chest x-rays are likely to lead to earlier diagnosis and improve treatment in low-income environments.

Pelvis and Extremities

The musculoskeletal (MSK) system is the most common site of residual disability in trauma survivors (Mock and Cherian 2008). If there is one permanently disabled person for every road traffic death, each year RTIs alone would account for 1.25 million newly disabled persons (WHO 2013c). For LMICs, the literature contains many more studies on the prevention of injuries than on their treatment (Forjuoh 2003; Norse and Hyder 2009). In many LMICs, particularly in rural areas, the first, and often only, point of care is the traditional healer. Although these healers probably do more good than harm overall, avoidable sequelae of significant injuries are well documented (Dada and others 2009). Unfortunately, the preventable burden has never been quantified.

Management protocols and techniques for optimal outcomes of MSK injuries are in general well known and widely available in HICs. They most often involve some form of bone or soft tissue surgical procedure using high-end diagnostic and intraoperative imaging and monitoring technologies and expensive implants and products. LMICs have severe shortages of well-trained surgeons, anesthesiologists, nurses, rehabilitation specialists, and equipment. Providers often have no choice but to use conservative treatment with casts and splints or traction and bed rest, with predictably worse outcomes.

Most pelvic fractures heal uneventfully with conservative management; only a minority suffer significant deformity, shortening, or chronic pain. The upper extremity can tolerate a certain degree of shortening or deformity without affecting function, so conservative treatment of fractures of the humerus, forearm, wrist, or hand, which are almost routinely treated surgically in HICs, can still yield acceptable functional results. This is not true of displaced intra-articular fractures or neglected dislocations of the shoulder, elbow, or wrist joints. The economic repercussions of a useless upper extremity in a farmer or manual laborer are self-evident. The lower extremity is not as forgiving of negative outcomes as the upper one: shortening of more than 2 centimeters, angulation of more than 5–10 degrees in any plane, displaced intra- or periarticular fractures, or nonunions all lead to significant functional impairment and eventually chronic joint pain or low back pain. The superior results of surgical treatment over conservative management of hip fractures, femur fractures, severe knee ligament injuries, many tibia fractures, and ankle and foot fractures and dislocations have all been well established in HICs during the past half century. However, to this day, most of these fractures are treated conservatively with cast or traction in LMICs. The long-term advantages of surgical management of some tibial shaft fractures over cast treatment are still debated, but not so for hip or femur fractures.

Yet it has been longstanding dogma that, even if all necessary resources are available, surgery for MSK injuries would be too expensive in LMICs. However, the Surgical Implant Generation Network (SIGN) intramedullary nailing system was designed specifically for austere environments. SIGN is a nonprofit, nongovernmental organization that provides the implants at no cost to patients. As long as all cases are reported in an electronic central database, all implants are replaced for free. This user-friendly system has seen remarkable growth; during a period of approximately 15 years, more than 110,000 patients were treated by more than 5,000 surgeons in more than 200 hospitals in 53 LMICs, with results comparable to those in HICs (Sekimpi and others 2011). This system was introduced in Cambodia in 2007. A study comparing the first 50 patients who received nails for their femur fractures to the last 50 patients who were treated by traction showed that surgery had better clinical outcomes and was more cost-effective than traction (US$888 versus US$1,107 per DALY averted, respectively) (Gosselin, Heitto, and Zirkle 2009).

Cross-Cutting Issue for Care of Injuries to All Body Regions: Bleeding

Tranexamic acid has been found to be effective in lowering mortality in bleeding trauma patients. It is a low-cost, generic medication. One cost-effectiveness analysis estimated that the cost per year of life gained by administering tranexamic acid was US$48–US$66, depending on the geographic location (Guerriero and others 2011).

BURNS

Burden of Disease

Burn injuries are among the most devastating of all injuries and a major global public health concern (Forjuoh 2006). Each year, more than 265,000 people die from fire-related burn injuries. Millions more suffer from burn-related disabilities and disfigurements, which have psychological, social, and economic effects on the survivors and their families. Fire-related burns account for 17 million DALYs lost worldwide annually (WHO 2013b). Strikingly, fires rank third worldwide for DALYs lost because of unintentional injury in Sub-Saharan Africa, second in Eastern Mediterranean and South-East Asian countries, and fifth in HICs.

Burn is a disease of poverty; the burden of burn injury falls predominantly on the world's poor, with 95 percent of fire-related burn deaths occurring in LMICs. Not only are burn deaths and injuries more common in people of lower socioeconomic status, but the survivors find that their poverty levels worsen after recovery (Peck, Molnar, and Swart 2009). The high incidence of burns in this population is driven by negative impact factors, including the influx of people to urban areas, haphazard urban development, inadequate electrification of homes, paraffin used as a primary energy source, and lack of preventive programs.

The worldwide incidence of death from fire-related injuries in 2004 was estimated to be 3.8 per 100,000 population, with the highest rates in Southeast Asia and Sub-Saharan Africa. The incidence of burns in LMICs is 4.4 per 100,000 population, compared with an incidence of 0.84 per 100,000 population in HICs (WHO 2013b). In Bangladesh, the incidence of nonfatal burn injury is 166.3 per 100,000 per year (Mashreky and others 2009).

In addition, the epidemiology of burn injuries is also different in LMICs, where it is predominantly a pediatric and geriatric disease (Ahuja and Bhattacharya 2002). Children, especially those under age five, have been shown to constitute the highest risk group of burn victims, followed by those ages 20–29. Of the studies that reported data on childhood burns, children under age four had a disproportionately higher number of burns; they accounted for nearly one-third of the total number of burn cases, all age groups considered. In many settings, including Brazil, Côte d'Ivoire, India, and Malawi, this age group accounts for nearly half of all childhood burns (Forjuoh 2006).

Burn centers are usually part of large urban hospitals and act as referral centers for patients from smaller first-level hospitals and health centers. Burn units are dedicated units within hospital structures that manage care for patients of all ages; burn units typically have dedicated nurses and staff. In LMICs, most existing burn centers are situated in large cities and are insufficient for the high incidence of injuries. Although management in these centers is based primarily on standard principles, hospitals are ill-equipped with staff and support facilities. In addition to inadequate physical structures, these centers are invariably plagued by lack of resources, lack of operating time, and shortages of blood. Often, no dedicated burn surgeons are available; general surgeons without formal burn training are involved in burn care. Burn nursing is also not a recognized concept. Resuscitation is often delayed because patients have to travel long distances and transport facilities are poor. Ambulance and prehospital services are practically nonexistent (Atiyeh, Masellis, and

Conte 2009). Furthermore, coordination between first-level hospitals and third-level burn centers is limited.

Cost-Effectiveness of Burn Care

Burn care requires a significant number of dedicated expert personnel and is resource intensive. When choosing between different treatment options, the available funds, personnel, and required expertise must be weighed. Reliable information relating costs to clinical outcomes is needed. Burn-care costs have been the subject of very few investigations and are among the least studied topics by health services researchers, particularly in LMICs (Atiyeh and others 2002). In a prospective study by Ahachi and others, the direct hospitalization cost of managing major acute burns in Lagos, Nigeria, was examined to identify the factors that influenced cost. The researchers found that the average daily cost of treating a burn patient was approximately US$6, and that the average overall cost for a burn admission was approximately US$62; the costs of wound dressings, hospital admission, and surgery constituted 29.5 percent, 25.7 percent, and 19.1 percent, respectively, of the total amount spent (Ahachi and others 2011). In a similar study in Bangladesh, the average cost for serious and major burns was US$166 and US$58 per burn injury, respectively. For the treatment of a severe burn, a family spent an average of US$462 (Mashreky and others 2009).

Prehospital care of burn victims using simple measures, such as irrigation with clean cool water and clean dressings, is of particular importance where access to hospital care is commonly delayed. Prehospital care is discussed at greater length in chapter 14.

Cost-Effectiveness of Hospital Management

Although very little literature exists on the effectiveness of burn centers compared with smaller local burn units, data suggest that the early burn excision frequently done in burn centers improves the survival of patients (Church and others 2006). Patients with burns exceeding 90 percent of total body surface area (TBSA) regularly survive in the world's best centers; this rate is in stark contrast to the mortality for burns exceeding 40 percent of TBSA in most LMICs, which approaches 100 percent (WHO 2002b). Cost-effective burn treatment to conserve scarce resources includes emphasizing early fluid resuscitation and ensuring proper compliance with established resuscitation protocols, such as the Parkland formula.

Increasingly aggressive surgical approaches, with early tangential excision and wound closure, are standard practice in burn units in HICs. Such approaches likely represent the most significant change in recent years and have led to improvements in mortality rates of burn victims at substantially lower costs than waiting for the eschar—the dead burned skin that forms a scab over the burned area—to peel off. In the absence of proper burn-care facilities, blood supply, and other resources such as dressings, and with inadequately trained personnel, such aggressive therapy in burn victims can induce further trauma and result in suboptimal outcomes (Munster, Smith-Meek, and Sharkey 1994). Smaller burns over critical areas such as joints are better suited to this technique (WHO 2011). However, for a large percentage of patients with extensive burns in most LMICs, early excisional surgery is not available.

Triage. With the realities of inadequate access to surgical facilities in the LMIC environment, closed burn wound dressing, eschar separation, and delayed skin grafting will help to separate patients with less extensive injuries (less than 40 percent of TBSA) with the potential to survive from those patients with extensive wounds exceeding 50 percent of TBSA with poor survival who should be triaged to palliative care (Ahuja and Bhattacharya 2004).

Wound Care. Local wound care in developing countries is one of the greatest barriers to effective burn wound management; wound-care products and dressing supplies are not easily obtainable or are too expensive. Cool running water at a temperature between 10 and 15 degrees centigrade for 20–30 minutes is considered adequate burn first aid treatment (Skinner and Peat 2002). In one study of burn treatment in LMICs that included all countries in Latin America and the Caribbean, the Middle East and North Africa, and Sub-Saharan Africa, plus China, India, and other countries in Asia and adjoining islands, cool water was applied to the burned area as a first aid therapy in one-third of the cases, a ratio comparable to that observed in some HICs (Forjuoh 2006). Silver-based dressing and ointment should be used, if available. However, the use of locally available and effective wound-care alternatives, amniotic membrane in particular, is cost-effective and ideal as a biological dressing. Amniotic membrane remarkably reduces the cost of dressing changes and the periods of stay in hospitals. It also significantly reduces nursing time and thereby nursing costs (Atiyeh, Gunn, and Hayek 2005). It is often in ample supply if the facility has a busy obstetrics department. However, other considerations, such as cultural acceptability or the risk of HIV or hepatitis infections, also need to be considered.

The medicinal properties of honey and other hive products have been well described for a variety of medicinal and nutritional purposes, including the treatment of burn wounds. The beneficial effects of honey include the cleansing of wounds, absorption of edema fluids, antimicrobial activity, promotion of granulation tissue, epithelialization, and the improvement of nutrition. Another cost-effective, locally available burn dressing is the banana leaf dressing (BLD). Its preparation is very simple: a banana leaf is washed, pasted to bandage cloth with flour paste, dried for 24 hours, rolled, packed into a paper bag, and autoclaved. This process can be easily taught to previously treated patients, relatives of patients, and literate as well as illiterate individuals. Banana leaves are readily available in most cities, towns, and villages in LMICs. It is even possible to have a patch of land with a banana plantation within the hospital premises in a busy burn unit. BLD, being totally nonadherent, tends to slip. BLD is 160 times cheaper than Soframycin-impregnated gauze, 1,750 times cheaper than collagen sheet, and 5,200 times cheaper than biosynthetic dressing (Atiyeh, Masellis, and Conte 2009). More recently, moist exposed burn ointment (MEBO), a traditional Chinese burn remedy, was reported to provide an adequate moist environment for optimal healing without the need for a cumbersome and expensive protective dressing. Its main active component is beta-sitosterol in a base of beeswax and sesame oil. MEBO has been found to be a useful alternative in the treatment of partial-thickness burns because of its convenient method of application; it could be a valuable treatment modality in LMICs (Atiyeh and others 2003).

Exposure therapy is often the method of choice because gauze dressings are considered expensive. The exposure method is particularly suitable for the treatment of pediatric burn injuries, especially in a tropical climate where patients are nursed under mosquito nets to keep flies and other insects away from open burn wounds. In an observational study by Gosselin and Kuppers comparing open and closed dressing in burn wounds, the open method had as good or better early outcomes than the closed method, at significantly lower cost; it is the recommended treatment for burns in environments similar to the one in this study (Gosselin and Kuppers 2008).

Pain Management. Pain management, particularly in children, is another factor that divides the developed from the developing world. Provision of pain relief in the face of limited resources and a limited spectrum of analgesics, if any are available, is a challenge. In a study of the patterns of pediatric analgesic use in Sub-Saharan Africa, paracetamol and ibuprofen were widely employed, constituting approximately 60 percent of all analgesics, while morphine was used in only 0.2 percent of cases. This falls short of the WHO standards (Madadi and others 2012).

Antibiotic Use. Because of the paucity of studies, whether the use of prophylactic systemic antibiotics is effective and cost-effective in preventing infective complications remains unclear; however, the available evidence does not support its use for prophylaxis (ICHRC 2013).

Adequate Nutrition. Healing a burn injury demands a great deal of energy from the body. Adequate nourishment, including adequate protein, calories, vitamins, and micronutrients, is essential to support healing. Some burn units have started to introduce "Plumpy'nut," a high-protein and high-energy peanut-based food that is readily available as a nutritional supplement for malnourished children, to the burn nutrition regimen. A two-month Plumpy'nut regimen for a child costs US$60.

Rehabilitation. In addition to burn-related mortality, burn-related disabilities have substantial functional and economic impacts. Functional disability is defined in the Global Burden of Disease report as disability-adjusted life years (DALYs), or the number of years lost due to poor health, disability, or early death (Murray and Lopez 1996). Worldwide, burns covering more than 20 percent of TBSA rank first among injury types causing short- or long-term disability. The WHO estimates that 116 million people have suffered such burns—approximately four times the number of people with HIV/AIDS at 31 million people (WHO 2008).

Rehabilitation of burn patients must begin immediately after the injury; the delay between inpatient and outpatient therapy should be minimized to facilitate a quick return of functional patients to society (Takayanagi, Kawai, and Aoki 1999). Part of the rehabilitation process is the prevention and treatment of postburn scarring, the most common and frustrating complication because of its aesthetic and functional consequences (van den Kerckhove 2001). The lack of available personnel significantly limits inpatients and outpatient postburn rehabilitation. The ability to train family members in basic physical and occupational therapy skills, such as range of motion exercises, is a cost-effective way to reduce the extent of disabilities. Effective rehabilitation can minimize the need for reconstruction. Local surgeons, where available, need to be trained in basic plastic surgical techniques, such as contracture release (see chapter 13).

Burn prevention strategies are well recognized as being very cost-effective, more so than burn treatment (see chapter 20).

Future Developments in the Treatment of Burns

Mandatory reporting of burn admissions to a central registry can generate data invaluable for evaluating strategies and prevention programs. Optimizing the current information system is achievable by customizing coding developments already underway; combining data from the various agencies to form a national burn injury database will provide the best national overview of burns.

Large-scale awareness programs aimed at policy makers, politicians, professionals, the general public, and the media are required to communicate the burden, impact, and losses due to burn-related injuries. Recognizing that burns are a public health problem, and making burn prevention and management a national programmatic priority, can ensure that sufficient funds are available for such programs.

Telemedicine is an effective tool for accurately evaluating the condition of patients with burns. This tool can reduce undertriage or overtriage for transport, improve resource utilization, and enhance and extend burn center expertise to many rural communities at low cost (Saffle and others 2009). Data specific to burn assessment and diagnosis using telemedicine suggest that this is a safe, reliable, and cost-effective means to attain consultation from specialists for patients in underserved areas (Kiser and others 2013). As this technology has evolved, it has become only slightly more expensive than a standard computer with a high-speed Internet connection.

ORTHOPEDICS

In many HICs, orthopedic surgeons manage acute MSK injuries and their more chronic sequelae, as well as nontrauma-related MSK conditions ("cold" orthopedics). Congenital and hereditary MSK conditions are addressed in chapter 8; this section considers only acquired MSK diseases and conditions.

The world population is aging: the global life-expectancy-adjusted median age will increase from 26.6 years as of 2014 to 31.1 years by 2050 (Lutz, Sanderson, and Scherbov 2008). The burden of age-related conditions, such as osteoporosis, will rise accordingly with the increase in prevalence of known risk factors, such as menopause, physical inactivity, tobacco and alcohol abuse, nutritional deficiencies such as for calcium and vitamin D, and the wider use of medications such as corticosteroids (Lunenfeld and Stratton 2013).

Osteoporosis predisposes people to insufficiency fractures—trauma-related fractures that would not cause failure of normal bone. Females are affected more than males and suffer more disability than males (Guralnik and others 1997). One study in Thailand showed that life expectancy at age 60 is 20.3 years for males and 23.9 years for females, yet disability-free life expectancy is 16.4 and 18.2 years, respectively (Jitapunkul and others 2003).

Traumatic Injuries

It has long been an orthopedic maxim that displaced fractures, particularly if intra-articular, have a better functional outcome if reduced and fixed, surgically if necessary. The shoulder, wrist, spine, and pelvis are common insufficiency fracture sites; although acutely disabling, most such fractures will heal without significant long-term disability without surgical treatment, even if displaced.

This outcome is not true for fractures of the lower extremity, in particular the hip. The personal, familial, and societal burden of hip fractures in elderly patients is well documented in HICs. Such information is lacking for most LMICs, but it is estimated that worldwide, there were 1.7 million hip fractures in 1990. This incidence is forecast to grow fourfold to 6 million by 2050 (WHO 2003). The mortality rate is approximately 20 percent, and the lifetime risk for a 50-year-old female is estimated to be 40 percent, the same as for coronary heart disease.

Early surgery to repair or replace the hip prevents the complications related to prolonged bed rest, including pressure sores, deep vein thrombosis, and urinary or pulmonary infections. It also leads to better functional outcomes with less mal-unions or painful nonunions than conservative bed treatment. However, even in the best-case scenario, one of every two patients suffers some form of permanent disability (WHO 2003). A study in Singapore reported that overall costs for surgical care of hip fractures were actually less than for conservative management (Lee and others 2012). Hip fractures have doubled or tripled in the past 30 years in Asia. If the same trend persists, the societal and economic burden will be nearly unsustainable by 2050 (Mithal and Kaur 2012).

Nontraumatic Conditions

Global aging will also increase acquired chronic MSK conditions, such as degenerative osteoarthritis (OA), inflammatory arthropathies (IA), and neoplasms (primary or metastatic).

A decade ago, OA was estimated to be the fourth leading cause of disability worldwide, most of it attributable to the involvement of the hip and knee (WHO 2002a). The GHE study estimates it accounts for approximately 16 percent of all MSK-related DALYs (WHO 2013b); it is strongly associated with aging and heavy physical occupational activity. In HICs, end-stage OA is most commonly treated with total joint replacement (TJR), a procedure unavailable for the vast majority of sufferers in LMICs. It is estimated that the Asian population older than age 65 will double between 2010 and 2040, and the OA burden will increase accordingly (Fransen and others 2011). Because surgical treatment will remain out of reach for most people, prevention strategies targeting such risk factors as obesity will have the greatest impact. In China, for example, each year only about 50,000 (0.05 percent) of the estimated 120 million OA sufferers receive TJRs (Huang, He, and Wang 2012). Although this number has increased by approximately 15 percent every year in the past 10 years, the unmet need will clearly remain enormous for the foreseeable future.

IAs include rheumatoid arthritis (RA), gout, sero-negative arthropathies, and a myriad of mono- or polyarthropathies associated with autoimmune diseases. According to the GHE, RA and gout account for approximately 5 percent of the burden attributable to MSK disorders (WHO 2013b). Although data on the IA burden in LMICs are unavailable, inadequate rheumatology services suggest that it is likely to be quite high. It is estimated that for the more than 4 billion people in LMICs, the prevalence of RA is between 8 million and 12 million (Chopra and Abdel-Nasser 2008). The WHO has devised the Community Oriented Program for the Control of Rheumatic Diseases, which is being implemented in many LMICs with the goal of collecting community-based data on pain and disability from rheumatic conditions (Chopra and Abdel-Nasser 2008).

The need for surgery for IA (synovectomy, tendon transfers, fusion, or arthroplasty) is less common than for OA. Medical management can be quite effective for many years, but depends on early and accurate diagnosis and the availability of human and technological resources, appropriate medications, and rehabilitative services (Woolf, Erwin, and March 2012). Many of these resources remain unavailable in LMICs, making educating the public and raising awareness of preventive strategies crucial. Such strategies include weight control, regular exercise, balanced diet, avoidance of tobacco and alcohol use, and modification of the work environment (Mody and Cardiel 2008). The higher prevalence of chronic infections, such as tuberculosis, HIV/AIDS, and hepatitis B or C, makes the medical management of IA even more challenging.

MSK tumors are rare. Primary MSK malignancies are not even on the neoplasm list of the GHE framework. Secondary, or metastatic, disease is more common, particularly with common primary cancers, such as those of the lung, breast, or prostate. A combination of chemotherapy, radiation, and surgery is often standard in HICs. No data are available from LMICs, but late presentation (often pathologic fracture) and lack of adjuvant therapies preclude any attempt at limb-saving surgery. Palliative amputation is often the only option. When limb-saving surgery is available and indicated, procedures such as autoclaving and then re-implanting diseased bone can be an acceptable alternative to prohibitively expensive prosthetic replacement (Khattak and others 2006).

Although rarely requiring surgery, low back pain (LBP) and neck pain are extremely common. They encompass a variety of etiologies: mechanical pain, perivertebral soft tissue problems, disk disease, degenerative conditions, and even malingering. The worldwide prevalence of LBP is estimated to be 10 percent; even if only 1 percent of those cases require surgical treatment, the unmet need is tremendous. Depending on duration and the presence or absence of leg pain, the disability weight for LBP in the Global Burden of Disease 2010 ranges from 0.269 to 0.374 (profound intellectual disability has a disability weight of 0.157; severe chronic obstructive pulmonary disease has a disability weight of 0.383), which reflects the significance of perceived impairment by the survey responders (Salomon and others 2012). Personal, societal, and economic burden are high and well documented in HICs; it is unlikely that the burden would be substantially different in LMICs, although no reliable data exist.

Table 3.3 summarizes the changes in rates between 2000 and 2011 for the above conditions.

INFECTIONS

Soft Tissue Infections

General surgical cases, including incision and drainage of abscesses, represent a high proportion of overall procedures at hospitals in LMICs (Ivers and others 2008). Surgical site infections are the second most commonly reported nosocomial infections in Sub-Saharan Africa, following urinary tract infections. In obstetric patients, surgical site infections were higher in LMICs than in HICs and were the most frequent nosocomial infection

Table 3.3 Change in Rates of Nontraumatic Musculoskeletal YLDs and DALYs, 2000–2011

Condition		Change in rates per 100,000 population (percent)
Osteoarthritis	YLDs	14.8
	DALYs	14.8
Rheumatoid arthritis	YLDs	7.2
	DALYs	9.2
Back and neck pain	YLDs	5.4
	DALYs	5.5
Other musculoskeletal conditions	YLDs	6.3
	DALYs	9.5

Source: Data based on Global Health Estimates (WHO 2013b).
Note: DALYs = disability-adjusted life years; YLDs = years lost to disability.

(Amenu, Belachew, and Araya 2011; Chalya and others 2012). Independent risk factors for increased nosocomial infections included age greater than 40 years, length of hospital stay, and an admitting diagnosis of trauma.

However, geographic variables present important barriers to timely access to health services (Spiegel and others 2011). Delayed presentation, inadequate antibiotic treatment before admission, shock on admission, compromised immune status with HIV positivity and low CD4 counts, and malnutrition lead to higher morbidity and mortality rates and may be part of the underlying increased risk in trauma patients. In obstetric patients, the omission of even one dose of antibiotics was associated with increased wound infection rates in Ethiopia (Amenu, Belachew, and Araya 2011).

Surveys employing the WHO Tool for Situational Analysis to Assess Emergency and Essential Surgical Care have identified significant gaps in infrastructure, human resources, life-saving and disability-preventing surgical interventions, and essential equipment in many LMICs (Kushner and others 2010; Spiegel and others 2011). Incision and drainage capabilities seem to exist in 75–100 percent of first-level facilities (local dispensaries, first-level health care facilities, and local hospitals), and general practitioners and nonphysician clinicians without significant surgical training perform the majority of procedures. Lack of supplies is the most common reason cited when patients are referred to higher-level facilities for incision and drainage. A coordinated countrywide initiative to strengthen surgical services at the first-level hospitals in Mongolia documented significantly increased capabilities to perform incision and drainage of abscesses, wound suturing, and wound debridement (Henry and others 2012) (figure 3.2). Additionally, the development of formal emergency rooms with adequate supplies and the implementation of basic standards and guidelines for emergency care have dramatically improved timely access to and availability of these basic procedures (figure 3.3).

Bone Infections

Osteomyelitis, literally the infection of bone or its marrow, is most often due to hematogenous (via the blood vessels) seeding in children, or as a complication of open fractures or orthopedic surgical procedures in patients of all ages. There is a paucity of information in the literature concerning the epidemiology, burden of disease, and cost-effectiveness of treatment for osteomyelitis.

Recognizing the complexity, labor intensiveness, complications, and anticipated costs of treating this condition when chronic, it is clearly better to prevent the condition by performing a select number of simple and cost-effective surgical procedures in the acute phase. These procedures may be considered to be preventive strategies aimed at reducing the risks of developing a chronically infected state; they include drainage of an abscess or debridement of an area of bone destruction, and prompt irrigation, debridement, and stabilization of open fractures. A literature search identified no reliable information on cost-effectiveness; we hypothesize but cannot prove that a multistage, resource-intensive treatment course of chronic osteomyelitis would not be cost-effective. However, preventive surgical strategies are much simpler, can be delivered at the first-level or referral level in most cases, and are likely to be more cost-effective.

Figure 3.2 Surgical Procedures Performed before and after Training at First-Level Facilities

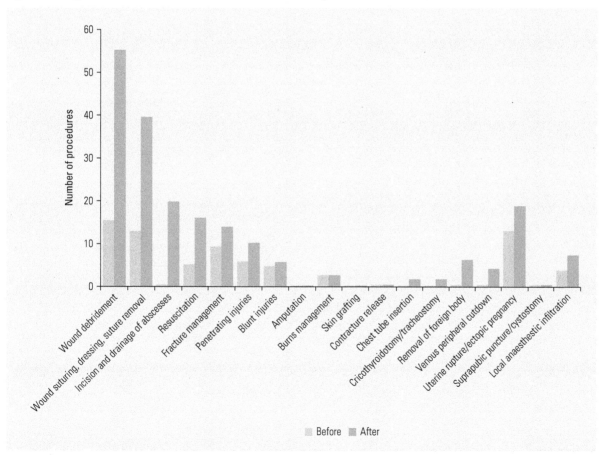

Before   After

Source: Henry and others 2012, figure 6. With permission from Springer Science and Business Media.
Note: Before = prior to training; after = two years posttraining, first-level health care workers.

Figure 3.3 Pilot at First-Level Facilities: Evaluation before and after Two Years Countrywide Training

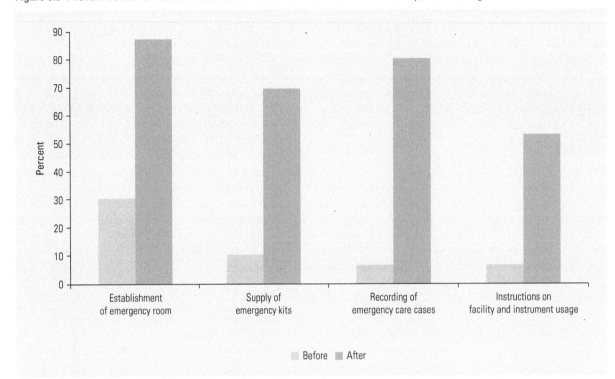

Source: Henry and others 2012, figure 5. With permission from Springer Science and Business Media.
Note: Before = prior to training; after = two years posttraining, first-level health care workers.

CONCLUSION

Throughout LMICs, the rates of trauma-related death and disability are increasing, a trend that is projected to continue. Timely access to surgical care can play a key role in improving outcomes; such access has been shown to be effective and cost-effective. Too often, however, the lack of access to surgical care means that medically preventable deaths occur and avoidable disabilities are incurred.

The toll in human terms is clear and cries out to be addressed. The toll in economic terms is no less clear: Societies lose the present and future contributions of productive members; poor families suffer increased poverty because of the relatively high costs of medical care as well as the loss or disability of members. Poor families are limited in their coping mechanisms, and paying for medical care may involve the liquidation of essential assets or heavy borrowing. Families might not be able to afford to send children to school or must send them to work to replace the contribution of the deceased or disabled family member.

Reliable data, particularly data obtained through improved surveillance and monitoring systems, are needed to better inform the decisions of policy makers as they make difficult choices in allocating scarce resources.

The international community can assist policy makers by developing and implementing guidelines and by regularly monitoring and evaluating them. Appropriate education and training programs, combined with the infusion of basic material and technical resources, may partially alleviate the brain drain crisis.

The creation and strengthening of trauma systems would also reinforce both the human and the material resources of existing health care systems.

NOTES

The World Bank classifies countries according to four income groupings. Income is measured using gross national income (GNI) per capita, in U.S. dollars, converted from local currency using the *World Bank Atlas* method. Classifications as of July 2014 are as follows:

- Low-income countries (LICs) = US$1,045 or less in 2013
- Middle-income countries (MICs) are subdivided:
  - Lower-middle-income = US$1,046 to US$4,125
  - Upper-middle-income (UMICs) = US$4,126 to US$12,745
- High-income countries (HICs) = US$12,746 or more

This chapter used the World Health Organization's geographical classification for six regions: African Region, Region of the Americas, South-East Asia Region, European Region, Eastern Mediterranean Region, and Western Pacific Region.

1. Healing Hands for Haiti. http://www.healinghandsforhaiti.org/Home/tabid/38/language/en-US/Default.aspx.

2. WHO and VIP (Violence and Injury Prevention). "Violence and Injury Prevention and Disability (VIP): Uganda." http://www.who.int/violence_injury_prevention/surveillance/countries/uga/en/index.html.

REFERENCES

ACS (American College of Surgeons). 2006. *Resources for Optimal Care of the Injured Patient.* Chicago: American College of Surgeons.

Ahachi, C. N., I. O. Fadeyibi, F. O. Abikoye, M. K. Chira, A. O. Ugburo, and S. A. Ademiluyi. 2011. "The Direct Hospitalization Cost of Care for Acute Burns in Lagos, Nigeria: A One-Year Prospective Study." *Annals of Burns and Fire Disasters* 24 (2): 94–101.

Ahuja, R. B., and S. Bhattacharya. 2002. "An Analysis of 11,196 Burn Admissions and Evaluation of Conservative Management Techniques." *Burns* 28 (6): 555–61.

———. 2004. "Burns in the Developing World and Burn Disasters." *British Medical Journal* 329: 447–49.

Alexander, T., G. Fuller, P. Hargovan, D. L. Clarke, D. J. Muckart, and S. R. Thomson. 2009. "An Audit of the Quality of Care of Traumatic Brain Injury at a Busy Regional Hospital in South Africa." *South African Journal of Surgery* 47 (4): 120–26.

Amenu, D., T. Belachew, and F. Araya. 2011. "Surgical Site Infection Rate and Risk Factors among Obstetric Cases of Jimma University Specialized Hospital, Southwest Ethiopia." *Ethiopian Journal of Health Sciences* 21 (2): 91–100.

Ameratunga, S., M. Hijar, and R. Norton. 2006. "Road-Traffic Injuries: Confronting Disparities to Address a Global Health Problem." *The Lancet* 367 (9521): 1533–40.

Atiyeh, B. S., R. Dham, M. Kadry, A. F. Abdallah, M. Al-Oteify, and others. 2002. "Benefit-Cost Analysis of Moist Exposed Burn Ointment." *Burns* 28: 659.

Atiyeh, B. S., S. Gunn, and S. N. Hayek. 2005. "New Technologies for Burn Wound Closure and Healing: Review of the Literature." *Burns* 31: 944–56.

Atiyeh, B. S., J. Ioannovich, G. Magliacani, M. Masellis, M. Costagliola, and others. 2003. "A New Approach to Local Burn Wound Care: Moist Exposed Therapy: A Multiphase, Multicenter Study." *Journal of Surgical Wound Care* 2 (1): 18–27.

Atiyeh, B. S., A. Masellis, and C. Conte. 2009. "Optimizing Burn Treatment in Developing Low- and Middle-Income Countries with Limited Health Care Resources (Part 1)." *Annals of Burns and Fire Disasters* 22 (3): 121–25.

Atiyeh, B., A. Masellis, and C. Conte. 2009. "Optimizing Burn Treatment in Developing Low-and Middle-Income Countries with Limited Health Care Resources (Part 2)." *Annals of Burns and Fire Disasters* 22 (4): 189–95.

Chalya, P. L., J. B. Mabula, M. Koy, J. B. Kataraihya, H. Jaka, and others. 2012. "Typhoid Intestinal Perforations at a University Teaching Hospital in Northwestern Tanzania: A Surgical Experience of 104 Cases in a Resource-Limited Setting." *World Journal of Emergency Surgery* 7: 4.

Chichom Mefire, A., P. E. Weledji, V. S. Verla, and N. M. Lidwine. 2014. "Diagnostic and Therapeutic Challenges of Isolated Small Bowel Perforations after Blunt Abdominal Injury in Low Income Settings: Analysis of Twenty-Three New Cases." *Injury* 45 (1): 141–45. doi:10.1016/j.injury.2013.02.022.

Choo, S., H. Perry, A. A. Hesse, F. Abantanga, E. Sory, and others. 2010. "Assessment of Capacity for Surgery, Obstetrics and Anaesthesia in 17 Ghanaian Hospitals Using a WHO Assessment Tool." *Tropical Medicine and International Health* 15 (9): 1109–15.

Chopra, A., and A. Abdel-Nasser. 2008. "Epidemiology of Rheumatic Musculoskeletal Disorders in the Developing World." *Best Practice and Research in Clinical Rheumatology* 22 (4): 583–604.

Church, D., S. Elsayed, O. Reid, B. Winston, and R. Lindsay. 2006. "Burn Wound Infections." *Clinical Microbiology Reviews* 19: 403–34.

Dada, A., S. O. Giwa, W. Yinusa, M. Ugbeye, and S. Gbadegesin. 2009. "Complications of Treatment of Musculoskeletal Injuries by Bone Setters." *West African Journal of Medicine* 28 (1): 43–47.

Forjuoh, S. N. 2003. "Traffic-Related Injury Prevention Interventions for Low-Income Countries." *Injury Control and Safety Promotion* 10 (1–2): 109–18.

———. 2006. "Burns in Low- and Middle-Income Countries: A Review of Available Literature on Descriptive Epidemiology, Risk Factors, Treatment, and Prevention." *Burns* 32 (5): 529–37.

Fransen, M., L. Bridgett, L. March, D. Hoy, E. Penserga, and P. Brooks. 2011. "The Epidemiology of Osteoarthritis in Asia." *International Journal of Rheumatic Diseases* 14 (2): 113–21.

Gabbe, B., P. Simpson, A. Sutherland, R. Wolfe, M. C. Fitzgerald, and others. 2012. "Improved Functional Outcomes for Major Trauma Patients in a Regionalized, Inclusive Trauma System." *Annals of Surgery* 255 (6): 1009–15.

Gosselin, R. A., and C. Coppotelli. 2005. "A Follow-Up Study of Patients with Spinal Cord Injury in Sierra Leone." *International Orthopedics* 29 (5): 330–32.

Gosselin, R. A., and M. Heitto. 2008. "Cost-Effectiveness of a District Trauma Hospital in Battambang, Cambodia." *World Journal of Surgery* 32 (11): 2450–53.

———, and L. G. Zirkle. 2009. "Cost-Effectiveness of Replacing Skeletal Traction by Interlocked Intramedullary Nailing for Femoral Shaft Fractures in a Provincial Trauma Hospital in Cambodia." *International Orthopedics* 33 (5): 1445–51.

Gosselin, R. A., and B. Kuppers. 2008. "Open versus Closed Management of Burn Wounds in a Low-Income Developing Country." *Burns* 34 (5): 644–47.

Gosselin, R. A., A. Maldonado, and G. Elder. 2010. "Comparative Cost-Effectiveness Analysis of Two MSF Surgical Trauma Centers." *World Journal of Surgery* 34 (3): 415–19.

Gruen, R. L., B. J. Gabbe, H. T. Stelfox, and P. A. Cameron. 2012. "Indicators of the Quality of Trauma Care and the Performance of Trauma Systems." *British Journal of Surgery* 99 (Suppl1): 97–104.

Guerriero, C., J. Cairns, P. Perel, H. Shakur, I. Roberts, and CRASH-2 trial collaborators. 2011. "Cost-Effectiveness Analysis of Administering Tranexamic Acid to Bleeding Trauma Patients Using Evidence from the CRASH-2 Trial." *PLoS One* 6 (5): e18987. doi:10.1371/journal .pone.0018987.

Guralnik, J. M., S. G. Leveille, R. Hirsch, L. Ferrucci, and L. P. Fried. 1997. "The Impact of Disability in Older Women." *Journal of the American Medical Association* 52 (3): 113–20.

Henry, J. A., S. Orgoi, S. Govind, R. R. Price, G. Lundeg, and B. Kehrer. 2012. "Strengthening Surgical Services at the Soum (First-Referral) Hospital: The WHO Emergency and Essential Surgical Care (EESC) Program in Mongolia." *World Journal of Surgery* 36 (10): 2359–70.

Huang, S. L., X. J. He, and K. Z. Wang. 2012. "Joint Replacement in China: Progress and Challenges." *Rheumatology* 51 (9): 1525–56.

Hulme, P. 2010. "Mechanisms of Trauma at a Rural Hospital in Uganda." *Pan African Medical Journal* 7: 5.

Hyder, A. A. 2013. "Injuries in Low- and Middle-Income Countries: A Neglected Disease in Global Public Health." *Injury* 44 (5): 579–80.

ICHRC (International Child Health Review Collaboration). 2013. "What Is the Role of Prophylactic Antibiotics in the Management of Burns?" http://www.ichrc.org/sites/www .ichrc.org/files/antibioticburns.pdf.

Ivers, L. C., E. S. Garfein, J. Augustin, M. Raymonville, A. T. Yang, and others. 2008. "Increasing Access to Surgical Services for the Poor in Rural Haiti: Surgery as a Public Good for Public Health." *World Journal of Surgery* 32 (4): 537–42.

Jamison, D. T., J. G. Breman, A. R. Measham, G. Alleyne, M. Claeson, D. B. Evans, P. Jha, A. Mills, and P. Musgrove, eds. 2006. *Disease Control Priorities in Developing Countries*. 2nd ed. Washington, DC: World Bank and Oxford University Press.

Jayaraman, S., J. R. Mabweijano, M. S. Lipnick, N. Caldwell, J. Miyamoto, and others. 2009. "First Things First: Effectiveness and Scalability of a Basic Prehospital Trauma Care Program for Lay First-Responders in Kampala, Uganda." *PLoS One* 4 (9): e6955.

Jitapunkul, S., C. Kunanusont, W. Phoolcharoen, P. Suriyawongpaisal, and S. Ebrahim. 2003. "Disability-Free Life Expectancy of Elderly People in a Population Undergoing Demographic and Epidemiologic Transition." *Age and Ageing* 32 (4): 401–05.

Khattak, M. J., M. Umer, R. Haroon-ur-Rasheed, and M. Umar. 2006. "Autoclaved Tumor Bone for Reconstruction: An Alternative in Developing Countries." *Clinical Orthopedics and Related Research* 447: 138–44.

Kiser, M., G. Beijer, S. Mjuweni, A. Muyco, B. Cairns, and A. Charles. 2013. "Photographic Assessment of Burn Wounds: A Simple Strategy in a Resource-Poor Setting." *Burns* 39 (1): 155–61.

Kushner, A. L., M. N. Cherian, L. Noel, D. A. Spiegel, S. Groth, and C. Etienne. 2010. "Addressing the Millennium Development Goals from a Surgical Perspective: Essential Surgery and Anesthesia in 8 Low- and Middle-Income Countries." *Archives of Surgery* 145 (2): 154–59.

Lee, A. Y., J. Tan, J. Koh, S. M. Fook-Chong, N. N. Lo, and T. S. Howe. 2012. "Five-Year Outcome of Individuals with Hip Fracture Admitted to a Singapore Hospital: Quality of Life and Survival Rates after Treatment." *Journal of the American Geriatric Society* 60 (5): 994–96.

Lunenfeld, B., and P. Stratton. 2013. "The Clinical Consequences of an Ageing World and Preventive Strategies." *Best Practice and Research in Clinical Obstetrics and Gynaecology* 27 (5): 643–49. doi:10.1016/j.bpobgyn.2013.02.005.

Lutz, W., W. Sanderson, and S. Scherbov. 2008. "The Coming Acceleration of Global Population Ageing." *Nature* 451 (7179): 716–19.

MacKenzie, E. J., F. P. Rivara, G. J. Jurkovich, A. B. Nathens, K. P. Frey, and others. 2006. "A National Evaluation of the Effect of Trauma-Center Care on Mortality." *New England Journal of Medicine* 354 (4): 366–78.

Madadi, P., E. F. Enato, S. Fulga, C. C. Umeoduagu, S. M. MacLeod, and others. 2012. "Patterns of Paediatric Analgesic Use in Africa: A Systematic Review." *Archives of Diseases in Childhood* 97 (12): 1086–91.

Mashreky, S. R., A. Rahman, S. M. Chowdhury, T. F. Khan, L. Svanstrom, and F. Rahman. 2009. "Non-fatal Burn Is a Major Cause of Illness: Findings from the Largest Community-Based National Survey in Bangladesh." *Injury Prevention* 15 (6): 397–402.

Mathew, G., and B. P. Hanson. 2009. "Global Burden of Trauma: Need for Effective Fracture Therapies." *Indian Journal of Orthopedics* 43 (2): 111–16.

McCord, C., and Q. Chowdhury. 2003. "A Cost Effective Small Hospital in Bangladesh: What It Can Mean for Emergency Obstetric Care." *International Journal of Gynaecology and Obstetrics* 81 (1): 83–92.

Mithal, A., and P. Kaur. 2012. "Osteoporosis in Asia: A Call to Action." *Current Osteoporosis Reports* 10 (4): 245–47.

Mock, C. N. 2007. "WHA Resolution on Trauma and Emergency Care Services." *Injury Prevention* 13 (4): 285–56.

———. 2011. "Strengthening Care of the Injured Globally." *Journal of Trauma* 270 (6): 1307–16.

———, and M. N. Cherian. 2008: "The Global Burden of Musculoskeletal Injuries: Challenges and Solutions." *Clinical Orthopedics and Related Research* 466 (10): 2306–16.

Mock, C. N., M. Joshipura, C. Arreola-Risa, and R. Quansah. 2012. "An Estimate of the Number of Lives That Could Be Saved through Improvements in Trauma Care Globally." *World Journal of Surgery* 36 (5): 959–63.

Mock, C. N., M. Joshipura, J. Goosen, and R. Maier. 2006. "Overview of the Essential Trauma Care Project." *World Journal of Surgery* 30 (6): 919–29.

Mock, C. N., G. J. Jurkovich, D. nii-Amon-Koti, C. Arreola-Risa, and R. V. Maier. 1998. "Trauma Mortality Patterns in Three Nations at Different Economic Levels: Implications for Global Trauma System Development." *Journal of Trauma* 44 (5): 804–12; discussion 812–4.

Mock, C. N., J. D. Lormand, J. Goosen, M. Joshipura, and M. Peden. 2004. *Guidelines for Essential Trauma Care*. Geneva: World Health Organization.

Mock, C. N., R. Quansah, L. Addae-Mensah, and P. Donkor. 2005. "The Development of Continuing Education for Trauma Care in an African Nation." *Injury* 36 (6): 725–32.

Mody, G. M., and M. H. Cardiel. 2008. "Challenges in the Management of Rheumatoid Arthritis in Developing Countries." *Best Practice and Research in Clinical Rheumatology* 22 (4): 621–41.

Munster, A. M., M. Smith-Meek, and P. Sharkey. 1994. "The Effect of Early Surgical Intervention on Mortality and Cost-Effectiveness in Burn Care (1978–1991)." *Burns* 20: 61–64.

Murray, C. J. L., and A. D. Lopez, eds. 1996. The Global Burden of Disease: A Comprehensive Assessment of Mortality and Disability from Diseases, Injuries, and Risk Factors in 1990 and Projected to 2020. Cambridge, MA: Harvard University Press.

Nakahara, S., S. Saint, S. Sann, M. Ichikawa, A. Kimura, and others. 2010. "Exploring Referral Systems for Injured Patients in Low-Income Countries: A Case Study from Cambodia." *Health Policy and Planning* 25 (4): 319–27.

Nielsen, K., C. N. Mock, M. Joshipura, A. M. Rubiano, A. Zakariah, and F. Rivera. 2012. "Assessment of the Status of Prehospital Care in 13 Low- and Middle-Income Countries." *Prehospital Emergency Care* 16 (3): 381–89.

Norse, N. N., and A. A. Hyder. 2009. "Call for More Research on Injury from the Developing World: Results of a Bibliometric Analysis." *Indian Journal of Medical Research* 129 (3): 321–26.

O'Reilly, G. M., M. Joshipura, P. A. Cameron, and R. Gruen. 2013. "Trauma Registries in Developing Countries: A Review of the Published Experience." *Injury* 44 (6): 713–21.

Ozgediz, D., D. T. Jamison, M. Cherian, and K. McQueen. 2008. "The Burden of Surgical Conditions and Access to Surgical Care in Low- and Middle-Income Countries." *Bulletin of the World Health Organization* 86 (8): 646–47.

Peck, M., J. Molnar, and D. Swart. 2009. "A Global Plan for Burn Prevention and Care." *Bulletin of the World Health Organization* 87 (10): 802–03.

Price, R. R. 2013. "Investigating the Causes of Trauma: Critical Initial Steps to Designing Sustainable Interventions in Sierra Leone: Comment on 'Traumatic Injuries in Developing Countries.'" *Journal of the American Medical Association Surgery* 148 (5): 469–70.

Qureshi, J. S., R. Ohm, H. Rajala, C. Mabedi, O. Sadr-Azodi, and others. 2013. "Head Injury Triage in a Sub-Saharan African Urban Population." *International Journal of Surgery* 11 (3): 265–69.

Rubiano, A. M., J. C. Puyana, C. N. Mock, M. R. Bullock, and P. D. Adelson. 2013. "Strengthening Neurotrauma Care Systems in Low and Middle Income Countries." *Brain Injury* 27 (3): 262–72.

Saffle, J. R., L. Edelman, L. Theurer, S. E. Morris, and A. Cochran. 2009. "Telemedicine Evaluation of Acute Burns Is Accurate and Cost-Effective." *Journal of Trauma* 67 (2): 358–65.

Salomon, J. A., T. Vos, D. R. Hogan, M. Gagnon, M. Naghavi, and others. 2012. "Common Values in Assessing Health Outcomes from Disease and Injury: Disability Weights Measurement Study for the Global Burden of Disease Study 2010." *The Lancet* 380 (9859): 2129–43.

Sekimpi, P., K. Okike, L. G. Zirkle, and A. Jawa. 2011. "Femoral Fracture Fixation in Developing Countries: An Evaluation of the Surgical Implant Generation Network (SIGN) Intramedullary Nail." *Journal of Bone and Joint Surgery (American)* 93(19): 1811–18.

Shamim, M. S., S. F. Ali, and S. A. Enam. 2011. "Non-operative Management Is Superior to Surgical Stabilization in Spine Injury Patients with Complete Neurological Deficits: A Perspective Study from a Developing World Country, Pakistan." *Surgical Neurology International* 2: 166.

Siman-Tov, M., I. Radomislensky, and K. Peleg. 2012. "Reduction in Trauma Mortality in Israel during the Last Decade (2000–2010): The Impact of Changes in the Trauma System." *Injury* 44 (11): 1448–52. http://www.ncbi .nlm.nih.gov/pubmed/23021368.

Sitsapesan, H. A., T. P. Lawrence, C. Sweasey, and K. Wester. 2013. "Neurotrauma Outside the High-Income Setting: A Review of Audit and Data-Collection Strategies." *World Neurosurgery* 79 (3–4): 568–75.

Skinner, A., and B. Peat. 2002. "Burns Treatment for Children and Adults: A Study of Initial Burns First Aid and Hospital Care." *New Zealand Medical Journal* 115: 199.

Solagberu, B. A. 2002. "Spinal Cord Injuries in Ilorin, Nigeria." *West African Journal of Medicine* 21 (3): 230–32.

Spiegel, D. A., S. Choo, M. Cherian, S. Orgoi, B. Kehrer, and others. 2011. "Quantifying Surgical and Anesthetic Availability at Primary Health Facilities in Mongolia." *World Journal of Surgery* 35 (2): 272–79.

Spiegel, D. A., R. A. Gosselin, R. R. Coughlin, M. Joshipura, B. D. Browner, and J. P. Dormans. 2008. "The Burden of Musculoskeletal Injury in Low- and Middle-Income Countries: Challenges and Opportunities." *Journal of Bone and Joint Surgery (American)* 90 (4): 15–23.

Stelfox, H. T., M. Joshipura, W. Chadbunchachai, R. N. Ellawala, G. O'Reilly, and others. 2012. "Trauma Quality Improvement in Low and Middle Income Countries of the Asia-Pacific Region: A Mixed Methods Study." *World Journal of Surgery* 36 (8): 1978–92.

Stewart, K. A., R. S. Groen, T. B. Kamara, M. M. Farhzad, M. Samai, and others. 2013. "Traumatic Injuries in Developing Countries: Report from a Nationwide Cross-Sectional Survey of Sierra Leone." *Journal of the American Medical Association Surgery* 148 (5): 463–69.

Takayanagi, K., S. Kawai, and R. Aoki. 1999. "The Cost of Burn Care and Implications for Efficient Care." *Clinical Performance and Quality Health Care* 7 (2): 70–73.

Tallon, J. M., S. A. Karim, S. Ackroydstolarz, and D. Petrie. 2012. "Influence of a Province-Wide Trauma System on Motor Vehicle Collision Process of Trauma Care and Mortality:

A 10-Year Follow-Up Evaluation." *Canadian Journal of Surgery* 55: 8–14.

Tollefson, T. T., and W. F. Larrabee, Jr. 2012. "Global Surgical Initiatives to Reduce the Surgical Burden of Disease." *Journal of the American Medical Association* 307 (7): 667–68.

U.S. DHHS (United States Department of Health and Human Services). 2006. "Model Trauma System Planning and Evaluation." Health Resources and Services Administration 9, U.S. DHHS.

van den Kerckhove, E., K. Stappaerts, W. Boeckx, B. van den Hof, S. Monstrey, and others. 2001. "Silicones in the Rehabilitation of Burns: A Review and Overview." *Burns* 27 (3): 205–14.

Vos, T. 2009. "Improving the Quantitative Basis of the Surgical Burden in Low-Income Countries." *PLoS Med* 6 (9): e1000149.

WHO (World Health Organization). 2002a. *World Health Report 2002*. Geneva: WHO.

———. 2002b. *The Injury Chartbook: A Graphical Overview of the Global Burden of Injuries*. Geneva: WHO.

———. 2003. *Prevention and Management of Osteoporosis*. Technical Report Series 921: 1–164, Geneva.

———. 2008. "Annex Tables." In *Global Burden of Disease: 2004 Update*. Geneva.

———. 2010. Strengthening Care for the Injured: Success Stories and Lessons Learned from around the World. Geneva: WHO.

———. 2011. Burn Prevention: Success Stories, Lessons Learned. Geneva: WHO.

———. 2013a. Disabilities and Rehabilitation: Better Health for People with Disabilities. Geneva. http://www.who.int/disabilities/en/.

———. 2013b. *Global Health Estimates for Deaths by Cause, Age, and Sex for Years 2000–2011*. Geneva. http://www.who.int/healthinfo/global_burden_disease/en/

———. 2013c. Global Status Report on Road Safety. Geneva: WHO.

Woolf, A. D., J. Erwin, and L. March. 2012. "The Need to Address the Burden of Musculoskeletal Conditions." *Best Practice and Research in Clinical Rheumatology* 26 (2): 183–224.

Zong, Z. W., N. Li, T. M. Cheng, X. Z. Ran, Y. Shen, and others. 2011. "Current State and Future Perspectives of Trauma Care System in Mainland China." *Injury* 42 (9): 874–78.

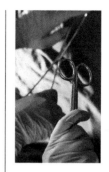

Chapter 4

General Surgical Emergencies

Colin McCord, Doruk Ozgediz, Jessica H. Beard,
and Haile T. Debas

INTRODUCTION

In low- and middle-income countries (LMICs), at least 60 percent of the surgical operations performed are for emergencies. Contrary to widespread belief, it has been shown that the provision of treatment, which is often lifesaving for these patients, can be inexpensive. The staff and equipment required at first-level facilities for all categories of surgical emergency, including trauma (chapter 3) and obstetrics (chapter 5), are essentially the same. Accordingly, the treatment of general surgical emergencies requires little additional cost and should be part of the services offered at first-level facilities. This chapter

- Describes the common types of general surgical emergencies that can be treated at first-level hospitals in LMICs
- Provides the best available estimates of disease burden for the conditions for which these facilities are responsible
- Considers the cost and cost-effectiveness of providing this essential surgical service
- Describes the basic systems and the major bottlenecks to access
- Discusses the training and distribution of appropriately skilled staff.

The chapter is written for two primary audiences, health planners and surgeons in LMICs, to show each group how much can be provided and accomplished in very simple facilities, given adequate training and support.

Burden of Disease

The annual death rate from acute abdominal conditions in the United States in 1935 was 38 per 100,000 population, or 3 percent of all deaths in that year. General practitioners performed most surgeries; formal surgical training did not begin until 1937, when the American Board of Surgery was formed. By 1990, the death rate for acute abdominal conditions had fallen to 4 per 100,000 (CDC 1990; U.S. Department of Commerce 1935). The 90 percent reduction in mortality was due to increased access to operations, made possible by new facilities and more skilled staff in combination with the availability of antibiotics for infection, safer anesthesia, and blood for transfusions. The operations were not complicated. They are available today in LMICs, as are low-cost antibiotics, competent anesthesia, and blood; however, as in the United States in 1935, access to these operations is very limited. In the United States and in many other high-income countries (HICs) in 1935, all general surgical emergencies were responsible for 3 percent to 5 percent of deaths. This estimate may be as good as any other estimate of the burden of disease from these causes in LMICs, where there is little or no available surgical treatment.

Corresponding author: Colin McCord, MD, Columbia University (retired), cwm1@columbia.edu

The problems that limit access to surgical services in most LMICs are correctible, although serious and not easily overcome. They include the following:

- Insufficient number of surgically trained personnel, and the concentration of these personnel in major urban areas
- Lack of ongoing training and supervision in peripheral surgical units to supplement and upgrade skills
- Lack of efficient supply systems to ensure the availability of medications and materials
- Lack of adequate maintenance systems and personnel for diagnostic and therapeutic equipment
- Lack of affordable and reliable transport for patients between facilities so they can receive the appropriate level of care in a timely manner

Despite these handicaps, much can be done and is being done in very simple facilities with minimal support. This progress is possible because many of the important surgical problems can be resolved with uncomplicated, well-standardized procedures. A fully equipped, modern hospital is not essential to remove an appendix, close a perforated ulcer, drain an abscess, or even resolve most causes of intestinal obstruction.

Levels of Hospital Care

Definitions of the levels of hospital care were delineated in *Disease Control Priorities in Developing Countries*, second edition (Jamison and others 2006); as adapted, these levels are shown in table 4.1.

TYPES OF GENERAL SURGICAL EMERGENCIES

The list of surgically treatable emergencies commonly seen in LMIC hospitals is not long, but it includes problems that fall within the purview of several different specialties (Abdullah and others 2011; Curci 2012; Lavy and others 2007; McCord and Chowdhury 2003). Fortunately, 90 percent of the operations can be mastered by a person without full specialty qualification, so it is not necessary to have fully qualified surgeons, obstetricians, and traumatologists in every first-level hospital. With even a very limited ability to refer patients and intermittent supervision by qualified specialists, a very productive network for surgical care can be established (box 4.1).

Acute Abdominal Emergencies

Incarcerated and Strangulated Inguinal Hernias. Incarcerated hernia, a cause of intestinal obstruction,

Table 4.1 Definitions of Levels of Hospital Care

Terminology and definitions	Alternative terms commonly found in the literature
First-level hospital	Primary-level hospital
Few specialties—mainly internal medicine, obstetrics and gynecology, pediatrics, and general surgery	District hospital
	Rural hospital
Often only one general practice physician or a nonphysician clinician	Community hospital
Limited laboratory services available for general analysis but not for specialized pathological analysis	General hospital
50–250 beds	
Second-level hospital	Regional hospital
More differentiated by function, with as many as 5 to 10 clinical specialties	Provincial (or equivalent administrative area, such as county) hospital
200–800 beds	
	General hospital
Third-level hospital	National hospital
Highly specialized staff and technical equipment—for example, cardiology, intensive care unit, and specialized imaging units	Central hospital
Clinical services highly differentiated by function	Academic, teaching, or university hospital
Teaching activities in some facilities	
300–1,500 beds	

Source: Mulligan and others 2003.

is very common in Sub-Saharan Africa (Shillcutt, Clarke, and Kingsnorth 2010). About 4 in 1,000 hernias per year will become incarcerated, with a segment of intestine trapped inside the hernia sac; if untreated, these hernias can become gangrenous within several days. In 85 percent of the cases in a large review of incarcerated hernias, the bowel within the hernia sac was viable: it could be returned to the abdomen and the hernia repaired (van den Heuvel and others 2011). If the intestine is not viable, it must be removed and the divided bowel repaired. This is not a complicated procedure for an adequately trained surgeon. If bowel resection is not indicated, 99 percent of patients should survive; if bowel resection is required, 80 percent or more should survive, depending on the experience of the surgeon (Nilsson and others 2007).

Appendicitis. This condition is rare in isolated villages but increasingly common with development and a more "western" diet containing less fiber and more meat (Burkitt, Walker, and Painter 1972). Appendicitis is common in cities, towns, and more developed rural areas in many LMICs. Removal of an inflamed appendix is a straightforward procedure. Even in late cases complicated by perforation and abscess formation, drainage will resolve the acute problem unless generalized peritonitis has developed. Overall, including the late-presenting cases with perforation or a gangrenous appendix, 95 percent of patients can be expected to survive; this number reaches 99 percent in the hands of experienced surgeons (Mason and others 2012; Ohene-Yeboah 2006).

Intestinal Obstructions Caused by Adhesions, Volvulus, Worm Infection, or Intussusception. The most common cause of intestinal obstruction in LMICs is incarcerated hernia, but if no inguinal hernia is visible, then several other conditions should be considered. If treated early, all cases can be successfully managed with conservative measures or very simple abdominal operations; these conditions can become difficult problems if allowed to progress to a later stage.

Twisting (volvulus) of the intestine around an adhesion or scar from a previous operation or infection is becoming increasingly common. In many LMICs, it is the second most common cause of blocked intestine. Seen early, it will often resolve with tube decompression of the stomach and intravenous fluids. If an operation is necessary, simple division of the adhesion and untwisting of the intestine will resolve the problem at an early stage; at later stages, the twist can interfere with the blood supply, the intestine will die, and only removal of the dead intestine will prevent death of the patient (Adesunkanmi and Agbakwuru 1996; Madziga and Nuhu 2008).

Less commonly, the lower end of the large intestine can spontaneously twist on itself (sigmoid volvulus), producing an obstructed bowel. In late cases, the twisted intestine can cut off its own blood supply, leading to gangrene and requiring resection and repair. The probability of gangrene cannot be predicted, and early surgery must be the rule. In complicated cases in which no qualified surgeon is available, simple procedures like colostomy (transferring the dead intestine outside of the abdomen by creating a usually temporary artificial anus, without reconstruction of the intestine) will resolve the acute problem, so that patients can be referred for a second operation that restores normal function. An uncomplicated sigmoid volvulus can be untwisted without opening the abdomen, by gently inserting a well-lubricated large rubber tube through an instrument (a proctoscope) inserted into the rectum. Overall survival should exceed 80 percent (Mnguni and others 2012; Nuhu and Jah 2010).

Two conditions in children are common causes of intestinal obstruction:

- Heavy infestation with *Ascaris* worms can lead to balls of living worms large enough to obstruct the lumen. In about 80 percent of cases, this condition will resolve spontaneously if the intestine is decompressed with a stomach tube. If an operation is needed, the worms can be removed through a small incision; in rare cases, the segment of intestine containing the worm ball may have to be removed. Overall mortality should be 1 percent to 2 percent (Wani and others 2010).

- Less commonly, usually in infants under age one, a segment of intestine can invaginate on itself (intussusception), leading to obstruction. This condition can occur spontaneously and is a relatively rare complication of the rotavirus vaccine immunization. In a hospital with a fairly sophisticated radiologist, it will be treated with a moderately high pressure enema, using a dye that can be seen on a fluoroscope as the pressure reduces the invagination. If the skills and equipment for this are not available, the invagination can be relieved by an operation. The procedure is to push on the invaginated segment, never to pull on the distal end. Removal of the invaginated segment is rarely needed. Overall mortality in infants should be 1 percent to 2 percent or less, given early treatment and competent management of anesthesia and fluid replacement. Because of inexperience in infant surgery in many first-level hospitals in LMICs most patients are referred, but referrals can delay treatment and increase mortality (Jiang and others 2013; Ngendahayo and others 2014).

Pelvic Infections with Abscesses. Sexually acquired infections of the fallopian tubes and adjacent organs are common and can usually be successfully treated with antibiotics and without surgery. If an abscess forms and does not respond to medication, simple drainage is usually adequate. In early cases, a trial of antibiotic treatment is the best course; exploratory laparotomy may be necessary for severe, nonresponsive cases. Overall survival should exceed 95 percent. When antibiotic treatment is late or inadequate, death is rare, but infertility and recurrent pelvic pain can ensue, as well as increased incidence of subsequent ectopic pregnancy (Soper 2010).

Peptic Ulcer Complications. Three major advances have reduced the incidence of and mortality rates for peptic ulcers: the discovery that *Helicobacter*, which can be treated with antibiotics, is a primary cause of ulcers; the development of powerful acid-reducing drugs; and the successful endoscopic control of bleeding from ulcers.

Helicobacter infection is widespread and difficult to prevent, and ulcerogenic medicines like nonsteroidal anti-inflammatory drugs (NSAIDs) are widely available and overused, with and without prescription.

Perforation of a peptic ulcer allows a flood of gastric juice to flow into the peritoneal cavity, resulting in diffuse peritonitis that is almost always fatal if untreated. Surgery within 24 hours, with closure of the perforation and washout of the abdominal cavity, is simple and is almost always successful; if followed by appropriate anti-ulcer medical treatment, it leads to a permanent cure for 95 percent of patients. Delayed operations carry higher risks, with a possibility of subsequent abscesses. Overall, 80 percent to 90 percent of patients are likely to survive (Chalya and others 2011; Ugochukwu and others 2013).

Bleeding ulcers pose more serious problems. Severe bleeding requires surgery, transfusions, and skilled anesthetic support, which are often unavailable in smaller hospitals. The old standard operation of pyloroplasty, suture of the bleeding blood vessel, and vagotomy (cutting the vagus nerve that stimulates acid production) is effective; 90 percent of patients will survive, but usually only a fully qualified surgeon will be able to perform the procedure. If possible, these patients should be transferred. If they can go to a third-level center that offers endoscopy services, it is likely that they can be successfully treated without surgery (Simon and others 2013). Younger patients with less than massive bleeding can usually be managed conservatively and transferred, if necessary, after the bleeding has stopped.

Bleeding from Esophageal Varices. In HICs, varicose veins at the lower end of the esophagus are usually complications of alcoholic cirrhosis of the liver. In many LMICs, they are commonly due to a scarred liver caused by *Schistosoma* infestation. The difference is that liver function is very poor in alcoholic cirrhosis patients but is relatively good in patients with varices due to schistosomiasis. When varices from any cause bleed, they almost always bleed massively, requiring multiple transfusions. Alcoholic cirrhosis patients do not do well with operations for varices, but those with schistosomiasis survive and do well with operations and with endoscopic treatments. However, the operations are major undertakings, and the endoscopic treatment requires expensive equipment and skilled personnel. This option is increasingly available in third-level hospitals; these patients are rarely seen in first- or second-level hospitals, probably because they so often die before they reach any hospital.

Perforated Typhoid Ulcers. Perforation is a very serious complication of advanced typhoid infection that causes ulcers of the small intestine. Ulcers can also erode blood vessels to produce major bleeding. Diagnosis of perforation is often late, even when it occurs in hospitalized patients. These ulcers develop in approximately 5 percent of hospitalized patients, and almost always in patients whose antibiotic treatment started late or had not yet become effective (Chalya and others 2012).

Perforated typhoid ulcer 40 years ago was considered to have a hopeless outcome. It is gratifying that several recent reports from Sub-Saharan African hospitals indicate survival rates of 80 percent to 90 percent after operative repair of a typhoid perforation (Chalya and others 2012; Mock and others 1995; Nasir, Abdur-Rahman, and Adeniran 2011).

Amebic Liver Abscess. Amebic liver abscess responds so well to antibiotics that it rarely needs surgical treatment, but surgeons are usually called to examine these patients and so must understand the proper diagnosis and treatment. The diagnosis is straightforward if ultrasound or computed tomography (CT) scan is available, but this equipment is usually not available in hospitals below the third level.

A trial of antibiotics can be a simple way to resolve the question. If pain and fever persist, indicating that rupture into the abdomen is imminent, the best approach is needle drainage or percutaneous catheter drainage, in combination with antibiotics. In the absence of ultrasound or other localization, surgery may be necessary to ensure proper placement of drainage.

The rupture of such an abscess through the diaphragm and into the pleural space requires urgent surgical intervention. Simple insertion of a large-bore chest tube, combined with appropriate antibiotics, is almost always sufficient.

In low-income countries (LICs), amebic abscesses are more common; in middle-income countries (MICs) and HICs, about 50 percent of the cases of liver abscess are bacterial, requiring intensive antibiotics and drainage (Conter and others 1986). Untreated amebic liver abscesses are often fatal, but even in complicated cases, 95 percent survival can be expected with appropriate treatment (Chavez-Tapia and others 2009; Jha and others 2012).

Gall Bladder and Bile Duct Disease. Acute inflammation of the gall bladder (acute cholecystitis) is very rare in rural parts of LICs but increasingly common in cities and MICs. Experienced surgeons treat most patients with antibiotics and prompt removal of the gall bladder, but antibiotics alone will control infection temporarily so that an operation can be done later. First-level hospitals choose the second option unless they have a fully trained surgeon on staff. Patients with jaundice caused by gallstones passing into and obstructing the common bile duct are referred.

Respiratory Obstructions, Foreign Bodies, and Pleural Disease

Obstruction has many causes, including head and neck infections, bleeding, trauma, tumors, improper positioning of an unconscious person and aspiration. A simple change of position, with or without the insertion of an oral airway or a tube into the trachea, may resolve the problem; often, an incision in the neck is needed to perform cricothyroidotomy or tracheostomy. All surgical staff members should be trained to intubate, perform these simple operations, and correctly position unconscious patients.

Foreign Bodies. If located in the ear, nose, or eye, foreign bodies are usually easy to remove; however, the failure to remove them can result in serious infections. In the larynx and trachea, they can obstruct respiration and cause death. If a foreign body goes beyond the trachea into the bronchial tree, it will produce a pneumonia that is unresponsive to treatment unless the foreign body is removed. The removal of foreign bodies in the bronchi requires referral for bronchoscopy. Swallowed material in the esophagus usually passes through or, if stuck at a high level (the cricopharyngeus), can be extracted with a balloon catheter.

Pneumothorax, Hemothorax, and Empyema. Pneumothorax, hemothorax, and empyema are collections of, respectively, air, blood, or pus in the pleural space that compresses the lungs, leading to respiratory insufficiency; they often produce scarring with permanent disability. Infected fluid is serious and can lead to death. In almost all cases, early drainage with a chest tube, combined with antibiotics as needed, resolves the problem. This simple procedure is easily learned (King and others 1986; WHO 2003).

Urinary Obstructions

Infection can cause scarring of the urethra, stones in the bladder can obstruct the outlet, and an enlarged prostate gland can compress the urethra. In any of these cases, the urethra can be blocked, making urination impossible. Often, an instrument can be passed through the obstruction, followed by a rubber catheter, to relieve the acute problem. However, because the obstruction often recurs, subsequent referral may be needed to remove the prostate or the stone or to more radically dilate the urethra. If the urethra cannot be dilated, a bladder catheter can be inserted above the pubic bone (suprapubic cystostomy) as an emergency procedure. Removal of bladder stones and cystostomy are practical operations at a first-level hospital, and prostatectomy can be performed there, if the skills are available. Stones can also form in the kidney itself. Small ones will pass without surgical treatment; if they do not pass, referral is necessary.

Infections of the Skin, Muscles, Bones, and Joints

Antibiotics have changed the course of infections of the skin, muscles, bones, and joints, which are often associated with bloodstream infections and were important causes of death and disability before the availability of antibiotics. In HICs, serious infections are often treated with aspiration of pus, culturing, and intensive use of antibiotics. In most LMICs, however, access to bacterial culturing is not available; antibiotic choice is limited by availability and cost; and long-term, high-dose antibiotic treatment is impractical.

Fortunately, early treatment with incision and drainage, in combination with a regimen of antibiotics for one to two weeks, is generally successful in locations with limited resources. In late-presenting cases, deaths from sepsis are usually preventable, but bone and joint infections, in particular, can require long-term treatment and subsequent surgery. Because acute infections are common, often occur in children, and do not require complicated surgery, this treatment option is an important and very cost-effective part of the work of a first-level hospital (King and others 1986; WHO 2003). Surgical infections are covered in more detail in chapter 3.

Other General Surgical Emergencies

Although this list of emergency conditions is not exhaustive, it covers at least 95 percent of the emergency problems faced in first- and second-level hospitals. Staff members who treat these patients must be prepared to deal with the common problems, including the traumatic and obstetric emergencies discussed in chapters 3 and 5. Facilities should be equipped and supplied to support this treatment. Referral is necessary for less common and more complicated conditions, but it should be kept to a minimum because of the weakness of existing referral systems.

Certain other surgical emergencies common in HICs but not in LMICs are not discussed in this chapter—notably, diverticulitis, intestinal obstruction or perforation resulting from colon cancer, and complications of arteriosclerosis (such as ruptured abdominal aortic aneurism and gangrene of extremities). These conditions will undoubtedly become more important as LMICs progress through the epidemiological transition, in which the complications of a western diet, arteriosclerosis, and cancer increase. Planners in LMICs must be aware of these changes in the disease spectrum, which will increase the cost and reduce the potential benefits of surgical treatment in the future (Stewart and others 2014).

Congenital surgical emergencies are covered in detail in chapter 8. Some of these, especially pyloric stenosis and colostomy for imperforate anus, are completely within the competence of a well-trained general surgeon in a first- or second-level hospital, although it is rare to find a general surgeon who does these operations.

Almost all of the conditions listed in box 4.1 can be treated in first-level hospitals (see table 4.1), although many of these facilities would refer most or all of these patients to a higher level. The public quickly comes to know if referral is likely and learns to bypass the closer hospital and go directly to a larger center. If bypassing is not possible, patients simply stay home. Patients often do not reach the higher-level hospitals to which they are referred, usually for economic reasons (Urassa and others 2005). The important factor limiting the capacity of first-level hospitals is training (Abdullah and others 2011). The shortage of qualified surgeons and anesthetists can be corrected in the short term by training general practitioners, nonphysician clinicians, and nurses to care for most of the common conditions; in the long term, the shortage can be corrected by training appropriate specialists. Approaches to these options are discussed briefly in this chapter and in more detail in chapters 12 and 17.

DISEASE BURDEN OF GENERAL SURGICAL EMERGENCIES

The World Health Organization's (WHO's) Global Health Estimates report global disability-adjusted life years (DALYs) lost from 163 specified disease causes (WHO 2013a); DALYs are a measure of the years of life lost or seriously impaired by disease, both overall and from specified disease entities.

The Global Health Estimates do not specifically identify general surgical emergencies, but by combining the estimates for three categories (peptic ulcer disease, appendicitis, other digestive diseases) out of the 163, in which death or disability usually results from a general surgical emergency, an estimate of the worldwide rate of DALYs lost from these conditions can be created. At 596 per 100,000 population, this constitutes 1.5 percent of DALYs from all causes, in all parts of the world (table 4.3). The estimates for injuries, maternal, neonatal, and three general surgical emergencies in LMICs were considerably higher than those in HICs.

Diagnoses for cause of death in LMICs are usually rough estimates, especially for the acute abdominal conditions lumped together under *other digestive diseases*.

Not included because they were not listed separately in this DALY calculation are respiratory obstruction, pneumothorax, and surgical infections (including empyema, osteomyelitis, abscesses, pelvic infections, and perforated typhoid ulcers).

Debas and others (2006) do not consider general surgical emergencies separately, but they estimate that 11 percent of all lost DALYs worldwide were due to surgically correctable conditions. They make it clear that this is a very rough estimate, based on "best guesses" by 18 surgical experts of the percentage of patients who could be successfully treated within a list of conditions considered surgically treatable. These estimates were then applied to the DALY numbers provided by WHO (2002) for each category of potential surgical conditions; the estimates are based on hospital experiences, not on population surveys.

Vital registers are inaccurate or nonexistent in almost all LMICs. Only three population-based surveys have tried to estimate the incidence and mortality rates from all surgical emergencies, using family members' recall of disease and death. One set of surveys, conducted in a remote, mountainous part of Pakistan, found death rates from nontraumatic surgical emergencies to be only moderately higher than in the United States in 1935: 55 and 61 per 100,000, respectively, depending on the sample surveyed (Ahmed and others 1999). The other two surveys, from rural parts of Sierra Leone and Rwanda, calculated much higher death rates for acute abdominal emergencies (825 per 100,000 per year for acute abdominal conditions), but the surveys probably encountered problems with the recall method. In one, the surveyors calculated a total (all diagnoses) crude death rate of 59.7 per 1,000, which is more than three times the total crude death rate estimated for Sub-Saharan Africa by WHO (Groen and others 2012; Petroze and others 2013).

Compiling these data can yield a rough estimate of the disease burden from general surgical emergencies in LMICs, from 1 percent to 3 percent of all deaths and all DALYs—more than 10 percent of all surgical DALYs. At that rate, these conditions are not unimportant, and several factors combine to make them even more so:

- Reasonably early treatment will achieve good results, usually with complete cures.
- Without treatment, mortality rates are high.
- All of the general surgical emergencies are common in children and young adults.
- Human and other resources needed for effective treatment are the same as those needed to treat the other important surgically treatable conditions, including trauma and maternal and perinatal mortality.

EFFECTIVENESS OF SURGICAL TREATMENT

In Germany in 1926, when surgery for acute peritonitis was considered contraindicated, Kirschner (1926) reported a peritonitis hospital mortality rate of 85 percent. Although established peritonitis is still a serious condition, mortality rates of less than 10 percent would be expected today in LMICs, with appropriate surgery combined with intravenous fluids and antibiotics. If surgery can be performed within 24 hours of disease onset, mortality should be much lower than 10 percent.

Meta-analysis of all available operative mortality statistics worldwide has shown that the overall decline in mortality has been slower in LMICs than in HICs (Bainbridge and others 2012). The problems that have led to this slower rate clearly need to be addressed, but the progress that has been achieved in perioperative mortality is not inconsiderable and seems to be increasing. Comparing 1970–90 with 1990–2010, the same meta-analysis shows a decline in perioperative mortality in LMICs from 0.73 percent in the first 20-year period to 0.25 percent in the second period.

The overall survival rates of higher than 95 percent cited for most of the four common categories of emergencies in table 4.2 are based on reports from hospitals in LICs, primarily in Sub-Saharan Africa. These results have been achieved despite the late arrival of many patients and the high prevalence of comorbid conditions, such as malaria and HIV infection. Médecins Sans Frontières reported on 16,377 major operations in LMICs, most performed for emergencies in the very basic, first-level hospitals they operated, with a hospital mortality rate of 0.2 percent (Chu, Ford, and Trelles 2010). Staff without formal surgical training performed many of these operations, but trained surgeons were almost always available for consultation and assistance. A report of 1,976

Table 4.2 Global DALYs, by Cause, 2011
per 100,000 population

Disease	DALYs	Percent
All causes	39,553	100.0
AIDS and tuberculosis	1,372	3.5
Cardiovascular disease	5,461	13.8
Injuries	4,278	10.8
Maternal	273	0.7
Neonatal	3,338	8.4
General surgical emergencies[a]	596	1.5

Source: WHO 2013a.
Note: DALYs = disability-adjusted life years.
a. Peptic ulcer disease, appendicitis, other digestive diseases.

operations for acute abdominal conditions in a Sub-Saharan African public hospital finds a hospital mortality rate of less than 10 percent (Ohene-Yeboah 2006). A small Sub-Saharan African hospital with no trained surgeon on staff and very limited capacity for referral reports a hospital mortality rate of 10 percent for 173 patients with acute abdominal emergencies (McConkey 2002). The operations were performed by general practitioners.

In most cases, if patients are discharged alive, they are discharged cured and will need no further treatment. Exceptions occur, with late problems requiring additional treatment in fewer than 10 percent of cases.

COST OF SURGICAL TREATMENT

Calculating the cost of individual surgical procedures in any setting involves multiple assumptions. The calculation becomes even more complicated in LMICs, where hospitals have multiple sources of income, including gifts in kind; records are poor; and corruption is commonplace. The overall cost per admission or procedure varies greatly between first- and third-level hospitals; third-level hospitals are much more expensive (see chapter 12).

Within regional income classifications, there is considerable variation between regions in per patient hospital expenditure. Latin American countries generally spend more, but even there the costs of major surgical procedures are very low, especially in first-level hospitals. One review compares the recurrent cost per major operation in six district hospitals in Mozambique, Tanzania, and Uganda, all three LICs. Results indicate that the cost per operation was US$42–US$98 in five of the six. At one low-volume Ugandan hospital, the cost was US$308 per operation (Kruk and others 2010). If these low-cost estimates were grouped with other estimates of DALYs averted by emergency operations (nine per general surgical operation in box 4.2), the cost per DALY would be very low indeed.

The calculation of the marginal cost-benefit of a particular operation is clearly not the first consideration for health policy makers and planners in LMICs. Political considerations will—and should—nearly always lead them to construct general first- and second-level hospitals that have the ability to manage or refer all emergency conditions, whether surgical, medical, or pediatric. The questions for policy makers and planners are how much the total cost of such facilities will be; what populations they can serve; what services will be most or least cost-effective; and what conditions, if any, can be referred.

The cost and effectiveness of first-level hospitals, the systems to support them, and the role of surgery within

---

Box 4.2

DALYs Averted by Kind of Surgery at Gonoshasthaya Kendra Hospital, Bangladesh, 1995

Table B4.2.1 reports the estimated DALYs averted by surgical treatment in a 50-bed hospital in Bangladesh. In the three-month period studied, 154 operations were performed; 80 percent were emergencies. A qualified surgeon and an obstetrician were available for most of these procedures. Anesthesia was provided by a locally trained paramedic with no formal hospital training. All nurses and operating room staff were locally trained without formal qualifications. One obstetric death and one general surgical operative death occurred. All other patients were discharged well. There were no referrals.

DALY estimates were based on local experience and are believed to be conservative, for example, acute appendicitis was considered to have a 10 percent risk of a fatal outcome without surgery if there was no perforation or gangrene; the risk estimate rose to 95 percent if perforation and peritonitis had occurred.

The list of operations is typical for small, first-level hospitals in LICs with trained specialists available.

- 27 percent of operations were general surgical; almost all of these were emergencies.
- 15 percent of DALYs averted came from general surgical emergencies.
- The hospital was rural but adjacent to a major highway. The relatively small number of trauma cases reflects the absence of any referral system to bring injured patients to the hospital.

box continues next page

Box 4.2 (continued)

Table B4.2.1 DALYs Averted in Three Months, First-Level Hospital, Bangladesh, 1995

	Number of operations	Total DALYs averted	DALYs averted per operation
Obstetrics and gynecology			
Cesarean section	40	1,588	40
Dilation and curettage	24	44	2
Ectopic pregnancy	2	72	36
Extraction of placenta	4	26	7
Cervical tear	1	3	3
Other gynecological	20	149	7
All obstetrics and gynecology	91	1,882	21
General surgery			
Appendectomy	10	49	5
Cancer	1	13	13
Gall bladder	4	30	8
Hernia	6	47	8
Other acute abdomen	4	64	16
Chest (tube drainage)	3	76	25
Incision and drainage of infection	13	91	7
All general surgery	41	370	9
Trauma			
Closed fractures	11	43	4
Major wounds and compound fractures	6	81	14
Burns	5	53	11
All trauma	22	177	8
All surgical procedures	154	2,429	16

Source: Data from McCord and Chowdhury 2003.
Note: DALY = disabilty-adjusted life year.

them is discussed in chapters 12, 18, and 19. First-level hospitals have been shown to best serve the needs of the population and to be cost-effective. Their surgical services are usually the most effective component (Debas and others 2006; Gosselin, Thind, and Bellardinelli 2006; McCord and Chowdhury 2003). At first-level facilities, the same staff can provide services for most general surgical, obstetric, and trauma emergencies. With minor adjustments, the same structure, equipment, and supplies can serve all three components at very low cost. At higher referral levels, increasingly specialized services combined with other inefficiencies can increase costs enormously.

BASIC SYSTEMS FOR SURGICAL EMERGENCIES

Although several types of operations can be done in less-than-ideal conditions, the availability of basic facilities and supporting systems makes procedures simpler, safer, and more efficient. Controlling cost and making optimal use of resources are important everywhere, especially in LMICs. Hence, it is essential to define the basic needs for a functioning surgical system. Fortunately, these essentials do not need to be expensive. Some hospitals in LMICs provide good, lifesaving service for a total cost of less than US$50 per patient day, compared with more than US$1,000 per patient day for hospitals in HICs (Kruk and others 2010). A well-equipped operating theater can be created in LMICs for less than the cost of a small diner or restaurant in a HIC.

Almost all of the surgical emergencies listed in table 4.2 can be managed successfully in a first-level hospital, but the basic elements must be in place:

- *Functioning hospital:* The hospital should have wards, an outpatient area, a receiving area for emergency patients, a pharmacy, and a laboratory. Ideally, the hospital would also have a blood bank and adequate staff quarters. Usually, these small facilities will have 50–250 beds.
- *Operating room:* The operating room should have appropriate surgical and anesthetic equipment and supplies.
- *Capacity to administer anesthesia:* It is important for first-level hospitals to have the capability to administer anesthesia (see chapter 15). Most general surgical emergencies can be managed with local, spinal, or ketamine anesthesia, but some require general anesthesia, with induced paralysis and tracheal intubation.
- *Resuscitation:* Many of the most severe emergency patients arrive at hospitals unconscious, in shock, with respiratory obstructions or other urgent problems that must be resolved before surgical treatment can be considered. The essentials of resuscitation are not complicated and are usually very effective: managing the airway, controlling bleeding, and providing adequate fluid replacement. Blood for transfusion can be useful but usually is not essential. Resuscitation, which is often not managed well, is one of the most important training needs in the hospital systems of LMICs. Staff members at all levels should be trained and equipped to provide this service, and areas should be set aside where equipment and trained staff are available (see chapters 14 and 15).
- *Supplies:* Adequate quantities of basic supplies are essential; in addition to gauze and linen, intravenous fluids and antibiotics are the most important. Complicated intravenous fluid preparations are not essential, but the basic dextrose with water and dextrose with saline must be available, along with the means to add potassium when needed. Appropriate use of high-dose antibiotics can be lifesaving in cases with established infections that require adequate drainage and debridement. Prophylactic antibiotics can be useful when there has been contamination without established infection (as in an operation requiring the opening of the intestine) but should not be continued beyond 24 hours. Almost all patients can be managed with inexpensive, long-established antibiotics. Guidelines for the appropriate use of antibiotics should be available at all levels. WHO's essential medicine list can be a basis for these guidelines (WHO 2013b).
- *Referral system:* A referral system, with health centers that refer, as well as larger hospitals that receive more complicated cases, should complement the hospital. This model requires some sort of transport system to move patients between these units.

Most countries have second-level facilities with fully trained surgeons. Budgetary, staffing, and transport constraints usually require that all hospitals, including at the second and third levels, have a first-level function for the local geographic area.

Training and Distribution of Staff Members

Training. Effective training programs for staff members are essential. It is not realistic to expect that all surgical staff will be fully qualified specialists or certified operating room nurses; general practitioners, nonphysician clinicians, and nurses can be trained to manage most of the surgical emergencies seen in first-level hospitals. Variation in surgical capability is an important factor that can limit the number of general surgical emergencies treated, as well as the quality of the outcomes.

Because first-level facilities need to perform emergency obstetrical and trauma surgery, training programs should create the capacity to manage all three categories of surgical emergencies: general surgical, traumatic, and obstetric. Programs in Sub-Saharan Africa and elsewhere have demonstrated that training can be done at low cost and without stationing qualified specialists at every location (Mkandawire, Ngulube, and Lavy 2008; Nyamtema and others 2011; Sani and others 2009; van Amelsfoort and others 2010).

Surgical societies, such as the West African College of Surgeons and the College of Surgeons of East, Central, and Southern Africa, have developed training and education programs for surgeons in most LMICs; these programs are modeled on the programs of similar societies in HICs. Most LMICs have a nucleus of well-trained surgical specialists; in some countries, large numbers of trained specialists are available. To date, qualified specialists and surgical societies have not had an important role in the training and supervision of those who perform surgery in the smaller, first-level hospitals. If these surgical societies could take a major interest in the creation of the surgical networks and in monitoring performance, surgical care in LMICs would be significantly improved.

Distribution. The effective distribution of skilled personnel is an additional challenge. All LMICs have difficulty inducing qualified medical personnel to work outside of major cities, largely because private patients are few and public facilities that serve poor people pay low salaries.

Most LMICs partially resolve this problem by sending recent medical graduates to staff first-level hospitals (general practitioner surgeons), training nurses or other staff to administer anesthesia, and staffing operating rooms with nurses or others without special training. A few countries have trained nonphysician clinicians to perform surgery (see chapters 17 and 19). Because 90 percent or more of the essential operations are within the potential competence of a general practitioner or nonphysician clinician surgeon with a nonphysician anesthetist, short-course training before assignment and periodic skills improvement courses can greatly improve the quantity and the quality of surgical treatment in these places. Regular visits by supervising specialists will serve to maintain and expand the skills, as well as to evaluate quality through audits. Regular supervision of this sort is extremely rare in LMICs.

The shortage of trained staff members results in costly inefficiency in facilities that are working at less than capacity (Kruk and others 2010). Many very poor countries are only beginning to train doctors to qualify as surgeons and anesthetists. General practitioner and nonphysician clinician surgeons in first-level hospitals usually become competent at managing obstetrical emergencies with nurse-midwives and nurse-anesthetists. However, they are less confident with general surgical emergencies and trauma, so that these patients are often referred. Because of financial and other barriers, this practice often means that the patients do not receive the treatment they need (Cannoodt, Mock, and Bucagu 2012; Grimes and others 2011).

Training programs, supply systems, and supervision should be designed to create and maintain the necessary capacity at each level and to facilitate transfers between facilities as much as is practical.

General Surgical Procedures in an Ideal System

Table 4.3 presents a list of procedures that should be available at different levels of the hospital system. For this system to function well, efficient patient transfers in and out are important. However, the realities of available transportation options, as well as the financial and other barriers faced by transferred patients and their families, make it essential to reduce the need

for transfers; common conditions must be managed locally to the extent possible. This need to diffuse services to smaller units may change as more specialists are trained, transportation improves, and economic growth increases the purchasing power of the population. But in most LICs for the next generation or more, most people will be treated in public hospitals. General practitioner or nonphysician clinician surgeons will provide much, if not most, of the surgical services available, and they will work in small, first-level facilities, serving populations from 50,000 to 250,000. Larger urban hospitals also need to provide first-level services in many cases; ideally, to avoid congestion in facilities that often serve several million people, networks of district first-level hospitals would be established even in cities.

NEW TECHNOLOGY

Two trends in the revolution in operative surgery in the past decade are particularly noteworthy. First is a general move to more conservative procedures to treat infections, malignancies, and biliary, vascular, and other diseases. Second, innovation and new technologies have facilitated this conservative trend. The intensive use of potent antibiotics has reduced the need for surgery. Video-assisted surgery and stapled suturing have simplified surgical techniques. Ultrasound, computerized radiographic technology, magnetic resonance imaging, and endoscopy have improved preoperative diagnoses; in some cases, they have eliminated the need for surgery.

Some of these advances, however, are very expensive; all of them increase the demand for technical expertise to operate and maintain the new equipment. Surgeons, policy makers, and planners should keep in mind that most of the improvements in surgical outcomes since the 1930s occurred before 1950, before any of these new techniques had been developed and become available.

It is important to address three limitations on the use of new technologies in the context of the limited budgetary and human resources in LMICs:

- *Cost:* Both the initial costs and the costs of maintenance and service should be reasonable.
- *Trained personnel:* Trained personnel should be available to perform the procedures, train assistants, and ensure that the equipment is adequately serviced and well maintained.
- *Disposable parts and supplies:* Parts and supplies are usually expensive, and they put an additional burden

Table 4.3 General Surgical Emergency Capacity in an Ideal System

Capacity	Health center	First-level hospitals with general practitioner surgeon or nonphysician clinician	First- or second-level hospitals with qualified surgeon	Third-level hospitals
Airway management, fluid replacement, bleeding control, antibiotics	X[a]	X	X	X
Blood transfusion		X[a]	X	X
Tube thoracostomy		X[a]	X	X
Tracheal tube		X[a]	X	X
Local anesthesia	X	X	X	X
Spinal and general anesthesia		X	X	X
Hernia and intestinal obstruction		X[a]	X	X
Appendicitis		X	X	X
Perforated peptic ulcer		X[a]	X	X
Bleeding peptic ulcer			X	X
Bleeding esophageal varices				X
Pelvic peritonitis		X	X	X
Perforated typhoid ulcer		X[a]	X	X
Colostomy		X[a]	X	X
Cystostomy		X[a]	X	X
Cricothyroidostomy		X[a]	X	X
Foreign body removal		X	X	X
Damage-control laparotomy[b]		X[a]	X[a]	X

a. Capacity (i.e., trained staff available 24 hours, with adequate equipment and supplies) should be there, but usually is not.
b. This procedure is usually a way to deal with severe trauma, but could be a way to deal with the intestine in a very sick patient, when intestine must be removed, but it is not possible to restore continuity by sewing the ends back together. The ends can simply be tied off and the patient referred for another operation.

on supply systems that are sometimes nonexistent and always under strain.

It may be possible to overcome these conditions in regional hospitals and in the major referral centers, but they are important barriers to the use of new technology in first- and second-level hospitals. Virtually no data are available to enable cost-effectiveness analysis.

Examples illustrating some of the complexities introduced by technical advances include the following:

- *Appendicitis* that has not progressed to perforation, abscess, gangrene, or generalized peritonitis can be successfully treated with high-dose, intensive antibiotics, but the condition will recur in 10 percent to 20 percent of patients who are treated without operation. Randomized controlled trials of antibiotic treatment for nonperforated, nongangrenous appendicitis are underway in HICs (Mason and others 2012); even if these trials favor nonsurgical treatment, they depend on a definitive determination that perforation or other complications have not occurred, which requires a CT scan. In LMICs, CT scanners generally are not available at first- or second-level hospitals and are only beginning to be introduced in third-level hospitals. Nonsurgical treatment of appendicitis is not likely to be practical for most people in LICs in the foreseeable future.

- *Bleeding peptic ulcer* can almost always be controlled without surgery using endoscopy. In one Indian hospital where mortality was very low, only 3 percent of patients required operations (Simon and others 2013). However, endoscopes and the skill to use them are rarely available at first-level hospitals, and the surgery to control a bleeding ulcer is considerably more complicated than that for an appendectomy. These patients should be referred, if possible.

One technological advance that can easily be made available in all hospital operating rooms is pulse oximetry.

The pulse oximeter, a simple, sturdy, and inexpensive device that continuously monitors oxygen levels in the blood, has increased the safety of general anesthesia. WHO has launched the Patient Safety Pulse Oximetry project to improve the safety of surgical anesthesia care in LMICs, testing the effect on patient outcome of providing a bundle consisting of the Surgical Safety Checklist, pulse oximeters, and training in a number of pilot hospitals globally. WHO, with the World Federation of Societies of Anaesthesiologists, the Association of Anaesthetists of Great Britain and Ireland, and others, has developed a training tool kit consisting of a manual, a video, and slide sets to improve provider responses to hypoxemia.

The results of "old-fashioned" surgery are generally comparable to those obtained with modern technology, so health policy makers and planners in LMICs may want to devote resources to other priorities. The first priority should be to provide the basic services that are the most cost-effective. Unfortunately, those patients who can pay often demand high technology, even in the poorest countries, which can influence the planning process. There is a real risk that basic surgery in first- and second-level hospitals will be considered second class and that qualified surgeons in private practice will encourage that opinion. That mindset needs to be avoided, or it could set back progress considerably.

BARRIERS TO EFFECTIVE SERVICE DELIVERY

Hospital and community surveys in LICs show that the proportion of patients with surgical emergencies who receive effective treatment is very low (Ahmed and others 1999; Grimes and others 2011; Kruk and others 2010; Mock and others 1998) and that many of those who are untreated die. Multiple barriers to delivery of surgical services exist in these countries. By far the most important are inadequate training of existing staff, lack of a referral system that can bring patients to referral hospitals from health centers and dispensaries, and the financial burden of a hospital stay for poor families (see chapter 12).

The financial burden for patients and families is very important. Even when services are free, a major operation can create a debt burden from which a family may not recover (Afsana 2004). Lost income; travel and maintenance costs for patients and those who accompany them; food, medications, and supplies not available in the hospital; and "informal charges" to obtain minimal services can add up to large sums. This reality is an important reason to avoid referrals as much as possible.

FUTURE DIRECTIONS

Research has underscored the magnitude of the burden of surgical disease in LMICs and the extent of the unmet need for surgical care. Although the estimates available are imprecise, most LMICs clearly have a substantial burden of surgically treatable disease, and the available surgical treatments reach only a fraction of the population in need. It is also clear that the needed services can be provided at remarkably low cost and that surgery in very simple settings can be effective.

- The urgent need today is to know more about the cost and cost-effectiveness of programs to expand services as well as to improve training, supervision, logistical support, and the referral system. This knowledge will be best acquired in the context of active programs to increase coverage, improve service delivery, and provide better support for service delivery in existing facilities, especially first-level hospitals.
- The standards for training and certification of all staff members providing surgical care need to be developed. These standards and certifications include specialists, but also general practitioner surgeons, nonphysician clinician surgeons, anesthetists, and operating theater staff.
- Monitored guidelines and checklists to organize and supervise treatment are needed. The active involvement of national and regional professional associations in these programs and investigations is essential.
- Monitoring and evaluating progress requires hospitals that provide surgical services to have databases. The databases need to be improved, but this improvement must acknowledge that too much paperwork can detract from service delivery. Nursing staff, in particular, already have a heavy recordkeeping burden. Improvements should be designed to reduce this burden, improve quality, and ensure that the data collected are used to improve service.

With commitment by the surgical leadership, progress could be rapid in coming years. The number of qualified surgeons and anesthetists in the poorest countries is growing exponentially, and ways can be found to persuade them to locate in or near first-level hospitals. In the interim, most of these conditions can be treated with relatively simple surgery, which means that general practitioners, nonphysician clinicians, and nurses can upgrade their skills with relatively short training aimed at those who will be assigned to first-level hospitals. Ideally, this training will be conducted in larger, high-volume hospitals by qualified surgeons who will follow up with in-service training and supervision conducted in the first-level hospitals where these short-course surgeons practice. Models exist for this sort of upgrading program in Malawi, Niger, and Tanzania (Mkandawire, Ngulube, and Lavy 2008; Nyamtema and others 2011; Sani and others 2009; van Amelsfoort and others 2010).

NOTE

The World Bank classifies countries according to four income groupings. Income is measured using gross national income (GNI) per capita, in U.S. dollars, converted from local currency using the *World Bank Atlas* method. Classifications as of July 2014 are as follows:

- Low-income countries (LICs) = US$1,045 or less in 2013
- Middle-income countries (MICs) are subdivided:
  - Lower-middle-income = US$1,046 to US$4,125
  - Upper-middle-income (UMICs) = US$4,126 to US$12,745
- High-income countries (HICs) = US$12,746 or more

REFERENCES

Abdullah, F., S. Choo, A. A. Hesse, F. Abantanga, E. Sory, and others. 2011. "Assessment of Surgical and Obstetrical Care at 10 District Hospitals in Ghana Using On-Site Interviews." *Journal of Surgical Research* 171 (2): 461–66. doi:10.1016/j.jss.2010.04.016.

Adesunkanmi, A. R., and E. A. Agbakwuru. 1996. "Changing Pattern of Acute Intestinal Obstruction in a Tropical African Population." *East African Medical Journal* 73 (11): 727–31.

Afsana, K. 2004. "The Tremendous Cost of Seeking Hospital Obstetric Care in Bangladesh." *Reproductive Health Matters* 12 (24): 171–80.

Ahmed, M., M. Shah, S. Luby, P. Drago-Johnson, and S. Wali. 1999. "Survey of Surgical Emergencies in a Rural Population in the Northern Areas of Pakistan." *Tropical Medicine and International Health* 4 (12): 846–57.

Bainbridge, D., J. Martin, M. Arango, and D. Cheng. 2012. "Perioperative and Anaesthetic-Related Mortality in Developed and Developing Countries: A Systematic Review and Meta-Analysis." *The Lancet* 380 (9847): 1075–81. doi:10.1016/s0140-6736(12)60990-8.

Burkitt, D. P., A. R. Walker, and N. S. Painter. 1972. "Effect of Dietary Fibre on Stools and the Transit-Times, and Its Role in the Causation of Disease." *The Lancet* 2 (7792): 1408–12.

Cannoodt, L., C. Mock, and M. Bucagu. 2012. "Identifying Barriers to Emergency Care Services." *International Journal of Health Planning and Management* 27 (2): e104–20. doi:10.1002/hpm.1098.

CDC (Centers for Disease Control). 1990. *Vital Statistics of the United States*, Vol. 2, *Mortality*, Part B. http://www.cdc.gov/nchs/data/vsus/mort90_2b.pdf.

Chalya, P. L., J. B. Mabula, M. Koy, J. B. Kataraihya, H. Jaka, and others. 2012. "Typhoid Intestinal Perforations at a University Teaching Hospital in Northwestern Tanzania: A Surgical Experience of 104 Cases in a Resource-Limited Setting." *World Journal of Emergency Surgery* 7: 4. doi:10.1186/1749-7922-7-4.

Chalya, P. L., J. B. Mabula, M. Koy, M. D. McHembe, H. Jaka, and others. 2011. "Clinical Profile and Outcome of Surgical Treatment of Perforated Peptic Ulcers in Northwestern Tanzania: A Tertiary Hospital Experience." *World Journal of Emergency Surgery* 6: 31. doi:10.1186/1749-7922-6-31.

Chavez-Tapia, N. C., J. Hernandez-Calleros, F. I. Tellez-Avila, A. Torre, and M. Uribe. 2009. "Image-Guided Percutaneous Procedure Plus Metronidazole versus Metronidazole Alone for Uncomplicated Amoebic Liver Abscess." *Cochrane Database of Systematic Reviews* 1: Cd004886. doi:10.1002/14651858.CD004886.pub2.

Chu, K. M., N. Ford, and M. Trelles. 2010. "Operative Mortality in Resource-Limited Settings: The Experience of Médecins Sans Frontiéres in 13 Countries." *Archives of Surgery* 145 (8): 721–25. doi:10.1001/archsurg.2010.137.

Conter, R. L., H. A. Pitt, R. K. Tompkins, and W. P. Longmire Jr. 1986. "Differentiation of Pyogenic from Amebic Hepatic Abscesses." *Surgery, Gynecology, and Obstetrics* 162 (2): 114–20.

Curci, M. 2012. "Task Shifting Overcomes the Limitations of Volunteerism in Developing Nations." *Bulletin of the American College of Surgeons* 97 (10): 9–14.

Debas, H. T., R. Gosselin, C. McCord, and A. Thind. 2006. "Surgery." In *Disease Control Priorities in Developing Countries*, 2nd ed., edited by D. T. Jamison, J. G. Breman, A. R. Measham, G. Alleyne, M. Claeson, D. B. Evans, P. Jha, A. Mills, and P. Musgrove, 1245–59. Washington, DC: World Bank and Oxford University Press.

Grimes, C. E., K. G. Bowman, C. M. Dodgion, and C. B. Lavy. 2011. "Systematic Review of Barriers to Surgical Care in Low-Income and Middle-Income Countries." *World Journal of Surgery* 35 (5): 941–50.

Gosselin, R. A., A. Thind, and A. Bellardinelli. 2006. "Cost/DALY Averted in a Small Hospital in Sierra Leone: What Is the Relative Contribution of Different Services?" *World Journal of Surgery* 30 (4): 505–11. doi:10.1007/s00268-005-0609-5.

Groen, R. S., M. Samai, K. A. Stewart, L. D. Cassidy, T. B. Kamara, and others. 2012. "Untreated Surgical Conditions in Sierra Leone: A Cluster Randomised, Cross-Sectional, Countrywide Survey." *The Lancet* 380 (9847): 1082–87. doi:10.1016/s0140-6736(12)61081-2.

Jamison, D. T., J. G. Breman, A. R. Measham, G. Alleyne, M. Claeson, D. B. Evans, P. Jha, A. Mills, and P. Musgrove, eds. 2006. *Disease Control Priorities in Developing Countries*, 2nd ed. Washington, DC: World Bank and Oxford University Press.

Jha, A. K., G. Das, S. Maitra, T. K. Sengupta, and S. Sen. 2012. "Management of Large Amoebic Liver Abscess— A Comparative Study of Needle Aspiration and

Catheter Drainage." *Journal of the Indian Medical Association* 110 (1): 13–15.

Jiang, J., B. Jiang, U. Parashar, T. Nguyen, J. Bines, and others. 2013. "Childhood Intussusception: A Literature Review." *PLoS One* 8 (7): e68482. doi:10.1371/journal.pone.0068482.

King, M., P. Bewes, J. Cairns, and J. Thornton, eds. 1986. Chapters 5, 6, and 7. In *Non-Trauma*. Vol. 1 of *Primary Surgery*, 52–103. Oxford: Oxford University Press.

Kirschner, M. 1926. "Die behandlung der akutren eitrigen freien Bauchfellentzundung." *Archivus Klinikum Chirurgicum* 142: 253.

Kruk, M. E., A. Wladis, N. Mbembati, S. K. Ndao-Brumblay, R. Y. Hsia, and others. 2010. "Human Resource and Funding Constraints for Essential Surgery in District Hospitals in Africa: A Retrospective Cross-Sectional Survey." *PLoS Med* 7 (3): e1000242. doi:10.1371/journal.pmed.1000242.

Lavy, C., A. Tindall, C. Steinlechner, N. Mkandawire, and S. Chimangeni. 2007. "Surgery in Malawi: A National Survey of Activity in Rural and Urban Hospitals." *Annals of the Royal College of Surgeons of England* 89 (7): 722–24. doi:10.1308/003588407x209329.

Madziga, A. G., and A. I. Nuhu. 2008. "Causes and Treatment Outcome of Mechanical Bowel Obstruction in North Eastern Nigeria." *West African Journal of Medicine* 27 (2): 101–05.

Mason, R. J., A. Moazzez, H. Sohn, and N. Katkhouda. 2012. "Meta-Analysis of Randomized Trials Comparing Antibiotic Therapy with Appendectomy for Acute Uncomplicated (No Abscess or Phlegmon) Appendicitis." *Surgical Infections* (Larchmt) 13 (2): 74–84. doi:10.1089/sur.2011.058.

McConkey, S. J. 2002. "Case Series of Acute Abdominal Surgery in Rural Sierra Leone." *World Journal of Surgery* 26 (4): 509–13. doi:10.1007/s00268-001-0258-2.

McCord, C., and Q. Chowdhury. 2003. "A Cost Effective Small Hospital in Bangladesh: What It Can Mean for Emergency Obstetric Care." *International Journal of Gynaecology and Obstetrics* 81 (1): 83–92.

Mkandawire, N., C. Ngulube, and C. Lavy. 2008. "Orthopaedic Clinical Officer Program in Malawi: A Model for Providing Orthopaedic Care." *Clinical Orthopaedics and Related Research* 466 (10): 2385–91. doi:10.1007/s11999-008-0366-5.

Mnguni, M. N., J. Islam, V. Manzini, V. Govindasamy, B. M. Zulu, and others. 2012. "How Far Has the Pendulum Swung in the Surgical Management of Sigmoid Volvulus? Experience from the KwaZulu-Natal Teaching Hospitals and Review of the Literature." *Colorectal Disease* 14 (12): 1531–37. doi:10.1111/j.1463-1318.2012.03046.x.

Mock, C. N., G. J. Jurkovich, D. nii-Amon-Kotei, C. Arreola-Risa, and R. V. Maier. 1998. "Trauma Mortality Patterns in Three Nations at Different Economic Levels: Implications for Global Trauma System Development." *Journal of Trauma* 44 (5): 804–12; discussion 812–4.

Mock, C. N., L. Visser, D. Denno, and R. Maier. 1995. "Aggressive Fluid Resuscitation and Broad Spectrum Antibiotics Decrease Mortality from Typhoid Ileal Perforation." *Tropical Doctor* 25 (3): 115–17.

Mulligan, J., J. Fox-Rushby, T. Adams, B. Johns, and A. Mills. 2003. "Unit Costs of Health Care Inputs in Low and Middle Income Regions." Working Paper 9, Disease Control Priorities. Fogarty International Center, National Institutes of Health, Bethesda, MD.

Nasir, A. A., L. O. Abdur-Rahman, and J. O. Adeniran. 2011. "Predictor of Mortality in Children with Typhoid Intestinal Perforation in a Tertiary Hospital in Nigeria." *Pediatric Surgery International* 27 (12): 1317–21. doi:10.1007/s00383-011-2924-2.

Ngendahayo, E., A. Bonane, G. Ntakiyiruta, A. Munyanshongore, N. Muganga, and others. 2014. "Preparing for Safety Monitoring after Rotavirus Vaccine Implementation: A Retrospective Review of Intussusception Cases among Children at a Large Teaching Hospital in Rwanda, 2009–2012." *Pediatric Infectious Disease Journal* 33 (Suppl 1): S99–103. doi:10.1097/inf.0000000000000093.

Nilsson, H., G. Stylianidis, M. Haapamaki, E. Nilsson, and P. Nordin. 2007. "Mortality after Groin Hernia Surgery." *Annals of Surgery* 245 (4): 656–60.

Nuhu, A., and A. Jah. 2010. "Acute Sigmoid Volvulus in a West African Population." *West African Journal of Medicine* 29 (2): 109–12.

Nyamtema, A. S., S. K. Pemba, G. Mbaruku, F. D. Rutasha, and J. van Roosmalen. 2011. "Tanzanian Lessons in Using Non-physician Clinicians to Scale up Comprehensive Emergency Obstetric Care in Remote and Rural Areas." *Human Resources for Health* 9: 28. doi:10.1186/1478-4491-9-28.

Ohene-Yeboah, M. 2006. "Acute Surgical Admissions for Abdominal Pain in Adults in Kumasi, Ghana." *ANZ Journal of Surgery* 76 (10): 898–903. doi:10.1111/j.1445-2197.2006.03905.x.

Petroze, R. T., R. S. Groen, F. Niyonkuru, M. Mallory, E. Ntaganda, and others. 2013. "Estimating Operative Disease Prevalence in a Low-Income Country: Results of a Nationwide Population Survey in Rwanda." *Surgery* 153 (4): 457–64. doi:10.1016/j.surg.2012.10.001.

Sani, R., B. Nameoua, A. Yahaya, I. Hassane, R. Adamou, and others. 2009. "The Impact of Launching Surgery at the District Level in Niger." *World Journal of Surgery* 33 (10): 2063–68. doi:10.1007/s00268-009-0160-x.

Shillcutt, S. D., M. G. Clarke, and A. N. Kingsnorth. 2010. "Cost-Effectiveness of Groin Hernia Surgery in the Western Region of Ghana." *Archives of Surgery* 145 (10): 954–61. doi:10.1001/archsurg.2010.208.

Simon, E. G., A. Chacko, A. K. Dutta, A. J. Joseph, and B. George. 2013. "Acute Nonvariceal Upper Gastrointestinal Bleeding: Experience of a Tertiary Care Center in Southern India." *Indian Journal of Gastroenterology* 32 (4): 236–41. doi:10.1007/s12664-013-0305-6.

Soper, D. E. 2010. "Pelvic Inflammatory Disease." *Obstetrics and Gynecology* 116 (2 Pt 1): 419–28. doi:10.1097/AOG.0b013e3181e92c54.

Stewart, B., P. Khanduri, C. McCord, M. Ohene-Yeboah, S. Uranues, and others. 2014. "Global Disease Burden of Conditions Requiring Emergency Surgery." *British Journal of Surgery* 101 (1): e9–22. doi:10.1002/bjs.9329.

Ugochukwu, A. I., O. C. Amu, M. A. Nzegwu, and U. C. Dilibe. 2013. "Acute Perforated Peptic Ulcer: On Clinical Experience in an Urban Tertiary Hospital in South East Nigeria." *International Journal of Surgery* 11 (3): 223–27. doi:10.1016/j.ijsu.2013.01.015.

Urassa, D. P., A. Carlstedt, L. Nystrom, S. N. Massawe, and G. Lindmark. 2005. "Are Process Indicators Adequate to Assess Essential Obstetric Care at District Level? A Case Study from Rufiji District, Tanzania." *African Journal of Reproductive Health* 9 (3): 100–11.

U.S. Department of Commerce, Bureau of the Census. 1935. *Mortality Statistics 1935: Thirty-Sixth Annual Report.* http://www.cdc.gov/nchs/data/vsushistorical/mortstatsh_1935.pdf/.

van Amelsfoort, J. J., P. A. van Leeuwen, P. Jiskoot, and Y. E. Ratsma. 2010. "Surgery in Malawi: The Training of Clinical Officers." *Tropical Doctor* 40 (2): 74–76. doi:10.1258/td.2009.090068.

van den Heuvel, B., B. J. Dwars, D. R. Klassen, and H. J. Bonjer. 2011. "Is Surgical Repair of an Asymptomatic Groin Hernia Appropriate? A Review." *Hernia* 15 (3): 251–59. doi:10.1007/s10029-011-0796-y.

Wani, I., M. Rather, G. Naikoo, A. Amin, S. Mushtaq, and others. 2010. "Intestinal Ascariasis in Children." *World Journal of Surgery* 34 (5): 963–68. doi:10.1007/s00268-010-0450-3.

WHO (World Health Organization). 2002. *World Health Report 2002: Reducing Risks, Promoting Healthy Life.* Geneva: WHO.

———. 2003. *Surgical Care at the District Hospital.* Geneva: WHO.

———. 2013a. "Global Health Estimates (GHE)." http://www.who.int/healthinfo/global_burden_disease/en/.

———. 2013b. "WHO Model List of Essential Medicines." http://www.who.int/medicines/publications/essentialmedicines/18th_EML_Final_web_8Jul13.pdf.

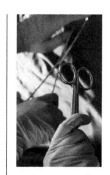

Chapter **5**

Obstetric Surgery

Clark T. Johnson, Timothy R. B. Johnson,
and Richard M. K. Adanu

GLOBAL BURDEN OF SURGICALLY TREATABLE OBSTETRIC CONDITIONS

Surgically Preventable or Treatable Conditions

Pregnancy is not a disease but a condition undertaken by most women during their reproductive lives. Pregnancy, however, is a time when health can be threatened. Any pregnancy carries the risk for hemorrhage, obstructed labor, or the need for a cesarean delivery. The sheer volume of maternal morbidity and mortality worldwide indicates that *every* pregnant woman is at risk for surgically preventable obstetric complications that can lead to death or disability.

Maternal morbidity and mortality are significantly increased by conditions that can be prevented by access to safe obstetric surgery. Obstructed labor, which can lead to fistula formation, uterine perforation, hemorrhage, sepsis, or death, can be avoided by observing labor for deviations from normal and providing access to nearby safe cesarean delivery. Most low- and middle-income countries (LMICs) do not have birth attendants present at deliveries to monitor for abnormalities; most of these countries also lack the capacity to provide access to nearby hospitals, where safe and timely cesarean deliveries can be undertaken. Hemorrhage during pregnancy and the postpartum period can be catastrophic; the occurrence of hemorrhage remote from access to surgical services, such as uterine curettage or lifesaving hysterectomy, drives avoidable maternal mortality rates worldwide.

This chapter uses the World Health Organization's (WHO's) six geographical regions: African Region, Region of the Americas, South-East Asia Region, European Region, Eastern Mediterranean Region, and Western Pacific Region.

Burden of Maternal Mortality

In 2000, total maternal mortality was 421,010; by 2011, worldwide maternal mortality had decreased significantly to 279,000. The maternal mortality ratio (MMR)—maternal deaths per 100,000 live births—improved from 321 in 2000 to 207 in 2011. In high-income countries (HICs), a small increase was noted, from 12 to 14; LMICs saw a marked improvement, from 352 to 227 (WHO 2013). This risk is much higher in adolescent pregnancies, which account for an increasing proportion of maternal mortality in LMICs (Patton and others 2009).

In LMICs, a woman has a 1:150 lifetime risk, on average, of dying from complications of pregnancy and childbirth (WHO 2012). In some areas of Sub-Saharan Africa, this risk is as high as 1:16; a woman who survives until childbearing years has a 6.25 percent chance that her life will be ended prematurely from the complications of pregnancy. These burdens are even higher in the underdeveloped regions of countries with high maternal morbidity and mortality rates (Liang and others 2011).

Corresponding author: Clark T. Johnson, MD, MPH, Johns Hopkins Medical Institutions, ctj@jhu.edu

The reduction of maternal mortality during pregnancy and up to six weeks postpartum was established as Millennium Development Goal (MDG) 5 (UN 2013). Although the world has yet to approach the MDG 5 goal of a 75 percent reduction in the MMR, there are reasons for optimism (Hogan and others 2010). Worldwide efforts to meet this goal have yielded dramatic improvements. Overall success has been attributed to improvements in the total fertility rate, per capita income, maternal education level, and presence of skilled birth attendants. However, the HIV epidemic has significantly added to MMRs; areas that could have been expected to see a reduction in maternal mortality have instead not seen significant differences. The tremendous disparity in MMRs between HICs on the one hand and LMICs on the other indicates the potential to reduce maternal morbidity and mortality on a worldwide scale.

Disability Burden

Assessments of disability-adjusted life years (DALYs) have been made for major obstetric complications worldwide (table 5.1). A DALY is a metric of the number of years lost due to ill health, disability, or early death for one individual. When summed for a population, it can assess the burden of a disease in a way that mortality assessments may miss. The significance of such assessments is that efforts to drive down MMRs succeed in part by creating permanent disabilities in lieu of maternal death. The societal costs of these DALYs can be significant, and a full assessment of the burden of disease should include an evaluation of DALYs.

In 2010, the collective disability for all measured maternal disorders reached 16 million DALYs (Murray and others 2012). Of this number, 3.3 million DALYs were attributed to maternal hemorrhage, 1.8 million to complications of obstructed labor, and 1.3 million to maternal sepsis. These numbers are indicative of the tremendous morbidity associated with surgically preventable obstetric complications that can be targeted worldwide.

As table 5.1 demonstrates, dramatic improvements in reducing MMRs have been made in the past 20 years. However, obstructed labor has lagged behind the other major maternal disorders (Murray and others 2012). This lag is partly due to the challenges in the treatment of this condition. Simply having access to safe and timely cesarean delivery can prevent the sequelae of obstructed labor. This simple procedure has been more difficult to implement in LMICs than have the medical treatments that can reduce morbidity from hemorrhage or hypertensive diseases, in large part because of the associated up-front infrastructural and systems costs of developing the environments

Table 5.1 The Global Disability Burden of Obstetric Disease in Terms of Disability-Adjusted Life Years, 1990–2010

	All ages DALYs (thousands)			DALYs (per 100,000 total population)		
	1990	2010	Difference (%)	1990	2010	Difference (%)
Maternal disorders	21,582 (18,000–25,720)	16,104 (12,972–18,912)	−25.4	407 (340–485)	234 (188–274)	−42.6
Maternal hemorrhage	4,784 (3,923–5,713)	3,289 (2,619–3,860)	−31.2	90 (74–108)	48 (38–56)	−47.1
Maternal sepsis	2,043 (1,701–2,508)	1,309 (1,059–1,585)	−35.9	39 (32–47)	19 (15–23)	−50.7
Hypertensive disorders of pregnancy	4,108 (3,406–4,986)	2,797 (2,254–3,357)	−31.9	77 (64–94)	41 (33–49)	−47.6
Obstructed labor	1,891 (1,451–2,625)	1,792 (1,249–2,806)	−5.2	36 (27–50)	26 (18–41)	−27.1
Abortion	3,218 (2,668–3,945)	2,138 (1,731–2,592)	−33.6	61 (50–74)	31 (25–38)	−48.9
Other maternal disorders	5,538 (4,576–6,538)	4,778 (3,819–5,512)	−13.7	104 (86–123)	69 (55–80)	−33.6

Source: Adapted from Murray and others 2012.
Note: 95 percent confident interval in parentheses.

in which patients can be referred and safe cesarean delivery performed.

Societal Impact of Maternal Mortality

A valid assessment of the health burden of obstetric complications should not be limited to maternal morbidity and mortality, but should also consider the effect of the morbidity and mortality rates in LMICs. Such assessments have included the effects that a maternal death can have on societies as well as on families (Yamin and others 2013). Children who are orphaned as the result of a maternal death suffer from hindered access to health care, poorer nutrition, and worse education. Female orphans particularly suffer because they are often expected to perform the household chores that their mothers would have performed. Their educational and economic opportunities become limited, and high-risk sexual behavior or early marriage can result. These developments, in turn, can lead to early pregnancies, putting daughters at risk for the same complications that led to their mothers' deaths.

In addition to the negative impacts on orphan children, maternal deaths affect the entire family structure (Yamin and others 2013). Economically, the loss of a mother is a loss of help around the house, a loss of a potentially important secondary income, and the loss of a caregiver. In these environments with high maternal mortality, high societal mortality rates often lead to women having multiple children with different fathers. It is uncommon for surviving fathers to care for non-biological children, potentially abandoning orphaned children without living fathers. The loss of mothers frequently can lead to the dissolution and permanent fragmentation of families, with children going to different homes or family members. Support structures for families that have lost mothers are uncommon and not well developed in countries where maternal death rates are high.

In sum, the global health burden of obstetric disease is tremendous, with essentially all women of reproductive age at risk for obstetric complications. Some percentage of pregnancies require some form of operative delivery; an estimated 15 percent of all deliveries require cesarean delivery to optimize maternal and neonatal outcomes (Gibbons and others 2012). Worldwide, 50 percent of countries have cesarean delivery rates that are less than 15 percent; 25 percent of countries have cesarean delivery rates of less than 5 percent. The WHO estimates that in LMICs, the cesarean rate should be at least 5 percent to 10 percent of deliveries to optimize maternal and neonatal outcomes (Gibbons and others 2012).

OVERVIEW OF SURGICAL OBSTETRICAL PROCEDURES

The successful management of labor and delivery requires a balanced use of medical and surgical practices. Most pregnancies end with uncomplicated vaginal deliveries. Pregnant women in labor have the right to attendants who can manage obstetric complications as they arise and who can transfer patients to a higher level of care as needed.

The presence of skilled birth attendants at all deliveries facilitates normal deliveries and the identification and referral of complications; but their effectiveness is limited by available referral resources. Although birth attendants may be able to accommodate minor complications, the benefit of their ability to identify major morbidity is limited if patients lack timely access to higher levels of care.

A majority of obstetric complications that require surgical intervention occurs peridelivery. Obstructed labor from a number of causes, including malpresentation and large fetal size, can necessitate one of a number of procedures to facilitate fetal delivery. Following delivery, hemorrhage from a number of etiologies, including lacerations and uterine atony, can similarly require one of a number of lifesaving procedures to help stop ongoing bleeding.

Operative Vaginal Delivery

Operative vaginal delivery, such as delivery assisted with forceps or a vacuum, requires trained providers as well as available instruments (Hale and Dennen 2001); its use in LMICs is often limited to the hospital setting. Vacuums require a fundamental level of training before routine use, and forceps require potentially more training, in addition to provision of the actual devices. The WHO is developing variations on a vacuum to provide a low-cost and easy-to-use device that can be widely implemented by birth attendants to reduce morbidity and mortality (FIGO 2012). Some devices are reusable; after the initial investment in the device, the subsequent cost largely consists of training providers to effectively and safely use it. The use of operative vaginal delivery techniques in the appropriate clinical circumstance might prevent the need for an inaccessible but otherwise necessary cesarean delivery. Additionally, manual or digital rotation of the fetal head without the use of forceps can help to guide the head through the pelvis to facilitate vaginal delivery (Le Ray and others 2007), but it requires a similar level of training. In sum, the minimal costs associated with providing the devices, as well as training for management of the second stage of labor, can help reduce morbidity and mortality without requiring the use of an operating theater.

Shoulder Dystocia

Shoulder dystocia and its association with poor fetal outcomes and brachial plexus injuries make it a feared obstetrical complication (Baskett, Calder, and Arulkumaran 2007; O'Grady and others 2008). Shoulder dystocia results from delivery of the fetal head, with a dystocia at the level of the shoulder that obstructs delivery. It is more common with large infants, particularly with relatively large shoulder widths born to mothers with diabetes. Attempts at delivery may cause permanent nerve injury, and delay in delivery may cause hypoxic injury or death.

Several maneuvers have been described for delivery. Most techniques involve rotation of the fetal shoulder from the anterior-posterior orientation to a more oblique position, where the more generous dimensions of the pelvis might permit shoulder delivery. Specific surgical instruments may be needed for operative management without successful resolution of the dystocia. Successful management of a shoulder dystocia depends primarily on the training of the attending providers.

Intentional pubic symphysiotomy, where the pubic bone is broken to facilitate fetal delivery, is controversial because it can cause significant maternal morbidity and chronic pain. Its implementation should be performed only by experienced providers when all other options have failed and cesarean delivery is not available. Significantly, it is only necessary without timely access to safe cesarean delivery.

Genital Tract Lacerations

Lacerations of the genital tract, which can occur spontaneously or result from an episiotomy, are the second most common cause of postpartum hemorrhage. They can occur at any level, including the perineum, sulci, cervix, or the broad ligament in the abdomen; without spontaneous hemostasis, they will require repair. The use of routine episiotomy in obstetrics has evolved, with studies demonstrating the cost-effectiveness of its selective rather than routine use (Borghi and others 2002). An attendant with available suture can repair a majority of perineal lacerations without referral, but severe lacerations can threaten or end a mother's life. Complicated lacerations can bleed profusely; ongoing bleeding can exhaust clotting factors, resulting in an inability to clot and death.

Similarly, hematomas can occur; even without visible bleeding, large volumes of blood can accumulate in the pelvis following vaginal delivery. Depending on their location, prompt identification and treatment can be life saving.

Abnormal Fetal Presentation

Breech Presentation. In most pregnancies, the fetus moves into the safest position of head down at approximately 36 weeks. However, this movement does not occur in 4 percent of cases, resulting in breech presentation (Baskett, Calder, and Arulkumaran 2007), and its incidence rises dramatically with prematurity. Breech presentation is associated with inferior fetal outcomes, as a result of both the antenatal risk factors and the perinatal risk of birth injury at delivery.

Ideally, a breech presentation is identified before delivery so that consideration can be given to attempting the external turning of the fetus. This technique is optimally performed near 36 weeks, when the success rate is generally better than 50 percent. Although external version can effectively make a mother a candidate for vaginal delivery and decrease morbidity, it carries the risk of manually traumatizing the placenta or the fetus, necessitating immediate delivery. It should only take place when the fetal status can be confirmed, and intervention, including cesarean delivery, is immediately available. Unfortunately, in LMICs where antenatal care is scant, breech presentation may not be identified until labor, and delivery has to be facilitated either by emergent cesarean or by unanticipated vaginal breech delivery.

Large studies have demonstrated improved fetal outcomes in breech presentation with cesarean delivery (Hannah and others 2000; Hannah and others 2002); safe cesarean delivery is preferred, when available, unless practitioners are trained to manage breech labor and its complications. Birth attendants should be trained in the maneuvers to assist intact delivery in cases in which breech delivery is inevitable or advisable. Particularly in the absence of antenatal care, a possible clinical scenario is a vaginal breech delivery in progress, and fetal outcome will depend on a present provider who can safely deliver the fetus.

Other Presentation. Malpresentation, in which neither the fetal vertex nor the breech is the presenting part, as with a transverse presenting fetus (where the fetus is sideways), is a universal indication for cesarean delivery. Without a safe and timely cesarean delivery, the pregnancy can end with obstructed labor and its sequelae, or fetal demise.

Multiple Gestation

Delivery of more than one fetus is inherently more complicated (Baskett, Calder, and Arulkumaran 2007). Contraindications to vaginal delivery include three or more fetuses, an exceedingly uncommon event in the absence of assisted reproductive technology. Fortunately, the presenting fetus will usually be head down in the pelvis and can be managed essentially as a singleton labor. Following delivery of the first twin, and if the second twin does not present vertex, attempts can be made to externally rotate the fetus to vertex and proceed with vaginal delivery. Otherwise, breech extraction of the second twin can be considered. In multifetal deliveries, vaginal delivery has lower maternal morbidity than cesarean delivery, but a combined vaginal delivery and cesarean delivery is more morbid than either. If vaginal delivery of a second twin is doubtful, particularly in the absence of a provider comfortable with breech extraction, cesarean delivery may be considered primarily.

Postpartum Hemorrhage

Postpartum hemorrhage is a dreaded complication akin to the most severe surgical trauma. The average blood losses for a routine vaginal delivery and a cesarean delivery are commonly accepted to be 500 mls and 1,000 mls, respectively; blood loss in excess of these values is considered to be hemorrhage. The causes of postpartum hemorrhage are as follows, in the order of frequency, with optimal management based on underlying etiology (O'Grady and others 2008):

- Uterine atony
- Lacerations
- Retained placenta, including abnormal placentation
- Uterine rupture
- Uterine inversion
- Coagulopathy

Uterine Atony. Uterine atony accounts for approximately 80 percent of all postpartum hemorrhage (O'Grady and others 2008). Risk factors include uterine overdistension, prolonged labor, multiparity, infection, and use of uterine relaxants. Medical uterotonics, where available, can be administered to assist uterine tone, including pitocin, misoprostol, and ergots or prostaglandins. Consideration may also be given to draining the bladder, given that a distended bladder can contribute to uterine atony. Mechanically, bimanual massage can at least temporize uterine atony. Without medical or surgical interventions, effective bimanual massage can be life saving. Research has suggested that effective bimanual massage is optimized when two parties coordinate to help compress the atonic uterus and stop maternal hemorrhage (Andreatta, Perosky, and Johnson 2012). Active management of the delivery of the placenta itself can significantly help prevent atonic hemorrhage and limit the need for additional uterotonics (Stanton and others 2009).

If hemorrhage continues despite these maneuvers, surgical management should be considered. Surgical management can include blunt or sharp curettage of the uterus, particularly with a large curette to minimize the risk of perforating the fragile peripartum uterus and necessitating abdominal surgery. Otherwise, laparotomy can be used to access the uterus and perform maneuvers such as compression sutures, ligation of uterine vessels, or ultimately hysterectomy for definitive management. Delays in or the unavailability of surgical interventions can lead to uncontrolled hemorrhage, disseminated intravascular coagulopathy, and death. For persistent hemorrhage, the uterus can be packed to tamponade and temporize the bleeding. This procedure can be done either with packing or with a balloon catheter to help drain the uterine cavity while providing tamponade. Surgical management may still be fundamentally needed, but maternal survival may depend on the ability to transport to provide abdominal surgery.

Retained Placenta. Following delivery of the placenta, any remnant of the products of conception can contribute to uterine atony and ongoing vaginal bleeding. Retained products may be suspected with difficult extrusion of the placental membranes. In any scenario in which retained products of conception are suspected, consideration should be given to the possibility of placenta accreta because further placental bed manipulation could contribute to catastrophic hemorrhage and death. Surgical curettage may be needed to remove persistent retained products and arrest hemorrhage if placental abnormalities are not present.

Uterine Inversion. Inversion of the uterus can occur as a result of overzealous traction on a placenta or from fundal pressure in the third stage of labor. With inversion, on examination, the fundus may be noted to have descended or prolapsed into the vagina. A skilled attendant can use gentle manual replacement of the fundus back to its appropriate station, and effort may be needed to avoid relapse of the prolapse. Without successful manual replacement, other techniques may be urgently needed in the face of ongoing hemorrhage or maternal shock (Baskett, Calder, and Arulkumaran 2007). Nonsurgically, intravaginal pressure can be increased with infusion of intravenous fluids while the introitus is blocked, which may reduce the inversion. Surgically, the abdomen can be entered with a Pfannenstiel incision or otherwise to gain exposure to the uterus. In the Huntington procedure, the round ligaments are elevated and followed medially, eventually restoring the inverted fundus. Alternatively, with the Haultian procedure, the inversion is incised vertically, permitting appropriate reapproximation of the fundus.

Blood Transfusion. The WHO considers access to safe blood transfusion be a key lifesaving intervention (WHO 2008). The availability of blood transfusions at the time of obstetric emergency can be life saving. Accordingly, blood transfusion services should be considered part of emergency obstetric management capacity. Blood transfusion availability is severely limited in LICs and LMICs, and efforts to make it available locally can save lives.

Cesarean Delivery

Prolonged labor can lead to uterine rupture, which can lead to rapid fetal or maternal exsanguination. In settings of prolonged and obstructed labor, eventual cesarean section has a significantly increased risk of maternal morbidity or potentially death, compared with timely cesarean delivery.

Indications. The indications for cesarean delivery are numerous, and its potential to reduce associated morbidity is significant. The decision to proceed is influenced by a number of factors, including the training of the operator, the operative and clinical resources, and the variables of the clinical presentation. The caveat is that cesarean delivery is a more morbid procedure: blood loss is increased, recovery time is lengthened, and potentially inferior fetal outcomes can occur. In certain scenarios, however, a cesarean is necessary and inevitable to save a life or lives. Efforts to develop evidence-based best practices for cesarean delivery are ongoing (Berghella, Baxter, and Chauhan 2005; Dahlke and others 2013).

Preoperative Preparation. Once the decision is made to proceed, the patient is moved to the operating theater, and the appropriate anesthesia, whether regional or general, is administered. The abdomen is prepared in a sterile manner. A Foley catheter may be placed to help minimize the presence of the bladder in the operative field and to provide an accurate assessment of urine output. A single dose of antibiotic prophylaxis within 30 minutes before incision is associated with decreased risk of infection. The risk of venous

thromboembolism during routine cesarean delivery is low in the absence of other risk factors, and routine medical thrombolytic prophylaxis is not recommended (Dahlke and others 2013).

Incision. The Pfannenstiel incision, transversely in the lower abdomen, has classically been described for cesarean delivery. A midline vertical incision may be considered for better exposure. Alternatives to the Pfannenstiel or midline vertical incisions include the Joel-Cohen technique and the Misgav-Ladach method in which blunt dissection is used and may decrease blood loss and operative time, although studies have not shown significant decreases in morbidity or mortality (CORONIS 2013).

The uterus is incised in the lower nonmuscular portion to facilitate fetal delivery. Occasionally, a contraction ring or "Bandl's ring" can be seen in prolonged obstructed labor at the time of cesarean delivery. Its treatment requires perpendicular incision, through the ring and muscle of the uterus, to relax the tension and permit delivery, with significant future morbidity associated with the incision. Notably, any uterine incision that extends up into the thick muscle significantly compromises the uterus and increases the risk of uterine rupture in a future pregnancy. It is considered a contraindication to a future trial of labor, sentencing the patient to indicated cesarean deliveries for all future pregnancies.

Delivery. The fetus is delivered through the uterine incision, with morbidity associated with cesarean delivery increasing if the fetal head has engaged in the pelvis and labor has taken longer, as with obstructed labor. Techniques to facilitate a challenging cesarean delivery may include breech extraction, use of the vacuum extractor, or use of one or two forceps blades to facilitate delivery through the hysterotomy. Morbidity includes hemorrhage, infection, or uterine excision extension into the nearby anatomy of either the major vasculature or the urinary tract.

If the placenta does not easily separate, occult placenta accreta may be considered. If accreta is suspected, manual removal should be avoided; if spontaneous delivery does not occur, then hysterectomy should be considered. The uterus may be exteriorized to facilitate exposure for closure, although this may increase patient discomfort and nausea, as well as risk of avulsion of adhesions to the uterus, if present.

Uterine closure then takes place quickly in the face of bleeding from the hysterotomy edges and from the uterus. Atony should be addressed while surgery continues with bimanual massage used as needed. If the patient desires an intrauterine device for contraception, it can be placed at this time directly at the level of the fundus, with the strings trimmed and introduced near or through the cervix.

Obstetric Hemorrhage at Time of Cesarean Delivery. Hemorrhage following cesarean differs from that following vaginal delivery in that there is already access to the abdominal cavity, improving the odds of successful definitive management. Conservative measures can also be taken, including medicines and bimanual massage. Without quick resolution, a stitch can be placed bilaterally around the large uterine vessels to decrease active hemorrhage from the uterus. Hypogastric artery ligation can similarly decrease the blood flow and rate of blood loss, although its dissection is technically challenging and should only be undertaken by an operator sufficiently trained in and comfortable with the procedure. Tamponade and packing can be performed and left in place to arrest bleeding as well.

If atony is the underlying issue and the outlined steps have not stopped the bleeding, compression sutures may be helpful in the scenario in which bimanual massage is effective, but as soon as the hands are removed uterine tone is lost.

When ongoing hemorrhage is significant and not easily abated, definitive management with hysterectomy should be strongly considered because delay will only increase morbidity. The B-Lynch suture is described as passing a stitch on a large needle across the hysterotomy about halfway toward the side (El-Hamamy, Wright, and Lynch 2009). The stitch is then taken to the posterior of the uterus, where it is passed transversely at approximately the level of the anterior low uterine segment hysterotomy. It is brought back anterior, where it is thrown vertically across the hysterotomy on the other side. The two ends of the suture are tied down while an assistant has maximally compressed and folded the uterus on itself, so that when the stitch is tied down, the uterus is as compressed as possible because any relaxation will contribute to bleeding from atony. Other types of compression sutures are described as passing anterior to posterior in the body of the uterus to tamponade sequential pockets throughout the cavity. If compression sutures are performed, care should be taken not to obstruct cavity outflow given that hematometra or pyometra can result.

Abnormal Placentation and Cesarean Hysterectomy

When the placenta grows into tissue beyond its normal boundaries, it can embed in that tissue and cause catastrophic hemorrhage with attempted removal.

The term *placenta accreta* encompasses *placenta increta* (where placenta grows into the uterine wall) and *percreta* (where placenta grows into nearby tissue including bowel and bladder). Risk factors include previous uterine scarring from surgical procedures, including previous cesarean section.

Antenatal diagnosis can be achieved with ultrasound imaging in combination with clinical history. With antenatal diagnosis, preparations should be made at the onset of labor to plan for delivery in a scheduled setting, ready for the probability of cesarean hysterectomy and the need for blood products, if available. Even in settings with full obstetric resources, placenta accreta can lead to poor maternal outcomes. The aggressive hemorrhage associated with incomplete placental separation can quickly lead to disseminated coagulopathy and require massive blood transfusions to maintain maternal life.

Suspicion of placenta percreta before delivery calls for the coordination of a team of surgeons in a facility with resources to maximize the likelihood of safe delivery. Cesarean delivery should be undertaken, with consideration for a midline vertical incision to facilitate a potential hysterectomy. Following exposure of the gravid uterus, a uterine incision may be made to avoid disruption of the placental bed if its location is known. In cases of diagnostic certainty, cesarean hysterectomy can be accomplished without attempting placental delivery, decreasing the risk of morbidity associated with hemorrhage. In cases in which accreta is not identified until the time of delivery, a balloon catheter can be used to tamponade the uterine cavity, potentially avoiding further surgical morbidity.

Following delivery, the hysterectomy is performed; in these cases, the caliber of the vasculature is significantly generous and the anatomy can be distorted. Care must be taken to skeletonize the engorged uterine vessels while ensuring safe distance from the ureters to prevent their injury.

There is no definitive answer for when to deliver suspected placenta accreta, although it is frequently done between 34 weeks and 36 weeks to balance neonatal survival against risk of onset of labor and emergent delivery in the setting of acute hemorrhage (ACOG 2013).

EFFECTIVENESS AND COST-EFFECTIVENESS OF OBSTETRIC SURGERY

The need to prove the cost-effectiveness of operative obstetrics to decrease the tragedy of preventable maternal mortality or morbidity may be offensive to some.

Regardless, the provision of safe cesarean delivery to prevent obstructed labor in LMICs has been demonstrated to be cost-effective, with a positive net economic return to those societies.

Safe Cesarean Delivery

Numerous studies have demonstrated the significant cost-effective benefits of providing access to safe cesarean delivery in countries where it is not currently available (table 5.2) (Grimes and others 2014). Separate analysis finds that the provision of cesarean for obstructed labor, malpresentation, or fetal distress in these countries would cost US$73 for each DALY averted in Sub-Saharan Africa, and US$2,638 in South-East Asia (Adam and others 2005).

A study in Guinea finds that the provision of cesarean delivery for obstructed labor was very cost-effective at US$18 per year of life saved (Jha, Bangoura, and Ranson 1998). A study in the Democratic Republic of Congo reinforces the challenges and the importance of providing emergency obstetric services during humanitarian crises; it further demonstrates that financial investments can significantly improve maternal and neonatal mortality (Deboutte and others 2013).

One of the major sequelae of not having access to safe cesarean delivery is obstetric fistula resulting from obstructed labor (see chapter 6). An estimated 3 million women suffer from obstetric fistula worldwide. Obstetric fistula can result in societal marginalization, in addition to significant medical morbidities that are frequently permanent (Wall 2006). One analysis that examines only the impact of obstructed labor sequelae finds that the provision of safe cesarean delivery where not available would avert 16,800 maternal deaths in one year (Alkire and others 2012). This study, which analyzes countries where the number of cesarean deliveries provided is inadequate to meet demand, finds that approximately 1 million DALYs would be saved by providing accessible cesarean delivery to 90 percent of the pregnancies complicated by obstructed labor

Table 5.2 Overview of Studies Evaluating the Cost-Effectiveness of Cesarean Delivery

Study	Country or region	Details of intervention analyzed	Cost-effectiveness	Measurement
Alkire and others 2012	49 countries with unmet demand for cesarean delivery	Evaluation of the unmet need for cesarean delivery indicated for obstructed labor	Median US$304 Range $251–$3,462	Cost per DALY averted
Adam and others 2005	High-risk areas of Sub-Saharan Africa and South-East Asia	Evaluation of the unmet need for cesarean delivery indicated for a composite of obstructed labor, malpresentation, and nonreassuring fetal status	Sub-Saharan Africa: US$1,576 South-East Asia: US$1,449	Cost per DALY averted
Jha, Bangoura, and Ranson 1998	Guinea	Evaluation of the unmet need for multiple surgical services, including cesarean delivery indicated for obstructed labor	US$18	Cost per YLS
Hu and others 2007	Mexico	Upgrading current obstetric practice to meet the WHO mother-baby standard of care package	US$550 US$390	Cost per YLS Cost per DALY
Erim, Resch, and Goldie 2012	Nigeria	Stepwise improvement in family planning; safe abortion provision; and intrapartum care, including cesarean delivery	US$3,930–US$4,481	Cost per maternal death averted
Goldie and others 2010	India	Stepwise improvement in family planning; safe abortion provision; and intrapartum care, including cesarean delivery	US$300 in rural India US$350 in urban India	Cost per YLS
Carvalho, Salehi, and Goldie 2013	Afghanistan	Stepwise improvement in family planning; safe abortion provision; and intrapartum care, including cesarean delivery	US$178	Cost per YLS
Deboutte and others 2013	Congo, Dem. Rep.	Investment in an NGO hospital in the postconflict environment to provide emergency obstetric care	US$9.2	Cost per health-adjusted YLS

Source: Adapted from Grimes and others 2014.
Note: NGO = nongovernmental organization; WHO = World Health Organization; YLS = year of life saved.

(Alkire and others 2012). The cost-effectiveness associated with providing cesarean delivery services at this level varies widely by country, from US$251 for each DALY averted in countries with higher maternal morbidity risks to US$3,462 per DALY averted in other countries analyzed.

Free or Subsidized Surgical Care

The provision of safe cesarean delivery services implies inherent costs to individuals without subsidized cesarean delivery that prevent implementation of indicated cesarean deliveries. This provision of free intrapartum services that include cesarean delivery is associated with increased rates of supervised labor and increased utilization of needed cesarean delivery (Lawn and others 2009). This scenario has been evaluated in Senegal, where the provision of free cesarean delivery helped to increase the rate to greater than 5 percent (Witter and Diadhiou 2008; Witter and others 2010). The US$461 cost associated with each additional cesarean delivery was judged to be beneficial, given that it represents a cesarean delivery that would otherwise not be provided. Similarly, in Ghana, a policy removing patient responsibility for costs at birth and postpartum was associated with an increase in attended births and institutional delivery (Lawn and others 2009; Witter and others 2007).

In India, Janani Suraksha Yojana, a cash incentive program to promote attended obstetric delivery, encouraged the practice, but it also raised concerns regarding the targeting of funding to the poorest in the population (Lim and others 2010). Subsidizing and encouraging safe obstetric delivery and free cesarean delivery in areas where the infrastructure exists to provide the services risks exacerbating disparities between areas where access to safe and timely cesarean delivery is available and areas where it is not available regardless of cost (Witter and others 2010).

In addition, care must be taken in auditing cesarean delivery rates in areas where costs are subsidized to ensure that the system does not develop a supratherapeutic cesarean rate. Overall, however, the evidence clearly indicates that the provision of financial incentives, or the removal of disincentives, can help improve access to emergency obstetric care (Briand and others 2012).

Synergy of Providing Obstetric Care with Family Planning Services

An analysis demonstrates that in Mexico, coupling effective family planning with emergency obstetric services saves costs of US$900,000 per 100,000 women compared with the current practice (Hu and others 2007).

The cost-effectiveness of safe cesarean delivery and emergency obstetric care can be significantly enhanced by effective family planning programs involving contraception and safe abortion (see chapter 7). An analysis in India suggests that combining the cost savings of effective family planning with the cost savings of providing emergency obstetric care could amount to savings of US$1.5 billion dollars per year and would help to reduce maternal mortality by as much as 75 percent (Goldie and others 2010). A similar analysis in Afghanistan finds that providing access to effective family planning services results in significant cost savings and reductions in maternal mortality (Carvalho, Salehi, and Goldie 2013). Additional reductions in maternal mortality depend on access to safe cesarean delivery and emergency obstetric care; in combination with family planning services, such access could help reduce maternal mortality by as much as 80 percent. In Nigeria, a similar analysis using a stepwise improvement package of family planning, abortion services, and emergency obstetric care demonstrates cost-effective improvements in public health (Erim, Resch, and Goldie 2012).

It is clear from these and other studies that the cost-effectiveness of cesarean delivery has synergy with other public health interventions involving family planning and abortion care (Souza and others 2013). The combination of these interventions will be far more effective than any single intervention in achieving the goals of substantial improvements in maternal mortality, as in MDG 5 (UN 2013).

An overview of studies evaluating the cost-effectiveness of obstetric interventions in different countries or areas is limited by the ability of the results from one setting to be generalized to another. The countries and areas in table 5.2 are widely variable, limiting this generalizability. A consistent theme, however, is that the provision of these fundamental obstetric packages is profoundly cost-effective or cost saving. The concept of areas where interventions can save a year of maternal life for less than US$20 or save the life of a reproductive-age woman for less than US$5,000 argues for the implementation of such programs to help save lives.

Other Obstetric Surgical Procedures

Little research has been conducted to justify the cost-effectiveness of other obstetric surgical procedures, in part because safe childbirth and prevention of unnecessary maternal and neonatal death may be considered goals without the need for cost justification.

Additional shared costs are involved when considering use of the techniques discussed in addition to cesarean delivery. Cost-effectiveness analysis of other operative obstetric techniques—including operative vaginal delivery and surgical treatment of postpartum hemorrhage—is limited in part by the difficulty of associating the costs and benefits of a single intervention. Although procedures may employ reusable equipment or sutures, these costs are relatively minor when compared with the cost of provider training to perform these procedures. Given the significant costs of developing a surgical center with providers trained to perform safe cesarean delivery, these same providers at these facilities—or elsewhere in the field—can be readily trained to perform the other obstetric surgical procedures.

Although the WHO estimates that the cesarean rate should be at least 5 percent to 10 percent of deliveries in LMICs to optimize maternal and neonatal outcomes, studies suggest that cesarean delivery rates higher than 15 percent to 20 percent in these countries may have greater associated maternal and neonatal surgical morbidity rates, compared with those for vaginal delivery, without providing significant health benefits (Gibbons and others 2012). The cost of excess cesarean rates in HICs has been estimated to be well over US$2 billion annually, suggesting the cost-saving utility of operative vaginal delivery to reduce the rate of unnecessary cesarean delivery in HICs (Gibbons and others 2012). The costs of both supplies and obstetric training must be considered in evaluating operative vaginal techniques, but both are likely to be cost saving compared with a cesarean delivery. This modeling has limitations when safe alternatives to vaginal delivery, including safe cesarean delivery, are not available.

Task-Shifting to Increase Skilled Providers

As countries attempt to meet the goal of providing safe cesarean delivery, expanding the pool of those who provide surgical services to providers other than obstetricians becomes an option. Mullan and Frehywot (2007) in an assessment of Sub-Saharan countries find that more than 50 percent use nonphysician clinicians in lieu of medical doctors to provide health care for communities. Task-shifting has been evaluated with non-obstetrician physicians, or even clinical officers, trained to perform cesarean deliveries.

In Tanzania, nonphysician clinicians have been an important asset in helping overcome the unmet need, which exceeds 70 percent, of emergency obstetric care (Nyamtema and others 2011). These nonphysician clinicians were given an effective three-month training

curriculum; upon completion, they have provided a majority of the emergency obstetric care in the area (Pereira and others 2011). The evaluation found no significant differences in the obstetric outcomes between the nonphysician clinicians and the physician providers (McCord and others 2009). Despite the implementation of these nonphysician clinician teams, most emergency obstetrical care needs remain unmet. Further gains appear to depend on access to hospital care centers rather than additional qualified obstetric providers.

The cost-effectiveness of using different providers has been evaluated in Burkina Faso (Hounton and others 2009). Clinical officers are trained nurses who undergo two additional years of surgical training; general practitioners in rural areas are trained in basic surgical techniques, including cesarean delivery. Obstetricians and general practitioners had significantly better maternal and neonatal outcomes compared with clinical officers. Obstetricians overall had moderately better neonatal outcomes than the general practitioners, but at significantly higher costs; the cost per cesarean delivery was twice as high with obstetricians compared with task-shifted providers. The benefit of using the trained general practitioners rather than clinical officers was associated with a cost of US$200 for each neonatal life saved.

A review in Ethiopia finds that more than 63 percent of obstetric procedures and cesarean deliveries are performed by nonphysician clinicians (Gessessew and others 2011). The study finds similar postoperative outcomes in the two groups. The review suggests that the nonphysician clinicians were more likely to remain in rural areas, providing a potential solution to the migration of more trained providers.

Unfortunately, the analysis of these clinical officers who perform emergency obstetric procedures in Malawi, Mozambique, and Tanzania finds that these officers are apt to leave their positions after training (McAuliffe and others 2013). Specifically, negative predictors of retention include an absence of oversight or supervision of the clinical providers in their roles, suggesting that formal supervision is correlated with job satisfaction and, in effect, with provider retention. Given the significant costs of training these individuals, attention to maintaining cohorts of trainees is important to maximize their benefit.

Diminishing returns were observed on investments in training providers to provide cesarean delivery in Burkina Faso (Hounton and others 2009) and Tanzania (Nyamtema and others 2011). Although these types of studies are difficult to perform and have limitations related to data collection, it is clearly more cost-effective to train lower-level providers to provide cesarean deliveries than fully trained obstetricians. In Sub-Saharan Africa, a small minority of countries (Ethiopia, Ghana, Malawi, Mozambique, and Tanzania) allow nonphysician providers to perform emergency obstetric surgery (Pereira and others 2011). In other areas, these nonphysician clinicians provide obstetric care but not cesarean delivery, limiting their utility.

Overall, clinical outcomes may be improved when a trained obstetrician performs the cesarean deliveries, but with significant cost. It is worth considering that trained obstetricians have the ability to train those around them and elevate the skills of other members of the team (Anderson and others 2014). Having supervisory forces for the nonphysician teams may assist in the retention of trained providers. Because of their lower up-front cost, however, task-shifted providers may solve short-term workforce problems.

When training a workforce, consideration needs to be given to training obstetric providers rather than medical practitioners to provide cesarean deliveries, depending on the resources and short- and long-term goals. It would be unreasonable in an HIC with an adequate supply of trained obstetric providers to fully revert to nonobstetricians to provide cesarean services and emergency obstetric care, because doing so would exacerbate negative maternal and neonatal outcomes. In LMICs attempting to establish fundamental obstetric care, task-shifting provides a short-term solution to unbearable circumstances (Hounton and others 2009). Given the tremendous burden of unmet need, however, implementation of task-shifting appears to be a reasonable step while infrastructure is developed (McCord and others 2009).

Challenges in Assessing the True Costs and Benefits of Obstetric Surgery

Cost analysis becomes difficult because of the wide number of variables across nations. In the long term, the common goal of reducing morbidity and mortality will be accomplished by establishing universally accessible first-level hospitals with mechanisms to refer to second- and third-level hospitals with fully trained providers to optimize maternal and neonatal outcomes. However, in the short term, in areas with limited resources for training an obstetric force, training task-shifted individuals can help mitigate maternal and neonatal morbidity and mortality rates.

Similar to the difficulty of assessing the cost-effectiveness of a single intervention, the difficulties of assessing the true costs associated with maternal morbidity or mortality hinder valid assessment.

As with obstetric fistula, obstetric morbidity has frequently been associated with social ostracism, the cost of which is difficult to measure (Wall 2006). The loss of a maternal life has far-reaching effects, including the impact on her family structure and downstream effects on that family and on society as a whole (Yamin and others 2013). This reality suggests that most assessments involving the cost of maternal deaths are likely to underestimate those costs. The cost of basic obstetric interventions widely used in HICs that can significantly reduce maternal morbidity in LMICs can be difficult to measure. Given the significant benefits to health that they offer, their potential implementation cost would have to be dramatic if they were to be not cost-effective in their lifesaving employment. Although cost-effectiveness data are lacking for some of these interventions, such as vaginal laceration repair to prevent hemorrhage, implementation costs are so minimal and health benefits are so significant that these data may not ever be produced.

The analyses examining the benefits of cesarean delivery focus on maternal morbidity and mortality, although neonatal morbidity and mortality are also directly related. The provision of cesarean delivery for obstructed labor, malpresentation, or intrauterine fetal distress often means the difference between neonatal intact survival, on the one hand, and fetal demise or permanent and significant injury, neurologic or otherwise, on the other hand (Hofmeyr and others 2009). The provision of neonatal resuscitation by birth attendants has been demonstrated to be cost-effective, at US$208 per neonatal life year saved and US$5 per neonatal DALY averted (Wall and others 2010). Full implementation of trained birth attendants to provide immediate neonatal care would avert 100 million DALYs at a cost of US$1.8 billion (Lawn and others 2009). In this analysis, the additional provision of emergency obstetric care to cover 90 percent of perceived need would cost US$2.8 billion and avert 150 million DALYs. Synergy was noted by bundling birth attendance, emergency obstetric care including cesarean delivery, and neonatal resuscitation, with resulting improved costs and cost-effectiveness of all the interventions. Overall, the universal provision of emergency obstetric services to 90 percent of women in need could avert approximately 500,000 neonatal deaths annually (Lawn and others 2009).

Beyond the provision of cesarean delivery, little evidence is available to guide cost-effective techniques, but common sense suggests that the provision of fundamental obstetrical services is a reproductive right. The fact that adolescent women in LMICs can have a higher risk of dying from pregnancy than other factors is not something that should be tolerated. The cost of birth attendants can vary, but their provision is accepted as fundamental to the amelioration of the status of women's health worldwide.

OBSTETRIC SURGICAL IMPLEMENTATION IN LOW- AND MIDDLE-INCOME COUNTRIES

Challenges to Provision of Safe Cesarean Delivery

Although access to safe and timely cesarean delivery should be a fundamental right guaranteed to all pregnant women, cesarean rates vary widely. The general consensus is that cesarean rates of less than 10 percent are low and inadequate to meet the obstetric needs of the population (Gibbons and others 2012). Cesarean rates of less than 5 percent, as throughout much of Sub-Saharan Africa, are considered extremely low. In these settings, most cesarean deliveries are undertaken intrapartum, frequently following failed labor.

A different problem has developed in countries with widely accessible cesarean delivery. Although many countries have rates well in excess of 20 percent, these higher rates are not associated with improvements in maternal or fetal outcomes (Gibbons and others 2012). Moreover, higher rates of cesarean delivery are associated with higher incidence of placenta accreta and surgical morbidity. Many factors influence increased cesarean delivery rates, including societal factors; some countries in South America have rates as high as 45 percent. Active discouragement of such high rates of cesarean delivery has not been successful. As further data are produced regarding the long-term morbidity and societal burden from these supratherapeutic cesarean rates, it is likely that the populations will start to respond.

Fundamental to the provision of safe cesarean delivery is an adequate triage system. In countries with the lowest rates of cesarean delivery, the many challenges faced in implementing skilled obstetric care include the following:

- The pervasive lack of trained obstetric providers— midwives, obstetricians, and anesthetists—especially in rural areas (Darmstadt and others 2009; Mavalankar and others 2009)
- The ineffective distribution of the available skilled providers, as well as difficulty retaining those who are dispersed
- The lack of support staff, infrastructure, equipment, and supplies (Koblinsky and others 2006).

Even when other factors are not an issue, transportation of patients can be limited because of poor roads and other impediments (Mehtsun and others 2012). These factors illustrate how a focus on relatively simple efforts in rural areas can have significant impacts on public health (You and others 2012).

Approaches to Improving Access to Surgical Care

More Widespread Technology. More widespread distribution of technology to access remote areas and link them to centers for emergency obstetric care will facilitate significant improvements to maternal health. The increasing availability of cell phones has the potential to improve women's health services networks while overcoming traditional obstacles to establishing effective health care systems (Fiander and Vanneste 2012). Low-cost cellular technology can connect birth attendants with regional obstetric officers, helping to guide management of intrapartum complications remotely, outside of health care centers, averting potential morbidity, and to coordinate access to emergency services. New methods of transferring funds using cell phones have been used to finance transport for patients to regional centers for advanced levels of care (Fiander and Vanneste 2012).

Improved Infrastructure. Infrastructural shortcomings and lack of provider motivation can prevent the full implementation of available obstetric resources to benefit maternal and child health in LMICs (Koblinsky and others 2006), as can societal reluctance to access available obstetric resources. Factors influencing this reluctance include financial costs and an unwelcome environment resulting from discriminatory or culturally insensitive practices. Any hesitation can delay presentation to permit the timely diagnosis and treatment of potential complications. Fundamentally, the establishment or development of first-level hospitals that can support safe cesarean delivery and obstetric care will be necessary to employ the trained providers and receive referred patients who require emergency obstetric care.

Increased Supply of Trained Providers. The education and training of obstetric providers need to be expanded to meet the needs of the populations in LMICs (Evans and others 2009; Hofmeyr and others 2009). Efforts to train large numbers of providers, which have been challenging without an established training infrastructure, must persist. An essential complement to initiatives to increase the numbers of skilled obstetric providers is the provision and maintenance of first-level hospitals or centers where the providers can perform cesarean deliveries and administer anesthesia (Anderson and others 2007).

Improved Patient Transport and Local Facilities. In HICs, the time to prepare to perform an indicated cesarean providing obstetric surgery is expected to be 30 minutes to optimize outcomes (ACOG 2009; Soltanifar and Russell 2012). This standard is ambitious for LMICs, but a realistic and reliable expectation of timely transport to such facilities would substantially reduce the burden of disease from obstructed labor (Spangler 2012).

The development of these locally accessible first-level hospitals would effectively make a network of these hospitals that would be universally accessible where cesarean deliveries could be performed. Such first-level obstetric institutions would require the availability of obstetric providers to perform the surgery and the capacity to administer anesthesia safely. Contributing to these structures would be the local network of skilled birth attendants at the bedside with mothers in labor— attendants with the ability to manage minor complications and successfully transfer patients in a timely manner when major complications arise or cesarean delivery is needed.

In developing these units, providing fully trained anesthesiologists and obstetricians for all deliveries will be a challenge (Evans and others 2009; Mavalankar and others 2009). Countries have examined the implementation of teams of nonspecialists trained to provide emergency obstetric care. Studies in Tanzania examining such nonphysician clinicians show good results (Nyamtema and others 2011; Pereira and others 2011). Despite the availability of trained nonspecialists, too many significant obstetric complications, particularly those requiring cesarean delivery, remained untreated.

CONCLUSION: FUTURE DIRECTIONS

Future efforts to reduce the global disease burden of obstetric complications requiring surgery will depend on interventions that have demonstrated equal effectiveness on small scales, and will implement those interventions on a universal scale.

Numbers of Skilled Birth Attendants

Significant progress has been seen with the provision of birth attendants; the next step is the universal provision of emergency obstetric providers who can perform safe cesarean delivery. These emergency obstetric providers will require additional training to acquire a more sophisticated skill set than that possessed by birth attendants. Societal and economic investments in successful outcomes will be critical, both in training and in retaining these providers. The effective retention of trained providers will require satisfactory facilities and resources to utilize their training. The provision of the resources for emergency obstetric care at local levels will dramatically improve worldwide maternal health in the coming decades.

Quality Care and Improvement Initiatives

Achieving the goal of universal provision of evidence-based obstetric care will take time and resources. Programs have examined established practice improvement techniques using educational outreach and morbidity and mortality reviews, as in the QUARITE (QUAlity of care, RIsk management and TEchnology in obstetrics) trial taking place in Senegal and Mali. The establishment of infrastructure to monitor outcomes will help improve care at local levels by focusing on unsatisfactory outcomes that can be improved in those areas (Dumont and others 2013; Pirkle and others 2013). Practice-based learning and morbidity and mortality reviews are established methods of improving care and maternal outcomes, and their application to nations working to establish or build up obstetric services will be significant (Choo and others 2013). Partnerships between programs in LMICs and HICs will help the former to develop the training infrastructure to cultivate and maintain an obstetric workforce (Klufio and others 2003).

Lessons from Ghana

Ghana has been a model for improvement in women's reproductive health. In 1989, a grant from the Carnegie Foundation established university-based training programs to help train obstetric providers; its goal was to maintain trained obstetricians in practice after they completed their training (Anderson and others 2014). Before this program, Ghana had significant difficulty retaining trained providers (Clinton, Anderson, and Kwawukume 2010); the retention rate of trained obstetric providers had been 10 percent. Since establishment of the program in 1989, over 95 percent of the trained obstetric providers have remained in country to practice (Anderson and others 2014).

With the exponential increase in obstetric providers in the country, the ability to train later generations of providers each year has increased; the country had 20 certified practicing obstetricians in 2000 and 85 in 2010.

With the increase in providers, some individuals have located to different periurban and more rural first-level hospitals, expanding the areas where safe emergency obstetric services are available. Although this program did not produce dedicated birth attendants, it produced certified obstetrical and gynecological providers who have the skills to manage a wide variety of women's health issues. Their wide variety of expertise encompasses contraception and obstetric care, including definitive delivery and management of obstetric complications. The influence of this program is difficult to assess because of the implementation of other programs to improve obstetric care. At one rural institution, however, the implementation of certified obstetrical and gynecological capacity reduced maternal mortality by 74 percent (Anderson and others 2014).

The establishment of this training program resulted from a concerted effort by the American College of Obstetrics and Gynecology and the Royal College of Obstetrics and Gynecology, in combination with the obstetrics and gynecology departments at The Johns Hopkins University and the University of Michigan (Anderson and others 2014). With the assistance of these institutions, Ghana was able to design the five-year program that has produced so many trained providers. The ongoing relationship between the university-based training programs in Ghana and the University of Michigan has caused the evolution of evidence-based obstetric training within the country. Practice-based learning and maternal mortality and morbidity reviews have guided improvements in obstetric training and management that have spread across the country as providers complete their training (Choo and others 2013). The provision of funding to establish this type of academic partnership, and the establishment of in-country training programs, will contribute significantly to the goal of providing universal access to emergency obstetric care services and cesarean delivery.

Future Goals of Global Operative Obstetrics

Future efforts to improve maternal mortality and morbidity will expand successful programs to areas where they have yet to be implemented, will scale up established programs to provide health care to a wider population, and will develop new methods to improve access to care and standards of care in LMICs. Self-reflection and evidence-based medicine will help identify programs that work and those that need to improve.

The numbers of skilled birth attendants, who constitute the front line in the ability to provide safe childbirth care, will continue to increase. Technological advances will help coordinate that front line with first-level hospitals that have essential emergency care capabilities, including cesarean delivery. Once cesarean delivery is available at the regional level, a wide variety of surgical interventions will be available to improve public health, using synergistic capabilities and therapies. These quantum units of referral and emergency care centers will become more widespread, making safe cesarean delivery a universally accessible reproductive right, available to women throughout all HICs and LMICs alike.

Regional and academic centers will assist in training and retaining the necessary workforces to provide care in these nations, and they will serve as referral centers for complicated cases beyond the first-level hospitals to second- and third-level hospitals where appropriate.

The common goal will be the prevention of unnecessary pregnancy-related morbidity and death through the provision of universal access to standard and emergency obstetric care that is safe and effective—with benefits to the mothers, their families, and their societies as a whole.

Consideration of Essential Obstetric Interventions to Improve Obstetric Outcomes

Surgical obstetric interventions—including operative vaginal delivery, cesarean delivery, and emergency obstetric care—are clearly effective at reducing morbidity and death. Sufficient evidence demonstrates that access to these services can improve the health of societies. As with any intervention, the costs must be weighed against the potential benefits. Whether these costs warrant investment is not easily answered with scientific study. We reviewed a number of studies that have evaluated a broad range of obstetric surgical interventions to improve the health of societies. These interventions appear universally cost-effective, albeit to different degrees, across different LMICs. We implore interested parties to consider the relatively small cost per individual of these interventions to save maternal and neonatal lives. We recommend consideration of the following goals to improve the health of reproductive-age women and their children worldwide.

Birth Attendants. Universal access to birth attendants who can help address obstetric emergencies that require emergent attention should be a goal. Training will ultimately include the management of postpartum hemorrhage, operative vaginal delivery, and facilitated emergency vaginal breech delivery. Most important, training will facilitate the identification of obstetric complications that require transfers to higher levels of care.

Hospital Units. Approximately 10 percent to 15 percent of deliveries need operative interventions that require access to a nearby hospital or center to provide these surgical services, including cesarean delivery. In the long term, transport to such centers within two hours for any woman in labor is desirable. In the short term, access to such centers within six hours would be a significant improvement.

These centers require the ability to perform safe cesarean delivery. An operating theater with anesthetic availability should be part of that center. Blood transfusion services could help improve maternal outcomes. These centers require staffing by individuals trained in cesarean delivery and management of obstetric emergencies, with the ability to transfer to higher levels of care, if needed.

Trained Obstetric Providers. Effectively trained obstetric providers could help train other providers, as well as the birth attendants present at time of delivery who may be in the best position to timely manage obstetric emergencies. Obstetric training partnerships, as in Ghana, can successfully train providers who can rapidly grow a nation's obstetric workforce to staff local centers for the management of obstetric emergencies and cesarean delivery. In the short term, nonphysician clinicians can participate in obstetric care to help quickly meet improvement goals. Involving these clinicians in all aspects of emergency obstetric care can help meet immediate health needs, depending on the population. Partnerships to train obstetric providers, along with financial support, will grow, as the obstetric workforce in Ghana has grown, thereby improving the worldwide supply of obstetric providers in local settings. These trainees can then help train other physician and nonphysician providers and provide ongoing supervision to help retention efforts. The training of these obstetric providers will affect all levels of obstetric care and improve overall reproductive health care in their individual nations.

Valuation of Maternal Health and Reproductive Rights

"When women thrive, all of society benefits, and succeeding generations are given a better start in life."

–Kofi Annan

Death or morbidity in childbirth is a preventable tragedy. As societies develop and improve maternal health, all levels of society will benefit. Future obstetric interventions will fully consider the value of these maternal lives and the societal costs of failing to provide these fundamental surgical services. Societal expectations will include the provision of obstetric care as a fundamental reproductive and human right. With this effective valuation of maternal health and consideration of obstetric and reproductive rights, maternal outcomes in particular and societal outcomes in general will improve.

NOTE

The World Bank classifies countries according to four income groupings. Income is measured using gross national income (GNI) per capita, in U.S. dollars, converted from local currency using the *World Bank Atlas* method. Classifications as of July 2014 are as follows:

- Low-income countries (LICs) = US$1,045 or less in 2013
- Middle-income countries (MICs) are subdivided:
  - Lower-middle-income = US$1,046 to US$4,125
  - Upper-middle-income (UMICs) = US$4,126 to US$12,745
- High-income countries (HICs) = US$12,746 or more

REFERENCES

ACOG (American Congress of Obstetricians and Gynecologists). 2009. "Optimal Goals for Anesthesia Care in Obstetrics." Committee Opinion No. 433, Committee on Obstetric Practice. *Obstetrics and Gynecology* 113: 1197–99.

———. 2013. "Medically Indicated Late-Preterm and Early-Term Deliveries." Committee Opinion No. 560, Committee on Obstetric Practice. *Obstetrics and Gynecology* 121 (4): 908–10.

Adam, T., S. S. Lim, S. Mehta, Z. A. Bhutta, H. Fogstad, and others. 2005. "Cost Effectiveness Analysis of Strategies for Maternal and Neonatal Health in Developing Countries." *British Medical Journal* 331 (7525): 1107.

Alkire, B. C., J. R. Vincent, C. T. Burns, I. S. Metzler, P. E. Farmer, and others. 2012. "Obstructed Labor and Caesarean Delivery: The Cost and Benefit of Surgical Intervention." *PloS One* 7 (4): e34595.

Anderson, F. W., I. Mutchnick, E. Y. Kwawukume, K. A. Danso, C. A. Klufio, and others. 2007. "Who Will Be There When Women Deliver? Assuring Retention of Obstetric Providers." *Obstetrics and Gynecology* 110 (5): 1012–16.

Anderson, F. W., S. A. Obed, E. L. Boothman, and H. Opare-Ado. 2014. "The Public Health Impact of Training Physicians to Become Obstetricians and Gynecologists in Ghana." *American Journal of Public Health* 104 (Suppl 1): S159–65.

Andreatta, P., J. Perosky, and T. R. Johnson. 2012. "Two-Provider Technique for Bimanual Uterine Compression to Control Postpartum Hemorrhage." *Journal of Midwifery and Women's Health* 57 (4): 371–75.

Baskett, T. F., A. A. Calder, and S. Arulkumaran. 2007. *Munro Kerr's Operative Obstetrics*. 11th ed. Philadelphia, PA: Saunders Elsevier.

Berghella, V., J. K. Baxter, and S. P. Chauhan. 2005. "Evidence-Based Surgery for Cesarean Delivery." *American Journal of Obstetrics and Gynecology* 193 (5): 1607–17.

Borghi, J., J. Fox-Rushby, E. Bergel, E. Abalos, G. Hutton, and others. 2002. "The Cost-Effectiveness of Routine versus Restrictive Episiotomy in Argentina." *American Journal of Obstetrics and Gynecology* 186 (2): 221–28.

Briand, V., A. Dumont, M. Abrahamowicz, M. Traore, L. Watier, and others. 2012. "Individual and Institutional Determinants of Caesarean Section in Referral Hospitals in Senegal and Mali: A Cross-Sectional Epidemiological Survey." *BMC Pregnancy and Childbirth* 12: 114. doi:10.1186/1471-2393-12-114.

Carvalho, N., A. S. Salehi, and S. J. Goldie. 2013. "National and Sub-national Analysis of the Health Benefits and Cost-Effectiveness of Strategies to Reduce Maternal Mortality in Afghanistan." *Health Policy and Planning* 28 (1): 62–74.

Choo, S., D. Papandria, S. D. Goldstein, H. Perry, A. A. Hesse, and others. 2013. "Quality Improvement Activities for Surgical Services at District Hospitals in Developing Countries and Perceived Barriers to Quality Improvement: Findings from Ghana and the Scientific Literature." *World Journal of Surgery* 37 (11): 2512–29.

Clinton, Y., F. W. Anderson, and E. Y. Kwawukume. 2010. "Factors Related to Retention of Postgraduate Trainees in Obstetrics-Gynecology at the Korle-Bu Teaching Hospital in Ghana." *Academic Medicine: Journal of the Association of American Medical Colleges* 85 (10): 1564–70.

CORONIS Collaborative Group, E. Abalos, V. Addo, P. Brocklehurst, M. E. Sheikh, and others. 2013. "Caesarean Section Surgical Techniques (CORONIS): A Fractional, Factorial, Unmasked, Randomised Controlled Trial." *The Lancet* 382 (9888): 234–48.

Dahlke, J. D., H. Mendez-Figueroa, D. J. Rouse, V. Berghella, J. K. Baxter, and others. 2013. "Evidence-Based Surgery for Cesarean Delivery: An Updated Systematic Review." *American Journal of Obstetrics and Gynecology* 209 (4): 294–306.

Darmstadt, G. L., A. C. Lee, S. Cousens, L. Sibley, Z. A. Bhutta, and others. 2009. "60 Million Non-facility Births: Who Can Deliver in Community Settings to Reduce Intrapartum-Related Deaths?" *International Journal of Gynaecology and Obstetrics* 107 (Suppl 1): S89–112.

Deboutte, D., T. O'Dempsey, G. Mann, and B. Faragher. 2013. "Cost-Effectiveness of Caesarean Sections in a Post-conflict Environment: A Case Study of Bunia, Democratic Republic of the Congo." *Disasters* 37 (Suppl 1): S105–20.

Dumont, A., P. Fournier, M. Abrahamowicz, M. Traore, S. Haddad, and others. 2013. "Quality of Care, Risk Management, and Technology in Obstetrics to Reduce Hospital-Based Maternal Mortality in Senegal and Mali (QUARITE): A Cluster-Randomised Trial." *The Lancet* 382 (9887): 146–57.

El-Hamamy, E., A. Wright, and C. B. Lynch. 2009. "The B-Lynch Suture Technique for Postpartum Haemorrhage: A Decade of Experience and Outcome." *Journal of the Institute of Obstetrics and Gynaecology* 29 (4): 278–83.

Erim, D. O., S. C. Resch, and S. J. Goldie. 2012. "Assessing Health and Economic Outcomes of Interventions to Reduce Pregnancy-Related Mortality in Nigeria." *BMC Public Health* 12 (786): 1–11.

Evans, C. L., D. Maine, L. McCloskey, F. G. Feeley, and H. Sanghvi. 2009. "Where There Is No Obstetrician: Increasing Capacity for Emergency Obstetric Care in Rural India: An Evaluation of a Pilot Program to Train General Doctors." *International Journal of Gynaecology and Obstetrics* 107 (3): 277–82.

Fiander, A. N., and T. Vanneste. 2012. "TransportMYpatient: An Initiative to Overcome the Barrier of Transport Costs for Patients Accessing Treatment for Obstetric Fistulae and Cleft Lip in Tanzania." *Tropical Doctor* 42 (2): 77–79.

FIGO (International Federation of Gynecology and Obstetrics). 2012. "Management of the Second Stage of Labor." Safe Motherhood and Newborn Health (SMNH) Committee. *International Journal of Gynaecology and Obstetrics* 119 (2): 111–16.

Gessessew, A., G. A. Barnabas, N. Prata, and K. Weidert. 2011. "Task Shifting and Sharing in Tigray, Ethiopia, to Achieve Comprehensive Emergency Obstetric Care." *International Journal of Gynaecology and Obstetrics* 113 (1): 28–31.

Gibbons, L., J. M. Belizan, J. A. Lauer, A. P. Betran, M. Merialdi, and others. 2012. "Inequities in the Use of Cesarean Section Deliveries in the World." *American Journal of Obstetrics and Gynecology* 206 (4): 331.e1, 331.19.

Goldie, S. J., S. Sweet, N. Carvalho, U. C. Natchu, and D. Hu. 2010. "Alternative Strategies to Reduce Maternal Mortality in India: A Cost-Effectiveness Analysis." *PLoS Medicine* 7 (4): e1000264.

Grimes, C. E., J. A. Henry, J. Maraka, N. C. Mkandawire, and C. Cotton. 2014. "Cost-Effectiveness of Surgery in Low- and Middle-Income Countries: A Systematic Review." *World Journal of Surgery* 38 (1): 252–63.

Hale, R. W., and E. H. Dennen. 2001. *Dennen's Forceps Deliveries*. 4th ed. Washington, DC: American College of Obstetricians and Gynecologists.

Hannah, M. E., W. J. Hannah, S. A. Hewson, E. D. Hodnett, S. Saigal, and others. 2000. "Planned Caesarean Section versus Planned Vaginal Birth for Breech Presentation at Term: A Randomised Multicentre Trial: Term Breech Trial Collaborative Group." *The Lancet* 356 (9239): 1375–83.

Hannah, M. E., W. J. Hannah, E. D. Hodnett, B. Chalmers, R. Kung, and others. 2002. "Outcomes at 3 Months after Planned Cesarean vs Planned Vaginal Delivery for Breech Presentation at Term: The International Randomized Term Breech Trial." *Journal of the American Medical Association* 287 (14): 1822–31.

Hofmeyr, G. J., R. A. Haws, S. Bergstrom, A. C. Lee, P. Okong, and others. 2009. "Obstetric Care in Low-Resource Settings: What, Who, and How to Overcome Challenges to Scale Up?" *International Journal of Gynaecology and Obstetrics* 107 (Suppl 1): S21, 44, 44–45.

Hogan, M. C., K. J. Foreman, M. Naghavi, S. Y. Ahn, M. Wang, and others. 2010. "Maternal Mortality for 181 Countries, 1980–2008: A Systematic Analysis of Progress towards Millennium Development Goal 5." *The Lancet* 375 (9726): 1609–23.

Hounton, S. H., D. Newlands, N. Meda, and V. De Brouwere. 2009. "A Cost-Effectiveness Study of Caesarean-Section Deliveries by Clinical Officers, General Practitioners and Obstetricians in Burkina Faso." *Human Resources for Health* 7 (34): 1–12.

Hu, D., S. M. Bertozzi, E. Gakidou, S. Sweet, and S. J. Goldie. 2007. "The Costs, Benefits, and Cost-Effectiveness of Interventions to Reduce Maternal Morbidity and Mortality in Mexico." *PloS One* 2 (8): e750.

Jha, P., O. Bangoura, and K. Ranson. 1998. "The Cost-Effectiveness of Forty Health Interventions in Guinea." *Health Policy and Planning* 13 (3): 249–62.

Klufio, C. A., E. Y. Kwawukume, K. A. Danso, J. J. Sciarra, and T. Johnson. 2003. "Ghana Postgraduate Obstetrics/Gynecology Collaborative Residency Training Program: Success Story and Model for Africa." *American Journal of Obstetrics and Gynecology* 189 (3): 692–96.

Koblinsky, M., Z. Matthews, J. Hussein, D. Mavalankar, M. K. Mridha, and others. 2006. "Going to Scale with Professional Skilled Care." *The Lancet* 368 (9544): 1377–86.

Lawn, J. E., M. Kinney, A. C. Lee, M. Chopra, F. Donnay, and others. 2009. "Reducing Intrapartum-Related Deaths and Disability: Can the Health System Deliver?" *International Journal of Gynaecology and Obstetrics* 107 (Suppl 1): S123–40, S140–42.

Le Ray, C., P. Serres, T. Schmitz, D. Cabrol, and F. Goffinet. 2007. "Manual Rotation in Occiput Posterior or Transverse Positions: Risk Factors and Consequences on the Cesarean Delivery Rate." *Obstetrics and Gynecology* 110 (4): 873–79.

Liang, J., L. Dai, J. Zhu, X. Li, W. Zeng, and others. 2011. "Preventable Maternal Mortality: Geographic/Rural-Urban Differences and Associated Factors from the Population-Based Maternal Mortality Surveillance System in China." *BMC Public Health* 11 (243): 1–9.

Lim, S. S., L. Dandona, J. A. Hoisington, S. L. James, M. C. Hogan, and others. 2010. "India's Janani Suraksha Yojana, a Conditional Cash Transfer Programme to Increase Births in Health Facilities: An Impact Evaluation." *The Lancet* 375 (9730): 2009–23.

Mavalankar, D., K. Callahan, V. Sriram, P. Singh, and A. Desai. 2009. "Where There Is No Anesthetist: Increasing Capacity for Emergency Obstetric Care in Rural India: An Evaluation of a Pilot Program to Train General Doctors." *International Journal of Gynaecology and Obstetrics* 107 (3): 283–88.

McAuliffe, E., M. Daly, F. Kamwendo, H. Masanja, M. Sidat, and others. 2013. "The Critical Role of Supervision in Retaining Staff in Obstetric Services: A Three Country Study." *PloS One* 8 (3): e58415.

McCord, C., G. Mbaruku, C. Pereira, C. Nzabuhakwa, and S. Bergstrom. 2009. "The Quality of Emergency Obstetrical Surgery by Assistant Medical Officers in Tanzanian District Hospitals." *Health Affairs* 28 (5): w876–85.

Mehtsun, W. T., K. Weatherspoon, L. McElrath, A. Chima, V. E. Torsu, and others. 2012. "Assessing the Surgical and Obstetrics-Gynecology Workload of Medical Officers: Findings from 10 District Hospitals in Ghana." *Archives of Surgery* 147 (6): 542–48.

Mullan, F., and S. Frehywot. 2007. "Non-physician Clinicians in 47 Sub-Saharan African Countries." *The Lancet* 370 (9605): 2158–63.

Murray, C. J., T. Vos, R. Lozano, M. Naghavi, A. D. Flaxman, and others. 2012. "Disability-Adjusted Life Years (DALYs) for 291 Diseases and Injuries in 21 Regions, 1990–2010: A Systematic Analysis for the Global Burden of Disease Study 2010." *The Lancet* 380 (9859): 2197–223.

Nyamtema, A. S., S. K. Pemba, G. Mbaruku, F. D. Rutasha, and J. van Roosmalen. 2011. "Tanzanian Lessons in Using Non-physician Clinicians to Scale Up Comprehensive Emergency Obstetric Care in Remote and Rural Areas." *Human Resources for Health* 9 (28): 1–8.

O'Grady, J. P., M. L. Gimovsky, L. A. Bayer-Zwirello, and K. Giordano. 2008. *Operative Obstetrics*. Baltimore: Williams & Wilkins.

Patton, G. C., C. Coffey, S. M. Sawyer, R. M. Viner, D. M. Haller, and others. 2009. "Global Patterns of Mortality in Young People: A Systematic Analysis of Population Health Data." *The Lancet* 374: 881–92.

Pereira, C., G. Mbaruku, C. Nzabuhakwa, S. Bergstrom, and C. McCord. 2011. "Emergency Obstetric Surgery by Non-physician Clinicians in Tanzania." *International Journal of Gynaecology and Obstetrics* 114 (2): 180–83.

Pirkle, C. M., A. Dumont, M. Traore, and M. V. Zunzunegui. 2013. "Effect of a Facility-Based Multifaceted Intervention on the Quality of Obstetrical Care: A Cluster Randomized Controlled Trial in Mali and Senegal." *BMC Pregnancy and Childbirth* 13 (24): 1–13.

Soltanifar, S., and R. Russell. 2012. "The National Institute for Health and Clinical Excellence (NICE) Guidelines for Caesarean Section, 2011 Update: Implications for the Anaesthetist." *International Journal of Obstetric Anesthesia* 21 (3): 264–72.

Souza, J. P., A. M. Gulmezoglu, J. Vogel, G. Carroli, P. Lumbiganon, and others. 2013. "Moving beyond Essential Interventions for Reduction of Maternal Mortality (The WHO Multicountry Survey on Maternal and Newborn Health): A Cross-Sectional Study." *The Lancet* 381 (9879): 1747–55.

Spangler, S. A. 2012. "Assessing Skilled Birth Attendants and Emergency Obstetric Care in Rural Tanzania: The Inadequacy of Using Global Standards and Indicators to Measure Local Realities." *Reproductive Health Matters* 20 (39): 133–41.

Stanton, C., D. Armbruster, R. Knight, I. Ariawan, S. Gbangbade, and others. 2009. "Use of Active Management of the Third Stage of Labour in Seven Developing Countries." *Bulletin of the World Health Organization* 87 (3): 207–15.

UN (United Nations). 2013. *The Millennium Development Goals Report 2013*. New York: United Nations.

Wall, L. L. 2006. "Obstetric Vesicovaginal Fistula as an International Public-Health Problem." *The Lancet* 368 (9542): 1201–19.

Wall, S. N., A. C. Lee, W. Carlo, R. Goldenberg, S. Niermeyer, and others. 2010. "Reducing Intrapartum-Related Neonatal Deaths in Low- and Middle-Income Countries: What Works?" *Seminars in Perinatology* 34 (6): 395–407.

WHO (World Health Organization). 2008. "Universal Access to Safe Blood Transfusion." WHO, Geneva.

———. 2012. *Trends in Maternal Mortality: 1990–2010—Estimates Developed by WHO, UNICEF, UNFPA, and the World Bank.* Geneva: WHO.

———. 2013. "Global Health Estimates for Deaths by Cause, Age, and Sex for Years 2000–2011." WHO, Geneva. http://www.who.int/healthinfo/global_health_estimates/en/.

Witter, S., D. K. Arhinful, A. Kusi, and S. Zakariah-Akoto. 2007. "The Experience of Ghana in Implementing a User Fee Exemption Policy to Provide Free Delivery Care." *Reproductive Health Matters* (30): 61–71.

Witter, S., and M. Diadhiou. 2008. "Key Informant Views of a Free Delivery and Caesarean Policy in Senegal." *African Journal of Reproductive Health* 12 (3): 93–111.

Witter, S., T. Dieng, D. Mbengue, I. Moreira, and V. De Brouwere. 2010. "The National Free Delivery and Caesarean Policy in Senegal: Evaluating Process and Outcomes." *Health Policy and Planning* 25 (5): 384–92.

Yamin, A. E., V. M. Boulanger, K. L. Falb, J. Shuma, and J. Leaning. 2013. "Costs of Inaction on Maternal Mortality: Qualitative Evidence of the Impacts of Maternal Deaths on Living Children in Tanzania." *PloS One* 8 (8): e71674.

You, F., K. Huo, R. Wang, D. Xu, J. Deng, and others. 2012. "Maternal Mortality in Henan Province, China: Changes between 1996 and 2009." *PLoS One* 7 (10): e47153.

Chapter 6

Obstetric Fistula

Mary Lake Polan, Ambereen Sleemi, Mulu Muleta Bedane,
Svjetlana Lozo, and Mark A. Morgan

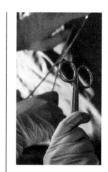

INTRODUCTION

Obstetric fistula is a serious and debilitating complication of childbirth affecting millions of women in
the developing world. A gynecologic fistula refers to
an abnormal communication between the urinary
tract or the gastrointestinal tract and the genital tract,
produced by obstetric causes, usually prolonged and
obstructed labor.

The earliest example of obstetric fistula was found in
2050 BC in Egypt, where an Eleventh Dynasty mummy,
Henhenit, appears to have had a vesico-vaginal fistula
(VVF). The relationship between obstructed labor and
fistula development was recognized and described by
the Persian physician, Avicenna, in 1037 AD (Zacharin
2000). Before the twentieth century, both urinary
and rectal fistulas were a common result of deliveries
throughout the world.

The unfortunate women who endure such
obstructed labors and resulting incontinence are often
young, undernourished, uneducated, and married
early (Wall and others 2004). They are usually from
rural, poor areas, often with an early first pregnancy.
However, a Tanzanian survey by the Women's Dignity
Project and Engender Health (2006) has shown that
fewer than half of the fistulas in that country resulted
from a first birth, suggesting that many fistulas occur
in subsequent pregnancies as well. The woman labors
at home, without the benefit of a trained birth

attendant and far from medical care capable of providing surgical intervention. In the absence of adequate communication or transportation services, labor
continues for several days; if delivery does not follow,
the baby dies and the mother often endures the long-
term complications of an obstetric fistula (IMPAC
2006). Figure 6.1 describes the clinical implications of
obstetric fistula.

The advent of anesthesia and safe, effective surgical
procedures for cesarean sections have made the occurrence of obstetric fistula a rare event in the developed
world; when they do occur, they are typically due to a
congenital anomaly, surgical complication, malignancy,
or radiation damage.

However, in the low- and middle-income regions
of Asia and Sub-Saharan Africa, the overwhelming cause of fistulas between the bladder and the
vagina (vesico-vaginal fistula, VVF) and between the
rectum and vagina (recto-vaginal fistula, RVF) is prolonged and obstructed labor. This is also the situation,
although less well documented, in Latin America and
the Caribbean. In prolonged labor, which frequently
results in delivery of a stillborn, the bladder and/or
rectal tissue is compressed between the pelvic bones
and the fetal head, cutting off blood flow and causing
ischemic pressure necrosis (Husain and others 2005).
In the hours or days following such a prolonged
labor, the fistula forms and leakage of urine, stool, or
both appears.

Corresponding author: Mary Lake Polan, MD, PhD, MPH, Columbia University, polan@stanford.edu

Figure 6.1 Worldwide Fistula Fund's Obstetric Fistula Pathway

Low socioeconomic status of women

Malnutrition   Limited social roles   Illiteracy and lack of formal education

Early marriage

Childbearing before pelvic growth is complete

Relatively large foetus or malpresentation → Cephalopelvic disproportion

Lack of emergency obstetric services

Obstructed labor

Harmful traditional practices

"Obstructed labor injury complex"

Fetal death
Fecal incontinence ← Fistula formation → Urinary incontinence
Complex urologic injury
Vaginal scarring and stenosis
Secondary infertility
Musculoskeletal injury
Foot drop
Chronic skin irritation
Offensive odor

Stigmatization
Isolation and loss of social support
Divorce or separation
Worsening poverty
Worsening malnutrition
Suffering, illness, and premature death

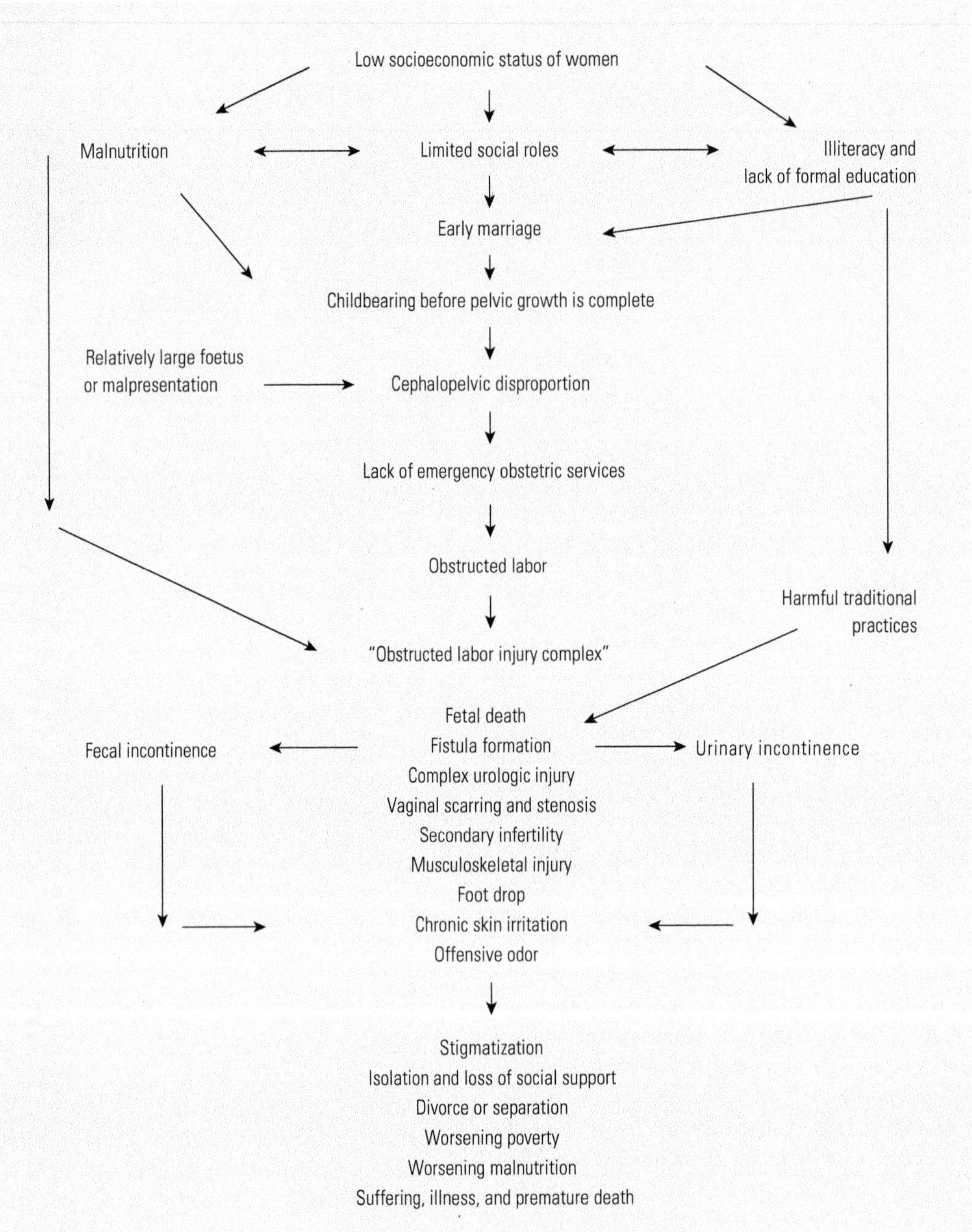

Source: "The Obstetric Fistula Pathway: Origins and Consequences" (Wall and others 2005), copyright Worldwide Fistula Fund. Used by permission.

Additional Complications

Additional major complications can include reproductive organ damage, such as uterine rupture, amenorrhea, and uterine scarring resulting in secondary infertility; dermatological conditions, resulting in excoriations and infections; neurological damage, resulting in weakness in the leg and foot drop (Arrowsmith, Hamlin, and Wall 1996); and renal damage, resulting in decreased kidney function. Women also report genital soreness; painful intercourse; constipation; and unpleasant odor, despite frequent washing and pad changes (Turan, Johnson, and Polan 2007).

As devastating as the physical outcomes of obstructed labor are, the emotional and social implications are equally tragic. A stillborn child is the most frequent result of such a delivery, and the woman may be abandoned by her husband and family to live as a social outcast without the ability to earn a living (Wall and others 2002). In many cultures, the woman either blames herself or is blamed by the community for the fistula, which is seen as a mark of punishment for some wrong-doing (Johnson and others 2010). She endures social isolation, economic deprivation, and depression (Turan, Johnson, and Polan 2007; Weston and others 2011).

Surgical Initiatives

Numerous surgical initiatives during the past 40 years have attempted to repair this obstetric damage and to rehabilitate these women. Among the first such initiatives was the establishment of the Addis Ababa Fistula Hospital in 1974 by Reginald and Catherine Hamlin. This hospital has cared for thousands of women and trained many surgeons in the techniques of fistula repair. Multiple surgical teams throughout Southeast Asia and Sub-Saharan Africa have reported successful closure of more than 80 percent of fistulas (Wall and others 2005).

However, successful closure of anatomic defects does not necessarily result in the absence of incontinence, which is an equally important criterion for a successful surgical outcome. The United Nations Population Fund (UNFPA) launched its Campaign to End Fistula in 2003. Awareness of the issues highlighted by this campaign, along with discussion of strategies to prevent and treat obstetric fistula, have resulted in increased interest in and knowledge of obstetric fistula, as well as the training of more fistula surgeons and additional reporting of the results of fistula surgeries (Husain and others 2005).

Chapter Goals

This chapter describes the present state of fistula surgery and the burden of death and disability, including the social and economic effects on women and their families. Although there is scant literature on both the cost of fistula surgeries and the quantitative impact on women's earnings in low- and middle-income countries (LMICs), we present what information is known. We describe current surgical procedures, as well as the skills and types of trained health workers necessary to perform these procedures. Clinical follow-up is complicated because most women return to their rural homes, making it difficult to contact them to assess long-term surgical outcomes. However, using the imperfect follow-up data available, we attempt to draw conclusions on the surgical outcomes and cost-effectiveness of the multiple surgical procedures used to repair obstetric fistula.

Finally, we offer comments on future directions and educational and surgical innovations to both prevent and treat the occurrence of obstructed labor and the resulting fistula.

BURDEN OF DISEASE DUE TO OBSTETRIC FISTULA

Beyond the actual physical and anatomic burdens of unrelenting urinary and fecal incontinence, the burden of disease encompasses many other physical and psychological consequences. Obstructed labor is a leading cause of maternal mortality and morbidity in LMICs. In these countries in the Middle East and North Africa, East Asia and Pacific, South Asia, and Sub-Saharan Africa, it is estimated that fistulas occur in one to three of every 1,000 deliveries (Wall 1998). An estimated 50,000 to 100,000 women worldwide develop obstetric fistula annually, 60,000 to 90,000 annually in Sub-Saharan Africa alone; more than 2 million women in Asia and Sub-Saharan Africa are living with an untreated obstetric fistula and the resulting urinary and/or rectal incontinence (UNFPA 2003).

Although obstetric fistulas in themselves rarely lead to immediate death, patients suffering with this disease have been referred to as the walking dead (Ahmed and others 2007). The women can also sustain long-term renal damage and eventually succumb to renal failure. In the words of expert fistula surgeon Dr. Kees Waaldijk of Katsina, Nigeria, "The poor woman survives the labor, and then the real problems begin" (personal communication). The physical disabilities include bladder and urethral damage, renal failure, and gynecologic and neurologic complications. The ischemic injury can lead to the damage and sloughing of bladder, urethral, rectal, and vaginal tissue, as well as tissue loss to the pelvic musculature and reproductive organs.

Reproductive Organ Damage

Vaginal, bladder, and rectal damage result from compression of the maternal tissue by the fetus during repeated uterine contractions that restrict blood flow, resulting in ischemia and tissue death. Vaginal strictures were noted in 17 percent of patients in one study (Raassen, Verdaasdonk, and Vierhout 2008), and a small Nigerian study reported vaginal scarring in up to 68 percent (Adetiloye and Dare 2000). Only 26.4 percent of women admitted for fistula repair surgery in this study were married, and these were the only women who reported regular sexual intercourse. Few studies to date have looked at sexual functioning in women who have such tissue damage or those who have had attempts such as vaginoplasty to repair the damage.

The widespread damage to the pelvis can lead to cervical and uterine scarring from both ischemia and subsequent infection, resulting in postpartum amenorrhea. Amenorrhea may also be caused by hypothalamic-pituitary dysfunction secondary to intra- or postpartum hemorrhage (Sheehan's syndrome). A study from Ethiopia reported amenorrhea in 63.1 percent of women with obstetric fistula (Arrowsmith, Hamlin, and Wall 1996). One high-volume expert surgeon in Nigeria reports amenorrhea rates of 12 percent to 15 percent if the fistula duration exceeds one year (Waaldijk 2008).

Although no long-term studies have examined the fecundity and birth rates of women with unrepaired fistulas, several papers have examined the reproductive performance in women who have had obstetric fistula surgery. No conclusive reproductive rates have been reported after repair; however, it is known from experiences at multiple sites that patients with repaired fistulas can conceive and subsequently deliver healthy infants, although the rates are presumed to be markedly diminished because of pelvic adhesions. The long-term social impact of infertility for young women in a poor country, where fistulas are endemic, includes the negative economic effect of not having offspring in societies in which government welfare programs are nonexistent and security in old age is directly linked to having children (Wall and others 2002).

Dermatological Conditions

Skin excoriations and ulcerations due to urinary ammonia deposition on the skin are a common complication of fistula. The chronic moisture and acidity of urine can cause the formation of uric acid crystals, and the skin may become infected. A review of 639 patients in East Africa found that almost 50 percent had evidence of excoriations of the labia and medial aspects of the thigh (Raassen, Verdaasdonk, and Vierhout 2008). Other studies report lower rates (20 percent) for similar skin damage (Gharoro and Agholor 2009). This skin condition is painful, and the constant contact with urine allows little relief from the discomfort. The ideal regimen for skin care remains to be determined; however, several salves and creams, including steroids and estrogens, have been proposed.

Neurological Disabilities

The extensive ischemic damage that leads to an obstetric fistula can also result in nerve damage. Foot drop may

be caused by compression injury or ischemic damage to the peroneal nerve, leading to the inability to dorsiflex the foot. The involvement of the L5 root is often noted, and severe pelvic ischemia can lead to postdelivery paraplegia that will recover (Hancock 2009a). Affected women tend to drag one or both legs, needing a stick or walls for support. Originally called "obstetric palsy," this lower extremity nerve damage has been associated with labor for hundreds of years. A prospective study of 947 Nigerian women with obstetric fistula found that approximately 27 percent had signs of peroneal nerve weakness, and approximately 38 percent had a history of relevant symptoms such as foot drop (Waaldijk and Elkins 1994).

In an East African study, unilateral or bilateral peroneal nerve damage was observed in 43.7 percent of first-time obstetrical fistula patients. On a scale of 0 (paralyzed) to 5 (normal strength), 7.1 percent had a score of ≤ 2 in one or both legs. When comparing routes of delivery, there was no statistically significant difference in peroneal paralysis frequency between women who eventually delivered vaginally (43.9 percent) and those who were delivered by cesarean section (43.5 percent) (Raassen, Verdaasdonk, and Vierhout 2008). Waaldijk and Elkins (1994) report that most women regain function after two years. Despite this, 13 percent remain with some residual nerve damage.

Renal Damage

The proximity of the ureters to the area where most obstetric fistulas occur puts them at risk of damage from obstructed labor. A radiology study in Nigeria looked at the incidence of renal and ureteric injury in 216 Nigerian women with obstetric fistula. Intravenous urographic studies found 48.6 percent of the patients evaluated had evidence of renal damage; 34 percent had evidence of unilateral or bilateral hydroureter with significant ureteral dilation. The most extreme damage was found in 4.6 percent of patients who had nonfunctioning bilateral kidneys (Lagundoye and others 1976). Long-term follow-up was not performed on these women.

Stillbirths

In cases in which the woman survives the obstruction, most of the pregnancies result in the birth of a stillborn fetus. After the traumatic ordeal of prolonged labor with associated pain and fear, this tragic outcome enhances the despair. In one study, 85 percent of women incurred fetal loss from deliveries resulting in fistula

(Raassen, Verdaasdonk, and Vierhout 2008). In another series of 899 fistula cases, fetal mortality was 92 percent; of the 75 infants who were live-born, an additional 14 died within the neonatal period (Wall and others 2004).

Mental and Emotional Issues

Obstetric fistula patients have been called the most dispossessed, outcast, powerless group of women in the world. For women in many cultures in which fistula is prevalent, the obstetrical problems that result in VVF are not only considered physiological events, they can also profoundly affect personal relationships with families and entire communities. Goh and others (2005) questioned women with obstetric fistula from Bangladesh and Ethiopia using a psychiatric disorders screening tool. They found that 97 percent of women screened positive for potential mental health dysfunctions. They estimated between 23 percent and 39 percent of women with fistula had major depression.

This finding is in contrast to controls surveyed during the same study in Bangladesh and Ethiopia, where only 32 percent screened positive with the same questionnaire, equating to a major depression prevalence of 8 percent to 13 percent (Goh and others 2005). A study of 70 women with fistula from Kenya reported depression in 72.9 percent, with 25.7 percent meeting the criteria for severe depression. Risk factors for depression appeared to be age older than 20 years, unemployment, lack of social support after fistula development, and living with fistula for more than three months (Weston and others 2011). Even though studies have suggested that some women commit suicide, no data have been published about the risk of murder or "honor killing." There is, however, anecdotal evidence of increased domestic violence.

One study found high levels of mental distress in women living with fistula resulting from long-time social isolation. The greatest distress and frustration appears to come from the inability to establish and maintain healthy social relationships. This same study reported that 14 percent of women attempted suicide while living with fistula (Nielsen and others 2009). Nearly all women suffered from isolation, shame, and stigma. Avoidance of public places due to the risk of being insulted or simply ignored was common. Patients have had community members hold their noses publicly and humiliate them with words of abuse.

In a survey of Eritrean fistula patients, self-imposed isolation during meal times and religious ceremonies was almost universal. A small cohort revealed that the smell of urine was the reason many felt unable to participate in routine activities that were a cornerstone of their social lives. The women would not go to church or be able to pray because of feeling "unclean" (ongoing survey of the quality of life of fistula patients, Eritrean MOH, personal communication, 2012).

From the social standpoint, the most traumatic aspects of VVF result from incontinence, distorted self-image, and childlessness. These factors can lead to divorce, depression, and exclusion from families and society. A review of 899 women with obstetrical fistula in central Nigeria found that approximately 50 percent of patients had been divorced as the result of fistula-related problems (Wall and others 2004). In a study from Bangladesh, 61.4 percent of women reported embarrassment in their social lives, 39.4 percent reported feeling constantly ill, and 33.3 percent reported difficulty in maintaining sexual relations. In addition, 67.4 percent reported the inability to perform their prayers, and 62 percent reported unhappiness in their married lives (Islam and Begum 1992).

Economic Burden

The obstetric fistula is an affliction of reproductive-age women who are primiparous in 31 percent to 66.7 percent of documented studies. The economic burden includes the patients' loss of the ability to work and perhaps the loss of a society's future workforce due to high rates of stillbirth and subsequent infertility (Tebeu and others 2012; Waaldijk 2008). In Nigeria, a study reported that women with fistula were 50 percent more economically impoverished by job loss. In many instances, such as in a study of women in Tanzania, they were farmers and were unable to perform hard manual labor after sustaining a fistula (Pope, Bangser, and Requejo 2011). All of the women had some form of occupation when the fistula developed; 92 percent were farmers, 5 percent were domestic workers, and one (3 percent) was a potter. While living with a fistula, 22 percent stopped working and remained at home. Following surgery, 75 percent of these women returned to their former occupations (Nielson and others 2009). Long hours of field labor may be difficult with injuries such as foot drop or pelvic trauma, and many women wait years before seeking help.

Research in Addis Ababa found that women affected by fistula and rejected by their husbands often had to depend on relatives for their food; some of the women were reduced to begging and lived on donations (Kelly 1995). A large number of women reported not having the means to afford soaps and clothes to stay clean and remain a productive part of working society. Most of the injured women were not able to continue employment and lost their ability to be contributing members of the household (Women's Dignity Project and Engender Health 2006). Families affected by fistula experience significant economic burdens that can be a factor in reducing families to poverty levels.

SURGICAL REPAIR AS EFFECTIVE TREATMENT

The surgical closure of an obstetric fistula is the most effective way to treat this condition. Evidence indicates that life improves dramatically for the majority of women after successful fistula repair. Women are able to return to their normal lives; interact freely with their families, friends, and communities; and play active roles in economic pursuits (Women's Dignity Project and Engender Health 2006).

A cross-sectional, prospective study sought to assess the quality of life of women with surgical repair of their VVF. Of the 150 women studied, only 20 percent felt satisfied with their general state of health and quality of life before the repair; this figure increased to 90 percent following successful repair. In the physical health domain, the mean quality of life score was significantly improved; this improvement was also seen in the mental health domain. In the social health domain, the mean score was 20.2 ± 2.7 before and 69.7 ± 2.3 after successful repair ($p < 0.001$). The conclusions suggest that successful repair of VVF is associated with significant improvement in the multidimensional quality of life among affected women (Umoiyoho and others 2011).

An Eritrea-based study of patients' postoperative experiences notes that patients described improvements in their conditions, but many continued to have problems with incontinence and sexual health (Turan, Johnson, and Polan 2007). The majority of women in another study were able to resume their household and farming responsibilities postrepair (Pope, Bangser, and Requejo 2011). By one year postrepair, 68 percent of the women who perceived themselves healed or mostly healed reported feeling "themselves again." Looking toward the future, most hoped that they could continue working in the fields, engage in small trade, bring their children to school, and "maybe build a home." Most treated women (99 percent) did not link their physical condition to economic problems. As one woman explained, "Life is tough, but that does not affect anything economically."

However, 60 percent of the women reported that being able to work again, principally in the fields doing agricultural labor, was the most important factor in their reintegration process. Those who experienced difficulties resuming their expected social roles after treatment mentioned that they were afraid that they would develop another fistula from physical exertion or sexual activity and/or experience a lot of pain and weakness while working (Pope, Bangser, and Requejo 2011).

Browning, Fentahun, and Goh (2007) report on the impact of surgical treatment on mental health. Closure of the fistula markedly improved mental health scores, despite the lack of any formal psychological or psychiatric input. Surgery improved quality of life and facilitated social reintegration to a level comparable to that experienced before fistula development for both women who were continent and those with residual incontinence. It was not surprising that no change was seen in those women still suffering from fistula (Nielson and others 2009).

COST-EFFECTIVENESS OF SURGERY

The cost-effectiveness of obstetric fistula repair is understudied, leading to a paucity of literature on this issue. Current research indicates that "[A]t the world's current capacity to repair fistula, it would take at least 400 years to clear the backlog of patients, provided that there are no more new cases" and that less than 1 percent of surgical needs for this disease is met (Browning and Patel 2004, 321). Prevention of the fistula is the ultimate goal. The mental, physical, and economic burden to women with obstetric fistula has been well documented. However, for those currently living with, and those who will develop, a fistula, the demonstrable benefit in economic terms must be studied further.

Estimated Costs

The UNFPA estimates that the average cost of fistula surgery is approximately US$400 (UNFPA 2012). According to the Fistula Foundation, costs vary depending on the sociopolitical situation in countries where wars, conflict, and political instability have significantly increased the cost of fistula repair; the estimated average cost of fistula surgery was US$1,000 (Church and Grant 2012). A Kenyan paper reports that the heavily subsidized cost of fistula repair is about 30,000 Kenya shillings (US$375) at the main referral center in Kenyatta National Hospital in Nairobi; the cost in a private hospital can be at least five times that amount. However, in Kenya, only 7.5 percent of women have access to treatment, and the majority cannot afford to travel to the fistula center.[1]

Disability-Adjusted Life Years

Research in Ethiopia finds that the average age of women at the time of fistula appearance is 22 years, and surgical treatment is initiated eight years later (Muleta 2009). The Fistula Foundation's Shaun Church and Kate Grant report that the life expectancy of women in Ethiopia is 58.8 years.[2] Therefore, it can be estimated that fistula surgery savings could be 28.8 disability-adjusted life years (DALYs). Using Ethiopia as an example and estimating the cost of fistula surgery to be US$1,163, dividing that cost by the estimated 28.8 DALYs results in a conservative savings of about US$40 per DALY averted with surgery. This suggests fistula surgery is a highly cost-effective intervention.

Prevention Strategies and Costs

The prevention of fistula requires significant social and economic attention. Investing in medical facilities that are able to provide adequate prenatal care as well as healthy deliveries needs to be a priority. Prenatal care, with early identification of at-risk pregnancies coupled with early referral to delivery centers capable of operative delivery, is essential for prevention. The cost of prenatal care varies by country, as well as by government-provided insurance plan, but all costs for these preventive strategies are significantly lower than the cost of later treatment.

Access to medical care in most of the countries where obstetric fistula is endemic is extremely limited. The economic cost of obtaining medical care at hospitals is beyond the budget of all but the wealthiest families. The costs of travel and accommodations for patients and family members are extremely high. Studies involving obstetrical costs in Benin, Ghana, and Pakistan concluded that vaginal delivery and cesarean sections in medical facilities were beyond the limits of what 75 percent of residents could afford (Lewis and de Bernis 2006).

Cesarean sections need to be more widely available as an option for the treatment of obstructed labor. A study in Kenya found that the cost of one cesarean section is about 3,000 Kenya shillings, or US$35 to US$40, in government hospitals; in rural Tanzania, the average cost is US$135.40 (Kowalewski, Mujinja, and Jahn 2002; Wanzala 2011). The patient population also needs to be educated about the natural progress of labor and to have the ability to be transported to the hospital when obstructed labor occurs.

One key factor in LMICs is the lack of transportation to medical facilities; women in prolonged labor often do not have adequate resources to reach medical facilities.

Once women develop fistulas, transportation to a medical facility is extremely difficult because of the cost of transportation and also because of the inadequate hygiene and leaking that women with fistulas exhibit. A 2001 UNFPA survey of fistula patients in Tanzania reports that some women travel as far as 500 kilometers to reach the nearest fistula center (UNFPA 2001). The survey notes that of 32 fistula centers, only 3 provide free surgery.

Education of the medical profession has been a challenge in LMICs, limiting access to doctors who are able to provide successful fistula repair. Sub-Saharan Africa, which accounts for about 24 percent of the global disease burden, has only 3 percent of the global health workforce (Anyangwe and Mtonga 2007). Insufficient numbers of medical schools, inadequate salaries, and poor working conditions account for this situation. There are an estimated 0.25 trained surgeons per 100,000 persons in East Africa, compared with 5.60 per 100,000 in the United States.

"Brain drain" exacerbates the shortage of trained medical personnel. Uganda's government spends an estimated US$21,000 and South Africa spends about US$59,000 to subsidize each medical doctor's training (Mills and others 2011). Sub-Saharan African countries spent about US$2 billion dollars to train doctors who later migrated to more stable, richer countries. Mills and others (2011) estimate that the United Kingdom benefited by about US$2.7 billion and the United States by about US$846 million from the immigration of Africa-trained physicians. Based on the impact of this loss of medical expertise, those countries that benefit the most from this drain of intellectual and surgical resources might consider investing in the source countries and strengthening their training systems.

PRESURGICAL PROCEDURES IN OBSTETRIC FISTULA REPAIR

Women with bladder fistulas can sometimes be treated conservatively if the injury is recent and the hole is small. Continuous bladder drainage with Foley catheters for four to six weeks has been reported to result in the spontaneous closure of small fistulas with fresh edges in 15 percent to 20 percent of cases (Waaldijk 1994). However, the majority of VVFs require surgical treatment.

General principles in obstetric fistula surgery include patient evaluation and preoperative care, maximum exposure of the repair site, adequate tissue mobilization, gentle tissue management, closure of the defect without tension, and meticulous postoperative care.

PATIENT SELECTION AND PREOPERATIVE CARE

A standard classification of obstetric fistula has not been agreed upon. However, urethral involvement, extent of scar, defect size, bladder capacity, and history of prior repair attempts are generally acknowledged as predictors of posttreatment continence (Nardos, Browning, and Chen 2009). The first attempt at fistula repair is likely to be the most successful; therefore, the woman should be provided the best available care and skill during the first surgery (Angioli and others 2003).

The timing of surgery after injury is controversial, but it should be delayed until the quality of the tissue needed for repair improves. This can take up to three months, although some surgeons advocate immediate repair and claim comparable results (Waaldijk 1994). Early repair might minimize the social neglect of the affected women; however, the evidence for this approach is limited. Physiotherapy and psychological counseling should begin preoperatively and should continue postoperatively. Malnutrition and anemia, ammonia dermatitis, and genital infections should be treated before surgery.

SURGICAL REPAIR

Repair Procedure

The surgical approach can be vaginal, abdominal, or combined, based on the location of the fistula and the preference and experience of the surgeon. The vaginal route seems to be associated with less blood loss and pain (Chigbu and others 2006). However, the evidence on the difference in operative complications and speed of recovery is limited. In some cases, the damage to the urethra and bladder is so severe that conventional repair methods are not successful. In specialized centers, these patients are sometimes offered urinary diversion in which the ureters are implanted in the lower bowel (Morgan and others 2009).

Maximizing the exposure of the defect is necessary to identify the location and size of the fistula, the extent of the tissue loss, the involved organs and tissues, and the amount of scar tissue in the vagina. The patient should be positioned in exaggerated lithotomy with a Trendelenburg tilt and the buttocks protruding on an adjustable operating table, if available. The use of bright and well-focused light over the field of surgery is essential.

An incision is made over the vaginal mucosa all around the fistula about 3 millimeters away from the junction of the bladder (rectum in RVF) and vaginal skin (epithelium). Lateral extension of the incision, at the 3:00 and 9:00 o'clock positions, is made bilaterally. These incisions over the vaginal mucosa should be just deep enough to cut only the vaginal mucosa. The bladder (rectum in RVF) should be mobilized adequately to avoid tension on the closure of the defect.

Bladder or rectal muscle should be approximated, avoiding the bladder or rectal mucosa. The closure of bladder fistulas can be in either a single or a double layer based on individual preference. Closure of rectal fistula is preferable in two layers, to avoid rectal mucosal interposition between the sutures. In patients who had had a diverting colostomy and repair of an RVF, a dye test must be done to confirm success of repair before planning for colostomy closure.

Postoperative Care

The main concern in VVF patients in the postoperative period is the maintenance of free and continuous bladder drainage. High fluid intake is widely advised; women should be encouraged to drink four to five liters a day (Hancock 2009b) and the color of the urine should be watched as the indicator of the adequacy of hydration. A blocked catheter signals an emergency. Transurethral drainage catheters are generally kept for an average of 14 days (up to 21 days following new urethral reconstruction) and should be removed without clamping. Some suggest that postoperative catheterization for 10 days may be sufficient for less complicated cases of VVF repair (Nardos, Browning, and Member 2008). Women are advised not to resume sexual contact for three months to give adequate time for the tissues to heal.

The most challenging situation in obstetric fistula management is post-VVF-repair incontinence. Although failure of fistula repair must be ruled out, incontinence is often due to stress incontinence or combined stress and urge incontinence (Murray and others 2002). Urodynamic studies of bladder and urethral function can be helpful, but the equipment is most often unavailable in settings where fistulas are frequently encountered.

POSTOPERATIVE TRAINING AND REINTEGRATION

For women who have lived with fistula for many years, reintegration into society involves redefinition of self and transition from being identified as filthy, dependent, and unworthy to being seen as clean, feminine, and active in family and community life. Thus, reintegration into family and community life is a major adjustment and goal after surgery. This need for reintegration requires that surgical programs dedicated to fistula repair consider and implement counseling for social integration and training in life skills to help these women return to gainful employment after repair.

Most women live an agrarian lifestyle, and returning to farming is important to them. One paper identifies the most important factor helping them feel normal again is the ability to return to farming after surgical repair (Pope, Bangser, and Requejo 2011). However, most women felt that they needed more time after surgery to fully recover their strength; the authors recommend having an alternate non-labor-intensive form of income for the first year after repair before most women return to their routine work. The full reintegration of a patient postrepair should also include her sexual and reproductive health needs (Mselle and others 2012). Preoperative and postoperative counseling for 47 Eritrean fistula patients was shown to increase their self-esteem (Johnson and others 2010).

After postsurgery counseling, women were significantly more likely to practice positive health behaviors, to use family planning, and to improve their nutritional intake. Following counseling, 91 percent of women expressed intentions to talk with family members and 77 percent intended to talk to other community members about fistula and fistula prevention, compared with 26 percent and 34 percent, respectively, before counseling. Counseling seems to have a marked impact on women's ability to resume their roles in their communities.

One Nigerian study calculated the cost of surgical treatment and rehabilitation to be US$2,300 per patient for a 10-month stay, and an additional US$340 for 12-month follow-up and reintegration (Mohammed 2007). To validate the long-term impact and sustainability of these programs, studies need to be performed in the community settings where patients settle after repair and after rehabilitation.

HEALTH SYSTEM CONSIDERATIONS

Obstetric fistula, a problem seen primarily in women from resource-poor countries, results from financial, cultural, political, and logistical obstacles. Although international efforts, such as the UNFPA's Campaign to End Fistula, have made some improvements in the number of fistulas treated, overall only a very small fraction of cases are ever repaired. The number of fistula treatment centers is especially low in countries that have the highest levels of maternal mortality

and fistulas. More than 50 percent of the reporting fistula treatment centers in the world provide surgery in fewer than 50 cases a year; only five centers report doing more than 500 a year (United Nations General Assembly 2012).

Models of Treatment

According to the World Health Organization (WHO), several models of treatment are currently in practice, but no convincing evidence is available with respect to which approach is superior. Many are supported by nongovernmental organizations and charitable donations; others are integrated into the country's reproductive health programs and are supported by the government, often with help from international organizations like the UNFPA.

The most famous standalone fistula center program is at Addis Ababa Fistula Hospital. The Women and Health Alliance International has integrated fistula repair centers into three university hospitals in Ethiopia, Somalia, and the Republic of the Sudan that are similar to centers in Eritrea (box 6.1), Niger, and Nigeria. Some centers are integrated into gynecology or urology departments in academic centers; others are satellite units that refer complicated cases to regional independent or national fistula centers.

Finally, there are "fistula camps" that are managed by national and international teams. International training centers are being selected and developed to serve as training sites for future fistula surgeons, using a *Global Competency-Based Fistula Surgery Training Manual* developed by the International Federation of Gynecology and Obstetrics (FIGO), the International Society of Obstetric Fistula Surgeons (ISOFS), and other international partners. The UNFPA funded development of the manual.

The WHO recommends that each country set up an obstetric fistula strategy committee as part of a national maternal-newborn health program. This program should include a needs assessment that is both facility and community based. It is important that the community understand the context in which fistulas develop so that cultural and logistical issues (for example, transportation) can be addressed. The program should include strategies for preventing fistula; for providing facilities for fistula repair and rehabilitation; and for training surgeons, nurses, and other health care personnel. The program should also include provisions for oversight and advocacy to ensure that the program continues to be funded and that the results are acceptable (Lewis and de Bernis 2006). Setting up this kind of model, however, is difficult in

Box 6.1

Case Study: Eritrean Women's Project 2000–13

Eritrea, a country of 5 million people, is located along the coast of the Red Sea and is bordered by Djibouti, Ethiopia, and the Republic of Sudan.

Eritrea's population is 20 percent urban and 80 percent rural; 55 percent of the people are farmers, and 30 percent are pastoralists who move across borders with their animals. There are nine main ethnic groups and religions, including Islam, Eastern Orthodoxy, and Catholicism.

The original goals of the Eritrean Women's Project, founded by Mary Lake Polan, MD, included repair of fistulas, training of Eritrean surgeons, implementation of interventions to educate women about the causes and treatment of fistulas, and establishment of the Fistulae Treatment Center for comprehensive care, education, and rehabilitation of women with fistulas.

Program Milestones:

- 2001–13: A small group of surgeons traveled to Eritrea two to three times a year for two weeks each time, scheduled by the Ministry of Health and UNFPA, to operate on women with fistulas. The trips were funded by the United Nations Population Fund (UNFPA) and private donations.
- 2005: The first class of medical students enrolled in Orotta School of Medicine in Asmara and was subsequently taught by the visiting surgeons.
- 2006: The project organized the perioperative counseling program.
- 2007: The community-based study of reproductive outcomes sponsored by the project showed that inclusion of the entire community in a fistula education program improved prenatal care.
- 2008: The Eritrean government established the National Fistula Center at Mendefera Referral Hospital.
- Two Eritrean fistula surgeons have been trained at the National Fistula Center since its opening in 2008 as part of the project.
- 2012: The first five residents in obstetrics and gynecology were trained in Eritrea.

- 2013: The 40-bed Fistula Waiting Home at Mendefera Referral Hospital opened.

Supportive Government Actions

The government of Eritrea and the Ministry of Health supported and amplified the project's goals for improving reproductive health by instituting a national campaign to promote the use of condoms, raising the legal age of marriage to 18, and prohibiting female genital mutilation. Most important, the Ministry of Health set a goal of ending fistula in Eritrea by 2013.

Outcomes

- More than 600 surgical procedures over 12 years were performed by the U.S. surgeons, with a continence rate of approximately 70 percent.
- More than 303 urinary and 49 recto-vaginal fistulas were repaired.
- More than 1,000 surgical procedures were performed by Eritrean and U.S. surgeons.
- Approximately 8 percent of patients required urinary diversion procedures because of irreparable fistulas; follow-up of one to nine years resulted in live births for five diversion patients and no perioperative mortality.
- Six articles on fistula issues were published in peer-reviewed journals.
- Three Eritrean residents' abstracts were accepted to attend the 2012 meeting of the International Federation of Gynecology and Obstetrics (FIGO) in Rome.
- Trained Eritrean surgeons now perform 80 percent of fistula repairs and treat more than 100 cases a year.
- The National Fistula Center now has dedicated and trained nursing staff.
- The 40-bed Fistula Waiting Home serving preoperative and postoperative patients and women with high-risk pregnancies in their third trimester was constructed on the grounds of the Mendefera Referral Hospital, with donations from Friends of UNFPA, and opened in April 2013.

box continues next page

Box 6.1 (continued)

Building a Sustainable Fistula Program: Lessons Learned

The considerable progress achieved in a relatively short time is the result of the widespread support and commitment of key organizations and partnerships, including the trained surgeons who treat patients and teach medical students and residents in obstetrics and gynecology, as well as the visiting physicians, nurses, physical therapists, and students from the United States who have donated their time and skills. The strong relationship with the Minister of

Health and staff members was an essential element, as was the support of the UNFPA and the Eritrean staff. The financial assistance of private donations to Friends of UNFPA in the United States supported the travel expenses of physicians, fellows, residents, and medical students. Moreover, the in-kind corporate donations of ultrasound equipment, sutures, retractors, catheters, and antibiotics allowed the surgeons to more effectively care for women with fistula.

Source: Data collected by Drs. Ambereen Sleemi and Mark Morgan.

many resource-poor countries, particularly in those with internal or external conflicts.

Health Workforce Requirements

The main obstacle in fistula care is the lack of trained medical personnel in surgery. The fistula surgeon must have basic surgical skills in abdominal, pelvic, and vaginal surgery. Training for this type of complex surgery is highly specialized and, until recently, was organized differently in different institutions. Recently, however, FIGO, ISOFS, and other partners developed a consensus-derived document that focuses on competency-based training in fistula surgery to three levels: standard, advanced, and expert (FIGO and Partners 2011).

Local gynecologists, urologists, general surgeons, and other professionals with basic surgical skills can be trained in fistula repair. Having a maximum number of trained local staff increases the number of locally managed fistula operations. A preferable strategy is to integrate fistula care and training into the services provided by local governmental institutions so that an adequate number of gynecology, urology, surgery, and other students with basic surgical skills are systematically trained to manage fistula cases. This approach is a sustainable way to dramatically increase the number of operations available in regions with the heaviest burden of fistula, and it offers a greater number of women the opportunity to return to normal and dignified lives. Good prenatal care, adequate transportation of patients in labor, and delivery facilities able to intervene with cesarean section for operative delivery would reduce the incidence of fistulas and, thereby, the specific need for fistula surgeons and specialized surgical care.

Good nursing care for patients with fistula is essential to the surgical outcome. Nurses often receive special training onsite; the training includes presurgery and postsurgery care, psychological support, and counseling and communication skills.

FUTURE DIRECTIONS

Centers providing obstetric fistula treatment are few, and patients must often undertake long and difficult journeys to access care. Many of these services operate outside the government health sector as part of campaigns involving surgeons who come for short visits.

A complete fistula treatment center includes surgical services (operating theaters, postoperative wards, and anesthetic services), investigation services (laboratory, radiology, and blood bank), and physiotherapy and social-reintegration services. The largest financial challenge of most fistula centers is the cost of consumables and salaries, renewal of equipment, and maintenance of the infrastructure. The less-than-optimal training and supervision of health workers and the very low wages for fistula surgeons have resulted in the uneven distribution of specialized health care providers. The long-term sustainability of such services depends on the strong commitment of health professionals, health management teams, governments, and local authorities (Donnay and Ramsey 2006).

Training facilities should be developed in districts with large numbers of untreated patients. The size of the health facility is determined by the magnitude of the problem in the area. Being part of a larger health institution provides access to and use of essential facilities, such as pharmacies, laboratories, laundries, sterilization services, and kitchens. Being part of a hospital offers other advantages as well, such as access to other aspects of health care, including prenatal health care services and emergency obstetric services.

A global consensus exists on the need for improved access to quality and sustainable fistula care and training services, as well as postoperative social-reintegration services. This goal can be attained by integrating fistula treatment and training into existing government health services (PMNCH 2006). Fistula centers do not need to be sophisticated, however, if they provide human resources with basic skills, facilities, and equipment to provide fistula-management services.

The UNFPA released a fistula map in 2013 to track fistula services internationally (http://www.globalfistulamap.org). It is hoped that these efforts will have a significant effect on the worldwide burden of obstetric fistula by combining prevention with treatment and rehabilitation services. Intensive advocacy for increased resource allocation to strengthen health systems to ensure prevention and treatment of obstetric fistula is equally important.

NOTES

The World Bank classifies countries according to four income groupings. Income is measured using gross national income (GNI) per capita, in U.S. dollars, converted from local currency using the *World Bank Atlas* method. Classifications as of July 2014 are as follows:

- Low-income countries (LICs) = US$1,045 or less in 2013
- Middle-income countries (MICs) are subdivided:
  - Lower-middle-income = US$1,046 to US$4,125
  - Upper-middle-income (UMICs) = US$4,126 to US$12,745
- High-income countries (HICs) = US$12,746 or more

1. Irin News. 2010. "Kenya Focus on Fistula," July. http://www.irinnews.org/Report/89886/KENYA-Focus-on-fistula.
2. Shaun Church and Kate Grant. 2012. "Fistula Foundation: Fistula Foundation Letter." February. http://www.givewell.org/files/DWDA%202009/Fistula%20Foundation/Fistula%20Foundation%20Letter%2002-09-12.pdf.

REFERENCES

Adetiloye, V. A., and F. O. Dare. 2000. "Obstetric Fistula: Evaluation with Ultrasonography." *Journal of Ultrasound Medicine* 19 (4): 243–49.

Ahmed, S., R. Genadry, C. Stanton, and A. B. Lalonde. 2007. "Dead Women Walking: Neglected Millions with Obstetric Fistula." *International Journal of Gynaecology and Obstetrics* 99 (Suppl 1): S1–3.

Angioli, R., M. Penalver, L. Muzii, L. Mendez, R. Mirhashemi, and others. 2003. "Guidelines of How to Manage Vesicovaginal Fistula." *Critical Reviews in Oncology and Hematology* 48 (3): 295–304.

Anyangwe, S. C., and C. Mtonga. 2007. "Inequities in the Global Health Workforce: The Greatest Impediment to Health in Sub-Saharan Africa." *International Journal of Environmental Research in Public Health* 4 (2): 93–100.

Arrowsmith, S., E. C. Hamlin, and L. L. Wall. 1996. "Obstetric Labor Injury Complex: Obstetric Fistula Formation and the Multifaceted Morbidity of Maternal Birth Trauma in the Developing World." *Obstetrical and Gynecological Survey* 51 (9): 568.

Browning, A., W. Fentahun, and J. Goh. 2007. "The Impact of Surgical Treatment on the Mental Health of Women with Obstetric Fistula." *BJOG* 114 (11): 1439–41.

Browning, A., and T. L. Patel. 2004. "FIGO Initiative for the Prevention and Treatment of Vaginal Fistula." *International Journal of Gynecology and Obstetrics* 86 (2): 317–22.

Chigbu, C. O., E. E. Nwogu-Ikojo, and H. E. Onah. 2006. "Juxta Cervical Vesicovaginal Fistulae: Outcome by Route of Repair." *Journal of Obstetrics and Gynaecology* 26 (8): 795–97.

Church, S., and K. Grant. 2012. "Fistula Foundation: Fistula Foundation Letter." February. http://www.givewell.org/files/DWDA%202009/Fistula%20Foundation/Fistula%20Foundation%20Letter%2002-09-12.pdf.

Donnay, F., and K. Ramsey. 2006. "Eliminating Obstetric Fistula: Progress in Partnerships." *International Journal of Gynaecology and Obstetrics* 94 (3): 256–61.

FIGO (International Federation of Gynecology and Obstetrics) and Partners. 2011. *Global Competency-Based Fistula Surgery Training Manual.* London: FIGO. http://www.figo.org/projects/fistula_initiative.

Gharoro, E. P., and K. N. Agholor. 2009. "Aspects of Psychosocial Problems of Patients with Vesico-Vaginal Fistula." *Journal of Obstetrics and Gynaecology* 29 (7): 644–47.

Goh, J. T. W., K. M. Sloane, H. G. Krause, A. Browning, and S. Akhter. 2005. "Mental Health Screening in Women with Genital Tract Fistulae." *British Journal of Obstetrics and Gynaecology* 112 (9): 1328–30.

Hancock, B. 2009a. "Obstetric Fistulae: Cause and Nature; The Obstetric Fistula Complex; Classification." In *Practical Obstetric Fistula Surgery*, edited by B. Hancock and A. Browning, 3–8. London: Royal Society of Medicine Ltd.

———. 2009b. "Post-operative Nursing Care of the Fistula Patient." In *Practical Obstetric Fistula Surgery*, edited by B. Hancock and A. Browning, 133–47. London: Royal Society of Medicine Ltd.

Husain, A., K. Johnson, C. A. Glowacki, J. Osias, C. R. Wheeless, and others. 2005. "Surgical Management of Complex Obstetric Fistula in Eritrea." *Journal of Women's Health* 14 (9): 839–44.

IMPAC (Integrated Management of Pregnancy and Childbirth). 2006. "Obstetric Fistula: Guiding Principles for Clinical Management of Programme Development." Department of Making Pregnancy Safer, World Health Organization, Geneva.

Islam, A. I., and A. Begum. 1992. "A Psycho-Social Study on Genito-Urinary Fistula." *Bangladesh Medical Research Council Bulletin* 18 (2): 82–94.

Johnson, K. A., J. M. Turan, L. Hailemariam, E. Mengsteab, D. Jena, and M. L. Polan. 2010. "The Role of Counseling for Obstetric Fistula Patients: Lessons Learned from Eritrea." *Patient Education and Counseling* 80 (2): 262–65.

Kelly J. 1995. "Ethiopia: An Epidemiological Study of Vesico-Vaginal Fistula in Addis Ababa." *World Health Statistics Quarterly* 48 (1): 15–17.

Kowalewski, M., P. Mujinja, and A. Jahn. 2002. "Can Mothers Afford Maternal Health Care Costs? User Costs of Maternity Services in Rural Tanzania." *African Journal of Reproductive Health* 6 (1): 65–73.

Lagundoye, S. B., D. Bell, G. Gill, and O. Ogunbode. 1976. "Urinary Tract Changes in Obstetric Vesico-Vaginal Fistulae: A Report of 216 Cases Studied by Intravenous Urography." *Clinical Radiology* 27 (4): 531–39.

Lewis, G., and L. de Bernis. 2006. *Obstetric Fistula: Guiding Principles for Clinical Management and Programme Development*. Geneva: World Health Organization.

Mills, E., S. Kanters, A. Hagopian, N. Bansback, J. Nachega, and others. 2011. "The Financial Cost of Doctors Emigrating from Sub-Saharan Africa: Human Capital Analysis." *British Medical Journal* 343: d7031.

Mohammed, R. H. 2007. "A Community Program for Women's Health and Development: Implications for the Long-Term Care of Women with Fistulas." *International Journal of Gynaecology and Obstetrics* 99: S137–42.

Morgan, M. A., M. L. Polan, H. H. Melecot, B. Debru, A. Sleemi, and others. 2009. "Experience with a Low-Pressure Colonic Pouch (Mainz II) Urinary Diversion for Irreparable Vesicovaginal Fistula and Bladder Extrophy in East Africa." *International Urogynecology Journal* 20 (10): 1163–68.

Murray, C., J. T. Goh, M. Fynes, and M. P. Carey. 2002. "Urinary and Faecal Incontinence Following Delayed Primary Repair of Obstetric Genital Fistula." *BJOG* 109 (7): 828–32.

Mselle, L. T., B. Evjen-Olsen, K. M. Moland, A. Mvungi, and T. W. Kohi. 2012. "Hoping for a Normal Life Again: Reintegration after Fistula Repair in Rural Tanzania." *Journal of Obstetetrics and Gynaecology* 34 (10): 927–38.

Muleta, Mulu. 2009. "Obstetric Fistula: Prevalence, Causes, Consequences and Associated Factors." University of Bergen.

Nardos, R., A. Browning, and C. C. Chen. 2009. "Risk Factors that Predict Failure after Vaginal Repair of Obstetric Vesico-Vaginal Fistulae." *American Journal of Obstetrics and Gynecology* 200 (5): 578.

Nardos, R., A. Browning, and B. Member. 2008. "Duration of Bladder Catheterization after Surgery for Obstetric Fistula." *International Journal of Gynaecology and Obstetrics* 103 (1): 30–32.

Nielsen, H. S., L. Lindberg, U. Nygaard, H. Aytenfisu, O. L. Johnston, and others. 2009. "A Community-Based Long-Term Follow Up of Women Undergoing Obstetric Fistula Repair in Rural Ethiopia." *British Journal of Obstetrics and Gynaecology* 116 (9): 1258–64.

PMNCH (Partnership for Maternal, Newborn, and Child Health). 2006. *Conceptual Institutional Framework*. Geneva: Partnership for Maternal, Newborn, and Child Health.

Pope, R., M. Bangser, and J. H. Requejo. 2011. "Restoring Dignity: Social Reintegration after Obstetric Fistula Repair in Ukerewe, Tanzania." *Global Public Health: International Journal for Research, Policy and Practice* 6 (8): 859–73.

Raassen, T. J., E. G. Verdaasdonk, and M. E. Vierhout. 2008. "Prospective Results after First-Time Surgery for Obstetric Fistulas in East African Women." *International Urogynecology Journal* 19 (1): 73–79.

Tebeu, P. M., J. N. Fomulu, S. Khaddaj, L. de Bernis, T. Delvaux, and C. H. Rochat. 2012. "Risk Factors for Obstetric Fistula: A Clinical Review." *International Urogynecology Journal* 23 (4): 387–94.

Turan, J. M., K. Johnson, and M. L. Polan. 2007. "Experiences of Women Seeking Medical Care for Obstetric Fistula in Eritrea: Implications for Prevention, Treatment and Social Reintegration." *Global Public Health* 2 (1): 64–77.

Umoiyoho, A. J., E. C. Inyang-Etoh, G. M. Abah, A. M. Abasiattaim, and O. E. Akaiso. 2011. "Quality of Life Following Successful Repair of Vesicovaginal Fistula in Nigeria." *Rural Remote Health* 11 (3): 1734.

UNFPA (United Nations Population Fund). 2001. "Tanzania: Campaign to End Fistula; Tanzania Fistula Survey 2001." New York. http://www.endfistula.org/webdav /site/endfistula/shared/documents/needs%20assessments /Tanzania%20OF%20Needs%20Assessment.pdf.

———. 2003. *Second Meeting of the Working Group for the Prevention and Treatment of Obstetric Fistula. Addis Ababa, 30 October–1 November, 2002*. New York: UNFPA.

———. 2012. "When Childbirth Harms: Obstetric Fistula." New York. https://www.unfpa.org/webdav/site/global/shared /factsheets/srh/EN-SRH%20fact%20sheet-Fistula.pdf.

United Nations General Assembly. 2012. "Supporting Efforts to End Obstetric Fistula: Report of the Secretary-General." New York.

Waaldijk, K. 1994. "The Immediate Surgical Management of Fresh Obstetric Fistulas with Catheter and/or Early Closure." *International Journal of Gynaecology and Obstetrics* 45 (1): 11–16.

———. 2008. *Obstetric Fistula Surgery, Art and Science: Basics*. Katsina, Nigeria: Babbar Ruga Fistula Teaching Hospital.

Waaldijk, K., and T. E. Elkins. 1994. "The Obstetric Fistula and Peroneal Nerve Injury: An Analysis of 947 Consecutive Patients." *International Urogynecology Journal* 5 (1): 12–14.

Wall, L. L. 1998. "Dead Mothers and Injured Wives: The Social Context of Maternal Morbidity and Mortality among the Hausa of Northern Nigeria." *Studies in Family Planning* 19 (4): 341–59.

Wall, L. L., S. D. Arrowsmith, N. D. Briggs, and A. Lassey. 2002. "Urinary Incontinence in the Developing World: The Obstetric Fistula." In *Incontinence*, second edition, edited by P. Abrams, L. Cardozo, S. Khoury, and A. Wein, 893–935. Plymouth, UK: Health Publications, Ltd.

Wall, L. L., S. D. Arrowsmith, N. D. Briggs, A. Browning, and A. Lassey. 2005. "The Obstetric Vesicovaginal Fistula in the Developing World." *Obstetric and Gynecologic Survey* 60 (7): S3–51.

Wall, L. L., J. A. Karshim, C. Kirschner, and S. D. Arrowsmith. 2004. "The Obstetric Vesicovaginal Fistula: Characteristics of 899 Patients from Jos, Nigeria." *American Journal of Obstetrics and Gynecology* 190 (4): 1011–19.

Wanzala, Ouma. 2011. "Thousands of Women Are Suffering in Silence." *All Africa News,* July 26. http://allafrica.com/stories/201107270191.html.

Weston, K., S. Mutiso, J. W. Mwangi, Z. Qureshi, J. Beard, and P. Venkat. 2011. "Depression among Women with Obstetric Fistula in Kenya." *International Journal of Gynaecology and Obstetrics* 115 (1): 31–33.

Women's Dignity Project and Engender Health. 2006. *Risk and Resilience: Obstetrical Fistula in Tanzania.* Dar es Salaam, Tanzania: Women's Dignity Project; New York: Engender Health.

Zacharin, R. F. 2000. "A History of Obstetric Vesico-Vaginal Fistula." *Australian and New Zealand Journal of Surgery* 70: 851.

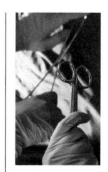

Chapter 7

Surgery for Family Planning, Abortion, and Postabortion Care

Joseph B. Babigumira, Michael Vlassoff,
Asa Ahimbisibwe, and Andy Stergachis

INTRODUCTION

This chapter discusses two related but conceptually distinct health concerns in low- and middle-income countries (LMICs): (a) voluntary family planning, and (b) abortion, including postabortion care. In the first section, on family planning, the health condition of interest is unmet need: the percentage of women who would like to either stop or delay childbearing but who are not using any contraceptive method to prevent pregnancy. The unmet need for family planning (to either limit family size or determine the intervals between children) results in unintended and unwanted pregnancies, which in turn lead to a broad range of maternal and child conditions that increase morbidity and mortality. Surgical procedures for family planning can help reduce this unmet need, particularly the need to limit childbirth.

The second section concerns surgery for induced abortion (as opposed to spontaneous abortion, or miscarriage) and the surgical management of the complications of induced, mostly unsafe, abortion.[1] Unsafe abortion is defined as abortion performed outside of health facilities (or any other place legally recognized for the procedure) or by an unskilled person (WHO 1992). The demand for abortion is high in many LMICs, and the illegality of the procedure in most of these countries increases the likelihood of postabortion

complications from clandestine, unsafe procedures (Grimes and others 2006; Shah and Ahman 2009; Singh and others 2006; Singh 2010). Therefore, postabortion care is a significant health issue in LMICs. Timely, safe surgical interventions can reduce the morbidity and mortality associated with unsafe abortions.

The same surgical procedures used for abortion are also used to manage incomplete abortion, which is one of the most common postabortion complications and is often accompanied by other complications such as bleeding, sepsis, and genital injury. The surgical procedures used to manage such complications include laparotomy for sepsis and uterine injury and a wide range of minor procedures to repair injuries to the proximal birth canal.

Both sections discuss the burden of reproductive health conditions, including morbidity, mortality, and other effects. We discuss surgical procedures (their performance, inputs, and implementation) and the health workforce implications of scaling up those procedures in LMICs. We also explore evidence on the procedures' effectiveness in reducing morbidity and mortality and improving quality of life as well as evidence on their cost-effectiveness. Finally, we outline future directions—including implementation challenges and considerations for increasing access to these surgical interventions—and conclude by summarizing the findings and recommendations.

Corresponding author: Joseph B. Babigumira, PhD, MS, MBChB, University of Washington, babijo@uw.edu

SURGERY FOR FAMILY PLANNING

Importance of Family Planning

Family planning is a pillar of reproductive and overall health in several ways:

- Reducing maternal mortality by reducing the number of times women are pregnant, including high-risk pregnancies associated with very young or older women (Ahmed and others 2012)
- Preventing high parity (among the potential factors leading to anemia in pregnancy)[2]
- Lengthening the intervals between pregnancies, which also improves perinatal outcomes and reduces child mortality (Cleland and others 2012)
- Decreasing the number of pregnancies that would have ended in induced, mostly unsafe, abortions in LMICs.

Recent data illustrate how high the stakes can be, although some trends have improved during the past two decades. The Global Burden of Disease (GBD) Study 2010 estimated that almost 254,700 deaths (4 per 100,000) globally were attributable to maternal conditions in 2010, a 29 percent decrease from 1990, when there were 358,600 maternal deaths (7 per 100,000) (Lozano and others 2013). Almost 1.8 million years lived with disability (YLDs) globally were attributable to maternal conditions in 2010, a 28 percent increase from 1990, when there were nearly 1.4 million YLDs (Vos and others 2013).[3]

Family planning is one of the most effective, and cost-effective, interventions against maternal mortality and disability. Increasing contraceptive coverage was primarily responsible for a substantial reduction in global fertility rates (from 3.63 births per woman in 1990 to 2.83 in 2005), also averting 1.2 million deaths (Stover and Ross 2010). Despite a 42 percent increase in the number of women of reproductive age (15–49 years old) between 1990 and 2008, the number of births per year remained constant, and the mortality risk per birth decreased (Ross and Blanc 2012). Meeting the need for family planning globally would further reduce maternal mortality by an estimated 29 percent, a reduction of more than 100,000 deaths annually (Ahmed and others 2012).

Moreover, family planning has both household and macroeconomic benefits. At the household level, it reduces fertility—an important attribute given that women in LMICs increasingly desire better-planned and better-spaced families (Darroch 2013; Darroch and Singh 2013). Family planning not only improves birth spacing but also increases women's earnings, assets, and body mass indexes, and improves children's schooling and body mass indexes (Canning and Schultz 2012). At the macroeconomic level, it reduces youth dependency and increases labor force participation by women, thereby enhancing economic growth (Canning and Schultz 2012). Increasing access to family planning will slow population growth, conveying environmental benefits such as substantial reductions in global carbon dioxide emissions (O'Neill and others 2012).

Conversely, when LMICs lack affordable, accessible, acceptable, and sustainable family planning methods, tangible economic development becomes more difficult: without low fertility, countries cannot attain the well-documented "demographic dividend" that has benefited several formerly low-income countries (Bloom, Canning, and Sevilla 2003).[4]

Family Planning Methods

Family planning comprises both traditional and modern methods of contraception. Traditional methods, including withdrawal and fertility awareness, have low efficacy; up to 24 percent of women who use them will have unintended pregnancies within one year (Trussell 2011a). Modern methods—including sterilization, intrauterine devices (IUDs), injections, implants, pills, and mechanical methods such as condoms—have higher effectiveness, resulting in lower rates of unintended pregnancies (Trussell 2011a).

Sterilization is the most common method of permanent family planning; most other methods are temporary. Permanent methods are indicated for couples who consider their families to be complete and would like to stop childbirth (limit the number of children). Temporary methods are indicated for couples who would like to delay childbirth to space children further apart or for other reasons.

Contraception can also be divided into surgical methods, methods that employ minor surgery (for insertion and removal), and nonsurgical methods (table 7.1). Methods involving surgery or minor surgery are generally more effective than the nonsurgical methods. Surgery is employed primarily for sterilization. The most common male sterilization procedure is vasectomy, and the most common female sterilization procedure is tubal ligation.

Vasectomy and tubal ligation are among the most effective of the modern contraceptive methods, having first-year failure rates of 0.15 percent and 0.5 percent, respectively (Trussell 2011b). Although some nonsurgical forms of female sterilization exist, they are either not available or not practicable for LMICs in the foreseeable future.[5] Therefore, this chapter focuses on tubal ligation and vasectomy.

Table 7.1 Primary Contraceptive Methods by Degree of Surgical Involvement

Surgery	Minor surgery	Nonsurgical
Female sterilization: tubal ligation	Intrauterine device (IUD) • Copper IUD • Hormonal IUD (for example, Mirena)	Fertility awareness • Standard days method[a] • Symptothermal[b] • Ovulation[c]
Male sterilization: vasectomy	Subdermal implant (for example, Implanon, Jadelle)	Barrier • Spermicide • Sponge • Male condom • Female condom • Diaphragm Hormonal • Injection (for example, Depo-Provera) • Birth control pill • Vaginal ring (for example, NuvaRing) • Transdermal patch (for example, Ortho Evra) Other • Lactational amenorrhea[d] • Withdrawal

a. In the "standard days" method, a calendar (using colored beads, for example) is used to track the menstrual cycle as an aid to abstinence from unprotected vaginal intercourse during peak fertility periods.
b. The symptothermal method usually combines a number of fertility awareness methods, including observation of primary fertility signs (such as basal body temperature and cervical mucus) and the calendar-based methods.
c. The ovulation method identifies patterns of relative fertility and infertility during the menstrual cycle based on vulvar sensation and the appearance of vaginal discharge.
d. Lactational amenorrhea is the temporary postnatal infertility that occurs when women are actively breastfeeding.

Contraceptive Prevalence and Unmet Need

Contraceptive Prevalence. Globally, total contraceptive prevalence is 63 percent, defined as the percentage of women of reproductive age who report that they or their partners use at least one traditional or modern contraceptive method. Countries vary widely in this estimate by development status: contraceptive prevalence is 72 percent in developed countries and 54 percent in developing countries (excluding China). In Africa, it is even lower, at 31 percent; some countries, such as Chad, Mali, Sierra Leone, and Republic of South Sudan, have a contraceptive prevalence of less than 10 percent (Alkema and others 2013).

In LMICs, more than 25 percent of almost 820 million sexually active women of reproductive age use low-efficacy traditional methods or no method at all. This percentage rises to 38 percent in Sub-Saharan Africa, South and Central Asia, and Southeast Asia. Among women in LMICs who use modern contraceptive methods, a substantial proportion report that they or their partners use male

or female sterilization: 10 percent in Sub-Saharan Africa, 64 percent in South and Central Asia, and 13 percent in Southeast Asia (Darroch, Sedgh, and Ball 2011; Singh and Darroch 2012).

Many factors, besides inadequate knowledge and poor-quality family planning services that are difficult to access, contribute to non-use of contraception:

- Ambivalence about pregnancy (Frost, Singh, and Finer 2007)
- Underestimation of the risk of pregnancy at the time of sexual intercourse (Nettleman and others 2007)
- Historical, cultural, and religious beliefs (Schuler, Choque, and Rance 1994; Thorburn and Bogart 2005; Wickstrom and Jacobstein 2011)
- Low levels of education (Ali and Okud 2013; Frost, Singh, and Finer 2007; Muyindike and others 2012; Tawiah 1997)
- Low income or poverty (Asiimwe, Ndugga, and Mushomi 2013; Muyindike and others 2012)

Other variables affecting contraceptive use or non-use include the number of children already born (Muyindike and others 2012), age (Muyindike and others 2012), and race (Frost, Singh, and Finer 2007). In LMICs overall, however, it is the most disadvantaged members of society who use contraceptives less often and have a higher unmet need for them.

Unmet Need for Contraception. Globally, at least 150 million women ages 15–49 years in a marriage or union have an unmet need for contraception, meaning that they want to either stop or delay childbearing but are using no contraceptive method to prevent pregnancy. This corresponds to 11–14 percent of these partnered women, varying widely by income status. In high-income countries (HICs), the unmet need is 9 percent and in developing countries, 13 percent (16 percent if China is excluded). In Africa, the unmet need is 23 percent, exceeding 35 percent in some countries, including Kenya, Rwanda, and Togo (Alkema and others 2013).

Among all women of childbearing age in developing countries who want to avoid pregnancy, more than 200 million, or 26 percent, have an unmet need for modern contraceptive methods. This unmet need varies widely by region: it is much higher in Africa (53 percent; 60 percent in Sub-Saharan Africa) than in Latin America and the Caribbean (22 percent) and Asia (21 percent) (Darroch and Singh 2013).

Among all women of reproductive age who want to either stop or delay childbearing but use no contraception, the proportion of those who want to have no (or no more) children is a crude indicator of potential demand for permanent contraception, that is, sterilization. This proportion varies substantially by geography: it is 32 percent in Sub-Saharan Africa, 41 percent in North Africa, 50 percent in Central America, 57 percent in the Caribbean, 63 percent in Asia (excluding China), and 64 percent in Southeast Asia (Clifton and Kaneda 2013). Despite substantial variation, many women would like to avoid all (or further) childbirth and could benefit from expanded access to sterilization methods, which are predominantly surgical.

Trends in Prevalence and Unmet Need. During the period 1990–2010, global contraceptive prevalence increased by 8 percentage points, from 55 percent to 63 percent. During the same period, unmet need for contraception decreased by 3 percentage points, from 15 percent to 12 percent (Alkema and others 2013).

However, prevalence has plateaued since 2000, especially in the use of modern contraceptives (Singh and Darroch 2012): Among all women of reproductive age in LMICs, 57 percent used modern contraceptives in 1990, 55 percent in 2000, and 55 percent in 2009. Among women in the poorest countries, use of modern contraception increased marginally, from 39 percent in 2008 to 40 percent in 2012.

Meanwhile, the unmet need for modern contraceptive methods in developing countries decreased from 29 percent in 2003 to 26 percent in 2012 (Darroch and Singh 2013). Although the unmet need decreased during this period in all LMICs, it remained far higher in Africa (despite a reduction from 60 percent to 53 percent), particularly in Sub-Saharan Africa, where it decreased from 68 percent to 60 percent (Darroch and Singh 2013).

Moreover, modern contraceptive users in developing countries shifted away from surgical contraception (sterilization) to other forms. The proportion using sterilization declined, on average, from 47 percent to 38 percent. In Africa overall, where sterilization use was already extremely low, it declined from 9 percent to 8 percent of modern contraceptive use, and in Sub-Saharan Africa, from 12 percent to 10 percent (Darroch and Singh 2013). This decline is, however, relative: sterilization use is increasing in absolute terms, but use of other modern methods is increasing at an even faster rate.

In addition to unwanted pregnancies, an unmet need for accessible, modern contraception has a variety of other consequences:

- Poorly timed and closely spaced pregnancies increase child mortality.
- Maternal deaths during childbirth also increase child mortality.
- Unwanted pregnancies lead to increased pregnancy complications, abortions (including unsafe, illegal abortions), childhood illnesses, and the overall disease burden.
- Excess fertility has negative economic and social results.

Surgical Contraception

Advantages of Sterilization. Sterilization is highly effective and offers permanent protection from unwanted pregnancy with none of the potential side effects of temporary contraceptive methods. Sterilization, whether of males or of females, eliminates the need for continuous involvement in family planning activities. It also spares couples and individuals some of the common worries associated with temporary methods, including partner compliance, domestic violence (arising from disagreements between partners about fertility goals), inconvenience, side effects, supply needs, and the consequences of forgetfulness (WHO 1999).

Convenience and the longer duration of effective action are often the overriding factors in choosing contraceptives, and sterilization provides both of these advantages (Steiner and others 2006). These positive factors may be even more attractive to couples in the lowest-income countries, where supplies may be irregular and health facilities may be substandard or far away from their homes. However, surgical contraception and other nonbarrier methods also have an important limitation: they do not protect against human immunodeficiency virus (HIV) and other sexually transmitted infections.

Barriers to Access. LMIC populations face a variety of demand- and supply-side barriers to access to surgical methods of family planning. Among the most important are individual attitudes and motivations: Some women want to have many children as a defense against high child mortality or as a source of future farm labor. Interpersonal factors may play a role—for example, women often reject long-acting or permanent surgical contraceptive methods in deference to their spouses' (or the community's) desire for fertility. Cultural and religious norms also impede access to surgical contraception. Some cultures value high fertility, and some religions prohibit any form of contraception.

In addition, lack of information leads to misunderstanding, misconceptions, and myths about tubal ligation and vasectomy. Generally, information on surgical contraception is limited, particularly among unmarried individuals. Myths about surgical methods of contraception are also common. For instance, in Uganda, some men equate vasectomy to castration or loss of manhood, and some women associate tubal ligation with laziness, disinterest in sex, loss of menstrual regularity, and weight gain (Kasedde 2000).

Other barriers include fear of surgery, poverty and other economic barriers, geographic impediments such as living in remote rural areas, and poor health services and facilities (Gaym 2012; Kasedde 2000). Studies also suggest that providers often have insufficient knowledge or motivation to provide surgical contraception (Gaym 2012).

Surgical Procedures. Surgical procedures for family planning include tubal ligation for female sterilization and vasectomy for male sterilization. Before either are performed, potential recipients should be carefully selected and counseled (ACOG 1996; Pollack and Soderstrom 1994). As part of the comprehensive consent process, clients should be informed about sterilization options (male or female sterilization) as well as other contraceptive methods. The reasons for choosing sterilization should be clear, and potential recipients should understand that the procedures are meant to be permanent methods of family planning, to be chosen only if they are certain they do not want more children. Clients should also receive information on the potential for reversal and chances of success. The most common reasons for sterilization regret—such as young age or marital instability—should be assessed and addressed before surgery.

The details of surgery, including the risks of anesthesia (particularly for tubal ligation), should be clearly communicated and informed consent obtained. Prospective tubal ligation recipients should understand the chance of procedure failure and the risk of ectopic pregnancy (estimated at 7.3 per 1,000 procedures [Peterson and others 1997]), which is quadruple the risk for women using oral contraceptives and triple the risk for women using barrier methods (Holt and others 1991). Women should be prepared for potential postsurgical physiological changes such as menstrual disorders, which may increase the chance of postprocedure hospitalization (Shy and others 1992). Potential recipients should also know that sterilization does not protect against sexually transmitted infections, including HIV and acquired immune deficiency syndrome (AIDS). Medical personnel and other providers should offer an opportunity to ask further questions regarding the procedure and its associated risks.

Female Sterilization: Tubal Ligation. Female sterilization (tubal ligation) prevents pregnancy by blocking the fallopian tubes so that the egg and sperm cannot unite. It involves surgery to (a) isolate the tubes and (b) achieve tubal occlusion (blockage) through a choice of methods.

Timing. The surgery can be performed postpartum, postabortion, or during time periods unrelated to pregnancy (interval tubal ligation). This timing affects the type of counseling, the type of surgery, and the method of tubal occlusion used, as described below (ACOG 1996):

Postpartum procedures. Postpartum tubal ligation may follow either (a) a cesarean section with the abdomen still open, or (b) a vaginal birth using minilaparotomy under local anesthesia with sedation, regional anesthesia, or general anesthesia. A postpartum minilaparotomy is conducted before full uterine involution but after a full assessment of mother and child. It uses a subumbilical incision, which allows easy access to the abdomen because the wall is thin at this point just above the uterine fundus. Laparoscopy should not be performed postpartum because of the nonoptimal orientation and the technical difficulty that may arise from the size and vascular nature of the postpartum uterus (WHO 1999).

Postabortion procedures. Following a first-trimester abortion, tubal ligation may be performed by either laparoscopy or minilaparotomy using a suprapubic incision. Following a second-trimester abortion, a minilaparotomy using a small vertical midline incision is preferred. The risk of perforating the soft uterus with the laparoscopic trocar may warrant either the use of open laparoscopy using the Hasson cannula or waiting for uterine inversion and performing an interval procedure.

Interval procedures. Interval sterilization procedures may be performed at any time during the menstrual cycle, preferably during the follicular phase to reduce the risk of a luteal-phase pregnancy (a pregnancy in which conception occurs before sterilization). However, because of nonoptimal uterine and tube positioning, tubal ligation should be avoided during pregnancy or between days 8 and 41 after delivery; it should be performed only with special care between days 3 and 7 postpartum (WHO 1999). On the day of the interval procedure, it is good practice to confirm that a woman is using contraception and to perform a pregnancy test. Interval procedures may be performed transvaginally (Kondo and others 2009) through posterior colpotomy (Ayhan, Boynukalin, and Salman 2006) or transcervically using hysteroscopy (Castano and Adekunle 2010).

Laparoscopy versus minilaparotomy. Laparoscopy emerged in the 1960s and 1970s; by 1990, one-third of all tubal ligations were performed using this method. Laparoscopic sterilization can be closed or open. In the closed procedure, the laparoscopic incision is made just below the umbilicus, through which the trocar is inserted into the peritoneum. In the open procedure, the incision goes through all abdominal wall layers, and the peritoneum is entered directly.

The advantages of laparoscopic sterilization include a quick recovery and minimal blood loss and postoperative pain; small, barely visible scars; and the opportunity to inspect internal organs. The disadvantage is that the trocar could injure organs.

Minilaparotomy became another option after its development in the 1970s, and most tubal ligations use this method. In minilaparotomy, an incision of 2–3 centimeters is placed in relation to the uterine fundus. For interval sterilization, a uterine manipulator is used to bring the uterine fundus close to the incision.

Both minilaparotomy and laparoscopy are safe and effective and can be performed in outpatient facilities and under local anesthesia and conscious sedation. Complications from female sterilization are rare and include immediate complications such as anesthetic issues, uterine injury and perforation, and organ injury. There is an increased chance of ectopic pregnancy (Holt and others 1991; Peterson and others 1996), which can be lethal, particularly in LMICs (Goyaux and others 2003).

On balance, minilaparotomy may be better suited to LMICs because it is simple and inexpensive, uses basic surgical equipment, may be performed by general practitioners and paramedics in maternity and health centers, and is recommended for both postpartum and interval procedures (WHO 1999). In contrast, laparoscopy—despite its smaller incision, lesser pain, smaller probability of complications, shorter recovery time, and smaller scar—requires specially trained surgeons; equipment that is sophisticated, expensive, and difficult to maintain; and fully equipped tertiary hospitals with sterile equipment and a surgical theater to reduce the risk of infections (WHO 1999).

Tubal occlusion methods. During female sterilization, tubal occlusion is achieved through electrical methods, mechanical methods, or ligation and excision as follows:

- *Monopolar and bipolar electrocoagulation* are the most commonly used tubal occlusion methods during laparoscopic procedures.
- *Tubal clips or rings* may be used to mechanically block the tubes. Similarly, in the Pomeroy method, a loop of tube is "strangled" with a suture, a cut, and the cauterization of the ends. Reversal of sterilization is easier with clips and rings than with electrocoagulation because clips destroy a smaller portion of the fallopian tube.
- *Ligation and excision*, severing of the tubes followed by ligation using a variety of techniques, is the most common procedure for tubal occlusion during laparotomy or at cesarean section.
- *Fimbriectomy*, which removes the part of the tube closest to the ovary, involves the modified Irving procedure in which ligatures are placed at two points on the tube, the segment between them is removed, and the ends are attached to the back of the uterus and connective tissue.
- *The Essure method*, a newer method, places small metal and fiber coils in the tubes to induce scarring and block the fallopian tubes.[6]

During interval sterilizations, ligation and mechanical devices can be used, but in the immediate postpartum period, ligation using clips, rings, or bands is preferred (WHO 1999). In the postabortion period, both blocking methods are acceptable (with special care when using mechanical devices to avoid injuring enlarged tubes) (WHO 1999).

Male Sterilization: Vasectomy. Vasectomy includes three steps: anesthesia, delivery and isolation of the vas deferens from the scrotal sac, and vas occlusion.

Anesthesia. The most common anesthesia is a local vasal block using lidocaine without epinephrine (Li and others 1992). Other techniques to improve anesthetic quality and comfort include the use of eutectic mixture of local anesthetics (EMLA) creams as an adjunct to the vasal block, buffered anesthesia, the spermatic cord block, the no-needle injector, and the mini-needle technique (Shih, Turok, and Parker 2011; Weiss and Li 2005). Vasectomy may be performed under general anesthesia in exceptional circumstances such as previous adverse reactions to local anesthesia, scarring or deformity that make local anesthesia difficult, current anticoagulation therapy (which increases the chance of hematoma formation), and when vasectomy is part of a series of procedures to be performed on the same day.

Isolation of vas deferens. In the traditional vasectomy, following anesthesia, two small incisions are made on each side of the scrotum with a scalpel, and both vas deferens are isolated for excision, followed by vassal occlusion (Cook, Pun, and others 2007). Alternatively, the no-scalpel method, or keyhole vasectomy, uses a sharp pair of forceps in lieu of a scalpel to puncture the scrotum. The no-scalpel method reduces bleeding and hematoma formation, reduces the probability of infection, removes the need for stitches, and increases healing time (Cook, Pun, and others 2007). The open-ended vasectomy leaves the testicular end of the vas open to allow a continuous stream of sperm into the scrotum. This procedure reduces the risk of postvasectomy pain syndrome and congestive epididymitis (Christiansen and Sandlow 2003; Moss 1992; Shapiro and Silber 1979).

Vas occlusion. The most common, but relatively less effective, method of vas occlusion is ligation and excision. (Vasectomy failure rates are estimated at less than 3 percent, but some studies suggest the rate is higher for ligation and excision [Aradhya, Best, and Sokal 2005]).[7] Other methods include electrical and thermal cautery, fascial interposition (FI), and vas irrigation (Shih, Turok, and Parker 2011). Both FI and vas irrigation are highly effective but rarely used (Cook, van Vliet, and others 2007). Reviews suggest that cautery combined with FI is the superior occlusion method (Cook, van Vliet, and others 2007; Labrecque and others 2004).

FI is commonly performed during vasectomy to prevent recanalization, a common cause of vasectomy failure. This procedure, which significantly increases the success rate of vasectomy, positions the prostatic end of the vas outside the fascial sheath of the scrotal sac, leaving the testicular side inside the fascia (Sokal and others 2004). Irrigation of the distal vas with sterile water or the spermicide euflavine is sometimes used to reduce time to achieve azoospermia (lack of measurable sperm in the semen).

Vas occlusive contraception also includes some newer, nontraditional methods. One of them—the use of clips without vas severance—has shown unacceptably high failure rates despite the procedure's higher potential for reversal (Levine, Abern, and Lux 2006). Another new, nonocclusive method involves insertion of a soft silicone or urethane intra vas device (IVD) that contains a set of tiny implants to block the flow of sperm, enabling the vas to remain intact and easing reversal. Although human clinical trials of the IVD have been conducted (for example, Song and others 2006), it has been neither marketed nor approved for general use as of this writing.

Safety and Effectiveness of Tubal Ligation and Vasectomy. Vasectomy is generally more effective and safer than tubal ligation (table 7.2). In addition, following attempted reversal, both procedures have similar success rates as measured by pregnancy after reversal (Cos and others 1983; Fox 1994; Henderson 1984; Lee 1986; Rock and others 1982; Spivak, Librach, and Rosenthal 1986). Tubal ligation is comparatively riskier, at least in part because either method (laparoscopy or minilaparotomy) could proceed to an open laparotomy if internal organs, especially major vessels, are injured, resulting in life-threatening hemorrhage (Hendrix, Chauhan, and Morrison 1999).

The vasectomy procedure is almost always performed under a local anesthetic and does not require as much technical expertise as tubal ligation does. Nurses in LMICs who are knowledgeable about anatomy can be trained to perform vasectomies because of their relatively less severe complications.

Costs and Cost-Effectiveness of Surgical versus Nonsurgical Contraception

Along with a higher success rate, surgical contraception generally costs more than nonsurgical interventions. In this section we evaluate evidence of the costs and cost-effectiveness of surgical versus nonsurgical methods of contraception. We also attempt to assess whether the added costs would represent value for money if scaled up in LMICs.

Table 7.2 Safety and Effectiveness of Surgical Sterilization, by Procedure

	Tubal ligation	Vasectomy
Failure rate (%)[a]		
Year 1	0.55	0.15
Year 2	0.29	0.01
Year 3	0.15	0.01
Year 4	0.19	0.01
Year 5	0.13	0.01
Cumulative probability of postprocedure failure (number per 1,000 procedures)[b]		
Year 1	7.4	5.5
Year 5	11.3	13.1
Pregnancy rate after reversal (%)[c]	40.0–60.0	42.0–74.0
Reversal requests after five years (%)[d]	6.0	6.0
Timing of efficacy[d]	Immediate	Delayed until azoospermia[e]
Relative rate of complications[f]	High (20 times that of vasectomy)	Low (1/20 that of tubal ligation)
Relative rate of mortality[f]	12 times that of vasectomy	1/12 that of tubal ligation

Sources:
a. Trussell 2011b.
b. Jamieson and others 2004; Peterson and others 1996.
c. Cos and others 1983; Fox 1994; Henderson 1984; Lee 1986; Spivak, Librach, and Rosenthal 1986.
d. Shih, Turok, and Parker 2011.
e. Azoospermia is lack of measurable sperm in the semen.
f. Hendrix, Chauhan, and Morrison 1999.
Note: The "failure rate" refers to the probability of pregnancy.

Costs. Surgical sterilization methods generally carry higher up-front or unit costs than nonsurgical methods. Notably, however, a single surgical set can be used for many years if well used and maintained, thus offsetting the up-front costs. However, the cost of continuously sterilizing and maintaining equipment is also important.

Among the surgical procedures, vasectomy, in addition to being more effective and safer, costs less than tubal ligation by either laparoscopy or laparotomy (Smith, Taylor, and Smith 1985). Increasing the number of vasectomies relative to tubal ligations would substantially reduce overall procedural costs and the costs of managing adverse events (Hendrix, Chauhan, and Morrison 1999).

Looking solely at *per use* commodity costs, the drugs and supplies for female sterilization cost $9.09 (in 2009 U.S. dollars) and, for male sterilization, $4.95. By comparison, oral contraceptives cost $0.21 per use; IUDs, $0.37; and injectable hormonal contraceptives, $0.87 (Ross, Weissman, and Stover 2009). However, some proprietary implants such as Implanon (an etonogestrel implant effective for three years) cost more ($24.09) than surgical methods (Ross,

Weissman, and Stover 2009). However, direct cost comparisons on this basis are difficult because contraceptive methods vary widely in duration of effectiveness.

The cost per couple-year of protection (CYP), is generally lower for surgical methods than for nonsurgical methods (the exception being IUDs, which have the lowest cost per CYP of all methods). Table 7.3 compares the total annual direct and indirect costs of contraceptive methods in four Sub-Saharan African countries: Burkina Faso, Cameroon, Ethiopia, and Uganda.

Cost-Effectiveness. Modern contraception as evaluated in program settings is highly cost-effective by various metrics including cost per life year and cost per disability-adjusted life year (DALY):

- In India, intensive efforts to improve family planning, control fertility, and provide safe abortions would save nearly 150,000 lives and save $1.5 billion over five years (Goldie and others 2010).
- In Uganda, universal access to contraception would reduce the average number of pregnancies per woman (15–50 years of age) by 1.6, reduce the fertility rate by 1.1 children per woman, improve

Table 7.3 Annual Cost per CYP of Contraceptive Methods in Selected African Countries
U.S. dollars per CYP

Method	Ethiopia (2008)	Uganda (2008)	Burkina Faso (2009)	Cameroon (2013)
Female sterilization	8.65	7.50	17.16	3.23
Male sterilization	8.26	7.24	3.07	2.42
Pill	31.43	23.66	28.51	17.00
IUD	5.24	4.14	6.51	23.35
Injectable or implant[a]	33.74	27.28	58.54	19.84
Condom	22.15	17.12	19.20	15.51
Other modern method[b]	23.14	18.05	18.66	16.26
Periodic abstinence	0.00	0.00	0.00	0.00
Withdrawal	0.00	0.00	0.00	0.00
Other traditional[c]	0.00	0.00	0.00	0.00

Sources: Vlassoff, Walker, and others 2009; Vlassoff and others 2011; Vlassoff and others 2012; Vlassoff, Jerman, and others 2014.
Note: CYP = couple-year of protection; IUD = intrauterine device.
a. Costs of injectables and implants were combined in the four studies.
b. The "other modern method" category includes other barrier methods such as spermicides, sponges, and diaphragms, as well as other hormonal methods such as the vaginal ring or transdermal patch.
c. The "other traditional" category includes fertility awareness methods that track the menstrual cycle or fertility signs and patterns.

maternal and child health outcomes, and save almost $40 per woman in societal costs (Babigumira and others 2012).[8]

• Satisfying unmet need for modern contraception through increased family planning that reduces mother and newborn care costs would save a net $112 million per year in Uganda (Vlassoff and others 2009). Similar studies found annual net savings of $35 million in Ethiopia (Sundaram and others 2010) and $32 million in Burkina Faso (Vlassoff and others 2011).

In the United States, one cost simulation found that the three most cost-effective contraceptive methods are vasectomy, the copper-T IUD, and a hormonal IUD (specifically, levonorgestrel [LNG]-20, marketed under brand names including Mirena). All other methods, including tubal ligation, were found to be less effective and more costly than the copper-T IUD (Trussell and others 2009).

A comprehensive review of the health economics of contraception supported the data presented above, finding that male and female sterilization and long-acting reversible methods such as IUDs and subdermal implants were the most cost-effective contraceptive options, followed by other hormonal methods such as oral contraceptives; the least cost-effective options were barrier and traditional behavioral methods (Mavranezouli 2009).

Future Directions

Goals, Trends, and Challenges. As noted at the outset of this section, family planning is important to the development aspirations of LMICs. Specifically, increasing access to the highly efficacious and convenient surgical methods of contraception can enhance important health, social welfare, educational, and other benefits (Canning and Schultz 2012).

To that end, universal access to reproductive health by 2015 is a target of the United Nations–led Millennium Development Goals (MDGs): MDG 5 is "to improve maternal health."[9] Increased access to reproductive health and family planning would also help to achieve most of the other MDGs: MDG 1 ("eradicate extreme poverty and hunger"); MDG 2 ("achieve universal primary education"); MDG 3 ("promote gender equality and empower women"); MDG 4 ("reduce child mortality"); MDG 6 ("combat HIV/AIDS, malaria and other diseases"); and MDG 7 ("ensure environmental sustainability").

Is access to family planning in the developing world expanding fast enough to contribute to those goals? Worldwide, sterilization is the most common form of modern family planning: 38 percent of women who used modern methods in 2012 chose sterilization. However, the reverse is true in LMICs, particularly in Africa, where contraceptive injections and pills dominate (Darroch and Singh 2013). Only 8 percent of women in Africa who use modern methods chose sterilization; among the four main groups of modern methods (sterilization, barriers, hormones, and IUDs), sterilization is the least common (Darroch and Singh 2013).

In Africa, a variety of factors have constrained expansion of sterilization: lack of planning tools; technical and programmatic difficulty; relatively high commodity and provision costs; health system constraints; overemphasis on short-term, commodity-based contraceptive methods instead of services; and social and cultural barriers (Wickstrom and Jacobstein 2011).

The Malawi Model. In contrast to the general pattern in Africa, the use of female sterilization (as a percentage of all modern contraceptive use) doubled in Malawi in the decade from 2000 to 2010. Sterilization use was relatively equitable, as measured by rural-urban or education status, although disparities existed by income status (wealthy women used sterilization more than poor women). Jacobstein (2013) attributed the overall increase to several factors:

- Increased demand due to increased knowledge of female sterilization
- Increased desire to limit childbearing
- Improved service delivery due to expanded service access within a supportive and enabling health care system characterized by strong public-private partnerships
- Provision of free and widespread outreach services by dedicated providers

This evidence suggests that LMICs with conditions such as Malawi's have great potential to scale up access to surgical sterilization. However, almost all sterilizations in Malawi are female sterilizations (about 150 tubal ligations for every vasectomy), so efficacy and savings could increase further if this gender gap could be closed.

To overcome human resource constraints such as severe physician shortages—an important collective barrier to increased access to surgical contraception in LMICs—programs in Malawi have developed dedicated nonphysician cadres (clinical officers) to provide mobile contraceptive services including tubal ligation (Jacobstein 2013). To succeed, the programs depend on task shifting (delegating or shifting some tasks to less-specialized health workers [WHO 2007]) and task sharing (in which providers of different levels do similar work, rather than leaving all provision of a service to less-credentialed workers [Janowitz, Stanback, and Boyer 2012]). Only if less-specialized health workers can be trained to perform selected clinical tasks

(such as sterilizations) competently will such efforts substantially increase access to contraception including surgical contraception (Janowitz, Stanback, and Boyer 2012; WHO 2012).

Agenda for Action. LMICs can increase access to surgical contraceptive methods to the extent that they achieve these goals (Wickstrom and Jacobstein 2011):

- Improve quality of services
- Increase public-policy advocacy as well as provider and population awareness of surgical contraception
- Increase financing to procure theater equipment; strengthen human resources; and ensure adequate supply of surgical contraceptive equipment, instruments, and national essential drugs and equipment
- Implement service-oriented instead of only commodity-oriented programs
- Expand and update resources and tools to support contraceptive security (for example, by including surgical contraception methods in health care logistics training)[10]
- Clarify definitions, goals, and success indicators for contraceptive security promotion

LMICs also need to change how their health workers and service providers promote contraception to people. Instead of stating, "You need to use family planning to reduce your fertility," they might ask the client, "What are your fertility desires, and how can we help you to have the number of children you can afford while also maintaining a productive lifestyle?" If LMIC populations receive enough information, education, and communication about the benefits of family planning and the available contraceptive methods, the planning of childbearing will begin to be their idea and they will start demanding family planning from their leaders as a basic need.

Moreover, ethical concerns about coerced sterilization have been raised, especially regarding women with HIV/AIDS (Mallet and Kalambi 2008). LMICs need to step up education and communication efforts to ensure that surgical contraceptive services are scaled up ethically to avoid coercion, particularly in countries with high HIV prevalence (Delvaux and Nostlinger 2007).

Conclusions and Recommendations

In this section, we have discussed the unmet need for modern surgical methods of contraception; the potential benefits of increasing access to contraception (particularly male and female sterilization); and both the effectiveness and cost-effectiveness of such an increase. Based on our findings, we offer the following conclusions and recommendations:

- The surgical methods of male and female sterilization (vasectomy and tubal ligation, respectively) are highly effective, cost-effective, and convenient. Although they constitute the most widely used contraceptive category worldwide, many LMICs, particularly in Sub-Saharan Africa, have not adopted them widely. We recommend that policy makers adopt policies to promote and ensure widespread access to surgical methods of family planning.
- As LMICs add, and expand access to, surgical facilities, equipment, and human resources, they should make increased access to surgical contraception a reproductive priority. Health workers should be trained to provide surgical family planning and, given the acute shortage of physicians, task shifting of surgical family planning to nurses and medical assistants should be encouraged.
- Contraception advocacy in LMICs needs to change such that the populations begin to own the idea of planning families and realize their ability to control their own fertility.
- Policy makers should advocate surgical methods of family planning because they provide value for money; despite relatively high up-front costs, they are among the most cost-effective contraceptive methods for LMICs in the long term.
- Policy dialogues on expansion of family planning programs should emphasize the greater effectiveness and cost-effectiveness of male sterilization (vasectomy) relative to female sterilization (tubal ligation).
- Policy makers and advocates in LMICs should encourage more qualitative and quantitative research on how to increase the quality, uptake, and impact of—and access to—surgical contraception.

SURGERY FOR ABORTION AND POSTABORTION CARE

Induced abortion is common in LMICs, particularly in those countries where the unmet need for family planning is high. Wherever abortion is legal, it can be performed safely in the first and second trimesters either medically or surgically. But in countries where abortion is legally restricted, most abortions are performed by poorly trained practitioners in clandestine locations using a variety of methods. Such abortions are, by the World Health Organization's definition, unsafe—that is, performed outside of health facilities or other places legally recognized for the procedure, or by an unskilled person (WHO 1992).

Incomplete Abortion

Incomplete abortion is one of the most common complications of induced abortion, particularly in the case of illegal induced abortion. It occurs when the products of conception have not been fully expelled through the cervix (Bottomley and Bourne 2009). The symptoms and signs of abortion complications—vaginal bleeding, abdominal pain, fever, purulent or foul-smelling vaginal discharge, and shock—are usually present with incomplete abortion. In one study, even after clinical assessments had suggested that no products were retained (in this case, following first-trimester spontaneous abortions, or miscarriages), ultrasounds showed that 45 percent of the women had retained tissue (Alcázar, Baldonado, and Laparte 1995).

Studies in Rwanda and Uganda (where abortion is legally restricted) showed that 65–75 percent of all postabortion complications involved incomplete abortions (Vlassoff and others 2014; Vlassoff and others 2009). Sepsis and hypovolemic shock were among the common complications, together making up about a quarter of all postabortion complications in these two countries.

Global Demand for Abortion

Globally, almost 44 million induced abortions were performed in 2008—86 percent of them in developing countries (Sedgh and others 2012). Although the worldwide total declined from about 46 million in 1995 to 44 million in 2008 (a 4 percent drop), the proportion of abortions that were unsafe increased by 4 percentage points during the same period, from 44 percent to 49 percent (Sedgh and others 2012). Moreover, almost all abortions performed in Africa (97 percent) were unsafe in 2008, only a slight decline from 99 percent in 1995 (Sedgh and others 2012).

Of the 185 million pregnancies that occurred in developing countries in 2008, 40 percent were unintended (Singh, Sedgh, and Hussain 2010). Most unintended pregnancies (82 percent) occur among couples using either no method or traditional methods of contraception (Darroch, Sedgh, and Ball 2011; Singh and Darroch 2012). Many unintended pregnancies result in induced abortions. In 2008, 37.8 million induced abortions were performed in developing countries, 6.4 million of them in Africa, almost all being unsafe (Sedgh and others 2012).

Driving the demand for induced abortion, particularly in low-income settings, are both individual factors (such as educational level, marital status, family size and composition, fertility expectations, and contraceptive use) and systemic factors (such as service availability and quality, social conditions, economic pressures, religious and cultural beliefs, and societal norms and values) (Warriner and Shah 2006).

Consequences of Unsafe Abortion

Abortions performed correctly by trained practitioners are safe, with minimal risk of complications (Bartlett and others 2004; Grimes and others 2006; Henshaw 1993). The occurrence of complications following induced abortion depends on both the type of procedure and the type of provider. In Uganda in 2003, for example, at least one complication occurred in 25 percent of abortions induced by doctors, 45 percent induced by clinical officers, 50 percent induced by pharmacy workers, 66 percent induced by traditional healers or lay practitioners, and 73 percent that were self-induced (Henshaw 1993; Prada and others 2005; Singh and others 2006).

The rates of unsafe abortion and abortion complications as well as the demand for postabortion care also vary remarkably by geographic region. The hospitalization rate for abortion complications per 1,000 women in 2005 was 8.8 in Africa, 4.1 in Asia, and 5.7 in Latin America and the Caribbean (Singh 2006). In that year alone, more than 5 million unsafe abortions in developing countries resulted in hospital admission, 1.7 million of them in Africa (Singh 2006).

That LMICs exhibit the world's highest demand for postabortion care is understandable given that, in most of them, induced abortion is either completely illegal, legal only to save the mother's life or after rape or incest, or legal but with limited access by women who need it. In such settings, the only option for women wishing to end their pregnancies is to procure clandestine, usually unsafe, abortions—with substantial negative consequences for themselves, their families, and their societies (Singh 2010):

- Increased death and disability (Murray and others 2013; Okonofua 2006)
- Increased health care costs (Babigumira and others 2011; Benson and others 2012; Shearer, Walker, and Vlassoff 2010; Vlassoff and others 2009)
- Decreased quality of life and social support (Lubinga and others 2013)
- Reduced economic productivity (Singh 2010; Sundaram and others 2010).

The GBD Study 2010 tells the global story in hard numbers, estimating that more than 37,000 abortion-related deaths occurred in 2010, a 39 percent decrease from 1990 and corresponding to almost 0.5 deaths per 100,000 women (Lozano and others 2013). Almost 32,000 YLDs, corresponding to 1 YLD per 100,000 women, were attributable to abortion in 2010, a 20 percent increase from 1990 and corresponding to fewer than 0.5 YLD per 100,000 women (Vos and others 2013).[11] During the same period, in a welcome downward trend, the burden of disease due to abortion declined by 33 percent (Murray and others 2013).[12]

Barriers to Access to Surgical Procedures for Abortion and Postabortion Care

Legal prohibition of abortion is the main barrier to access to surgical abortion and postabortion care in LMICs. Many countries have one or more legal barriers to abortion, ranging from complete criminalization to limitation of services to specific periods during pregnancy. Other legal barriers include requirements that abortions be provided by more than one physician, that abortion be provided only at licensed facilities, that parents consent (for young girls), that women receive preabortion counseling, or that abortions be delayed by mandated preabortion "reflection" periods.

Social and cultural norms constitute another important barrier to access to surgical abortion and postabortion care. In many LMICs, the culture so disapproves of sexual activity by young women that, when they get pregnant, they often travel long distances to ensure confidentiality. They are stigmatized for getting pregnant, seeking abortions, and seeking postabortion care. Pregnancy or abortion may also be associated with gender-based violence in some areas.

Low-quality health services present yet another barrier to access to surgical services for abortion and postabortion care. In LMICs that lack good health systems or quality of service, surgical methods are often unavailable as choices, health workers are rude or judgmental toward women who seek abortion or postabortion care, confidentiality is limited, and health workers are absent or poorly trained. Moreover, the health systems in many LMICs are unaffordable, limited in number and distribution, and lacking drugs and equipment.

Surgical Procedures

The long-standing standard for safe induced abortion is surgery through either dilation and curettage (D&C) or vacuum aspiration (VA). However, medical abortion (which induces abortion nonsurgically, using medicines) is now considered a safe and viable alternative (Neilson and others 2010, 2013; Ngo and others 2011).

In low-income settings, postabortion surgical intervention is most commonly a result of incomplete abortion, which presents with sepsis and hemorrhage. Management of incomplete abortion comprises three types:

- *Expectant management*, which allows products of conception to be spontaneously evacuated
- *Medical management*, which uses medications to induce evacuation
- *Surgical management*, which uses either sharp metal curettage (with or without cervical dilation) or VA (manual vacuum aspiration [MVA] or electric vacuum aspiration [EVA]).

Other surgical procedures are necessary to manage the complications of induced abortions, particularly those that are clandestine and unsafe. These include surgery to repair tears and perforations in the genital tract, laparotomy for reasons such as repairs and sepsis management, and hysterectomy.

Dilation and Curettage. Sharp metal curettage involves evacuation of the retained products of conception using forceps and a sharp metal curette. In most cases following incomplete abortion, the cervix is already open and no dilation is needed. If the cervix is open, curettage is preceded by evacuation.

Sharp metal curettage is usually performed in an operating room under general anesthesia, but in some countries it is performed under mild sedation with analgesics and in minor theaters. Some practitioners administer medications for presurgical preparation of the cervix, using prostaglandin gels or pessaries to reduce trauma to the cervix and uterus. Pessaries and gels also reduce the technical difficulties of performing the procedure, thereby reducing the procedure time and postprocedural pain and discomfort.

The curette has a handle at one end and a sharp loop at the other. After administering anesthesia, if the cervix is still closed, it is gently dilated by inserting serial Hegar's dilators until an appropriately sized curette can be introduced safely without force to avoid lacerating or tearing the cervix (which would create a false passage into the cervix and risk torrential bleeding and severe uterine perforation). The curette is then used to gently scrape the uterine wall and remove tissue in the uterus, which is examined to ensure the procedure is complete.

In addition to the complications of anesthesia, D&C may result in uterine perforation, infection, and

adhesions (Asherman's syndrome), the latter of which increases the risks of future ectopic pregnancy, miscarriage, or abnormal placentation (placenta previa and acreta) (Dalton and others 2006).

Vacuum Aspiration. VA uses suction to remove retained products of conception through the cervix. Generally performed in an outpatient setting under local anesthesia or with analgesics, VA has been documented in multiple studies to be safe (Greenslade and others 1993), although complications can include hemorrhage, infection, cervical and uterine injury, and adhesions (Dalton and others 2006).

The procedure was pioneered in 1958 by Chinese physicians Wu Yuantai and Wu Xianzhen (Wu and Wu 1958). Improvements in the West over the years led to the development of a soft, flexible device, the Karman cannula, which removed the need for cervical dilation and reduced uterine injury. MVA uses a manual vacuum syringe and cannula, and EVA uses an electric pump. In both methods, the pump mechanism creates a vacuum that empties the uterus.

Effectiveness of Methods

To avoid anesthesia and surgery, some women prefer medical (drug-induced) abortion. However, medical abortion is associated with more pain and bleeding, more distress after the procedure, and more side effects in general than surgical abortion (Grimes, Smith, and Witham 2004; Grossman, Blanchard, and Blumenthal 2008; Grossman and others 2011; Kelly and others 2010; Lohr, Hayes, and Gemzell-Danielsson 2008). In the first trimester, medical abortion is more painful, is associated with more negative experiences and complications after the procedure, and is both less effective and less acceptable than surgical abortion (Robson and others 2009; Say and others 2005). In the second trimester, surgical abortion is similar in efficacy to medical abortion (Grossman and others 2011; Grossman, Blanchard, and Blumenthal 2008; Lohr, Hayes, and Gemzell-Danielsson 2008; Kelly and others 2010).

Regarding the three methods for management of incomplete abortion—expectant, medical, and surgical—a 2005 meta-analysis found that surgical management was more likely to complete uterine evacuation than medical management, which in turn was more effective than expectant management (Sotiriadis and others 2005). However, studies report mixed results regarding the overall advantages and disadvantages of medical versus surgical management of incomplete abortion or miscarriage. One study reported that surgical management resulted in more infections but less pain, a lower chance of retained products, and greater satisfaction than medical management (Niinimaki and others 2006; Niinimaki and others 2009). A Cochrane review found that, compared with expectant management, surgical management reduced the risk of incomplete abortion or miscarriage, need for additional surgery, bleeding, and transfusion despite being less costly; however, the two methods carried similar risks of infection and psychological issues (Nanda and others 2012).

Specifically comparing surgical methods, a 2010 Cochrane review found that VA was safer, quicker, and less painful than sharp metal curettage and also led to less blood loss. However, differences were nonsignificant in the incidence of sepsis postprocedure, uterine perforation, or the need for reevacuation (Forna and Gulmezoglu 2001; Tuncalp, Gulmezoglu, and Souza 2010). MVA and EVA do not appear to differ substantially in efficacy (Mittal and others 2011).

Additionally, VA can be performed in the absence of a fully equipped facility and at secondary health facilities, with or without electricity, and without the capacity for general anesthesia. It is better suited for low-income settings because it is more accessible and reduces the consequences of blood loss and worsening infection associated with transportation to tertiary health facilities.

Despite its advantages over sharp metal curettage, VA has not been adopted in many LMICs, particularly in Sub-Saharan Africa, because practitioners generally lack the knowledge and training to perform it, lack the necessary equipment, or remain unconvinced of its effectiveness and safety.

Cost-Effectiveness of Methods

Relative to unsafe abortion, provision of safe abortion is highly cost-effective in LMICs (Hu and others 2009; Hu and others 2010). Studies that compare the cost-effectiveness of safe procedures break down their findings by trimester of the procedure, usually finding surgical management to be the most cost-effective method. The conclusions are far more mixed, however, concerning the distinct circumstances of spontaneous abortion (miscarriage).

First-trimester abortion. Clinic-based MVA is the most effective and most cost-effective method in Mexico, Nigeria, and the United States, far surpassing D&C and medical abortion (Hu and others 2009; Hu and others 2010; Rocconi and others 2005). In Ghana, however, medical abortion was found to be more cost-effective than clinic-based MVA (Hu and others 2010).[13]

Second-trimester abortion. D&C is less expensive and more effective than medical induction for second-trimester abortion (Cowett, Golub, and Grobman 2006). Others suggest that medical management is less preferable economically because its higher probability of abortion failure and bleeding increases costs (Xia, She, and Lam 2011).

Miscarriage. Medical management of miscarriage using the labor-induction medication misoprostol is less costly than expectant management, which in turn is less costly than surgical management of first-trimester miscarriage (You and Chung 2005). However, to treat first-trimester miscarriage or incomplete abortion, medical management is more efficacious and cost-effective (Tasnim and others 2011). Some studies indicate no clear preference concerning the cost-effectiveness of medical versus surgical management but cite other advantages associated with both (Niinimaki and others 2009). Others suggest that either expectant or medical management of first-trimester miscarriage would be more cost-effective than traditional surgical management (Petrou and others 2006). For first-trimester pregnancy loss, surgical management is more cost-effective and more efficacious than medical management when performed in the outpatient setting (Rausch and others 2012). For incomplete or inevitable abortion, medical management is cost-effective and more efficacious (Rausch and others 2012). Among the surgical procedures, MVA is more cost-effective than EVA because it costs less, does not require general anesthesia, and is more suited to LMICs (Tasnim and others 2011).

Future Directions

Surgical methods for safe abortion are unlikely to be used in most LMICs because prevailing legal restrictions force women to seek clandestine, usually unsafe, abortions. Therefore, surgical methods will likely play a more significant role in the management of abortion complications, particularly incomplete abortion.

Although medical management will probably constitute a substantial proportion of management of incomplete abortion in LMICs in the future, surgery will continue to be important as long as medical management remains inaccessible to many, if not most, women in need. To date, the use of medical management is limited because of high drug costs and health systems that lack adequate ability to provide careful follow-up and continuous access to medical care (Ballagh, Harris, and Demasio 1998).

Ultimately, comprehensive family planning would reduce unintended pregnancies and therefore the incidence of unsafe abortions. For example, universal access to contraceptives by women who express the need for them would reduce unintended pregnancies in developing countries by more than two-thirds—from 80 million to 26 million (Singh and Darroch 2012). Such a massive decline would reduce the number of induced abortions by an estimated 26 million, unsafe abortions by 14.5 million (from 20 million to 5.5 million), and unsafe-abortion-related deaths by more than four-fifths, from 46,000 to 8,000 (Guttmacher Institute 2010; Singh and Darroch 2012).

Conclusions and Recommendations

In this section, we discuss the burden of unintended pregnancy and the demand for both abortion and postabortion care in LMICs, the potential benefits of increased access to surgical services for abortion and postabortion care, and the potential health and economic results of such an increase. Based on our findings, we offer the following conclusions and recommendations:

- Surgical methods for abortion and the management of incomplete abortion are more effective and more cost-effective than medical management, particularly in LMICs where access to medical interventions might be limited. They are associated with fewer side effects such as pain and bleeding—a critical advantage in LMICs, where health facilities might be distant and transportation difficult.
- Access to VA and D&C should be increased by training more health workers and investing in surgical equipment in secondary health care settings.
- Although surgical management of incomplete abortion predominates where such services are available in LMICs, increased access should be a priority to improve postabortion care and reduce abortion-related morbidity and mortality.
- Safe surgical abortion is not a current option in most LMICs, given their legal restrictions; expanding access to it will be impossible for the foreseeable future. That these restrictions encourage women to seek unsafe abortions, with their higher complication rates, only heightens the need to expand access to surgical management of incomplete abortion.
- Increased investment in family planning will help satisfy the large unmet need for contraception in LMICs and, by reducing the number of unintended pregnancies, dramatically lower maternal mortality and morbidity as well as the number of unsafe abortions.

NOTES

The World Bank classifies countries according to four income groupings. Income is measured using gross national income (GNI) per capita, in U.S. dollars, converted from local currency using the *World Bank Atlas* method. Classifications as of July 2014 are as follows:

- Low-income countries (LICs) = US$1,045 or less in 2013
- Middle-income countries (MICs) are subdivided:
  - Lower-middle-income = US$1,046 to US$4,125
  - Upper-middle-income (UMICs) = US$4,126 to US$12,745
- High-income countries (HICs) = US$12,746 or more

1. This section considers surgery for induced abortion only. We do not consider induced abortion to be a method of family planning (although some people use it as such). In this regard, we follow the global policy community, which has considered family planning and induced abortion to be separate concerns.
2. There is no consensus on the definition of "high parity": some authors suggest a threshold of more than five viable pregnancies, and others suggest a threshold of more than eight births (Aliyu and others 2005).
3. Increased population and aging drove the seemingly paradoxical increase in YLDs during a decrease in the YLD rate. Although the absolute number of YLDs increased by 28 percent from 1990 through 2010, the number of YLDs per 100,000 declined by 1.2 percent (Vos and others 2013).
4. The "demographic dividend" refers to the increased economic growth that changes in the age structure of a country's population can generate as it transitions from high birth and death rates to low ones.
5. Nonsurgical female sterilization techniques include transcervical tubal occlusion, which emerged in 2003 (Bartz and Greenberg 2008; Zite and Borrero 2011), and chemical sterilization using the cytotoxic agent quinacrine sulfate, which has been proposed but not approved by the U.S. Food and Drug Administration (Zipper and Kessel 2003). Transcervical tubal occlusion is not feasible for LMICs in the near future because it requires high-technology (hysteroscopic) equipment, highly skilled surgeons, and high equipment maintenance costs.
6. A similar method, the Adiana method, which used silicone to induce scarring, was removed from the market for infringing on the Essure patent.
7. The "failure rate" of vasectomy is defined as the presence of motile sperm in the postvasectomy ejaculate. Early failure occurs within three to six months after the vasectomy, and late failure occurs if motile sperm appear in the ejaculate after documented azoospermia in two postvasectomy semen analyses.
8. "Societal costs" refers to an all-inclusive set of costs including direct medical costs, direct nonmedical costs (such as transportation to receive health services), indirect costs (such as lost productivity while seeking health services), and program-related costs.

9. For more information about the eight MDGs, see the United Nations website: http://www.un.org/millenniumgoals/.

10. "Contraceptive security" refers to individuals' ability to choose, obtain, and use reliable, high-quality contraceptives for family planning when they want them.

11. Increased population and aging drove the seemingly paradoxical 20 percent increase in YLDs from 1990 through 2010, even though, during the same 20-year period, the number of abortion-related deaths decreased by 39 percent (Vos and others 2013) and the burden of disease decreased by 33 percent (Murray and others 2013).

12. The World Health Organization (WHO) "burden of disease" refers to a time-based measure that combines the years of life lost from premature mortality and the years of life lost from being in less than full health (http://www.who.int/topics /global_burden_of_disease/en/). It is measured by disability-adjusted life years (DALYs).

13. The differences in the rank order of cost-effectiveness of medical abortion and MVA in the study by Hu and others (2010) were due to the country-specific and sector-specific variations in the baseline cost of service provision.

REFERENCES

ACOG (American College of Obstetricians and Gynecologists). 1996. "Technical Bulletin: Sterilization." *International Journal of Gynecology and Obstetrics* 53 (3): 281–88.

Ahmed, S., Q. Li, L. Liu, and A. O. Tsui. 2012. "Maternal Deaths Averted by Contraceptive Use: An Analysis of 172 Countries." *The Lancet* 380 (9837): 111–25.

Alcázar, J. L., C. Baldonado, and C. Laparte. 1995. "The Reliability of Transvaginal Ultrasonography to Detect Retained Tissue after Spontaneous First-Trimester Abortion, Clinically Thought to Be Complete." *Ultrasound in Obstetrics and Gynecology* 6 (2): 126–29.

Ali, A. A., and A. Okud. 2013. "Factors Affecting Unmet Need for Family Planning in Eastern Sudan." *BMC Public Health* 13 (1): 102.

Aliyu, M. H., P. E. Jolly, J. E. Ehiri, and H. M. Salihu. 2005. "High Parity and Adverse Birth Outcomes: Exploring the Maze." *Birth* 32 (1): 45–59.

Alkema, L., V. Kantorova, C. Menozzi, and A. Biddlecom. 2013. "National, Regional, and Global Rates and Trends in Contraceptive Prevalence and Unmet Need for Family Planning between 1990 and 2015: A Systematic and Comprehensive Analysis." *The Lancet* 381 (9878): 1642–52.

Aradhya, K. W., K. Best, and D. C. Sokal. 2005. "Recent Developments in Vasectomy." *BMJ* 330 (7486): 296–99.

Asiimwe, J. B., P. Ndugga, and J. Mushomi. 2013. "Socio-Demographic Factors Associated with Contraceptive Use among Young Women in Comparison with Older Women in Uganda." DHS (Demographic and Health Surveys) Working Paper 95, ICF International (for the United States Agency for International Development), Calverton, MD.

Ayhan, A., K. Boynukalin, and M. C. Salman. 2006. "Tubal Ligation via Posterior Colpotomy." *International Journal of Gynecology and Obstetrics* 93 (3): 254–55.

Babigumira, J. B., A. Stergachis, D. L. Veenstra, J. S. Gardner, J. Ngonzi, and others. 2011. "Estimating the Costs of Induced Abortion in Uganda: A Model-Based Analysis." *BMC Public Health* 11: 904.

Babigumira, J. B., A. Stergachis, D. L. Veenstra, J. S. Gardner, J. Ngonzi, P. Mukasa-Kivunike, and L. P. Garrison. 2012. "Potential Cost-Effectiveness of Universal Access to Modern Contraceptives in Uganda." *PLoS One* 7 (2): e30735.

Ballagh, S. A., H. A. Harris, and K. Demasio. 1998. "Is Curettage Needed for Uncomplicated Incomplete Spontaneous Abortion?" *American Journal of Obstetrics and Gynecology* 179 (5): 1279–82.

Bartlett, L. A., C. J. Berg, H. B. Shulman, S. B. Zane, C. A. Green, and others. 2004. "Risk Factors for Legal Induced Abortion-Related Mortality in the United States." *Obstetrics and Gynecology* 103 (4): 729–37.

Bartz, D., and J. A. Greenberg. 2008. "Sterilization in the United States." *Reviews in Obstetrics and Gynecology* 1 (1): 23–32.

Benson, J., M. Okoh, K. KrennHrubec, M. A. Lazzarino, and H. B. Johnston. 2012. "Public Hospital Costs of Treatment of Abortion Complications in Nigeria." *International Journal of Gynaecology and Obstetrics* 118 (Suppl 2): S134–40.

Bloom, D. E., D. Canning, and J. Sevilla. 2003. "The Demographic Dividend: A New Perspective on the Economic Consequences of Population Change." Population Matters Monograph MR-1274, RAND, Santa Monica, CA.

Bottomley, C., and T. Bourne. 2009. "Diagnosing Miscarriage." *Best Practice and Research Clinical Obstetrics and Gynaecology* 23 (4): 463–77.

Canning, D., and T. P. Schultz. 2012. "The Economic Consequences of Reproductive Health and Family Planning." *The Lancet* 380 (9837): 165–71.

Castano, P. M., and L. Adekunle. 2010. "Transcervical Sterilization." *Seminars in Reproductive Medicine* 28 (2): 103–09.

Christiansen, C. G., and J. I. Sandlow. 2003. "Testicular Pain Following Vasectomy: A Review of Postvasectomy Pain Syndrome." *Journal of Andrology* 24 (3): 293–98.

Cleland, J., A. Conde-Agudelo, H. Peterson, J. Ross, and A. Tsui. 2012. "Contraception and Health." *The Lancet* 380 (9837): 149–56. doi:10.1016/s0140-6736(12)60609-6.

Clifton, D., and T. Kaneda. 2013. "Family Planning Worldwide 2013 Data Sheet." Population Reference Bureau, Washington, DC.

Cook, L. A., A. Pun, H. van Vliet, M. F. Gallo, and L. M. Lopez. 2007. "Scalpel versus No-Scalpel Incision for Vasectomy." *Cochrane Database of Systematic Reviews* 18 (2): CD004112.

Cook, L. A., H. van Vliet, L. M. Lopez, A. Pun, and M. F. Gallo. 2007. "Vasectomy Occlusion Techniques for Male Sterilization." *Cochrane Database of Systematic Reviews* 18 (2): CD003991.

Cos, L. R., J. R. Valvo, R. S. Davis, and A. T. Cockett. 1983. "Vasovasostomy: Current State of the Art." *Urology* 22 (6): 567–75.

Cowett, A. A., R. M. Golub, and W. A. Grobman. 2006. "Cost-Effectiveness of Dilation and Evacuation versus the Induction of Labor for Second-Trimester Pregnancy Termination." *American Journal of Obstetrics and Gynecology* 194 (3): 768–73.

Dalton, V. K., N. A. Saunders, L. H. Harris, J. A. Williams, and D. I. Lebovic. 2006. "Intrauterine Adhesions after Manual Vacuum Aspiration for Early Pregnancy Failure." *Fertility and Sterility* 85 (6): 1823.e1–1823.e3.

Darroch, J. E. 2013. "Trends in Contraceptive Use." *Contraception* 87 (3): 259–63.

Darroch, J. E., G. Sedgh, and H. Ball. 2011. *Contraceptive Technologies: Responding to Women's Needs*. New York: Guttmacher Institute.

Darroch, J. E., and S. Singh. 2013. "Trends in Contraceptive Need and Use in Developing Countries in 2003, 2008, and 2012: An Analysis of National Surveys." *The Lancet* 381 (9879): 1756–62.

Delvaux, T., and C. Nostlinger. 2007. "Reproductive Choice for Women and Men Living with HIV: Contraception, Abortion and Fertility." *Reproductive Health Matters* 15 (29 Suppl): 46–66.

Forna, F., and A. M. Gulmezoglu. 2001. "Surgical Procedures to Evacuate Incomplete Abortion." *Cochrane Database of Systematic Reviews* 1 (1): CD001993.

Fox, M. 1994. "Vasectomy Reversal—Microsurgery for Best Results." *British Journal of Urology* 73 (4): 449–53.

Frost, J. J., S. Singh, and L. B. Finer. 2007. "Factors Associated with Contraceptive Use and Nonuse, United States, 2004." *Perspectives on Sexual and Reproductive Health* 39 (2): 90–99.

Gaym, A. 2012. "Current and Future Role of Voluntary Surgical Contraception in Increasing Access to and Utilization of Family Planning Services in Africa." *Ethiopian Medical Journal* 50 (4): 363–70.

Goldie, S. J., S. Sweet, N. Carvalho, U. C. Natchu, and D. Hu. 2010. "Alternative Strategies to Reduce Maternal Mortality in India: A Cost-Effectiveness Analysis." *PLoS Med* 7 (4): e1000264.

Goyaux, N., R. Leke, N. Keita, and P. Thonneau. 2003. "Ectopic Pregnancy in African Developing Countries." *Acta Obstetricia et Gynecologica Scandinavica* 82 (4): 305–12.

Greenslade, F. C., A. L. Leonard, J. Benson, J. Wunkler, and V. L. Henderson. 1993. *Manual Vacuum Aspiration: A Summary of Clinical and Programmatic Experience Worldwide*. Chapel Hill, NC: Ipas.

Grimes, D. A., J. Benson, S. Singh, M. Romero, B. Ganatra, and others. 2006. "Unsafe Abortion: The Preventable Pandemic." *The Lancet* 368 (9550): 1908–19.

Grimes, D. A., M. S. Smith, and A. D. Witham. 2004. "Mifepristone and Misoprostol versus Dilation and Evacuation for Midtrimester Abortion: A Pilot Randomised Controlled Trial." *BJOG: An International Journal of Obstetrics and Gynaecology* 111 (2): 148–53.

Grossman, D., K. Blanchard, and P. Blumenthal. 2008. "Complications after Second Trimester Surgical and Medical Abortion." *Reproductive Health Matters* 16 (31 Suppl): 173–82.

Grossman, D., D. Constant, N. Lince, M. Alblas, K. Blanchard, and others. 2011. "Surgical and Medical Second Trimester Abortion in South Africa: A Cross-Sectional Study." *BMC Health Services Research* 11: 224.

Guttmacher Institute. 2010. "Facts on Investing in Family Planning and Maternal and Newborn Health." In Brief update, November.

Henderson, S. R. 1984. "The Reversibility of Female Sterilization with the Use of Microsurgery: A Report on 102 Patients with More than One Year of Follow-Up." *American Journal of Obstetrics and Gynecology* 149 (1): 57–65.

Hendrix, N. W., S. P. Chauhan, and J. C. Morrison. 1999. "Sterilization and Its Consequences." *Obstetrical and Gynecological Survey* 54 (12): 766–77.

Henshaw, S. K. 1993. "How Safe Is Therapeutic Abortion?" In *The Current Status of Gynaecology and Obstetrics Series*, Vol. 5, edited by E. S. Teoh, S. S. Ratnam, and M. Macnaughton, 31–41. Carnforth, U.K.: Parthenon Publishing Group.

Holt, V. L., J. Chu, J. R. Daling, A. S. Stergachis, and N. S. Weiss. 1991. "Tubal Sterilization and Subsequent Ectopic Pregnancy. A Case-Control Study." *JAMA* 266 (2): 242–46.

Hu, D., D. Grossman, C. Levin, K. Blanchard, R. Adanu, and others. 2010. "Cost-Effectiveness Analysis of Unsafe Abortion and Alternative First-Trimester Pregnancy Termination Strategies in Nigeria and Ghana." *African Journal of Reproductive Health* 14 (2): 85–103.

Hu, D., D. Grossman, C. Levin, K. Blanchard, and S. J. Goldie. 2009. "Cost-Effectiveness Analysis of Alternative First-Trimester Pregnancy Termination Strategies in Mexico City." *BJOG: An International Journal of Obstetrics and Gynaecology* 116 (6): 768–79.

Jacobstein, R. 2013. "Lessons from the Recent Rise in Use of Female Sterilization in Malawi." *Studies in Family Planning* 44 (1): 85–95.

Jamieson, D. J., C. Costello, J. Trussell, S. D. Hillis, P. A. Marchbanks, and H. B. Peterson. 2004. "The Risk of Pregnancy after Vasectomy." *Obstetrics and Gynecology* 103 (5 Pt 1): 848–50.

Janowitz, B., J. Stanback, and B. Boyer. 2012. "Task Sharing in Family Planning." *Studies in Family Planning* 43 (1): 57–62.

Kasedde, S. 2000. "Long-Term and Permanent Family Planning Methods in Uganda: A Literature Review." Unpublished paper (USAID Cooperative Agreement 617-00-00-00001-00). http://www.ugandadish.org/best.shtml.

Kelly, T., J. Suddes, D. Howel, J. Hewison, and S. Robson. 2010. "Comparing Medical versus Surgical Termination of Pregnancy at 13–20 Weeks of Gestation: A Randomised Controlled Trial." *BJOG: An International Journal of Obstetrics and Gynaecology* 117 (12): 1512–20.

Kondo, W., R. W. Noda, A. W. Branco, M. Rangel, and A. J. Branco Filho. 2009. "Transvaginal Endoscopic Tubal Sterilization." *Journal of Laparoendoscopic and Advanced Surgical Techniques Part A* 19 (1): 59–61.

Labrecque, M., C. Dufresne, M. A. Barone, and K. St.-Hilaire. 2004. "Vasectomy Surgical Techniques: A Systematic Review." *BMC Medicine* 2 (21): 21.

Lee, H. Y. 1986. "A 20-Year Experience with Vasovasostomy." *Journal of Urology* 136 (2): 413–15.

Levine, L. A., M. R. Abern, and M. M. Lux. 2006. "Persistent Motile Sperm after Ligation Band Vasectomy." *Journal of Urology* 176 (5): 2146–48.

Li, P. S., S. Q. Li, P. N. Schlegel, and M. Goldstein. 1992. "External Spermatic Sheath Injection for Vasal Nerve Block." *Urology* 39 (2): 173–76.

Lohr, P. A., J. L. Hayes, and K. Gemzell-Danielsson. 2008. "Surgical versus Medical Methods for Second Trimester Induced Abortion." *Cochrane Database of Systematic Reviews* 23 (1): CD006714.

Lozano, R., M. Naghavi, K. Foreman, S. Lim, K. Shibuya, and others. 2013. "Global and Regional Mortality from 235 Causes of Death for 20 Age Groups in 1990 and 2010: A Systematic Analysis for the Global Burden of Disease Study 2010." *The Lancet* 380 (9859): 2095–128.

Lubinga, S. J., G. A. Levine, A. M. Jenny, J. Ngonzi, P. Mukasa-Kivunike, and others. 2013. "Health-Related Quality of Life and Social Support among Women Treated for Abortion Complications in Western Uganda." *Health and Quality of Life Outcomes* 11: 118.

Mallet, J., and V. Kalambi. 2008. "Coerced and Forced Sterilization of HIV-Positive Women in Namibia." *HIV/AIDS Policy and Law Review* 13 (2–3): 77–78.

Mavranezouli, I. 2009. "Health Economics of Contraception." *Best Practice and Research Clinical Obstetrics and Gynaecology* 23 (2): 187–98.

Mittal, S., R. Sehgal, S. Aggarwal, J. Aruna, A. Bahadur, and G. Kumar. 2011. "Cervical Priming with Misoprostol before Manual Vacuum Aspiration versus Electric Vacuum Aspiration for First-Trimester Surgical Abortion." *International Journal of Gynaecology and Obstetrics* 112 (1): 34–39.

Moss, W. M. 1992. "A Comparison of Open-End versus Closed-End Vasectomies: A Report on 6,220 Cases." *Contraception* 46 (6): 521–25.

Murray, C. J., T. Vos, R. Lozano, M. Naghavi, A. D. Flaxman, and others. 2013. "Disability-Adjusted Life Years (DALYs) for 291 Diseases and Injuries in 21 Regions, 1990–2010: A Systematic Analysis for the Global Burden of Disease Study 2010." *The Lancet* 380 (9859): 2197–223.

Muyindike, W., R. Fatch, R. Steinfield, L. T. Matthews, N. Musinguzi, and others. 2012. "Contraceptive Use and Associated Factors among Women Enrolling into HIV Care in Southwestern Uganda." *Infectious Diseases in Obstetrics and Gynecology* 2012: 340782.

Nanda, K., L. M. Lopez, D. A. Grimes, A. Peloggia, and G. Nanda. 2012. "Expectant Care versus Surgical Treatment for Miscarriage." *Cochrane Database of Systematic Reviews* 3 (14): CD003518.

Neilson, J. P., G. M. Gyte, M. Hickey, J. C. Vazquez, and L. Dou. 2010. "Medical Treatments for Incomplete Miscarriage (Less than 24 Weeks)." *Cochrane Database of Systematic Reviews* 20 (1): CD007223.

———. 2013. "Medical Treatments for Incomplete Miscarriage." *Cochrane Database of Systematic Reviews* 3 (28): CD007223.

Nettleman, M. D., H. Chung, J. Brewer, A. Ayoola, and P. L. Reed. 2007. "Reasons for Unprotected Intercourse: Analysis of the PRAMS Survey." *Contraception* 75 (5): 361–66.

Ngo, T. D., M. H. Park, H. Shakur, and C. Free. 2011. "Comparative Effectiveness, Safety and Acceptability of Medical Abortion at Home and in a Clinic: A Systematic Review." *Bulletin of the World Health Organization* 89 (5): 360–70.

Niinimaki, M., P. Jouppila, H. Martikainen, and A. Talvensaari-Mattila. 2006. "A Randomized Study Comparing Efficacy and Patient Satisfaction in Medical or Surgical Treatment of Miscarriage." *Fertility and Sterility* 86 (2): 367–72.

Niinimaki, M., P. Karinen, A. L. Hartikainen, and A. Pouta. 2009. "Treating Miscarriages: A Randomised Study of Cost-Effectiveness in Medical or Surgical Choice." *BJOG: An International Journal of Obstetrics and Gynaecology* 116 (7): 984–90.

O'Neill, B. C., B. Liddle, L. Jiang, K. R. Smith, S. Pachauri, and others. 2012. "Demographic Change and Carbon Dioxide Emissions." *Lancet* 380 (9837): 157–64.

Okonofua, F. 2006. "Abortion and Maternal Mortality in the Developing World." *Journal of Obstetrics and Gynaecology Canada* 28 (11): 974–79.

Peterson, H. B., Z. Xia, J. M. Hughes, L. S. Wilcox, L. R. Tylor, and others. 1996. "The Risk of Pregnancy after Tubal Sterilization: Findings from the U.S. Collaborative Review of Sterilization." *American Journal of Obstetrics and Gynecology* 174 (4): 1161–68; discussion 1168–70.

———. 1997. "The Risk of Ectopic Pregnancy after Tubal Sterilization." U.S. Collaborative Review of Sterilization Working Group. *New England Journal of Medicine* 336 (11): 762–67.

Petrou, S., J. Trinder, P. Brocklehurst, and L. Smith. 2006. "Economic Evaluation of Alternative Management Methods of First-Trimester Miscarriage Based on Results from the MIST Trial." *BJOG: An International Journal of Obstetrics and Gynaecology* 113 (8): 879–89.

Pollack, A. E., and R. M. Soderstrom. 1994. "Female Tubal Sterilization." In *Fertility Control*, 2nd ed., edited by S. L. Corson, R. J. Derman, and L. B. Tyrer, 293–318. London, ON: Goldin Publishers.

Prada, E., E. T. Mirembe, F. Ahmed, R. Nalwadda, and C. Kiggundu. 2005. *Abortion and Postabortion Care in Uganda: A Report from Health Care Professionals and Health Facilities*. Occasional Report No. 17. New York: The Alan Guttmacher Institute.

Rausch, M., S. Lorch, K. Chung, M. Frederick, J. Zhang, and others. 2012. "A Cost-Effectiveness Analysis of Surgical versus Medical Management of Early Pregnancy Loss." *Fertility and Sterility* 97 (2): 355–60.

Robson, S. C., T. Kelly, D. Howel, M. Deverill, J. Hewison, and others. 2009. "Randomised Preference Trial of Medical versus Surgical Termination of Pregnancy Less than 14 Weeks' Gestation (TOPS)." *Health Technology Assessment* 13 (53): 1–124, iii–iv.

Rocconi, R. P., S. Chiang, H. E. Richter, and J. M. Straughn Jr. 2005. "Management Strategies for Abnormal Early

Pregnancy: A Cost-Effectiveness Analysis." *Journal of Reproductive Medicine* 50 (7): 486–90.

Rock, J. A., C. A. Bergquist, H. A. Zacur, T. H. Parmley, D. S. Guzick, and others. 1982. "Tubal Anastomosis Following Unipolar Cautery." *Fertility and Sterility* 37 (5): 613–18.

Ross, J. A., and A. K. Blanc. 2012. "Why Aren't There More Maternal Deaths? A Decomposition Analysis." *Maternal and Child Health Journal* 16 (2): 456–63.

Ross, J., E. Weissman, and J. Stover. 2009. *Contraceptive Projections and the Donor Gap: Meeting the Challenge.* Brussels: Reproductive Health Supplies Coalition.

Say, L., R. Kulier, M. Gulmezoglu, and A. Campana. 2005. "Medical versus Surgical Methods for First Trimester Termination of Pregnancy." *Cochrane Database of Systematic Reviews* 25 (1): CD003037.

Schuler, S. R., M. E. Choque, and S. Rance. 1994. "Misinformation, Mistrust, and Mistreatment: Family Planning among Bolivian Market Women." *Studies in Family Planning* 25 (4): 211–21.

Sedgh, G., S. Singh, I. H. Shah, E. Ahman, S. K. Henshaw, and A. Bankole. 2012. "Induced Abortion: Incidence and Trends Worldwide from 1995 to 2008." *Lancet* 379 (9816): 625–32.

Shah, I., and E. Ahman. 2009. "Unsafe Abortion: Global and Regional Incidence, Trends, Consequences, and Challenges." *Journal of Obstetrics and Gynaecology Canada* 31 (12): 1149–58.

Shapiro, E. I., and S. J. Silber. 1979. "Open-Ended Vasectomy, Sperm Granuloma, and Postvasectomy Orchialgia." *Fertility and Sterility* 32 (5): 546–50.

Shearer, J. C., D. G. Walker, and M. Vlassoff. 2010. "Costs of Post-Abortion Care in Low- and Middle-Income Countries." *International Journal of Gynaecology and Obstetrics* 108 (2): 165–69.

Shih, G., D. K. Turok, and W. J. Parker. 2011. "Vasectomy: The Other (Better) Form of Sterilization." *Contraception* 83 (4): 310–15.

Shy, K. K., A. Stergachis, L. G. Grothaus, E. H. Wagner, J. Hecht, and others. 1992. "Tubal Sterilization and Risk of Subsequent Hospital Admission for Menstrual Disorders." *American Journal of Obstetrics and Gynecology* 166 (6 Pt 1):1698–1705; discussion 1705–06.

Singh, S. 2006. "Hospital Admissions Resulting from Unsafe Abortion: Estimates from 13 Developing Countries." *Lancet* 368 (9550): 1887–92.

———. 2010. "Global Consequences of Unsafe Abortion." *Womens Health (London, England)* 6 (6): 849–60.

Singh, S., and J. E. Darroch. 2012. "Adding It Up: Costs and Benefits of Contraceptive Services—Estimates for 2012." Guttmacher Institute and United Nations Population Fund (UNFPA), New York.

Singh, S., A. M. Moore, A. Bankole, F. Mirembe, D. Wulf, and E. Prada. 2006. *Unintended Pregnancy and Induced Abortion in Uganda: Causes and Consequences.* New York: Guttmacher Institute.

Singh, S., G. Sedgh, and R. Hussain. 2010. "Unintended Pregnancy: Worldwide Levels, Trends, and Outcomes." *Studies in Family Planning* 41 (4): 241–50.

Smith, G. L., G. P. Taylor, and K. F. Smith. 1985. "Comparative Risks and Costs of Male and Female Sterilization." *American Journal of Public Health* 75 (4): 370–74.

Sokal, D., B. Irsula, M. Hays, M. Chen-Mok, and M. A. Barone. 2004. "Vasectomy by Ligation and Excision, with or without Fascial Interposition: A Randomized Controlled Trial." *BMC Medicine* 2 (6): 6.

Song, L., Y. Gu, W. Lu, X. Liang, and Z. Chen. 2006. "A Phase II Randomized Controlled Trial of a Novel Male Contraception, an Intra-Vas Device." *International Journal of Andrology* 29 (4): 489-95. doi:10.1111/j.1365-2605.2006.00686.x.

Sotiriadis, A., G. Makrydimas, S. Papatheodorou, and J. P. Ioannidis. 2005. "Expectant, Medical, or Surgical Management of First-Trimester Miscarriage: A Meta-Analysis." *Obstetrics and Gynecology* 105 (5 Pt 1): 1104–13.

Spivak, M. M., C. L. Librach, and D. M. Rosenthal. 1986. "Microsurgical Reversal of Sterilization: A Six-Year Study." *American Journal of Obstetrics and Gynecology* 154 (2): 355–61.

Steiner, M. J., J. Trussell, N. Mehta, S. Condon, S. Subramaniam, and others. 2006. "Communicating Contraceptive Effectiveness: A Randomized Controlled Trial to Inform a World Health Organization Family Planning Handbook." *American Journal of Obstetrics and Gynecology* 195 (1): 85–91.

Stover, J., and J. Ross. 2010. "How Increased Contraceptive Use Has Reduced Maternal Mortality." *Maternal and Child Health Journal* 14 (5): 687–95.

Sundaram, A., M. Vlassoff, A. Bankole, L. Remez, and Y. Gebrehiwot. 2010. "Benefits of Meeting the Contraceptive Needs of Ethiopian Women." *Issues Brief* (Alan Guttmacher Institute) 1: 1–8.

Tasnim, N., G. Mahmud, S. Fatima, and M. Sultana. 2011. "Manual Vacuum Aspiration: A Safe and Cost-Effective Substitute of Electric Vacuum Aspiration for the Surgical Management of Early Pregnancy Loss." *Journal of Pakistan Medical Association* 61 (2): 149–53.

Tawiah, E. O. 1997. "Factors Affecting Contraceptive Use in Ghana." *Journal of Biosocial Science* 29 (2): 141–49.

Thorburn, S., and L. M. Bogart. 2005. "Conspiracy Beliefs about Birth Control: Barriers to Pregnancy Prevention among African Americans of Reproductive Age." *Health Education and Behavior* 32 (4): 474–87.

Trussell, J. 2011a. "Contraceptive Efficacy." In *Contraceptive Technology: Twentieth Revised Edition*, edited by R. A. Hatcher, J. Trussell, A. L. Nelson, W. Cates, D. Kowal, and others. New York: Ardent Media.

———. 2011b. "Contraceptive Failure in the United States." *Contraception* 83 (5): 397–404.

Trussell, J., A. M. Lalla, Q. V. Doan, E. Reyes, L. Pinto, and others. 2009. "Cost Effectiveness of Contraceptives in the United States." *Contraception* 79 (1): 5–14.

Tuncalp, O., A. M. Gulmezoglu, and J. P. Souza. 2010. "Surgical Procedures for Evacuating Incomplete Miscarriage." *Cochrane Database of Systematic Reviews* 8 (9): CD001993.

Vlassoff, M., G. Beninguisse, F. Kamgaing, F. Zinvi-Dossou, J. Jerman, and others. 2014. "Benefits of Meeting the

Contraceptive Needs of Cameroonian Women." *In Brief*, Guttmacher Institute, No. 1.

Vlassoff, M., T. Fetters, S. Kumbi, and S. Singh. 2012. "The Health System Cost of Postabortion Care in Ethiopia." *International Journal of Gynaecology and Obstetrics* 118 (Suppl 2): S127–33.

Vlassoff, M., S. Furere, I. R. Kalisa, F. Ngabo, F. Sayinzoga, and others. 2014. "The Health System Cost of Post-abortion Care in Rwanda." *Health Policy and Planning* (advance online access). doi:10.1093/heapol/czu006.

Vlassoff, M., J. Jerman, G. Beninguisse, F. Kamgaing, and F. Zinvi-Dossou. 2014. "Benefits of Meeting the Contraceptive Needs of Cameroonian Women." *Issues Brief* (Alan Guttmacher Institute) 1: 1–13.

Vlassoff, M., A. Sundaram, A. Bankole, L. Remez, and D. Belemsaga-Yugbare. 2011. "Benefits of Meeting Women's Contraceptive Needs in Burkina Faso." *Issues Brief* (Alan Guttmacher Institute) 1: 1–33.

Vlassoff, M., A. Sundaram, A. Bankole, L. Remez, and F. Mugisha. 2009. "Benefits of Meeting the Contraceptive Needs of Ugandan Women." *Issues Brief (Alan Guttmacher Institute)* 4 (4): 1–8.

Vlassoff, M., D. Walker, J. Shearer, D. Newlands, and S. Singh. 2009. "Estimates of Health Care System Costs of Unsafe Abortion in Africa and Latin America." *International Perspectives on Sexual and Reproductive Health* 35 (3): 114–21.

Vos, T., A. D. Flaxman, M. Naghavi, R. Lozano, C. Michaud, and others. 2013. "Years Lived with Disability (YLDs) for 1,160 Sequelae of 289 Diseases and Injuries 1990–2010: A Systematic Analysis for the Global Burden of Disease Study 2010." *Lancet* 380 (9859): 2163–96.

Warriner, I. K., and I. H. Shah. 2006. *Preventing Unsafe Abortion and Its Consequences: Priorities for Research and Action.* New York: Guttmacher Institute.

Weiss, R. S., and P. S. Li. 2005. "No-Needle Jet Anesthetic Technique for No-Scalpel Vasectomy." *Journal of Urology* 173 (5): 1677–80.

WHO (World Health Organization). 1992. *The Prevention and Management of Unsafe Abortion.* Report of a Technical Working Group (WHO/MSM/92.5). Geneva: WHO.

———. 1999. *Female Sterilization: What Health Workers Need to Know.* Geneva: WHO.

———. 2007. "Task Shifting to Tackle Health Worker Shortages." WHO, Geneva.

———. 2012. *Optimizing Health Worker Roles for Maternal and Newborn Health Interventions through Task Shifting.* Geneva: WHO.

Wickstrom, J., and R. Jacobstein. 2011. "Contraceptive Security: Incomplete without Long-Acting and Permanent Methods of Family Planning." *Studies in Family Planning* 42 (4): 291–98.

Wu, Y., and X. Wu. 1958. "A Report of 300 Cases Using Vacuum Aspiration for the Termination of Pregnancy." *Chinese Journal of Obstetrics and Gynaecology* (in English translation from *BMJ*): 447–49.

Xia, W., S. She, and T. H. Lam. 2011. "Medical versus Surgical Abortion Methods for Pregnancy in China: A Cost-Minimization Analysis." *Gynecologic and Obstetric Investigation* 72 (4): 257–63.

You, J. H., and T. K. Chung. 2005. "Expectant, Medical or Surgical Treatment for Spontaneous Abortion in First Trimester of Pregnancy: A Cost Analysis." *Human Reproduction* 20 (10): 2873–78.

Zipper, J., and E. Kessel. 2003. "Quinacrine Sterilization: A Retrospective." *International Journal of Gynaecology and Obstetrics* 83 (Suppl 2): S7–11.

Zite, N., and S. Borrero. 2011. "Female Sterilisation in the United States." *European Journal of Contraception and Reproductive Health Care* 16 (5): 336–40.

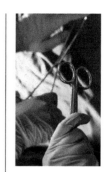

Chapter **8**

Surgical Interventions for Congenital Anomalies

Diana Farmer, Nicole Sitkin, Katrine Lofberg,
Peter Donkor, and Doruk Ozgediz

INTRODUCTION

Great strides have been made during the past 50 years in the diagnosis and management of congenital anomalies, once referred to as birth defects. Formally fatal conditions can now be treated with success rates exceeding 90 percent. Yet improvements in care have been largely limited to high-income countries (HICs), even though many anomalies can be cured with simple operations (Chirdan, Ngiloi, and Elhalaby 2012). If surgery is the neglected stepchild of global health (Farmer and Kim 2008), then pediatric surgery is the child not yet born.

Improving the accessibility and quality of pediatric surgical care in low-income (LICs) and lower-middle-income countries (LMICs) has the potential to substantially reduce childhood mortality and lifelong disability. Data on congenital anomalies in these countries are sparse, including on the incidence (conservatively estimated at 3 percent to 6 percent [CDC 2012; Christianson, Howson, and Modell 2006]), country-specific differences in disease burden, and cost-effective interventions. These areas of knowledge must be developed to identify implementation and surveillance priorities, and to advocate for resources.

This chapter briefly summarizes the growing body of knowledge on surgical congenital anomalies in LICs and LMICs, highlights prevalent anomalies that exemplify the

unrealized promise of pediatric surgery, and concludes with crucial future steps to reduce the burden of disease.

Chapter 21 addresses economic evaluation of cleft lip and palate repair.

MORBIDITY, MORTALITY, AND ADDITIONAL ADVERSE CONSEQUENCES

Congenital anomalies are one of the leading causes of global disease, responsible for a staggering 57.7 million disability-adjusted life years (DALYs) lost worldwide (WHO 2013b). DALYs—a measure of the number of healthy life years lost to premature death or disability—are an established metric for the burden of disease.

Current estimates of the surgical burden of disease are acknowledged to be a "best educated guess," given the "near total lack of pertinent data" (Jamison and others 2006, 1246). Even less is known about pediatric surgical disease (Bickler and Rode 2002). The studies that have begun to fill this knowledge gap paint a brutal picture. The burden of congenital anomalies falls most heavily on LICs and LMICs, where 94 percent of anomalies occur (WHO 2012). Higher fertility rates translate to higher birth rates and more children born with anomalies. Disease incidence (or frequency of disease occurring in the population) is also higher, a phenomenon attributed to higher micronutrient and macronutrient deficiencies,

Corresponding author: Diana Farmer, MD, University of California, Davis, diana.farmer@ucdmc.ucdavis.edu exposure to teratogens, prevalence of intrauterine infection, and self-medication with unsupervised drugs or traditional remedies (Christianson, Howson, and Modell 2006; Penchaszadeh 2002). Though decreased fertility may reduce incidence of anomalies, most are not otherwise preventable and are treated through surgical interventions.

Some anomalies are "quick fixes" that can be easily repaired; others require staged, or multioperation, surgical interventions, and delays in treatment may result in lifelong illness, disability, and poor quality of life. The paucity of surgical resources in LICs and LMICs means that anomalies attributed to the former category in HICs often fall into the latter in LICs and LMICs. Anomalies resulting in visible deformity—such as clubfoot and cleft lip—cause stigma, which can trigger abandonment or infanticide. Invisible deformities that result in chronic disability can lead to similar outcomes. A long-term, "incurable" anomaly may also endanger families' well-being because key resources are allocated to care for the afflicted child. Families may fracture, with one or both parents leaving the child with other family members.

Improving the pediatric surgical capabilities of LICs and LMICs will dramatically reduce this burden. Because children are the future economic engine powering the development of these countries, the value of investing in surgical care for children extends beyond DALYs averted to encompass the future socioeconomic well-being of LICs and LMICs themselves. It is critical to address the gaps in knowledge that impede the development of effective care systems.

Data Collection Challenges

Many LICs and LMICs lack rigorous congenital anomaly surveillance programs, making calculations of incidence and prevalence (the total number of individuals in the population with a given disease) difficult (Penchaszadeh 2002). Estimates, which range from 4 to 12 cases per 1,000 births, likely undervalue the problem because of stigma and exclusion (Bickler and others 2010; Goksan and others 2006; Wu and Poenaru 2013). LICs and LMICs often report incidence in cases over time, as opposed to using standard metrics, such as incidence per 10,000 live births. Incidence and prevalence data are also skewed by the survivability of the anomaly under consideration. Because children with anomalies that are not immediately life threatening are more likely to reach medical centers, the relative incidence and prevalence of immediately life-threatening impairments appears comparatively lower in hospital-based data (Nandi, Mungongo, and Lakhoo 2008). Population-based surveys—which directly collect data from noncentralized sites—are one

approach to addressing this challenge (Wu, Poenaru, and Poley 2013).

Mortality Rate Estimation Challenges

The burden of disease associated with congenital anomalies in LICs and LMICs is most often calculated as the mortality rate, including neither measures of morbidity nor the cost of ongoing illness (table 8.1). Analysis of mortality data in these countries can be challenging; for example, autopsies were performed in only 0.8 percent of nearly 1,100 neonatal deaths in Benin. In all examined cases, autopsies provided additional information on the cause of death (Ugiagbe and Osifo 2012). Furthermore, a high proportion of children with surgical diseases do not reach a health facility and die at home or in transit, suggesting a sizable hidden mortality (Mo Suwan and others 2009; Ozgediz and others 2008). Nonfatal anomalies can result in extensive, ongoing morbidity. The burden of disease is grossly underestimated if this measure of impairment is not included. Extant calculations do, however, highlight marked disparities in outcomes between HICs, on the one hand, and LICs and LMICs, on the other hand.

CHALLENGES TO PROVIDING CARE FOR CONGENITAL ANOMALIES

Despite the higher incidence of congenital anomalies in LICs and LMICs, lower population prevalence is seen compared with HICS, most likely indicating a high infant and child mortality rate (Christianson, Howson, and Modell 2006). *In LICs and LMICs, up to 10 percent of infants die during the neonatal period* (Zupan 2005); a considerable portion of this mortality can reasonably be attributed to congenital anomalies.

Treatment Delays

Heightened mortality rates stem from delays in treatment caused by the paucity of health professionals trained to identify and treat anomalies and by pejorative cultural beliefs surrounding anomalies. In LICs and LMICs, many births occur at home, either with no assistance or with traditional birth attendants (TBAs), and patients must often travel great distances to reach medical facilities. Hypothermia—a dangerous drop in body temperature—is common following medically unsupervised transport over long distances, with severe repercussions on patient outcomes (Agarwala and others 1996;

Table 8.1 Prevalence and Mortality of Selected Congenital Anomalies in Selected Countries

Congenital anomalies	High-income countries		Selected countries		
	Reference prevalence	Reference mortality (percent)	Country of reporting institution	Prevalence at reporting institution	Mortality (percent)
Anorectal malformations	1 per 5,000 live births[a]	<5[a]	Iran, Islamic Rep.[b]	22 (1993–96)	27.3 (1993–96)
				106 (2002–05)	13.2 (2002–05)
			Nigeria[c]	88 over 17 years	30.2
			India[d]	125 over 2 years	22.0
			Nigeria[e]	81 over 8 years (38 percent of neonatal obstructions)	32.0
			Nigeria[f]	54 over 10 years	20.4
			Ethiopia[g]	27 over 5 years	33.0
			India[h]	948 over 14 years	15.0–20.0 (staged repair)
					4.5 (primary repair)
			Nigeria[i]	55 over 10 years	20.0
Hirschsprung's disease	1 per 5,000 live births[a]	Less than 5–10[j, k]	Iran, Islamic Rep.[b]	8 (1993–96)	25.0 (1993–96)
				50 (2002–05)	4.0 (2002–05)
			Nigeria[e]	30 over 8 years (14 percent of neonatal obstructions)	20.0
			Nigeria[i]	24 over 10 years (18.7 percent of neonatal obstructions)	20.8
			Bangladesh[l]	1,273 over 5.5 years	14.3
			Burkina Faso[m]	52 over 7 years	16.0
			Eritrea[n]	11 over 5 years	9.1
			Nigeria[o]	78 over 10 years	22.6
Congenital heart disease	8.2 per 1,000 live births (Europe)[p]	3–7[q]	Guatemala[r]	1,215 over 8 years	10.7 (overall) 32.1 (highest-risk patients)
	6.9 per 1,000 live births (North America)[p]		India[s]	330 over 8 years	21.4 (1999–2001)
					4.3 (2002–06)
			Nepal[t]	5.8 per 1,000 children	20.2
			Sri Lanka[u]	102 over 1 year	18.6
Esophageal atresia	One per 3,500 live births[a]	5–15[a]	India[v]	50 over 2 years	30.0
			Barbados[w]	2.06 per 10,000 live births	30.8
			Saudi Arabia[x]	48 over 20 years	25.0
			Bangladesh[y]	21 over 2 years	47.6
			China[z]	15 over 10 years	46.7 following surgery
			Malaysia[aa]	52 over 10 years	23.0

table continues next page

Table 8.1 Prevalence and Mortality of Selected Congenital Anomalies in Selected Countries (continued)

| Congenital anomalies | High-income countries | | Selected countries | | |
	Reference prevalence	Reference mortality (percent)	Country of reporting institution	Prevalence at reporting institution	Mortality (percent)
			Pakistan[ab]	80 over 1 year, excluding isolated esophageal atresia patients	58.0
			Saudi Arabia[ac]	94 over 15 years	30.8
			Iran, Islamic Rep.[b]	22 (1993–96)	75.0 (1993–96)
				106 (2002–05)	58.8 (2002–05)
			Ethiopia[a]	12 over 5 years	91.7
Gastroschisis	3.3 to 5 per 10,000 live births[a, ad, ae]	1 (30-day mortality)[af]	Ghana; Nigeria; South Africa[af]	Over four years: 2 (Ghana) 5 (Nigeria) 19 (South Africa)	23.0 (30-day mortality)
			Iran, Islamic Rep.[b]	2 (1993–96)	100 (1993–96)
				7 (2002–05)	85.7 (2002–05)
			Iran, Islamic Rep.[ag]	0.65 per 1,000 births	80.0 (2005–07)
				10 per 15,321 live births (2005–07)	
			Nigeria[ah]	14 over 10 years	71.4
			Nigeria[ai]	12 over 11 years	33.0
			Colombia[aj]	32 over 9 years	18.8
			South Africa[ak]	106 over 6 years;	43.0 (total)
				6 neonatal surgical admissions (2003);	68.0 patients with staged, silo-assisted closure
				15 neonatal surgical admissions (2007)	
			Thailand[al]	49 over 3 years	14.0
			Nigeria[am]	7 of 2,381 patients treated at the pediatric surgery unit over eight years	57.1
Omphalocele	2.18–5 per 10,000 live births[a, ad, ae]	5[a]	Iran, Islamic Rep.[b]	12 (1993–96)	75.0 (1993–96)
				68 (2002–05)	58.8 (2002–05)
			Iran, Islamic Rep.[ag]	2.1 per 1,000 births	20.0 (2005–07)
				42 of 15,321 live newborn births (2005–07)	
			Nigeria[ai]	42 over 11 years	43.0
			Colombia[aj]	23 over 9 years	43.5
			Nigeria[am]	49 over 8 years	32.4 (patients with omphalocele major)

table continues next page

Table 8.1 Prevalence and Mortality of Selected Congenital Anomalies in Selected Countries (continued)

Congenital anomalies	High-income countries			Selected countries		
	Reference prevalence	Reference mortality (percent)	Country of reporting institution	Prevalence at reporting institution	Mortality (percent)
Congenital diaphragmatic hernia	1 per 2,000 to 1 per 5,000 live births[a]	≤ 10[an]	Turkey[ao]	10 over 4 years	50.0
			Tunisia[ap]	28 over 13 years	39.0
			Nigeria[aq]	64 over 24 years	35.5 (overall)
					60.0 in patients born in hospital
					28.5 in patients born outside hospital who survive until presentation
			Nigeria[ar]	7 over 6 years	43.0
			Malaysia[as]	21 over 6 years	47.6

Sources: Anorectal malformations, Ethiopia: Anorectal malformations, India: Anorectal malformations, Iran, Islamic Rep.: Anorectal malformations, Nigeria:
a. Coran and others 2012. b. Peyvasteh and others 2011. c. Adejuyigbe and others 2004. d. Chalapathi and others 2004. e. Adeyemi 1989. f. Archibong and Idika 2004. g. Tefera, Teka, and Derbew 2007. h. Gangopadhyay and others 2005. i. Ekenze, Ibeziako, and Ezomike 2007. j. Rescorla and others 1992. k. Swenson 2002. l. Banu and others 2009. m. Bandre and others 2010. n. Calisti and others 2011. o. Chirdan and Uba 2006. p. van der Linde and others 2011. q. Bernier and others 2010. r. Larrazabal and others 2007. s. Bakshi and others 2007. t. Shah and others 2008. u. Wickramasinghe, Lambabadusuriya, and Narenthiran 2001. v. Upadhyaya and others 2007. w. Singh and others 2012. x. Rayes 2010, y. Islam and Aziz 2011. z. Yang and others 2006. aa. Narasimman, Nallusamy, and Hassan 2013. ab. Anwar-ul-Haq and others 2009. ac. Al-Salem and others 2006. ad. Sadler 2010. ae. Canfield and others 2006. af. Manson and others 2012. ag. Askarpour and others 2012. ah. Ameh and Chirdan 2000b. ai. Uba and Chirdan 2003. aj. Toro, Rave, and Gomez 2010. ak. Sekabira and Hadley 2009. al. Saranrittichai 2008. am. Abdur-Rahman, Abdulrasheed, and Adeniran 2011. an. Chiu and Hedrick 2008. ao. Ozdogan and others 2010. ap. Khemakhem and others 2012. aq. Adegboye and others 2002. ar. Abubakar and others 2011. as. Rohana, Boo, and Thambidorai 2008.

Sekabira and Hadley 2009; Uba and Chirdan 2003). The misdiagnosis of anomalies as better-known infectious diseases, and added delays for invisible anomalies, may further hinder the provision of timely, appropriate services. These multifactorial delays are a crucial hurdle in treating both immediately and non-immediately life-threatening anomalies. While non-immediately life-threatening anomalies often require emergency interventions, the period before these conditions become emergencies can be better used to dramatically improve outcomes.

Scarcity of Skilled Surgeons

The scarcity of trained surgeons in LICs and LMICs also significantly contributes to the burden: one pediatric general surgeon may serve millions of children (Chirdan and others 2010), and physicians performing pediatric surgery may have little or no pediatric surgery training (Ekenze, Ibeziako, and Ezomike 2007; Mhando, Young, and Lakhoo 2008). Whereas North America has an estimated one pediatric cardiac surgeon per 3 million people, Sub-Saharan Africa has one per 38 million people (Bernier and others 2010); 75 percent of the world's population is estimated to have no access to cardiac surgery (Hoffman 2013). Similarly, 33 percent of the world's population is covered by 5 percent of its neurosurgeons (Warf 2013). Expanding the pool of specially trained

surgeons and surgery teams must be a fundamental goal of ongoing and future programs to address the pediatric surgical burden of disease.

ESTIMATING THE IMPACT OF PEDIATRIC SURGERY ON THE GLOBAL BURDEN OF DISEASE

In the World Health Organization's (WHO's) most recent Global Health Estimates, congenital anomalies constitute 2.1 percent of the total disease burden and rank eleventh in the causes of disease burden (WHO 2013b). Although impressive, these figures are likely to be underestimates because of the limited number of anomalies included in the analysis and the difficulties in evaluating incidence, morbidity, and mortality. Only six congenital surgical conditions had disability weights in the 2004 estimates, and congenital anomalies were not among the new disability weights estimated in 2012 (Saloman and others 2012; WHO 2008).

Some researchers have tried to fill the gap with evidence-based estimates of selected disability weights (Poenaru and others 2013). Of the conditions measured in the Global Health Estimates, cardiac anomalies represent the greatest overall burden (table 8.2), and, along with neural tube anomalies and cleft lip and palate, cause

32 million DALYs. Some 57 percent, or 18 million, of these DALYs are estimated to be surgically preventable if outcomes in HICs could be achieved in LICs and LMICs (Higashi, Barendregt, and Vos 2013). These anomalies typify the reservoir of unmet need that congenital anomalies in LICs and LMICs create (table 8.3).

Only a small body of literature evaluates the potential of surgery to reduce this burden in terms of DALYs averted or cost-effectiveness. Yet, these foundational studies have provided compelling evidence that pediatric surgery is a cost-effective intervention with the potential to avert more than 67 percent of the DALYs associated with congenital anomalies (Corlew 2010; Higashi, Barendregt, and Vos 2013; Ozgediz and Poenaru 2012; Poenaru 2013; Wu and Poenaru 2013; Wu, Poenaru, and Poley 2013). Favorable outcomes have been reported in HICs for such conditions as anorectal malformations (ARMs) and congenital diaphragmatic hernia (Poley and others 2008). In LICs and LMICs, the human capital approach to cleft lip and palate repair (see chapter 21) has provided very favorable cost-effectiveness analysis estimates. An extension of this methodology to treatment for congenital swelling of the brain in Uganda has also yielded favorable results, at a cost of US$59 to US$126 per DALY averted (Warf and others 2011). Surgical repair of congenital inguinal hernias in Uganda has been estimated to have an incremental cost-effectiveness of US$12 per DALY averted (Eason and others 2012). Another report from Cambodia estimates a cost-effectiveness of US$99 per DALY averted over three months for reconstructive surgery for an array of anomalies (Rattray and others 2013).

Table 8.2 Burden of Disease due to Congenital Anomalies

Anomaly	DALYs (thousand)	YLDs
Cardiac	20,760	565
Neural tube	10,075	759
Down syndrome	2,939	1,225
Cleft lip	709	254
Other chromosomal	2,941	694
Other congenital	20,272	1,835
Total	57,696	5,332

Source: WHO 2013b.
Note: DALYs = disability-adjusted life years; YLDs = years living with disability.

Table 8.3 Prevalent Congenital Anomalies and Avertable Disease Burden

Congenital anomaly	Brief description	Treatment opportunities
Cardiac anomalies	Most prevalent anomalies *Incidence:* Approximately 8 per 1,000 births *Most common:* Ventricular septal defect (hole between the lower chambers of the heart)	Backlog of 1 million to 2 million children need congenital cardiac surgery in India. Requires relatively resource-intensive treatment compared with other anomalies; estimated US$2,500 per operation in some programs (Hoffman 2013). Cost containment and capacity-building strategies have been described (Rao 2007).
Neural tube defects	*Incidence:* Nearly 1 per 1,000 births *Most common:* Spina bifida	Preventable through folate supplementation, a major public health strategy in many LICs and LMICs. ETV is an innovative, sustainable strategy to treat associated hydrocephalus, or swelling of the brain, with favorable results compared with traditional treatment. Longer-term follow-up confirms the feasibility and effectiveness of community-based strategies for ETV (Warf and others 2011; Warf 2011).
Cleft lip and palate	*Incidence:* 1 per 700 live births; slightly higher in some regions, like Sub-Saharan Africa (Poenaru 2013) Approximately 25 percent of cases associated with other anomalies	Global backlog of unrepaired cleft cases is between 400,000 and 2 million cases. Guidelines suggest that cleft lip should be repaired in the first six months of life; cleft palate, in the first year to 18 months. Average age at time of repair is nearly age 10 years in Sub-Saharan Africa (Poenaru 2013). Cleft lip may require a single corrective operation. Approximately 20 percent of palate repair cases may require subsequent surgery; postoperative speech therapy is essential (Semer 2001).

Sources: Hoffman 2013; Poenaru 2013; Rao 2007; Semer 2001; Warf and others 2011; Warf 2011.
Note: ETV = endoscopic third ventriculostomy; LICs = low-income countries; LMICs = lower-middle-income countries.

The benefits of improved pediatric surgical services in averted morbidity and cost extend across the lifespan. Treating congenital disease at its inception may result in a significantly greater reduction in the burden of disease. The following sections present examples of anomalies that are prime targets for intervention. Because of the lack of cost-effectiveness data, these anomalies are presented as case studies that highlight the preventable burden of disease and the potential of low-cost measures adapted to low-resource settings (i.e., low-income countries [LICs] and LMICs) to substantially improve outcomes. Further research is urgently needed to develop and evaluate cost-effective treatment programs to take advantage of the substantial DALY upside of treating congenital anomalies. Congenital heart conditions are discussed in more detail in volume 5, *Cardiovascular, Respiratory, Renal, and Endocrine Disorders.*

Case Study 1: Congenital Colorectal Disease— Anorectal Malformations and Hirschprung's Disease

Description. ARMs and Hirschsprung's disease (HD) are two of the most prevalent congenital anomalies.

- ARMs are physical anomalies that prevent the passage of fecal matter through a distinct anus. Examples include absence of an anus or fusion of the anus to other openings in the body (for example, the urethra).
- HD is a functional obstruction of the bowel caused by the absence of the nerve cells needed to stimulate normal contractile movement of the bowel. If food matter cannot move through the bowel, material collects in the preceding bowel and dilates it, causing megacolon. The intestinal tract may perforate, causing widespread infection and death.

HD and some ARMs are not immediately life threatening when partial passage of fecal material is possible. For example, female children in LICs and LMICs with the most common female ARM—vestibular fistula, whereby the rectum opens into the vagina—often remain undiagnosed until much later in life. Untreated, however, non-immediately life-threatening conditions can lead to substantial morbidity and eventual mortality due to intestinal rupture.

The etiology of ARMs is unclear, but both genetic and environmental factors have been implicated (Davies, Creighton, and Wilcox 2004). The incidence of ARMs is cited as one per 3,000 to 5,000 live births (Chalapathi and others 2004; Chowdhary and others 2004; Eltayeb 2010), but this incidence varies with ethnicity and geography (Moore and others 2008; van Heurn and others 2002). ARMs are reportedly more common in Sub-Saharan Africa and constitute a significant clinical load (Calisti and others 2011; Moore and others 2008). HD has been associated with a number of congenital syndromes and anomalies, and may have various genetic causes (Amiel and others 2008). The incidence of HD is comparable to that of ARMs (Coran and others 2012) and is one of the leading causes of pediatric intestinal obstruction in LICs and LMICs (Adeyemi 1989; Ameh and Chirdan 2000a; Saha and others 2012). Hidden mortality and traditional health practices (for example, enemas) mask prevalence (Bandre and others 2010), suggesting that the burden of disease may be significantly underestimated.

Diagnosis and Treatment in LICs and LMICs. ARMs are usually diagnosed on physical examination. HD is not visually identifiable, so must be diagnosed based on the symptoms—feeding intolerance, vomiting, abdominal distension, delayed passage of the meconium (the first stool passed by a newborn) and severe neonatal intestinal infection, or enterocolitis (Amiel and others 2008). Meconium passage may serve as a valuable screening tool for HD in HICs, LICs, and LMICs; 95 percent of children with HD do not pass the meconium within the first 24 hours of life, while only 1 percent of children without HD experience a comparable delay.

HD is definitively diagnosed via rectal biopsy[1] (Amiel and others 2008), but diagnostic ability may be limited in LICs and LMICs because of the cost of biopsy analysis and the scarcity of pathology services (Bandre and others 2010). Many practitioners are forced to provide definitive treatment without confirmation of the HD diagnosis. Analytic protocols for biopsy specimens can, however, be adapted to the resources of medical laboratories in LICs and LMICs (Babu and others 2003; Poenaru and others 2010), and inexpensive radiography can replace costly endoscopic technologies in preoperative planning (Pratap and others 2007).

In LICs and LMICs, late presentation for nonemergency congenital colorectal disease is the norm. More than 60 percent of patients with HD present late, as children, adolescents, and even adults (Ameh and Chirdan 2000a; Poenaru and others 2010; Sharma and Gupta 2012; Vincent and Jackman 2009). Delayed diagnosis results from a web of interacting societal, cultural, and socioeconomic factors that delay the diagnosis of other anomalies detailed in this chapter. Presentation and diagnosis are delayed by geographical and financial barriers to care, social taboo, cultural norms (for example, routine traditional enemas), lack of awareness among medical personnel in first- and second-level facilities, inaccurate medical advice, and failed or unwarranted procedures at other medical facilities (Al-Jazaeri and others 2012; Bandre and others 2010; Ekenze, Ngaikedi, and

Obasi 2011; Sharma and Gupta 2012; Sinha and others 2008; Vincent and Jackman 2009). Delayed diagnosis of ARMs leads to severe morbidities and elevated mortality, which are further heightened for infants in rural areas where delayed diagnosis is coupled with subsequent transport to distant medical facilities (Adejuyigbe and others 2004; Chalapathi and others 2004; Eltayeb 2010; Turowski, Dingemann, and Giilick 2010).

Delayed presentation of HD is characterized by chronic constipation, abdominal distension, bowel loops visible through the abdominal wall, failure to thrive, anemia, malnutrition, and fecal impaction (Al-Jazaeri and others 2012; Coran and Teitelbaum 2000; Ekenze, Ngaikedi, and Obasi 2011; Frykman and Short 2012; Prato and others 2011; Sharma and Gupta 2012). Some patients present with bloody diarrhea due to HD-associated enterocolitis, the leading cause of HD-related morbidity.

In HICs, mortality for ARMs is negligible. In LICs and LMICs, mortality reaches 20 percent to 30 percent (Adejuyigbe and others 2004; Adeyemi 1989; Archibong and Idika 2004; Chalapathi and others 2004; Ekenze, Ibeziako, and Ezomike 2007; Peyvasteh and others 2011; Tefera, Teka, and Derbew 2007). The mortality rate for HD is less than 5 percent to 10 percent in HICs (Rescorla and others 1992; Swenson 2002) but jumps to 20 percent to 43 percent in LICs and LMICs (Adeyemi 1989; Ameh and Chirdan 2000a; Bandre and others 2010; Ekenze, Ibeziako, and Ezomike 2007). These disparities are linked to delayed diagnosis and treatment, sepsis,[2] and the absence of critical care when patients present with advanced complications (Adeniran and Abdur-Rahman 2005; Chalapathi and others 2004; Chowdhary and others 2004).

Both ARMs and HD can be treated with either primary (one-step) or staged (multistep) surgical repair (Coran and others 2012). These operations generally do not require intensive postoperative care, but they do require general anesthesia. Delays in diagnosis often preclude primary repair because these repairs cannot be performed when the bowel is grossly distended. In such cases, a colostomy[3] is a life-saving first step in staged repair. Colostomy complications, however, are common in HICs, LICs, and LMICs (Chalya and others 2011; Chandramouli and others 2004; Patwardhan and others 2001). The risks are compounded in LICs and LMICs by the prohibitive cost of colostomy bags, cultural prejudice, and limited parental understanding (Adeniran and Abdur-Rahman 2005; Chandramouli and others 2004; Olivieri and others 2012). Although simple, inexpensive treatments may ameliorate some of these challenges (Chalya and others 2011), a significant burden remains. Many children live for years with colostomies without receiving definitive repair. The burden on families of caring for children with long-term colostomies has not yet been well captured.

Primary repair reduces the number of surgeries, minimizing treatment costs and averting colostomy-related morbidity and mortality. Good outcomes in LICs and LMICs have been reported (Adeniran and Abdur-Rahman 2005; Elhalaby 2006; Ibrahim 2007; Osifo and Okolo 2009; Pratap and others 2007), with mortality rates rivaling those in HICs (Ibrahim 2007; Osifo and Okolo 2009). However, the prevalence of delayed diagnosis and treatment render routine primary repair risky. Reducing delays is key to relieving the preventable burden of congenital colorectal disease. Suggestions include the following (Adeniran and Abdur-Rahman 2005; Al-Jazaeri and others 2012; Ameh and others 2006; Ekenze, Ngaikedi, and Obasi 2011; Olivieri and others 2012; Peyvestah 2011; Poenaru and others 2010):

- Increase the number of third-level facilities (major hospitals offering a full spectrum of services)
- Increase participation of existing third-level facilities in the training of community health centers in diagnosis and preoperative management
- Improve training at the level of the TBA, primary care provider, and community health worker
- Modify medical education curricula to encompass ARMs and HD
- Target surgeons at first-level hospitals to perform colostomies with available resources
- Institute low-cost modifications to standard repair procedures

Substantial loss to follow-up after colostomy formation in LICs and LMICs remains a challenge, and innovative approaches to ensuring patient return or local follow-up in home regions must be developed to overcome barriers to continuity of care.

Case Study 2: Abdominal Wall Defects—Omphalocele and Gastroschisis

Description. Omphalocele and gastroschisis are abdominal wall defects in which the internal organs, or viscera, protrude through the abdominal wall. In omphalocele, the gut and other abdominal organs, such as the liver, spleen, and gonads, protrude through the abdominal wall into a membranous sac. In gastroschisis, no sac is present and usually only the gut protrudes from the abdomen (Coran and others 2012). Patients with omphalocele can be fed if the sac is intact; those with gastroschisis cannot be fed and quickly perish without treatment.

The incidence of omphalocele is approximately 2.18 to 5 per 10,000 live births; that of gastroschisis is 3.3 to

5 per 10,000 live births (Canfield and others 2006; Coran and others 2012; Sadler 2010; Stoll and others 2001). The incidence of gastroschisis is on the rise and varies geographically (Andrew, Holland, and Badawi 2010; Arnold 2004; Benjamin and others 2010; Castilla, Mastroiacovo, and Orioli 2008; Laughon and others 2003; Loane, Dolk, and Bradbury 2007; Vu and others 2008).

Risk factors for omphalocele include chromosomal anomalies, very young and very advanced maternal age, lack of multivitamin and folic acid supplementation during pregnancy, and maternal history of fevered illness (Botto and others 2002; Botto, Mulinare, and Erickson 2002; Frolov, Alali, and Klein 2010; Mills and others 2012). Gastroschisis has not yet been associated with any particular genes. Risk factors for gastroschisis include young maternal age, low socioeconomic status, poor nutrition, and lack of vitamin supplementation during pregnancy (Coran and others 2012). Mothers in LICs and LMICs are more likely to have children at both younger and more advanced ages, to have limited family planning knowledge and resources, and to suffer nutritional deficiencies. Accordingly, their children are likely to be at greater risk for omphalocele and gastroschisis.

Diagnosis and Treatment in LICs and LMICs. Ultrasonography, a low-cost technology once in place, can detect omphalocele and gastroschisis before birth with high success (Richmond and Atkins 2005). This technology can inform decisions about pregnancy termination and mode of delivery, facilitating improvements in outcomes.

Several effective surgical strategies for omphalocele have been described. Gastroschisis necessitates greater attention to heat loss and moisture preservation because a larger surface area of viscera is exposed. Historically, primary closure has been the treatment of choice in that it limits damage incurred by exposure. Recent studies have shown that using a silo (a moisture-retaining bag that holds the viscera before they are returned to the abdomen) and postponing closure for hours to days can be equally effective (Coran and others 2012).

Treatment is highly effective in HICs; multiple series report survival rates of 70 percent to 95 percent for omphalocele and 90 percent or greater for gastroschisis (Coran and others 2012). In comparison, the mortality associated with omphalocele and gastroschisis in LICs and LMICs is shockingly elevated, with survival falling to less than 20 percent in some studies (Askarpour and others 2012; Richmond and Atkins 2005). Delayed presentation plays a key role because hypothermia and gangrenous bowel may develop in the interim (Ameh and Chirdan 2000b; Sekabira and Hadley 2009; Uba and Chirdan 2003). An additional challenge with gastroschisis is that bowel function can be impaired initially, necessitating the use of intravenous nutrition, often not available in poorer countries. It has been suggested that in-house birth at centers equipped to medically manage patients with abdominal wall defects is essential to improving outcomes, as is improving training for transport personnel, obstetricians, and primary care physicians (Sekabira and Hadley 2009). Training TBAs to recognize omphalocele and gastroschisis, and to place children from the shoulder down in clean polyethylene bags to protect the bowels during transport, is another viable option for reducing complications associated with delayed presentation (Ameh and Chirdan 2000b).

Surgical procedures commonly used in HICs may increase mortality in LICs and LMICs, largely as a result of infection and sepsis (Ameh and Chirdan 2000b; Uba and Chirdan 2003); nonsurgical or altered surgical procedures may be preferable. Uba and Chirdan (2003) report the successful treatment of unruptured omphalocele using daily application of scab-inducing topical ointments, leading to eventual skin growth over the defect. Bedside placement of a silo bag followed by gradual reduction of the viscera into the abdomen and sutureless repair is a potentially cost-effective treatment strategy worthy of additional evaluation in LICs and LMICs. Several studies have investigated low-cost alternatives to silos, including transfusion bags and female condoms (Bustorff-Silva and others 2008; Miranda and others 1999). The female condom is particularly intriguing because its use requires no sutures, surgery, or anesthesia; allows for easy preoperative observation; and allows gravity to gradually move the viscera into the abdomen (Bustorff-Silva and others 2008).

Once infants with omphalocele or gastroschisis survive the neonatal period, there is little to no associated disability or mortality. These anomalies are highly treatable and thus potentially highly DALY averting.

Case Study 3: Clubfoot

Description. Talipes equinovarus, or clubfoot, is a complex congenital anomaly in which the entire foot is rotated inward (van Bosse 2011). Clubfoot may be idiopathic—without an identifiable cause—or associated with other congenital anomalies. The etiology is unknown but likely involves genetic and environmental factors (Dobbs and Gurnett 2009). According to estimates from HICs, the incidence is approximately 1 per 1,000 live births (Coran and others 2012). However, incidence varies widely with ethnicity, and reports from LICs and LMICs have shown that incidence may be about 1 per 500 live births (Dobbs and Gurnett 2009; Mkandawire and Kaunda 2002); 80 percent of children with untreated clubfoot are born in LICs and LMICs (WHO 2013a). Untreated clubfoot leads to lifelong disability, social stigmatization, and decreased economic self-sufficiency in adulthood (Alavi and others 2012; Lourenço and Morcuende 2007).

Diagnosis and Treatment in LICs and LMICs. The most effective treatment for idiopathic clubfoot, the Ponseti method, is largely nonsurgical. We have included this anomaly for analysis because it exemplifies the importance of holistically approaching surgical disease to use both low-cost surgical and nonsurgical interventions to reduce the burden of disease.

The Ponseti method, in which a series of casts are applied between incremental manipulations of the foot by trained practitioners, is successful in up to 98 percent of patients (WHO 2013a). The Achilles tendon is often cut through the skin to correct lingering deformity, and corrective braces are worn for several years to prevent relapse (Dobbs and others 2000). The Ponseti method is also successful in treating neglected idiopathic clubfoot, in which the anomaly is not treated before walking age (Lourenço and Morcuende 2007). If surgery alone is used to correct this aggravated form of the deformity, functionality is low and may degrade into crippling pain and weakness in adolescence and adulthood (Gupta and others 2008).

The Ponseti procedure is well suited to use in LICs and LMICs; it is a low-cost intervention that can be performed by health and allied health professionals[4] (Janicki and others 2009; Lavy and others 2007; Mayo and others, n.d.), an advantageous attribute in contexts with few orthopedic surgeons. It requires no specialized surgical facilities and produces a functional foot (Gupta and others 2008).

Treatment programs using the Ponseti method have been set up in many LICs and LMICs, with success rates that regularly approximate those seen in HICs (Goksan and others 2006; Gupta and others 2008; Jawadi 2010; Makhdoom and others 2011; Mendez-Tompson and others 2012; Panjavi and others 2012; Sarrafan and others 2012). The Ponseti method is also successful in treating neglected clubfoot in LICs and LMICs, yielding superior outcomes and incurring significantly lower costs than purely surgical interventions (Adegbehingbe and others 2010; Hegazy, Nasef, and Abdel-Ghani 2009; Spiegel and others 2009).

The success of national clubfoot programs (box 8.1) provides strong evidence for the utility of task-shifting, that is, training paramedical practitioners to perform select health care tasks. Nonphysician practitioners trained in orthopedics and the Ponseti method can achieve results comparable to those of surgeons in HICs (Tindall and others 2005). Collaborations among diverse partners, including nongovernmental organizations, ministries of health, and academic institutions,

---

Box 8.1

The Uganda Sustainable Clubfoot Care Project

Clubfoot, the most common cause of locomotor disability in low-income countries leads to profound impairments in activities of daily life, social exclusion, and abandonment. After several years of pilot intervention, the Uganda Sustainable Clubfoot Care Project was implemented in 2000. Essential elements include the following:

- Development of a national strategic plan addressing all levels of the health system
- Endorsement by the Ministry of Health and incorporation into the National Health Policy
- Community awareness campaigns
- Sensitization of maternity units via education
- Training: Ponseti method trainers at the national hospital to train nonphysician orthopedic officers

in serial casting in rural hospitals and medical officers in tenotomy
- Development and distribution of locally made orthoses, or mechanical devices (for example, braces) to provide support and correct alignment of the clubfoot.

In 2006 and 2007, 872 children were treated, nearly 800 providers were trained, and services were made available in 21 hospitals. Using this experience in Uganda and a similar program in Malawi as a basis, interventions have been implemented in 10 other countries; early two-year follow-up data suggest similarly successful results.

Source: Pirani and others 2009; Tindall and others 2005.

are instrumental for increasing the number of trained paramedical practitioners, and thereby the availability of treatment (Owen and others 2012). To achieve these goals, it is critical to implement a coordinated, standardized program to decentralize care, and to integrate education, awareness, and service delivery into the public health sector.

IMPLEMENTATION AND SURVEILLANCE PRIORITIES

Addressing the Burden of Disease of Congenital Anomalies

Strategies to increase the accessibility of surgical care for children with congenital anomalies include development of treatment centers for specific conditions (niche hospitals), short-term surgical missions, partnerships to train local providers, and the transporting of patients to other countries for care. Interventions at the policy level may also play a role, as may novel tools such as telemedicine.

The strengths and weaknesses of these strategies are summarized in table 8.4. It is critical that local expertise and buy-in be integrated into all efforts to increase the accessibility of pediatric surgery so as to create sustainable systems that increase long-term capacity and take advantage of the substantial potential intellectual, creative, and personnel resources in LICs and LMICs.

Strategy 1. Cultivating Treatment Centers in LICs and LMICs

Recent humanitarian efforts have favored establishing sustainable surgical centers in LICs and LMICs, staffed by either local or foreign personnel. This approach maximizes the number of children treated and enables local trainees to learn to practice in their future professional environments, preventing later struggles to adapt protocols learned abroad to local resources (Larrazabal and others 2007). The entire surgical team can be concurrently trained, prepping both the surgeon and the center to operate independently (Larrazabal and others 2007; Loisance 2012).

Table 8.4 Increasing the Accessibility of Pediatric Surgery

Strategy	Advantages	Disadvantages
Treatment centers in LICs and LMICs	Creates infrastructure and expertise to broadly affect the burden of disease caused by congenital anomalies	Streamlined centers often not integrated with local training programs and public health care systems
	Streamlines care if center focuses on one pathology or organ system	
	Provides treatment in home countries	
Surgical missions	Minimizes costs and culture shock for patients	Episodic
	Streamlines care if missions focus on one condition	Limited time window restricts number of patients treated
	Offers opportunity to train local personnel	Pressure to deliver care in limited period may restrict training efforts
	Are well suited for nonemergency conditions with backlogs	Follow-up limited
		Integration with existing services may be limited
		Not designed to treat emergency life-threatening conditions
Academic partnerships	Provides coordinated interface for students and professionals from HICs, LICs, and LMICs to learn from and collaborate with each other	Not as focused on delivery of care
		Research may not be truly collaborative
	Opportunity for training and resource sharing	Potential for medical tourism by HIC practitioners, especially if training not provided to LIC and LMIC partners
	Facilitates scholarly approach to intervention and evaluation	Financial sustainability may be limited by availability of institutional funding
Human resources and policy changes Telemedicine	Task-shifting increases health care access	Necessitates rigorous regulation and standardization

table continues next page

Table 8.4 Increasing the Accessibility of Pediatric Surgery (continued)

Strategy	Advantages	Disadvantages
	Potentially reduces transport risks and costs	No opportunity for hands-on training
	Builds local capacity through consultation	
	Improves communication between different points of health care access	
Health care delivery outside of LICs and LMICs	Increases level of care compared with local systems	Costly
		Benefits only a few patients
		Does not contribute to developing capacity in LICs and LMICs

Note: HICs = high-income countries; LICs = low-income countries; LMICs = lower-middle-income countries.

Successful centers have developed from international partnerships, foreign humanitarian initiatives, and home-grown efforts in LICs and LMICs (Bode-Thomas 2012), with evidence that continuous support through development programs can build pediatric surgery capacity. Networks of faith-based hospitals also provide specialized surgical services, such as the CURE network, which focuses primarily on neurosurgery and orthopedics; CBM International, which supports an array of surgical services; and the Pan-African Academy of Christian Surgeons network, which has developed training programs in association with BethanyKids, a faith-based pediatric surgical organization. Surgical mission–oriented organizations may also develop treatment centers, as has been done by Operation Smile, a mission program specializing in cleft lip and palate repairs (Patel and others 2013).

Treatment at these centers can be tailored to available resources. Less-expensive, but effective, diagnostic and therapeutic modalities can be used. Simple, palliative surgeries may predominate in the neonatal period if early definitive repair is too risky. Cheaper surgical materials are produced by countries like Brazil and China; medical equipment companies may be persuaded to make donations; and some disposable surgical materials can be sterilized and reused (Rao 2007; Senga and others 2013).

The few cost-effectiveness analyses that have been published support the feasibility of developing local treatment centers. For example, at the CURE Children's Hospital in Mbale, Uganda, children with hydrocephalus are treated at an estimated cost of US$59 to US$126 per DALY averted, with US$3 million to US$5 million saved to Uganda, and US$5 million to US$188 million saved based on statistical calculations of the value of a life (Warf and others 2011).

Strategy 2. Surgical Missions

The short-term surgical mission, also commonly referred to as humanitarian assistance or a volunteer trip, is an established health care delivery model that is becoming increasingly popular. Individual providers or organized teams travel from HICs to deliver surgical care in LICs and LMICs (Martiniuk and others 2012). Smile Train and Operation Smile, the two largest global cleft lip and palate charities, exemplify two different models of successful, long-running surgical missions. Operation Smile primarily funds teams from HICs to provide short-term health care delivery and training in LICs and LMICs; Smile Train[5] funds local providers to offer outreach and training (Poenaru 2013). In some regions, these teams provide the only surgical services for children (Walker and others 2010). In recent years, Operation Smile has also developed treatment centers as a more sustainable approach (Magee and others 2012).

Sustainability, follow-up for postsurgical complications, and integration with existing health systems are significant challenges for the inherently episodic surgical mission model. Perhaps most important, surgical missions are better suited for "prevalent" rather than "incident" conditions. Prevalent conditions incur increasing morbidity, whereas incident conditions are surgical emergencies. A greater proportion of the burden of disease may be averted by targeting emergency conditions, but emergency treatment cannot be improved without improving capacity at the systems level (Bickler and others 2010).

Strategy 3. Partnerships between Academic Organizations and Development Programs

Academic organizations have increasingly focused on augmenting surgical capacity in LICs and LMICs through partnerships (Calland and others 2013; Qureshi and others 2011). Some organizations subsidize academic surgeons, who then deliver care, train providers, and conduct research in LICs and LMICs. Partnerships also provide mechanisms by which practitioners from LICs can obtain foreign training in middle-income countries (MICs) (for example, a Sub-Saharan African practitioner training in India) or HICs. Training outside of the home environment has the disadvantage that the trainee may not return for practice. Funding the training of local practitioners by underwriting the presence of visiting surgeons in partnered development programs may be an effective alternative. For example, during the course of a four-year project funded by the Italian Cooperation in Eritrea, local Eritrean surgeons achieved independence and favorable outcomes in the treatment of a wide range of congenital anomalies (Calisti and others 2011). Overall, the scope of activities undertaken by academic organizations in these partnerships varies widely, and outcomes of many permutations of partnership are not yet well characterized.

Strategy 4. Human Resources and Policy Changes

Policy changes, such as the provision of free health care to children, may increase access to pediatric surgery (Groen and others 2013). The expansion of training programs is key to ensuring that children with anomalies are diagnosed in a timely manner and can access appropriate surgical services. Regional professional societies offer a limited number of training spots and scholarships, and training programs need support (Elhalaby and others 2012). More training positions are required to meet the need for trained pediatric surgeons and the interest level of general surgery trainees. To date, only limited analyses of the cost-effectiveness of such programs have been conducted.

Specially trained paramedical practitioners may be a viable solution to the scarcity of providers, as demonstrated by the success of clubfoot programs; however, the scope of treatment may be limited to select conditions (Mayo and others, n.d.; Pirani and others 2009; Tindall and others 2005). The scope of practice for a pediatric general surgeon includes congenital anomalies, acquired surgical diseases, and a high proportion of emergencies. This breadth has made it challenging to design and implement intervention packages in hospitals and health care systems. Other surgical providers may do their best to meet the need, but the shortfall is tremendous. Pediatric anesthesia providers are similarly few, as are trained pediatric neurosurgeons, cardiac surgeons, orthopedic surgeons, and other surgical subspecialists. Although task-shifting has been promoted to meet the need for essential surgery in adults, its applicability to

pediatric surgical conditions has not been specifically analyzed.

Strategy 5. Telemedicine

Telemedicine[6] may increase the accessibility of limited surgical specialists to large populations requiring care. Chaotic roads and a lack of medical transport complicate the great distances that patients in LICs and LMICs must travel to reach care. Children seeking treatment may present in critical and sometimes unsalvageable condition following such physiologically stressful transit (Rao 2007). With telemedicine, physicians at local or regional medical centers can interact with experts at centralized third-level facilities to guide patient treatment, potentially circumventing the need for patients to undergo life-threatening journeys. The cost burden of travel and treatment for families is decreased, and unspecialized providers can receive training from specialized peers (Sekar and Vilvanathan 2007). Telemedicine can also link medical centers for educational or research purposes (Hadley and Mars 2008). This developing technology has the potential to beneficially decentralize specialized care and education in LICs and LMICs.

Strategy 6. Health Services Delivery Outside of Local Systems

Families may seek care in foreign treatment centers, funded out of pocket, through community fundraising, or by humanitarian organizations. Increased access to advanced treatment methods saves lives that would otherwise be lost. However, transporting children to foreign centers limits the number of children treated. Because the cost of surgery abroad often surpasses a family's annual income in LICs and LMICs, even the highest-earning families must rely on limited governmental and nongovernmental agency funds (Sadoh, Nwaneri, and Owobu 2011). If patients require multiple surgeries, financial sponsors must decide whether to perform the surgery at all, abstain from follow-up surgeries, or fly the patient back for additional surgeries. If patients die abroad, the families must wrestle with substantial financial and emotional challenges in coordinating burial arrangements (Bode-Thomas 2012). Furthermore, this approach does not build local surgical capacity. The social and economic costs for patients and families who seek care abroad are likely significant but have not been estimated; an estimate may provide incentives for governments and funders to invest in local care.

These strategies are not mutually exclusive; they may coexist or evolve into different models.

Although the development of health care capacity within LICs and LMICs is crucial to the long-term reduction of the burden of disease associated with congenital anomalies, other intervention strategies provide additional and immediate opportunities to improve pediatric surgical care and outcomes.

ACTION PLAN

Clinical Intervention at Every Level

Given that platforms for delivery vary by setting, we propose only general guidelines for congenital anomalies

(table 8.5). Robust data from LICs and LMICs are sparse; therefore, the following recommendations—based on the available literature—should be understood as the best available at this time. Future research will undoubtedly lead to more precise, substantiated recommendations.

- The village health center should have health providers trained to identify anomalies. In Tanzania, educating TBAs and using a birth card to register and record birth data are being evaluated as tools for improving identification of treatable anomalies (Norgrove Penny, personal communication) and may be useful in other practice settings. Public education

Table 8.5 Pediatric Surgery Capacity in an Ideal System

Capacity	Village health center	First-level hospital	Second-level hospital	Third-level hospital
Airway management, fluid replacement, bleeding control, antibiotic therapy	X[a]	X	X	X
Blood transfusion		X[a]	X	X
Tracheal tube		X[a]	X	X
Local anesthesia	X	X	X	X
Spinal and general anesthesia		X	X	X
Pediatric hernia		X	X	X
Pediatric hernia (infant)			X[a]	X
Umbilical hernia		X	X	X
Pyloric stenosis			X[a]	X
Colostomy		X[a]	X	X
Neonatal bowel obstruction (atresia, stenosis, malrotation)				X
Tracheoesophageal fistula repair				X[a]
Clubfoot		X	X	X
Cleft lip		X	X	X
Anorectal malformations or Hirschsprung's disease (first stage; often colostomy)		X	X	X
Anorectal malformations or Hirschsprung's disease (definitive treatment)			X	X
Abdominal wall defects			X[a]	X
Hydrocephalus			X[a]	X
Congenital cardiac anomalies			X[a]	X
Spina bifida				X
Bladder extrophy				X
Undescended testicles			X	X
Hypospadias				X

Note: "Capacity" is defined as trained staff available 24 hours, seven days a week, with adequate equipment and supplies.
a. Capacity should already be there but usually is not.

is important for raising awareness that congenital anomalies are treatable and not a death sentence; this vital information prompts families to seek care.

- The first-level hospital should have the ability to stabilize pediatric patients with surgical emergencies and to definitively treat conditions for which the capacity exists. In-depth guidelines have been suggested for first-level hospitals but have not yet been tested or validated (Bickler and Ameh 2011).
- The second-level hospital should provide life-saving surgical treatments, especially those that are part of staged repair procedures, and should house at least one specialist surgeon with training in pediatric general surgery.
- The third-level hospital must be able to provide treatment for a broader range of neonatal emergencies and more complex urgent conditions. The availability of specialist pediatric surgeons and anesthesia providers with expertise in infants and children is critical.

Research Priorities

Improved data collection and identification of disparities will fuel advocacy and inform targeted intervention programs for congenital anomalies. Research priorities include the following:

Data Expansion for Further Evaluation. Epidemiology, prevalence, and incidence of disease in various health contexts need further evaluation. Epidemiology may vary locally, but additional data are needed (Bickler 2000). Registries for selected anomalies may assist in improving surveillance (for example, via participation in the International Clearinghouse for Birth Defects Surveillance and Research). The evaluation of hidden mortality and morbidity will better approximate the true burden of disease.

Capacity Assessment and Guideline Development. The capacity for pediatric surgical care at various levels of the health system must be assessed, and guidelines for minimum human resources and infrastructure for countries at different stages of development should be created. The WHO Tool for Situational Analysis to Assess Emergency and Essential Surgical Care includes only two items pertaining to pediatric surgical care, and an alternative capacity tool has been proposed (Nacul and others 2013). This tool could be refined and further evaluated as it is piloted in different countries. Although surgical outreach programs can tackle the backlog of nonemergency conditions, emergency conditions require development of the whole health system. More work is needed to define and develop

the mechanisms to strengthen systems for pediatric surgery.

Metric Optimization. The quantitative metrics of disease burden should be optimized. Although DALYs are an accepted metric, they are difficult to apply practically. Surgical backlogs can be calculated for congenital anomalies and can be a useful advocacy tool for estimating the resources needed to treat prevalent, nonfatal anomalies. Improved measurements of the burden imposed by delayed access to care have not yet been developed. In middle- and high-income countries, many prevalent congenital anomalies are treated in the first year of life; in LICs, they are never treated or are treated years later, after children have suffered unnecessary complications. Many diseases with 100 percent survivability in HICs result in death or permanent disability in LICs and LMICs. Improved measurement of disparities must be highlighted as an advocacy tool for health equity.

Integration Model Evaluation. Models for the integration of pediatric surgical services within existing child health initiatives should be evaluated. Large-scale child health initiatives exist (such as the WHO's Integrated Management of Childhood Illness but have not historically included surgical care. Providers of children's surgical services share a general concern that if the particular needs of children are not specifically addressed, then they are often neglected. Although congenital anomalies are sometimes considered noncommunicable diseases (as in the Global Burden of Disease study), the agenda of the noncommunicable disease movement has not addressed them. Furthermore, greater planning is needed between networks of specialty organizations and providers treating a broad range of congenital anomalies to collaborate where possible.

Cost-Effectiveness Data Generation. Cost-effectiveness data should be generated to evaluate and select models to improve access to care. Although cost-effectiveness has been estimated for adult general surgery wards in selected hospitals (Gosselin, Thind, and Bellardinelli 2006), only one attempt has been made for pediatric surgical wards (Rattray and others 2013). Low-cost technological innovations and modification of surgical procedures hold great promise to improve perioperative care (Hadley 2008). Cost-effectiveness analysis of training programs could also aid advocacy for greater resources for training.

Marketing and Advocacy Alignment. Marketing and advocacy should become more aligned. Congenital anomalies vary greatly in scope and severity. Some treatable visible anomalies have received greater emphasis than those invisible anomalies for which it has been more difficult to engage donor programs for targeted support. Improved multidimensional measurements of the burden may help to make children and families suffering from all treatable anomalies more visible to the public health community. Development of innovative strategies for this process is needed.

CONCLUSIONS

This chapter highlights the considerable burden of disease associated with congenital anomalies and outlines key strategies for intervention. The consequences of nonintervention are readily apparent. It is both an economic and a moral imperative that global partners invest in pediatric surgery as a vital component of reducing the burden of disease and improving the public health and economic fortunes of LICs and LMICs.

NOTES

The World Bank classifies countries according to four income groupings. Income is measured using gross national income (GNI) per capita, in U.S. dollars, converted from local currency using the *World Bank Atlas* method. Classifications as of July 2014 are as follows:

- Low-income countries (LICs) = US$1,045 or less in 2013
- Middle-income countries (MICs) are subdivided:
  - Lower-middle-income (LMICs) = US$1,046 to US$4,125
  - Upper-middle-income (UMICs) = US$4,126 to US$12,745
- High-income countries (HICs) = US$12,746 or more

1. Rectal biopsy: A surgeon removes small samples of tissue from the patient's rectum. These samples are subjected to laboratory tests that lead to a diagnosis.
2. Sepsis: Severe widespread infection within the body that can lead to death.
3. Colostomy: Temporary creation of an opening in the abdomen that is connected to the intestine; fecal material exits the opening into a colostomy bag.
4. Allied health or paramedical practitioners: Nonphysician health professionals who provide supplementary or emergency health services.
5. Smile Train. "Smile Train Report Card." http://www .smiletrain.org/our-model/.
6. Telemedicine: Using technology to exchange information between different locations to improve training or clinical care.

REFERENCES

Abdur-Rahman, L. O., N. A. Abdulrasheed, and J. O. Adeniran. 2011. "Challenges and Outcomes of Management of Anterior Abdominal Wall Defects in a Nigerian Tertiary Hospital." *African Journal of Paediatric Surgery* 8 (2): 159–63.

Abubakar, A. M., M. A. Bello, D. Y. Chinda, K. Danladi, and I. M. Umar. 2011. "Challenges in the Management of Early versus Late Presenting Congenital Diaphragmatic Hernia in a Poor Resource Setting." *African Journal of Paediatric Surgery* 8 (1): 29–33.

Adegbehingbe, O. O., L. M. Oginni, O. J. Ogundele, A. L. Ariyibi, P. O. Abiola, and O. D. Ojo. 2010. "Ponseti Clubfoot Management: Changing Surgical Trends in Nigeria." *Iowa Orthopaedic Journal* 30: 7–14.

Adegboye, V., S. Omokhodion, O. Ogunkunle, M. Obajimi, A. Brimmo, and O. Adebo. 2002. "Experience with the Management of Congenital Diaphragmatic Hernia at the University College Hospital, Ibadan." *Nigerian Journal of Paediatrics* 29 (2): 40–46.

Adejuyigbe, O., A. M. Abubakar, O. A. Sowande, O. S. Olayinka, and A. F. Uba. 2004. "Experience with Anorectal Malformations in Ile-Ife, Nigeria." *Pediatric Surgery International* 20 (11–12): 855–58.

Adeniran, J. O., and L. Abdur-Rahman. 2005. "Late-Stage Correction of Intermediate Imperforate Anus in Males." *Pediatric Surgery International* 21 (2): 88–90.

Adeyemi, D. 1989. "Neonatal Intestinal Obstruction in a Developing Tropical Country: Patterns, Problems, and Prognosis." *Journal of Tropical Pediatrics* 35 (2): 66–70.

Agarwala, S., V. Bhatnagar, M. Bajpai, D. Gupta, and D. Mitra. 1996. "Factors Contributing to Poor Results of Treatment of Esophageal Atresia in Developing Countries." *Pediatric Surgery International* 11 (5–6): 312–15.

Alavi, Y., V. Jumbe, S. Hartley, S. Smith, D. Lamping, and others. 2012. "Indignity, Exclusion, Pain and Hunger: The Impact of Musculoskeletal Impairments in the Lives of Children in Malawi." *Disability and Rehabilitation* 34 (20): 1736–46.

Al-Jazaeri, A., S. Al-Shanafey, M. Zamakhshary, W. Al-Jarbou, E. Hajr, and others. 2012. "The Impact of Variation in Access to Care on the Management of Hirschsprung Disease." *Journal of Pediatric Surgery* 47 (5): 952–55.

Al-Salem, A. H., M. Tayeb, S. Khogair, A. Roy, N. Al-Jishi, and others. 2006. "Esophageal Atresia with or without Tracheoesophageal Fistula: Success and Failure in 94 Cases." *Annals of Saudi Medicine* 26 (2): 116–19.

Ameh, E. A., and L. B. Chirdan. 2000a. "Neonatal Intestinal Obstruction in Zaria, Nigeria." *East African Medical Journal* 77 (9): 510–13.

———. 2000b. "Ruptured Exomphalos and Gastroschisis: A Retrospective Analysis of Morbidity and Mortality in Nigerian Children." *Pediatric Surgery International* 16 (1–2): 23–25.

Ameh, E. A., P. M. Mshelbwala, L. Sabiu, and L. B. Chirdan. 2006. "Colostomy in Children—An Evaluation of Acceptance among Mothers and Caregivers in a Developing Country." *South African Journal of Surgery* 44 (4): 138–39.

Amiel, J., E. Sproat-Emison, M. Garcia-Barcelo, F. Lantieri, G. Burzynski, and others. 2008. "Hirschsprung Disease, Associated Syndromes, and Genetics: A Review." *Journal of Medical Genetics* 45 (1): 1–14.

Andrew, J. A., K. W. Holland, and N. Badawi. 2011. "Gastroschisis: An Update." *Pediatric Surgery International* 26 (9): 871–78.

Anwar-ul-Haq, N. Akhter, Ubaidullah, Javeria, Samiullah, and others. 2009. "Factors Affecting Survival in Patients with Oesophageal Atresia and Tracheo-Oesophageal Fistula." *Journal of Ayub Medical College Abbottabad* 21 (4): 129–33.

Archibong, A. E., and I. M. Idika. 2004. "Results of Treatment in Children with Anorectal Malformations in Calabar, Nigeria." *South African Journal of Surgery* 42 (3): 88–90.

Arnold, M. 2004. "Is the Incidence of Gastroschisis Rising in South Africa in Accordance with International Trends? A Retrospective Analysis at Pretoria Academic and Kalafong Hospitals, 1981–2001." *South African Journal of Surgery* 42 (3): 86–88.

Askarpour, S., N. Ostadian, H. Javaherizadeh, and S. Chabi. 2012. "Omphalocele, Gastroschisis: Epidemiology, Survival, and Mortality in Imam Khomeini Hospital, Ahvaz-Iran." *Polski Przeglad Chirurgiczny* 84 (2): 82–85.

Babu, M. K., U. Kini, K. Das, A. Alladi, and A. D'Cruz. 2003. "A Modified Technique for the Diagnosis of Hirschsprung Disease from Rectal Biopsies." *National Medical Journal of India* 16 (5): 245–48.

Bakshi, K. D., B. Vaidyanathan, K. R. Sundaram, S. J. Roth, K. Shivaprakasha, and others. 2007. "Determinants of Early Outcome after Neontal Cardiac Surgery in a Developing Country." *Journal of Thoracic and Cardiovascular Surgery* 134 (3): 765–71.

Bandre, E., R. A. Kabore, I. Ouedraogo, O. Sore, T. Tapsoba, and others. 2010. "Hirschsprung's Disease: Management Problem in a Developing Country." *African Journal of Paediatric Surgery* 7 (3): 166–68.

Banu, T., M. Hoque, K. Laila, H. Ashraf Ul, and A. Hanif. 2009. "Management of Male H-Type Anorectal Malformations." *Pediatric Surgery International* 25 (10): 857–61.

Benjamin, B. G., M. K. Ethen, C. L. Van Hook, C. A. Myers, and M. A. Canfield. 2010. "Gastroschisis Prevalence in Texas 1999–2003." *Birth Defects Research Part A: Clinical and Molecular Teratology* 88 (3): 178–85.

Bernier, P. L., A. Stefanescu, G. Samoukovic, and C. Tchervenkov. 2010. "The Challenge of Congenital Heart Disease Worldwide: Epidemiologic and Demographic Facts." *Pediatric Cardiac Surgery Annual of the Seminars in Thoracic and Cardiovascular Surgery* 13 (1): 26–34.

Bickler, S. W. 2000. "Non-Communicable Diseases: Is Their Emergence in Industrialized Societies Related to Changes in Neuroendocrine Function?" *Medical Hypotheses* 54 (5): 825–28.

Bickler, S. W., and E. Ameh. 2011. *Surgical Care for Children: A Guide for Primary Referral Hospitals*. London: Macmillan.

Bickler, S., D. Ozgediz, R. Gosselin, T. Weiser, D. Spiegel, and others. 2010. "Key Concepts for Estimating the Burden of Surgical Conditions and the Unmet Need for Surgical Care." *World Journal of Surgery* 34 (3): 374–80.

Bickler, S. W., and H. Rode. 2002. "Surgical Services for Children in Developing Countries." *Bulletin of the World Health Organization* 80 (10): 829–35.

Bode-Thomas, F. 2012. "Challenges in the Management of Congenital Heart Disease in Developing Countries." In *Congenital Heart Disease: Selected Aspects*, edited by P. Syamasundar Rao, 263–72. Rijeka, Croatia: Intech. http://www.intechopen.com/books/congenital-heart-disease-selectedaspects/challenges-in-the-management-of-congenital-heart-disease-in-developing-countries.

Botto, L. D., J. D. Erickson, J. Mulinare, M. C. Lynberg, and Y. Liu. 2002. "Maternal Fever, Multivitamin Use, and Selected Birth Defects: Evidence of Interaction?" *Epidemiology* 13 (4): 485–88.

Botto, L. D., J. Mulinare, and J. D. Erickson. 2002. "Occurrence of Omphalocele in Relation to Maternal Multivitamin Use: A Population-Based Study." *Pediatrics* 109 (5): 904–08.

Bustorff-Silva, J. M., A. F. S. Schmidt, A. Goncalves, S. Marba, and L. Sbragia. 2008. "The Female Condom as a Temporary Silo: A Simple and Inexpensive Tool in the Initial Management of the Newborn with Gastroschisis." *Journal of Maternal-Fetal and Neonatal Medicine* 21 (9): 648–51.

Calisti, A., K. Belay, G. Mazzoni, G. Fiocca, G. Retrosi, and others. 2011. "Promoting Major Pediatric Surgical Care in a Low-Income Country: A 4-Year Experience in Eritrea." *World Journal of Surgery* 35 (4): 760–66.

Calland, J. F., R. T. Petroze, J. Abelson, and E. Kraus. 2013. "Engaging Academic Surgery in Global Health: Challenges and Opportunities in the Development of an Academic Track in Global Surgery." *Surgery* 153 (3): 316–20.

Canfield, M. A., M. A. Honein, N. Yuskiv, J. Xing, C. T. Mai, and others. 2006. "National Estimates and Race/Ethnic-Specific Variation of Selected Birth Defects in the United States, 1999–2001." *Birth Defects Research Part A: Clinical and Molecular Teratology* 76 (11): 747–56.

Castilla, E. E., P. Mastroiacovo, and I. M. Orioli. 2008. "Gastroschisis: International Epidemiology and Public Health Perspectives." *American Journal of Medical Genetics Part C: Seminars in Medical Genetics* 148C (3): 162–79.

CDC (Centers for Disease Control). 2012. Birth defects.

Chalapathi, G., S. K. Chowdhary, K. L. Rao, R. Samujh, K. L. Narasimhan, and others. 2004. "Risk Factors in the Primary Management of Anorectal Malformations in Northern India." *Pediatric Surgery International* 20 (6): 408–11.

Chalya, P. L., J. B. Mabula, E. S. Kanumba, G. Giit, A. B. Chandika, and others. 2011. "Experiences with Childhood Colostomy at a Tertiary Hospital in Mwanza, Tanzania." *Tanzania Journal of Health Research* 13 (3): 1–12.

Chandramouli, B., K. Srinivasan, J. Jagdish, and N. Ananthakrishnan. 2004. "Morbidity and Mortality of Colostomy and Its Closure in Children." *Journal of Pediatric Surgery* 39 (4): 596–99.

Chirdan, L. B., E. A. Ameh, F. A. Abantanga, D. Sidler, and E. A. Elhalaby. 2010. "Challenges of Training and Delivery of Pediatric Surgical Services in Africa." *Journal of Pediatric Surgery* 45 (3): 610–18.

Chirdan, L. B., P. J. Ngiloi, and E. A. Elhalaby. 2012. "Neonatal Surgery in Africa." *Seminars in Pediatric Surgery* 21 (2): 151–59.

Chirdan, L. B., and A. F. Uba. 2006. "Hirschsprung's Disease Presenting in the Neonatal Period in Jos, Nigeria." *Nigerian Journal of Surgical Research* 8 (1–2): 62–64.

Chiu, P., and H. L. Hedrick. 2008. "Postnatal Management and Long-Term Outcome for Survivors with Congenital Diaphragmatic Hernia." *Prenatal Diagnosis* 28 (7): 592–603.

Chowdhary, S. K., G. Chalapathi, K. L. Narasimhan, R. Samujh, J. K. Mahajan, and others. 2004. "An Audit of Neonatal Colostomy for High Anorectal Malformation: The Developing World Perspective." *Pediatric Surgery International* 20 (2): 111–13.

Christianson, A. L., C. P. Howson, and B. Modell. 2006. *Global Report on Birth Defects: The Hidden Toll of Dying and Disabled Children.* White Plains, NY: March of Dimes Birth Defects Foundation.

Coran, A. G., A. Caldamone, N. S. Adzick, T. M. Krummel, J.-M. Laberge, and others. 2012. *Pediatric Surgery: Expert Consult (2 volumes).* 7th ed. London: Elsevier Health Sciences.

Coran, A. G., and D. H. Teitelbaum. 2000. "Recent Advances in the Management of Hirschsprung's Disease." *American Journal of Surgery* 180 (5): 382–87.

Corlew, D. S. 2010. "Estimation of Impact of Surgical Disease through Economic Modeling of Cleft Lip and Palate Care." *World Journal of Surgery* 34 (3): 391–96.

Davies, M. C., S. M. Creighton, and D. T. Wilcox. 2004. "Long-Term Outcomes of Anorectal Malformations." *Pediatric Surgery International* 20 (8): 567–72.

Dobbs, M. B., and C. A. Gurnett. 2009. "Update on Clubfoot: Etiology and Treatment." *Clinical Orthopaedics and Related Research* 467 (5): 1146–53.

Dobbs, M. B., J. A. Morcuende, C. A. Gurnett, and I. V. Ponseti. 2000. "Treatment of Idiopathic Clubfoot: An Historical Review." *Iowa Orthopedic Journal* 20: 59–64.

Eason, G., M. Langer, D. Birabwa-Male, E. Reimer, M. Pennington, and others. 2012. "Costs and Cost-Effectiveness of Pediatric Inguinal Hernia Repair in Uganda." Abstract presented at the European Paediatric Surgeons Association and British Association of Paediatric Surgeons Joint Congress, Rome, June.

Ekenze, S. O., S. N. Ibeziako, and U. O. Ezomike. 2007. "Trends in Neonatal Intestinal Obstruction in a Developing Country, 1996–2005." *World Journal of Surgery* 31 (12): 2405–09.

Ekenze, S. O., C. Ngaikedi, and A. A. Obasi. 2011. "Problems and Outcome of Hirschsprung's Disease Presenting after 1 Year of Age in a Developing Country." *World Journal of Surgery* 35 (1): 22–26.

Elhalaby, E. A. 2006. "Primary Repair of High and Intermediate Anorectal Malformations in the Neonates." *Annals of Pediatric Surgery* 2 (2): 117–22.

Elhalaby, E. A., F. A. Uba, E. S. Borgstein, H. Rode, and A. J. Millar. 2012. "Training and Practice of Pediatric Surgery in Africa: Past, Present, and Future." *Seminars in Pediatric Surgery* 21 (2): 103–10.

Eltayeb, A. A. 2010. "Delayed Presentation of Anorectal Malformations: The Possible Associated Morbidity and Mortality." *Pediatric Surgery International* 26 (8): 801–06.

Farmer, P., and J. Kim. 2008. "Surgery and Global Health: A View from beyond the OR." *World Journal of Surgery* 32 (4): 533–36.

Frolov, P., J. Alali, and M. D. Klein. 2010. "Clinical Risk Factors for Gastroschisis and Omphalocele in Humans: A Review of the Literature." *Pediatric Surgery International* 26 (12): 1135–48.

Frykman, P. K., and S. S. Short. 2012. "Hirschsprung-Associated Enterocolitis: Prevention and Therapy." *Seminars in Pediatric Surgery* 21 (4): 328–35.

Gangopadhyay, A. N., S. Shilpa, T. V. Mohan, and S. C. Gopal. 2005. "Single-Stage Management of All Pouch Colon (Anorectal Malformation) in Newborns." *Journal of Pediatric Surgery* 40 (7): 1151–55.

Goksan, S. B., A. Bursali, F. Bilgili, S. Sivacioglu, and S. Ayanoglu. 2006. "Ponseti Technique for the Correction of Idiopathic Clubfeet Presenting up to 1 Year of Age: A Preliminary Study in Children with Untreated or Complex Deformities." *Archives of Orthopedic Trauma Surgery* 126 (1): 15–21.

Gosselin, R. A., A. Thind, and A. Bellardinelli. 2006. "Cost/DALY Averted in a Small Hospital in Sierra Leone: What Is the Relative Contribution of Different Services?" *World Journal of Surgery* 30 (4): 505–11.

Groen, R. S., M. Samai, R. T. Petroze, T. B. Kamara, L. D. Cassidy, and others. 2013. "Household Survey in Sierra Leone Reveals High Prevalence of Surgical Conditions in Children." *World Journal of Surgery* 37 (6): 1220–26.

Gupta, A., S. Singh, P. Patel, J. Patel, and M. K. Varshney. 2008. "Evaluation of the Utility of the Ponseti Method of Correction of Clubfoot Deformity in a Developing Nation." *International Orthopaedics* 32 (1): 75–79.

Hadley, G. P. 2008. "Perspectives on Congenital Abnormalities in the Third World." *African Journal of Paediatric Surgery* 5 (1): 1–2.

———, and M. Mars. 2008. "Postgraduate Medical Education in Paediatric Surgery: Videoconferencing—A Possible Solution for Africa?" *Pediatric Surgery International* 24 (2): 223–26.

Hegazy, M., N. M. Nasef, and H. Abdel-Ghani. 2009. "Results of Treatment of Idiopathic Clubfoot in Older Infants Using the Ponseti Method: A Preliminary Report." *Journal of Pediatric Orthopaedics. Part B* 18 (2): 76–78.

Higashi, H., J. J. Barendregt, and T. Vos. 2013. "The Burden of Congenital Anomalies Amenable to Surgeries in Low-Income and Middle-Income Countries: A Modeled Analysis." *The Lancet* 381: S62.

Hoffman, J. 2013. "The Global Burden of Congenital Heart Disease." *Cardiovascular Journal of Africa* 24 (4): 141–45.

Ibrahim, A. I. 2007. "One Stage Posterior Sagittal Anorectoplasty for Treatment of High and Intermediate Anorectal Anomalies at Birth." *Annals of Pediatric Surgery* 3 (3–4): 11–124.

Islam, M., and M. A. Aziz. 2011. "Esophageal Atresia: Outcome in 21 Cases." *Bangladesh Armed Forces Medical Journal* 44 (1): 47–50.

Jamison, D. T., J. G. Breman, A. R. Measham, G. Alleyne, M. Claeson, D. B. Evans, P. Jha. A. Mills, and P. Musgrove, eds. 2006. *Disease Control Priorities in Developing Countries*, 2nd ed. Washington, DC: World Bank and Oxford University Press.

Janicki, J. A., U. G. Narayanan, B. J. Harvey, A. Roy, S. Weir, and others. 2009. "Comparison of Surgeon and Physiotherapist-Directed Ponseti Treatment of Idiopathic Clubfoot." *Journal of Bone and Joint Surgery* 91 (5): 1101–08.

Jawadi, A. H. 2010. "Clubfoot Management by the Ponseti Technique in Saudi Patients." *Saudi Medical Journal* 31 (1): 49–52.

Khemakhem, R., B. Haggui, H. Rahay, F. Nouira, A. Charieg, and others. 2012. "Congenital Diaphragmatic Hernia in Neonate: A Retrospective Study about 28 Observations." *African Journal of Paediatric Surgery* 9 (3): 217–22.

Larrazabal, L. A., K. J. Jenkins, K. Gauvreau, V. L. Vida, O. J. Benavidez, and others. 2007. "Improvement in Congenital Heart Surgery in a Developing Country: The Guatemalan Experience." *Circulation* 116 (17): 1882–87.

Laughon, M., R. Meyer, C. Bose, A. Wall, E. Otero, and others. 2003. "Rising Birth Prevalence of Gastroschisis." *Journal of Perinatology: Official Journal of the California Perinatal Association* 23 (4): 291–93.

Lavy, C. B. D., S. J. Mannion, N. C. Mkandawire, A. Tindall, C. Steinlechner, and others. 2007. "Club Foot Treatment in Malawi: A Public Health Approach." *Disability and Rehabilitation* 29 (11–12): 857–62.

Loane, M., H. Dolk, and I. Bradbury. 2007. "Increasing Prevalence of Gastroschisis in Europe 1980–2002: A Phenomenon Restricted to Younger Mothers?" *Paediatric and Perinatal Epidemiology* 21 (4): 363–69.

Loisance, D. Y. 2012. "Training Young Cardiac Surgeons in Developing Countries." *Asian Cardiovascular and Thoracic Annals* 20 (4): 384–86.

Lourenço, A., and J. Morcuende. 2007. "Correction of Neglected Idiopathic Club Foot by the Ponseti Method." *Journal of Bone and Joint Surgery. British Volume* 89 (3): 378–81.

Magee, W., H. M. Raimondi, M. Beers, and M. C. Koech. 2012. "Effectiveness of International Surgical Program Model to Build Local Sustainability." *Plastic Surgery International* 2012: 185725. doi:10.1155/2012/185725.

Makhdoom, A., M. A. Laghari, M. K. Pahore, P. A. L. Qureshi, I. A. Bhutto, and others. 2011. "Clubfoot Treatment by Ponseti Method." *Journal of the Liaquat University of Medical and Health Sciences* 10 (2): 71–74.

Manson, J., E. Ameh, N. Canvassar, T. Chen, A. V. den Hoeve, and others. 2012. "Gastroschisis: A Multi-centre Comparison of Management and Outcome." *African Journal of Paediatric Surgery* 9 (1): 17–21.

Martiniuk, A. L. C., M. Manouchehiran, J. A. Negin, and A. B. Zwi. 2012. "Brain Gains: A Literature Review of Medical Missions to Low and Middle-Income Countries." *BMC Health Services Research* 12: 134.

Mayo, E., A. Cuthel, J. Macharia, C. Lavy, and T. Mead. n.d. "Creating a Countrywide Program Model for Implementation of a Ponseti Method Clubfoot Treatment Program in Developing Countries." Unpublished. http://cure.org/downloads/site/clubfoot/ccw-creating_a_countrywide_program_model.pdf.

Mendez-Tompson, M., O. Olivares-Becerril, M. Preciado-Salgado, I. Quezada-Daniel, and J. G. Vega-Sanchez. 2012. "Management of Congenital Adduct Clubfoot with the Ponseti Technique. Experience at La Perla General Hospital." *Acta Ortopedica Mexicana* 26 (4): 228–30.

Mhando, S., B. Young, and K. Lakhoo. 2008. "The Scope of Emergency Paediatric Surgery in Tanzania." *Pediatric Surgery International* 24 (2): 219–22.

Mills, J. L., T. C. Carter, D. M. Kay, M. L. Browne, L. C. Brody, and others. 2012. "Folate and Vitamin B12–Related Genes and Risk for Omphalocele." *Human Genetics* 131 (5): 739–46.

Miranda, M. E., E. D. Tatsuo, J. T. Guimaraes, R. M. Paixao, and J. C. B. D. Lanna. 1999. "Use of a Plastic Hemoderivative Bag in the Treatment of Gastroschisis." *Pediatric Surgery International* 15 (5–6): 442–44.

Mkandawire, M., and E. Kaunda. 2002. "An Audit of Congenital Anomalies in the Neonatal Unit of Queen Elizabeth Central Hospital. One-Year Study Period: 1st November 2000 to 31st October 2001." *East and Central African Journal of Surgery* 7 (1): 29–33.

Mo Suwan, L., S. Isaranurug, P. Chanvitan, W. Techasena, S. Sutra, and others. 2009. "Perinatal Death Pattern in the Four Districts of Thailand: Findings from the Prospective Cohort Study of Thai Children." *Journal of the Medical Association of Thailand* 92 (5): 660–66.

Moore, S. W., A. Alexander, D. Sidler, J. Alves, G. P. Hadley, and others. 2008. "The Spectrum of Anorectal Malformations in Africa." *Pediatric Surgery International* 24 (6): 677–83.

Nacul, L. C., A. Stewart, C. Alberg, S. Chowdhury, M. W. Darlison, and others. 2013. "A Toolkit to Assess Health Needs for Congenital Disorders in Low- and Middle-Income Countries: An Instrument for Public Health Action." *Journal of Public Health.* Advance online publication. doi:10.1093/pubmed/fdt048.

Nandi, B., C. Mungongo, and K. Lakhoo. 2008. "A Comparison of Neonatal Surgical Admissions between Two Linked Surgical Departments in Africa and Europe." *Pediatric Surgery International* 24 (8): 939–42.

Narasimman, S., M. Nallusamy, and S. Hassan. 2013. "Review of Oesophageal Atresia and Tracheoesophageal Fistula in Hospital Sultanah Bahiyah, Alor Star. Malaysia from January 2000 to December 2009." *Medical Journal of Malaysia* 68 (1): 48–51.

Olivieri, C., K. Belay, R. Coletta, G. Retrosi, P. Molle, and A. Calisti. 2012. "Preventing Posterior Sagittal Anoplasty 'Cripples' in Areas with Limited Medical Resources: A Few Modifications to Surgical Approach in Anorectal Malformations." *African Journal of Paediatric Surgery* 9 (3): 223–26.

Osifo, O. D., and C. J. Okolo. 2009. "Outcome of Trans-anal Posterior Anorectal Myectomy for the Ultrashort Segment Hirschprung's Disease—Benin City Experience in 5 Years." *Nigerian Postgraduate Medical Journal* 16 (3): 213–17.

Owen, R. M., J. N. Penny, A. Mayo, J. Morcuende, and C. B. Lavy. 2012. "A Collaborative Public Health Approach to Clubfoot Intervention in 10 Low-Income and Middle-Income Countries: 2-Year Outcomes and Lessons Learnt." *Journal of Pediatric Orthopaedics. Part B* 21 (4): 361–65.

Ozdogan, T., C. Durakbasa, M. Mutus, and M. Iscen. 2010. "Congenital Diaphragmatic Hernia: A 4-Year Experience in a Single Centre." *African Journal of Paediatric Surgery* 7 (2): 105–06.

Ozgediz, D., D. T. Jamison, M. Cherian, and K. McQueen. 2008. "The Burden of Surgical Conditions and Access to Surgical Care in Low- and Middle-Income Countries." *Bulletin of the World Health Organization* 86 (8): 646–47.

Ozgediz, D., and D. Poenaru. 2012. "The Burden of Pediatric Surgical Conditions in Low and Middle Income Countries: A Call to Action." *Journal of Pediatric Surgery* 47 (12): 2305–11.

Panjavi, B., A. Sharafatvaziri, R. H. Zargarbashi, and S. Mehrpour. 2012. "Use of the Ponseti Method in the Iranian Population." *Journal of Pediatric Orthopaedics* 32 (3): e11–14.

Patel, A., J. E. Clune, D. M. Steinbacher, and J. A. Persing. 2013. "Comprehensive Cleft Center: A Paradigm Shift in Cleft Care." *Plastic and Reconstructive Surgery* 131 (2): 312e–13e.

Patwardhan, N., E. Kiely, D. P. Drake, L. Spitz, and A. Pierro. 2001. "Colostomy for Anorectal Anomalies: High Incidence of Complications." *Journal of Pediatric Surgery* 36 (5): 795–98.

Penchaszadeh, V. B. 2002. "Preventing Congenital Anomalies in Developing Countries." *Community Genetics* 5 (1): 61–69.

Peyvasteh, M., S. Askarpour, H. Javaherizadeh, and T. Fatahian. 2011. "Evaluation of Epidemiologic Indices of Neonate's Diseases in the Pediatric Surgery Ward of the Ahvaz Jundishapur University Hospitals during the Period 1993–1996 and 2002–2005." *Annals of Pediatric Surgery* 7 (1): 7–9.

Pirani, S., E. Naddumba, R. Mathias, J. Konde-Lule, J. N. Penny, and others. 2009. "Towards Effective Ponseti Clubfoot Care: The Uganda Sustainable Clubfoot Care Project." *Clinical Orthopaedics and Related Research* 467 (5): 1154–63.

Poenaru, D. 2013. "Getting the Job Done: Analysis of the Impact and Effectiveness of the Smile Train Program in Alleviating the Global Burden of Cleft Disease." *World Journal of Surgery* 37 (7): 1562–70.

Poenaru, D., E. Borgstein, A. Numanoglu, and G. Azzie. 2010. "Caring for Children with Colorectal Disease in the Context of Limited Resources." *Seminars in Pediatric Surgery* 19 (2): 118–27.

Poenaru, D., J. Pemberton, C. Frankfurter, and B. Cameron. 2013. "Establishing Disability Weights for Congenital Pediatric Surgical Disease: A Multi-modal Study." *The Lancet* 381: S3115.

Poley, M. J., W. F. B. Brouwer, J. J. V. Busschbach, F. W. J. Hazebroek, D. Tibboel, and others. 2008. "Cost-Effectiveness of Neonatal Surgery: First Greeted with Skepticism, Now Increasingly Accepted." *Pediatric Surgery International* 24 (2): 119–27.

Pratap, A., D. K. Gupta, A. Tiwari, A. Sinha, N. Bhatta, and others. 2007. "Application of a Plain Abdominal Radiograph Transition Zone (PARTZ) in Hirschsprung's Disease." *BMC Pediatrics* 7: 5.

Prato, A. P., V. Rossi, S. Avanzini, G. Mattioli, N. Disma, and others. 2011. "Hirschsprung's Disease: What about Mortality?" *Pediatric Surgery International* 27 (5): 473–78.

Qureshi, J. S., J. Samuel, C. Lee, B. Cairns, C. Shores, and others. 2011. "Surgery and Global Public Health: The UNC-Malawi Initiative as a Model for Sustainable Collaboration." *World Journal of Surgery* 35 (1): 17–21.

Rao, S. G. 2007. "Pediatric Cardiac Surgery in Developing Countries." *Pediatric Cardiology* 28 (2): 144–48.

Rattray, K. W., T. C. Harrop, J. Aird, M. Beveridge, J. G. Gollogly, and others. 2013. "The Cost Effectiveness of Reconstructive Surgery in Cambodia." *Asian Biomedicine* 7 (3): 319–24.

Rayes, O. M. 2010. "Congenital Tracheoesophageal Fistula with or without Esophageal Atresia, King Abdulaziz University Hospital Experience over 15 Years." *Journal of King Abdulaziz University-Medical Sciences* 17 (4): 59–72.

Rescorla, F. J., A. M. Morrison, D. Engles, J. W. West, and J. L. Grosfeld. 1992. "Hirschsprung's Disease: Evaluation of Mortality and Long-Term Function in 260 Cases." *Archives of Surgery* 127 (8): 934.

Richmond, S., and J. Atkins. 2005. "A Population-Based Study of the Prenatal Diagnosis of Congenital Malformation over 16 Years." *BJOG: An International Journal of Obstetrics and Gynaecology* 112 (10): 1349–57.

Rohana, J., N. Y. Boo, and C. R. Thambidorai. 2008. "Early Outcome of Congenital Diaphragmatic Hernia in a Malaysian Tertiary Centre." *Singapore Medical Journal* 49 (2): 142–44.

Sadler, T. W. 2010. "The Embryologic Origin of Ventral Body Wall Defects." *Seminars in Pediatric Surgery* 19 (3): 209–14.

Sadoh, W. E., D. U. Nwaneri, and A. C. Owobu. 2011. "The Cost of Out-Patient Management of Chronic Heart Failure in Children with Congenital Heart Disease." *Nigerian Journal of Clinical Practice* 14 (1): 65–69.

Saha, A. K., M. B. Ali, S. K. Biswas, H. M. Z. Sharif, and A. Azim. 2012. "Neonatal Intestinal Obstruction: Patterns, Problems and Outcomes." *Bangladesh Medical Journal (Kulna)* 45 (1-2): 6–10.

Salomon, J. A., T. Vos, D. R. Hogan, M. Gagnon, M. Naghavi, and others. 2012. "Common Values in Assessing Health Outcomes from Disease and Injury: Disability Weights Measurement Study for the Global Burden of Disease Study 2010." *The Lancet* 380 (9859): 2129–43.

Saranrittichai, S. 2008. "Gastroschisis: Delivery and Immediate Repair in the Operating Room." *Journal of the Medical Association of Thailand* 91 (5): 686–92.

Sarrafan, N., S. A. M. Nasab, M. Fakoor, and A. Zakeri. 2012. "Short Term Outcome of Congenital Clubfoot Treated by Ponseti Method." *Pakistan Journal of Medical Sciences* 28 (3): 459–62.

Sekabira, J., and G. P. Hadley. 2009. "Gastroschisis: A Third World Perspective." *Pediatric Surgery International* 25 (4): 327–29.

Sekar, P., and V. Vilvanathan. 2007. "Telecardiology: Effective Means of Delivering Cardiac Care to Rural Children." *Asian Cardiovascular and Thoracic Annals* 15 (4): 320–23.

Semer, N. 2001. *Practical Plastic Surgery for Nonsurgeons.* Philadelphia, PA: Hanley and Belfus.

Senga, J., E. Rusingiza, J. Mucumbitsi, A. Binagwaho, B. Suys, and others. 2013. "Catheter Interventions in Congenital Heart Disease without Regular Catheterization Laboratory Equipment: The Chain of Hope Experience in Rwanda." *Pediatric Cardiology* 34 (1): 39–45.

Shah, G., M. Singh, T. Pandey, B. Kalakheti, and G. Bhandari. 2008. "Incidence of Congenital Heart Disease in a Tertiary Care Hospital." *Kathmandu University Medical Journal* 6 (1): 33–36.

Sharma, S., and D. K. Gupta. 2012. "Hirschsprung's Disease Presenting beyond Infancy: Surgical Options and Postoperative Outcome." *Pediatric Surgery International* 28 (1): 5–8.

Singh, K., C. Greaves, L. Mohammed, and A. Kumar. 2012. "Epidemiology of Treacheoesophageal Fistula and Other Major Congenital Malformations of the Digestive System among Newborns in an English Speaking Caribbean Country: A Population Based Study." *British Journal of Medical Sciences* 1 (3): 16–25.

Sinha, S. K., R. P. Kanojia, A. Wakhlu, J. D. Rawat, S. N. Kureel, and others. 2008. "Delayed Presentation of Anorectal Malformations." *Journal of the Indian Association of Pediatric Surgery* 13 (2): 64–68.

Spiegel, D. A., O. P. Shrestha, P. Sitoula, T. Rajbhandary, B. Bijukachhe, and others. 2009. "Ponseti Method for Untreated Idiopathic Clubfeet in Nepalese Patients from 1 to 6 Years of Age." *Clinical Orthopaedics and Related Research* 467 (5): 1164–70.

Stoll, C., Y. Alembik, B. Dott, and M. P. Roth. 2001. "Risk Factors in Congenital Abdominal Wall Defects (Omphalocele and Gastroschisi): A Study in a Series of 265,858 Consecutive Births." *Annales De Genetique* 44 (4): 201–08.

Swenson, O. 2002. "Hirschsprung's Disease: A Review." *Pediatrics* 109 (5): 914–18.

Tefera, E., T. Teka, and M. Derbew. 2007. "Neonatal Gastrointestinal Surgical Emergencies: A 5-Year Review in a Teaching Hospital in Addis Ababa, Ethiopia." *Ethiopian Medical Journal* 45 (3): 251–56.

Tindall, A. J., C. W. E. Steinlechner, C. B. D. Lavy, S. Mannion, and N. Mkandawire. 2005. "Results of Manipulation of Idiopathic Clubfoot Deformity in Malawi by Orthopaedic Clinical Officers Using the Ponseti Method: A Realistic Alternative for the Developing World?" *Journal of Pediatric Orthopaedics* 25 (5): 627–29.

Toro, M. N. H., M. E. A. Rave, and P. M. J. Gomez. 2010. "Management of Abdominal Wall Defects (Gastroschisis and Omphalocele) at Hospital Universitario San Vicente de Paúl, in Medellín, Colombia, 1998–2006." [Spanish]. *Iatreia* 23 (3): 220–26.

Turowski, C., J. Dingemann, and J. Giilick. 2010. "Delayed Diagnosis of Imperforate Anus: An Unacceptable Morbidity." *Pediatric Surgery International* 26 (11): 1083–86.

Uba, A. F., and L. B. Chirdan. 2003. "Omphalocoele and Gastroschisis: Management in a Developing Country." *Nigerian Journal of Surgical Research* 5 (1): 57–61.

Ugiagbe, E. E., and O. D. Osifo. 2012. "Postmortem Examinations on Deceased Neonates: A Rarely Utilized Procedure in an African Referral Center." *Pediatric and Developmental Pathology* 15 (1): 1–4.

Upadhyaya, V. D., A. N. Gangopadhyaya, D. K. Gupta, S. P. Sharma, V. Kumar, and others. 2007. "Prognosis of Congenital Tracheoesophageal Fistula with Esophageal Atresia on the Basis of Gap Length." *Pediatric Surgery International* 23 (8): 767–71.

van Bosse, H. J. 2011. "Ponseti Treatment for Clubfeet, An International Perspective." *Current Opinion in Pediatrics* 23 (1): 41–45.

van der Linde, D., E. E. M. Konings, M. A. Slager, M. Witsenburg, W. A. Helbing, and others. 2011. "Birth Prevalanece of Congenital Heart Disease Worldwide." *Journal of the American College of Cardiology* 58 (21): 2241–47.

van Heurn, L. W. E., W. Cheng, B. de Vries, H. Saing, N. J. G. Jansen, and others. 2002. "Anomalies Associated with Oesophageal Atresia in Asians and Europeans." *Pediatric Surgery International* 18 (4): 241–43.

Vincent, M. V., and S. U. Jackman. 2009. "Hirschsprung's Disease in Barbados—A 16-Year Review." *West Indian Medical Journal* 58 (4): 347–51.

Vu, L. T., K. K. Nobuhara, C. Laurent, and G. M. Shaw. 2008. "Increasing Prevalence of Gastroschisis: Population-Based Study in California." *Journal of Pediatrics* 152 (6): 807–11.

Walker, I. A., A. D. Obua, F. Mouton, S. Ttendo, and I. H. Wilson. 2010. "Paediatric Surgery and Anaesthesia in South-Western Uganda: A Cross-Sectional Survey." *Bulletin of the World Health Organization* 88 (12): 897–906.

Warf, B. C. 2011. "Hydrocephalus Associated with Neural Tube Defects: Characteristics, Management, and Outcomes in Sub-Saharan Africa." *Child's Nervous System* 27 (10): 1589–94.

———. 2013. "Educate One to Save A Few. Educate Few to Save Many." *World Neurosurgery* 79 (2 Suppl.): e15–8.

Warf, B. C., B. C. Alkire, S. Bhai, C. Hughes, S. J. Schiff, and others. 2011. "Costs and Benefits of Neurosurgical Intervention for Infant Hydrocephalus in Sub-Saharan Africa." *Journal of Neurosurgical Pediatrics* 8 (5): 509–21.

WHO (World Health Organization). 2008. "Global Burden of Disease 2004 Update: Disability Weights for Diseases and Conditions." WHO, Geneva.

———. 2012. "Congenital Anomalies," Fact Sheet No. 370, WHO, Geneva. http://www.who.int/mediacentre/factsheets/fs370/en/.

———. 2013a. "Emergency and Essential Surgical Care: Congenital Anomalies." http://www.who.int/surgery/challenges/esc_congenital_nomalies/en/.

———. 2013b. "Global Health Estimates for Deaths by Cause, Age, and Sex for Years 2000–2011." WHO, Geneva.

Wickramasinghe, P., S. P. Lambabadusuriya, and S. Narenthiran. 2001. "Prospective Study of Congenital Heart Disease in Children." *Ceylon Medical Journal* 46 (3): 96–98.

Wu, V., and D. Poenaru. 2013. "Burden of Surgically Correctable Disabilities among Children in the Dadaab Refugee Camp." *World Journal of Surgery* 37 (7): 1536–43.

Wu, V., D. Poenaru, and M. J. Poley. 2013. "Burden of Surgical Congenital Anomalies in Kenya: A Population-Based Study." *Journal of Tropical Pediatrics* 59 (3): 195–220.

Yang, C. F., W. J. Soong, M. J. Jeng, S. J. Chen, Y. S. Lee, and others. 2006. "Esophageal Atresia with Tracheoesophageal Fistula: Ten Years of Experience in an Institute." *Journal of the Chinese Medical Association* 69 (7): 317–21.

Zupan, J. 2005. "Perinantal Mortality in Developing Countries." *New England Journal of Medicine* 352 (20): 2047–48.

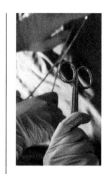

Chapter 9

Hernia and Hydrocele

Jessica H. Beard, Michael Ohene-Yeboah,
Catherine R. deVries, and William P. Schecter

INTRODUCTION

Groin hernia and hydrocele are two of the most common surgical conditions globally. This chapter summarizes the literature on the pathogenesis, clinical presentation, and treatment for groin hernia and hydrocele, focusing on unique clinical characteristics and management strategies for these conditions in low- and middle-income countries (LMICs).

We present our estimate of the global and regional burden of disease from groin hernia, the first of its kind in the literature. In addition, we highlight the existing data on the cost-effectiveness of surgical treatment for groin hernia and hydrocele. We document the successful global efforts of Operation Hernia and the Global Programme to Eliminate Lymphatic Filariasis (GPELF) in combating hernia and lymphatic filariasis, a common cause of hydrocele in LMICs.

Groin hernia repair and hydrocelectomy are cost-effective curative therapies that can improve the quality of life. In addition, herniorrhaphy can prevent life-threatening complications associated with groin hernia. Unfortunately, many people do not have access to safe and effective surgical care for these common conditions.

The treatment of groin hernia and hydrocele should be a high priority on any global surgery agenda. Basic surgical care for these conditions is a crucial part of health care services that should be available at first-level hospitals. Training programs to improve the skills of surgical-care providers in LMICs, in combination with infrastructure investment to build hospital capacity, are urgently needed to increase access to these essential surgical procedures.

GROIN HERNIA

Definitions of Groin Hernia

A hernia is a protrusion of a body part through a defect in the anatomic structure that normally contains it. A groin hernia is a specific type of hernia involving the bulging of abdominal contents through the inguinal or femoral canal. The inguinal canal is a "corridor" in the abdominal wall that, in men, houses the spermatic cord as it passes on its way to the testicle. Inguinal hernias may be caused either by a failure in the normal closure of the abdominal wall lining in the inguinal canal during fetal development, or by an acquired weakening of the abdominal wall, often later in life. In either case, the hernia sac, a pouch made of the membrane lining the abdomen and containing fat, ovary, bowel, or bladder, protrudes into the inguinal canal.

A scrotal hernia is a type of inguinal hernia in which the hernia sac, often containing bowel, follows the path of the spermatic cord into the scrotum. Femoral hernias occur rarely and involve the protrusion of abdominal contents through the femoral canal, a space

Corresponding author: Jessica H. Beard, MD, MPH, University of California, San Francisco, Jessica.Beard@ucsfmedctr.org adjacent to the femoral vein in the upper thigh. This type of hernia occurs most commonly in women (Nilsson and others 2007).

Groin hernias may be further classified as reducible, incarcerated, or strangulated.

- A reducible hernia is one in which the hernia contents can be gently pushed back into the abdominal cavity.
- An incarcerated hernia is irreducible, meaning that the hernia sac contents are "stuck" outside the abdomen.
- A strangulated hernia refers to an incarcerated hernia in which the entrance to the hernia sac or "neck" is constricted, limiting blood supply to the sac contents and ultimately resulting in tissue necrosis, bowel infarction, and perforation. This condition is a life-threatening emergency requiring immediate surgery.

Scrotal and femoral hernias are more likely to become incarcerated and cause complications.

Risk Factors and Natural History of Groin Hernia

In a study of hernias in adults (5,316 men and 8,136 women) in the United States participating in the First National Health and Nutrition Examination Survey (NHANES) between 1971–75 and followed up in 1993, male gender and increasing age were identified as important groin hernia risk factors. Black race and obesity were independently associated with a lower incidence of inguinal hernia in the cohort (Ruhl and Everhart 2007).

Increased intra-abdominal pressure has long been implicated in the pathogenesis of inguinal hernia; however, data on physical activity as a risk factor for groin hernia are inconclusive. NHANES found no evidence of association between physical activity and hernia risk, but two case-control studies from Spain suggest that strenuous activity may play a role in hernia development (Carbonell and others 1993; Flich and others 1992; Ruhl and Everhart 2007). It is likely that different types of physical activity are associated with different levels of risk, and further study is needed. Other risk factors for groin hernia include a family history of hernia and the presence of a hiatal hernia (Ruhl and Everhart 2007). Prematurity is an important risk factor in children (Lau and others 2007).

The natural history of inguinal hernia is poorly understood. Population-based studies of inguinal hernia's natural history are nearly impossible today because inguinal hernia repair is at least somewhat available in most settings. The little contemporary data that exist are limited by selection bias (Gallegos and others 1991).

The key question in determining the natural history of hernia centers on the identification of the annual risk of hernia accident (that is, bowel obstruction, incarceration, or strangulation) without hernia repair. To address this question, Neuhauser (1977) examined data in two settings in which herniorrhaphy was generally not practiced: Paul Berger's Paris truss clinic (circa 1880) and Cali, Colombia (circa 1970). He found that the probabilities of hernia accident per year were 0.0037 and 0.00291 in the Berger and Colombia data, respectively.

Using Neuhauser's figures and U.S. life-table analysis, Turaga, Fitzgibbons, and Puri (2008) calculated a hernia accident lifetime incidence of 19.4 percent in 18-year-old men with inguinal hernia in the United States. They found only a 4.4 percent lifetime incidence of hernia accident in 72-year-old men with hernia. These calculations suggest that hernia accident is a relatively common lifetime event in younger patients with unrepaired inguinal hernia.

Clinical Features of Groin Hernia in LMICs

Patients with inguinal hernia generally present with a bulge in the groin, which may have associated symptoms. Limited access to surgical care in LMICs leads to a clinical picture of groin hernia that is distinct from that in high-income countries (HICs). In fact, most cases of inguinal hernia in LMICs go untreated, resulting in large painful hernias that often limit physical activity (Herszage 2004; Sanders and others 2008; Shillcutt, Clarke, and Kingsnorth 2010). In a prospective study from Ghana, 67 percent of patients presenting for repair had scrotal hernias, placing them at increased risk of hernia complications. When the Ghanaian cohort was compared with a similar group of patients from the United Kingdom, the Ghanaians were found to be younger and have larger hernias (Sanders and others 2008).

Groin hernias are often longstanding in LMICs. In Tanzania, nearly 50 percent of hernia patients in one study presented for repair more than five years after disease onset (Mabula and Chalya 2012). Groin hernias also have negative effects on patients' well-being and productivity in LMICs. For example, in another Ghanaian hernia cohort, 16 percent of hernia patients were unable to work, and 64 percent reported limited daily activity (Sanders and others 2008).

Most symptomatic groin hernias in HICs are treated with elective surgery before complications such as obstruction or strangulation occur. In a prospective study of 6,895 patients in the Swedish Hernia Register, only 5 percent of groin herniorrhaphies in men were classified as emergencies (Koch and others 2005).

In contrast, patients with groin hernias in LMICs often present for medical care with complications. More than two-thirds of inguinal hernia repairs at a third-level center in Kumasi, Ghana, were emergency operations (Ohene-Yeboah and others 2009). In a study from Bugando Medical Center in Tanzania, more than half of presenting groin hernias were incarcerated, while 18.6 percent and 11.1 percent of patients, respectively, had obstructed and strangulated hernias (Mabula and Chalya 2012). The unique clinical features of groin hernias in LMICs, including large size, longer disease duration, physical limitations, and complicated hospital presentation, result in high morbidity and mortality rates.

Epidemiology and Burden of Disease

Prevalence and Incidence of Inguinal Hernia in HICs.
Inguinal hernia is one of the most common surgical conditions globally. An estimated 20 million groin hernias are repaired annually worldwide (Bay-Nielsen and others 2001). Despite the high disease prevalence, relatively few studies of inguinal hernia epidemiology have been undertaken, even in HICs. Data from World War II cohorts demonstrate an inguinal hernia prevalence of between 6.5 percent and 8.0 percent in American soldiers (Everhart 1994). A study from the United Kingdom found a 27 percent lifetime risk for inguinal hernia repair in men and 3 percent in women (Primatesta and Goldacre 1996). A rigorous community-based survey demonstrated an inguinal hernia prevalence of 18.3 percent among men in an ethnically diverse Jerusalem neighborhood (Abramson and others 1978). Of note, 7.6 percent of men had "obvious" groin hernias in this study, while the remaining 10.7 percent had hernia diagnosed as a palpable impulse at the external inguinal canal by physician examination. These data suggest that the actual hernia prevalence in Jerusalem may be less than 18.3 percent.

Studies of groin hernia incidence are particularly limited. Data from the NHANES study have been used to make the most reliable assessment of inguinal hernia incidence in the United States. In their analysis of the NHANES cohort, Ruhl and Everhart (2007) found an annual incidence of inguinal hernia of 315 per 100,000 population in adults in the United States.

Not surprisingly, the incidence of inguinal hernia repair is lower than disease incidence. A retrospective review of all inguinal hernia repairs in Minnesota during a 20-year period found an incidence of hernia repair of 217 per 100,000 person-years (Zendejas and others 2013). This finding means that approximately 670,000

inguinal hernia repairs are performed annually in the United States.

The annual inguinal hernia repair rate in the United Kingdom (130 per 100,000 population) is lower than the rate of repair in the United States (Primatesta and Goldacre 1996). Differing practice patterns among surgeons and referring primary care physicians may explain regional differences in the incidence of inguinal herniorrhaphy in HICs (Hair and others 2001).

Epidemiology of Inguinal Hernia in LICs and MICs.
Published information on inguinal hernia epidemiology in low-resource settings is limited to two studies of hernia prevalence in Sub-Saharan Africa from the 1960s and 1970s (Belcher, Nyame, and Wurapa 1978; Yardov and Stoyanov 1969). Inguinal hernia prevalence in men in these studies ranged from 7.7 percent in rural Ghana to 25 percent on the island of Pemba in East Africa. Given poor access to surgical care in LMICs, it makes sense that inguinal hernia prevalence would be higher in LMICs than in HICs. However, only limited evidence supports this thesis.

A rigorous population-based investigation of groin hernia prevalence has been recently conducted in eastern Uganda (Löfgren and others 2014). This study demonstrated a prevalence of untreated hernia of 6.6 percent in men, with an overall hernia prevalence (including repaired hernias) of 9.4 percent. Although this study is an important contribution to the literature on hernia epidemiology, contemporary data on the incidence of inguinal hernia in LMICs is notably lacking.

To fill this gap in knowledge, Beard and colleagues created a method to estimate inguinal hernia incidence and prevalence in LMICs, carrying out their analysis in both the Ghanaian and Tanzanian contexts (Beard, Oresanya, Akoko, and others 2013; Beard, Oresanya, Ohene-Yeboah, and others 2013). In their Tanzanian analysis, they adjusted incidence data from the NHANES study for the population age and gender structure of the country, and calculated an annual incidence of new hernias in Tanzanian adults of 244 per 100,000 population. This number is lower than the inguinal hernia incidence of 315 per 100,000 person-years calculated in the NHANES study (Ruhl and Everhart 2007). The authors attribute the lower incidence of inguinal hernia in Tanzania to the relative youth of the population compared with that of the United States.

Despite demonstrating a lower incidence of inguinal hernia, Beard and others estimated a relatively high prevalence of inguinal hernia in Tanzanian men at 12.1 percent (Beard, Oresanya, Akoko, and others 2013). Because heavy labor and racial factors have not been clearly substantiated as significant inguinal hernia risk factors in the literature, the authors attribute the higher prevalence of hernia in Sub-Saharan Africa to lack of access to surgery in the region (Lau and others 2007; Ruhl and Everhart 2007).

Global Burden of Inguinal Hernia

Estimates of the global burden of inguinal hernia are rough at best. Yang and others (2011) calculated that 58.7 million disability-adjusted life years (DALYs) would be averted by repair of all adult hernias in Sub-Saharan Africa. This figure is more than double the estimates of the total surgical disease burden for Sub-Saharan Africa calculated by Debas and others (2006). The discrepancy could be caused either by a previous underestimation of the burden of surgical disease or, more likely, by different methods used to calculate surgical DALYs. A standard metric for measuring the surgical burden of disease is urgently needed to accurately identify global surgical priorities and guide resource allocation and advocacy efforts.

In the 2010 Global Burden of Disease study (referred to as GBD 2010), Murray and others (2012) found that 11 DALYs per 100,000 population per year were attributable to groin hernia worldwide. This figure is less than their estimates for non-life-threatening conditions like premenstrual syndrome (18 DALYs per 100,000 population) and scabies (23 per 100,000 population). We believe that GBD 2010 underestimated the disease burden of groin hernia, and we present our estimates of inguinal hernia epidemiology and global disease burden.

To test our hypothesis, we recalculated the DALYs attributable to inguinal hernia using the method described by Beard, Oresanya, Akoko, and others (2013). We adjusted the NHANES incidence figures to the population age structures of the six World Health Organization (WHO) regions.[1] We then calculated incidence and prevalence accordingly. Deaths were estimated by using Neuhauser's figure of 0.0037 probability of hernia accident per year, along with our own estimates of death from hernia complications in the various WHO regions (Neuhauser 1977).

For our DALY calculation, we assumed that hernia patients in the Sub-Saharan African region present for surgical treatment at an average age of 45 years, whereas patients in other regions present at an older age (60 years in North and South America, the Eastern Mediterranean, Southeast Asia, and the Western Pacific; 70 years in Europe) (Mabula and Chalya 2012; Nilsson and others 2007). We used the GBD 2010 inguinal hernia disability weight of 0.012 to calculate years of life lost due to disability.

The results of our epidemiologic analysis are presented in table 9.1. We estimate that inguinal hernia prevalence in the general population ranges from 4.06 percent in Europe to 6.05 percent in the Western Pacific. Prevalence differences across regions are likely to be caused by variations in population age structure, access to surgical care, and risk of death from hernia accident. We estimate a global inguinal hernia prevalence of 5.85 percent, meaning that about 223 million people globally have hernias. The global mortality from inguinal hernia is significant; according to our calculations, nearly 44,000 people die from hernia each year.

Our analysis indicates that hernia prevalence is highest in the Sub-Saharan African and Western Pacific regions. Although the literature on hernia epidemiology in Africa is relatively well developed, studies of hernia disease burden and treatment in the Western Pacific are notably quite limited. More research on the burden of hernia in this region is needed in light of these findings.

Table 9.2 presents our estimate of global and regional inguinal hernia disease burden. The figures suggest that

Table 9.1 Estimated Global and Regional Inguinal Hernia Epidemiologic Figures

Region	Prevalence (%)	Yearly incidence (per 100,000 people)	Number of people with inguinal hernia (million)	Estimated deaths per year
World	5.85	293	223	43,689
Africa	5.35	250	22.7	8,396
Americas	4.36	307	28.2	4,173
Eastern Mediterranean	4.70	251	15.4	2,857
Europe	4.06	336	27.1	3,010
Southeast Asia	4.88	278	54.9	10,159
Western Pacific	6.05	310	81.6	15,094

Sources: Authors' estimates based on Beard, Oresanya, Akoko, and others (2013) and United States Census Bureau International Database (http://www.census.gov/population /international/data/idb/region.php).

Table 9.2 Estimated Burden of Inguinal Hernia by Region

Region	Total DALYs (100,000)	Estimated surgical DALYs (100,000)	Estimated inguinal hernia DALYs (100,000)	Estimated inguinal hernia DALYs as a percentage of surgical DALYs	Estimated inguinal hernia DALYs per 100,000 population per year
World	1,5230	1,640	38.4	2.3	85
Africa	3,770	250	5.8	2.3	136
Americas	1,430	180	4.3	2.4	67
Eastern Mediterranean	1,420	150	2.5	1.7	76
Europe	1,510	220	3.7	1.7	55
Southeast Asia	4,430	480	8.9	1.9	79
Western Pacific	2,650	370	13.2	3.6	98

Sources: Authors' estimates based on Beard, Oresanya, Akoko, and others (2013); Debas and others (2006); and United States Census Bureau International Database (http://www.census.gov/population/international/data/idb/region.php).
Note: DALY = disability-adjusted life year.

inguinal hernia accounts for a small but measureable proportion of the surgical DALYs, as estimated by Debas and others (2006). Most important, we demonstrate that the disease burden of hernia is likely to be higher than the GBD 2010 calculations suggest. According to our method, inguinal hernia accounts for an average of 85 DALYs per 100,000 population per year, almost eight times the disease burden calculated by GBD 2010 (Murray and others 2012). This finding places the disease burden of hernia on par with that of other surgical diseases such as benign prostatic hypertrophy and ovarian cancer. Notably, the burden of inguinal hernia is highest in the most impoverished regions of the world, where access to surgical care and surgical outcomes are likely to be the poorest.

Met and Unmet Need for Inguinal Hernia Repair in LMICs

Mock and others (2010) have identified improved access to safe inguinal hernia repair as a high global health priority. Studies indicate that inguinal herniorrhaphy is the most frequently performed general surgical procedure at many first-level hospitals throughout Sub-Saharan Africa (Galukande and others 2010; Nordberg 1984).

There is general consensus that the unmet need for inguinal herniorrhaphy in LMICs is significant. Estimates of need range from 163 to 357 hernia repairs per 100,000 population per year, depending on whether incident only or incident and prevalent cases are to be addressed (Beard, Oresanya, Akoko, and others 2013; Beard, Oresanya, Ohene-Yeboah, and others 2013; Nordberg 1984). Grimes and others (2012) reported that the average first-level hospital in Sub-Saharan Africa

performs only 30 hernia repairs per 100,000 population per year, illustrating the vast unmet need for herniorrhaphy in the region.

Beard and colleagues in an unpublished study investigated surgical activity at all seven first-level hospitals in the Pwani Region of Tanzania. Despite its proximity to Dar es Salaam, Pwani is one of the poorest regions in Tanzania. According to estimates by the Tanzanian government, Pwani ranks fourteenth out of 21 regions in measures of GDP per capita (National Bureau of Statistics and Coast Regional Commissioners Office 2007).

Table 9.3 presents data from this study, specifically focusing on rates of both elective and emergency repairs in each of the Pwani districts. Our analysis found that first-level hospitals in Pwani performed a population-weighted average of 34.5 elective and emergency herniorrhaphies per 100,000 population, a number similar to the hernia repair rate calculated by Grimes and others (2012). These findings further document the surgical capacity crisis in first-level hospitals in Sub-Saharan Africa.

There also appears to be a significant disparity in the number of inguinal hernia repairs by district in the Pwani region. In Kibaha, only 10.5 inguinal hernia repairs were performed per 100,000 population in 2012, compared with nearly 67 repairs per 100,000 population in Kisarawe. Additional operations are possibly performed in other health dispensaries, which may account for variations in hernia repair rates. Patients from one district may also be seeking care in a neighboring district. Further research is needed to more accurately characterize surgical capacity and the need for essential surgical services in low-resource settings.

Table 9.3 Rates of Elective and Emergency Inguinal Hernia Repair in the Pwani Region, Tanzania, 2012

District	Elective hernia repair per 100,000 population	Emergency hernia repair per 100,000 population	Performed by nonphysicians, number (percent)	Performed by surgeons, number (percent)
Bagamoyo	18.5	12.1	76 (100)	0 (0)
Kibaha	7.8	2.7	8 (29.6)	11 (40.7)
Kisarawe	46.2	20.7	38 (55.9)	0 (0)
Mafia	23.3	0	4 (40.0)	6 (60.0)
Mkuranga	23.8	6.7	58 (98.3)	0 (0)
Rufiji	47.9	9.6	73 (57.9)	6 (4.8)
Weighted average	25.8	8.7		

Management of Inguinal Hernia

Nonsurgical Management. Nonsurgical management is appropriate for small, minimally symptomatic or asymptomatic inguinal hernias in HICs. In a randomized controlled trial comparing a "watchful waiting" approach with routine herniorrhaphy for minimally symptomatic inguinal hernias, the risk of hernia accident was low (1.8 accidents per 1,000 patient-years during the 2- to 4.5-year follow-up period); outcomes were similar between groups (Fitzgibbons and others 2006). In LMICs, this watchful waiting approach to inguinal hernia may not be safe (and is generally not practiced) because patients have limited access to routine follow-up and emergency surgery.

Surgical Management. Various techniques are available for surgical reconstruction of the posterior wall of the inguinal canal. The most common procedures are the Bassini, McVay, and Shouldice repairs, all of which involve different methods of suturing together components of the abdominal wall through an inguinal incision. The problem with these repairs is that groin tissues are sutured together under tension. The tension results in a relatively high risk of postoperative hernia recurrence, in the range of 10 percent to 30 percent (RAND Corporation 1983).

In 1986, Lichtenstein introduced a tension-free repair technique, using prosthetic mesh to reinforce weakness in the posterior wall of the inguinal canal. A randomized trial demonstrated a recurrence rate of only 1 percent to 2 percent with the Lichtenstein technique (Fitzgibbons and others 2006). Although some studies suggest that the mesh technique may increase the risk of chronic postoperative groin pain, the results of the Lichtenstein repair represent a significant improvement over traditional tissue repair (Hakeem and Shanmugam 2011).

First described in 2001, the Desarda repair, which uses an undetached strip of external oblique aponeurosis to reconstruct the posterior wall of the inguinal canal, is an example of a tension-free tissue repair. This technique has been shown to have rates of recurrence and postoperative pain similar to that of the Lichtenstein technique (Szopinski and others 2012).

Laparoscopic approaches to inguinal herniorrhaphy were introduced in the 1990s. Although the risk of postoperative complications is slightly higher after laparoscopic repair, laparoscopy is associated with decreased recovery time and less postoperative pain than open mesh techniques (McCormack and others 2003; Neumayer and others 2004). Cost-effectiveness studies comparing laparoscopic with open inguinal hernia repair techniques have been inconclusive (Heikkinen and others 1997; Schneider and others 2003).

Although the tension-free repair has become the gold standard in HICs, most inguinal hernias are still repaired with the Bassini method in LMICs because of the high cost of prosthetic mesh and the lack of training in mesh repair (Ohene-Yeboah and Abantanga 2011). However, a report from Nigeria found that the mesh repair was well tolerated, with few complications at one-year follow-up (Arowolo and others 2011). In India, mesh repairs are more common than in other LMICs, and laparoscopic inguinal hernia repair is becoming more widely practiced (Krishna and others 2012; Swadia 2011). Nevertheless, the cost of the prosthetic mesh remains prohibitive for most patients in LMICs. A study from Uganda comparing patients randomized to receive the Desarda tension-free tissue hernia repair and the Lichtenstein mesh repair demonstrated similar short-term clinical outcomes. Of note, the operating time for the Desarda repair was shorter in this study (Manyilirah and others 2012). The Desarda technique is a promising and potentially effective low-cost method to repair hernias in LMICs, and its applicability in this context merits further investigation.

Anesthesia Considerations. Open inguinal hernia repair may be performed using local, spinal, or general anesthesia, depending on both patient status and surgeon preference. All three anesthetic techniques are safe in healthy young patients when administered by skilled practitioners in HICs. However, spinal and general anesthesia are associated with higher rates of myocardial infarction and urinary retention, respectively, in patients older than age 65 years (Bay-Nielsen and Kehlet 2008).

A meta-analysis demonstrated the incredible disparity in anesthesia-related mortality in LMICs when compared with HICs (Bainbridge and others 2012). Factors associated with this disparity included few qualified anesthetists, lack of appropriate training of anesthesia practitioners, and limited supplies for safe monitoring and administration of anesthesia in many LMICs (Walker and Wilson 2008). No pulse oximeters were found in any of the 14 government hospitals surveyed in a study from Uganda (Linden and others 2012). Given these limitations in anesthesia care and the inherently higher risk associated with a general anesthetic, we recommend that groin hernia repairs in LMICs be carried out under local or spinal anesthesia whenever possible.

Mosquito-Net Mesh Hernia Repair. Mosquito netting has been introduced as a prosthesis for inguinal hernia repair to address the high cost of industry mesh. In the 1990s, sterilized mosquito-net mesh was first used to repair inguinal hernias in India. Tongaonkar and others (2003) reported a series of 359 hernias that were repaired with a copolymer mosquito-net mesh (polyethylene and polypropylene) in multiple hospitals throughout India. On short-term follow-up, the minor wound infection rate was less than 5 percent; there were no mesh infections and one hernia recurrence.

These promising preliminary findings in India have prompted further investigation into the use of non-insecticide-treated mosquito-net mesh for inguinal hernia repair in other low-resource settings, specifically, Africa. The feasibility and safety of this technique have been demonstrated for nylon and polyester mosquito-net mesh in Burkina Faso, Ghana, and India (Clarke and others 2009; Freudenberg and others 2006; Gundre, Iyer, and Subramaniyan 2012). In addition, experimental research in goats has shown that nylon mesh leads to a similar amount of tissue fibrosis when compared with standard polypropylene industry mesh (Wilhelm and others 2007). Effective sterilization techniques have been described for both copolymer and polyester mosquito-net meshes (Stephenson and Kingsnorth 2011).

Newer studies have investigated the molecular characteristics and associated infection risk of mosquito-net mesh compared with commercial hernia prosthetics. In one study, Sanders and others (2013) inoculated polyethylene mosquito-net and industry meshes with staphylococcus epidermidis and staphylococcus aureus. They found no difference in the mean number of adherent bacteria to mosquito-net mesh when compared with commercial polypropylene-based meshes. These results suggest that implantation of mosquito-net mesh should not increase the risk of surgical site infection. Sanders, Kingsnorth, and Stephenson (2013) investigated the macromolecular structure of polyethylene mosquito-net mesh using electron microscopy and spectroscopy, demonstrating that the material and mechanical properties of mosquito net, including tensile strength, are equivalent to those of common lightweight commercial meshes.

Although the results of these studies are promising, sample sizes are small and follow-up is limited. Further investigation into the efficacy and safety of mosquito-net mesh for inguinal hernia repair is needed before widespread implementation. The United Kingdom's nonprofit organization Operation Hernia (see box 9.1) is planning an audit of outcomes of copolymer mosquito-net mesh purchased from India for use during humanitarian surgical repair camps (Stephenson and Kingsnorth 2011). (See box 9.2 for a description of a successful local initiative.)

If the safety of mosquito-net mesh is demonstrated, steps should be taken to make it more widely available for hernia repair in LMICs. Potential challenges to widespread implementation include inadequate training in the mesh technique, barriers to acceptance of mosquito netting as a surgical tool by care providers, and complexities of acquisition and distribution of the mosquito-net mesh. A comprehensive program that addresses these issues is needed to ensure equitable access to mesh inguinal hernia repair in LMICs.

Complications Associated with Groin Hernia Repair

Repair Complications in HICs. Complications after elective herniorrhaphy in HICs include wound hematoma (6.1 percent), scrotal hematoma (4.5 percent), urinary tract infection (2.1 percent), wound infection (1.8 percent), and testicular swelling (1.6 percent) (Fitzgibbons and others 2006). Another important and increasingly recognized complication is chronic postoperative groin pain. Postoperative pain syndrome may occur in up to 53 percent of patients and is often difficult to prevent and treat (Poobalan and others 2003).

Mortality following groin herniorrhaphy is difficult to measure. Primatesta and Goldacre (1996) observed the rate of postoperative deaths following elective and

Effective Global Health Program: Operation Hernia

Operation Hernia, a nonprofit organization based in the United Kingdom, is an effective program aimed at combating inguinal hernia in low- and middle-income countries (LMICs). Years before Operation Hernia began, a "sister city" relationship was established between Takoradi, Ghana, and Plymouth, United Kingdom. In 2005, Andrew Kingsnorth and Chris Oppong, surgeons from Plymouth Hospital, initiated the first Operation Hernia mission to Ghana. With support from the British High Commissioner and the European Hernia Society, the team of surgeons repaired 130 hernias during their first one-week mission (Kingsnorth and others 2006). Since then, Operation Hernia has established a Hernia Treatment Center in Takoradi and expanded its services to 10 countries in Africa, Asia, Eastern Europe, and Latin America. This organization has supported more than 85 humanitarian missions and treated more than 9,000 patients with hernias worldwide.[a]

Operation Hernia has been instrumental in advocacy for recognition of the global public health significance of groin hernia. In addition, leaders of the organization have spearheaded much of the research on hernia epidemiology in LMICs, along with safety and efficacy studies of mosquito net mesh repair. Much of the literature on cost-effectiveness of groin hernia repair in low-resource settings was funded and carried out by Operation Hernia.

One of Operation Hernia's stated goals is to teach mesh hernia repair techniques to local surgical care providers (Kingsnorth and others 2006). If this aspect of the mission were to be systemized and expanded, it would make the humanitarian model for the delivery of hernia surgical care more sustainable. Although some might criticize Operation Hernia for being a disease-focused vertical intervention, this organization has demonstrated that its model is scalable and effective.

a. Operation Hernia Website 2013. http://www.operationhernia.org.uk.

Local Solutions: The Ghana Hernia Society's Comprehensive Approach to Groin Hernia Care

During the past decade, local surgeons have become increasingly interested in improving hernia care and increasing access to groin hernia repair throughout Ghana. Initially, a core group of surgeons engaged independently in surgical outreach programs focused on hernia care, working with the Apridec Medical Outreach Group, a Ghanaian nongovernmental organization whose mission is to provide free specialist care in northern Ghana.

To better coordinate their individual hernia treatment efforts, Michael Ohene-Yeboah and F. A. Abantanga (professors at Kwame Nkrumah University of Science and Technology in Kumasi, Ghana) along with Stephen Tabiri (Department of Surgery, Tamale Teaching Hospital in Tamale, Ghana) and others founded the Ghana Hernia Society (GHS) in February 2013. Since its inception, the GHS has held two teaching workshops on groin anatomy and mesh hernia repair techniques in Kumasi and Tamale.

Figure B9.2.1 demonstrates the current structure of activities of the GHS. The GHS employs a comprehensive public health approach to the treatment of groin hernia in Ghana, partnering with key actors in the Ghanaian government, the Ghana Health Service, and local hospitals to address hernia at multiple levels. The GHS coordinates groin hernia community education programs, advocacy efforts for the prioritization of hernia care, surgical skills training in mesh techniques, and hernia epidemiology research. The GHS's ultimate goals include the development of a Pan-African Hernia Society and partnership with other international hernia organizations.

box continues next page

Figure B9.2.1 Activity Flowchart of the Ghana Hernia Society

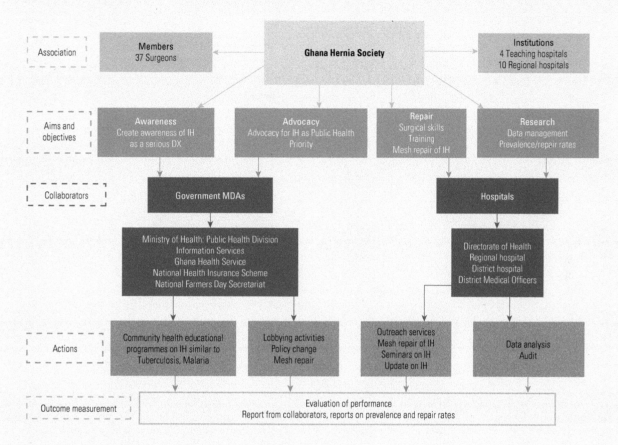

Source: Correspondence to authors from S. Tabiri and M. Ohene-Yeboah of the Ghana Hernia Society, 2013.
Note: IH = inguinal hernia; MDA = ministries, departments, and agencies.

The GHS's plan could easily be adapted for use in the establishment of hernia societies with similar goals in other low-resource settings. In addition, this four-pronged approach including community education, advocacy, surgical intervention and education, and research could serve as a model for the development of local solutions for other common surgical conditions such as hydrocele, traumatic injury, and obstetric fistula. Although in its early stages, the GHS is an excellent example of a local public health solution to a common and important surgical issue.

emergency inguinal hernia repairs during a 10-year period in the United Kingdom. They found a significantly increased risk of death after emergency compared with elective herniorrhaphy (1.6 percent and 0.1 percent, respectively). Inguinal hernia was listed as the cause of death in only 17 percent of cases of early postoperative mortality after emergency hernia repair, suggesting underestimation of the risk of death from this condition in the United Kingdom (Primatesta and Goldacre 1996).

A study of the mortality rate after groin hernia surgery in Sweden found similar results. The mortality rate after elective hernia repair was similar to that of the background population, but it increased 7-fold after emergency operations and 20-fold if bowel resection was required (Nilsson and others 2007).

Repair Complications in LMICs. Although the literature on the subject is sparse, complications after groin hernia repair in LMICs appear to be higher than in HICs. In Senegal, Fall and others (2005) reported a complication rate of more than 20 percent after elective groin herniorrhaphy. Some of the most serious postoperative complications found in this study, such as bladder injury and immediate hernia recurrence, were likely to be related to surgical technique. In Jos, Nigeria, rates of wound infections after elective inguinal hernia repair approach 8 percent, significantly higher than the rate of less than 2 percent reported in the United States (Ramyil and others 2000). Reliable data on the rate of hernia recurrence are not available in LMICs.

A review of the literature on inguinal hernia epidemiology and management in Africa found in-hospital inguinal hernia–related mortality rates ranging from 0.48 percent to 40.0 percent in six studies (Ohene-Yeboah and Abantanga 2011). A retrospective investigation of morbidity and mortality associated with inguinal hernia in Nigeria demonstrated an overall hernia mortality rate of 5.3 percent (Mbah 2007). Of note, although there were no deaths among patients with hernias treated electively in the Nigerian study, the mortality rate of patients with obstructed or strangulated hernias was greater than 21 percent (Mbah 2007). In Niger, mortality from hernia strangulation with small bowel necrosis may be as high as 40 percent (Harouna and others 2000).

Figure 9.1 demonstrates the pronounced disparity in outcomes after inguinal hernia repair in HICs and LMICs found in our review of the literature. This increased risk

of postoperative morbidity and mortality in LMICs is likely due to delayed presentation of large scrotal hernias; inadequate training of surgical, anesthetic, and nursing staff; and limitations in preoperative and postoperative care, hospital infrastructure, and supplies.

Task-Shifting in Hernia Surgery: A Targeted Way to Improve Quality of Care

LMICs face a severe shortage of skilled health care providers. The global workforce crisis is especially pronounced in the fields of surgery and anesthesia. In their analysis of surgical care provided at the hospitals in Pwani, Tanzania, Beard and others (2014) found only two staff general surgeons providing care in the region with a population of more than 1.1 million people (table 9.3). At Bagamoyo and Mkuranga District Hospitals, nearly all hernia repairs in 2012 were done by nonphysician clinicians (NPCs). Mafia District Hospital, located on a remote island off the coast of southern Tanzania, has no surgical specialist on staff; surgeons performing hernia repairs at this hospital during the study period were flown in by the nonprofit organization African Medical and Research Foundation. In Kibaha, the presence of a general surgeon did not increase surgical output in the district in 2012.

NPCs and nonsurgeon physicians clearly play a key role in the delivery of surgical care for inguinal hernia in Tanzania. Reports from other countries in Africa, including Malawi, Mozambique, and Niger, indicate a similar function for NPCs in the provision of surgical care (Kruk and others 2010; Sani and others 2009; Wilhelm and others 2011). Several studies document the safety of task-shifting of emergency obstetric procedures to nonphysicians in Ethiopia, Mozambique, and Tanzania (Gessessew and others 2011; McCord and others 2009; Pereira and others 1996).

Studies on outcomes after general surgical procedures performed by nonsurgeons, specifically hernia, are notably lacking in the literature. Wilhelm and others (2011) found similar outcomes after repair of strangulated inguinal hernia with bowel resection performed by surgeons and clinical officers at Zomba Central Hospital, a large teaching center in Malawi. Although promising, these results may not be generalizable to other LMICs. At Zomba Central Hospital, clinical officers were often directly proctored by fully qualified surgeons, which may explain the good results. In other Sub-Saharan African countries, NPCs and nonsurgeon physicians often operate independently with no oversight from a surgical specialist. Although one retrospective study showed similar outcomes after major surgery performed by NPCs and physicians in

Figure 9.1 Disparity in Outcomes in Inguinal Hernia Repair in HICs and LICs and MICs

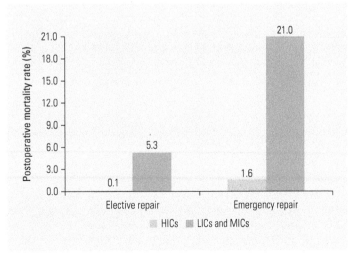

Sources: Mbah 2007; Primatesta and Goldacre 1996.
Note: HICs = high-income countries; LICs = low- income countries; MICs = middle-income countries.

Tanzania, more studies on outcomes after nonobstetric general surgical procedures performed by NPCs are urgently needed to guide policy and program planning (Beard and others 2014).

First-level hospitals in LMICs offer few continuing education programs in surgical care. This would be an ideal level at which to intervene with an inguinal hernia educational program targeted to nonsurgeons providing surgical care. Tension-free mesh repair techniques with mosquito net could be taught through short courses at first-level hospitals. The introduction of these educational programs and tension-free techniques should improve outcomes.

Cost-Effectiveness of Groin Hernia Repair

Inguinal hernia repair is one of the most cost-effective general surgical procedures performed in HICs. Data from a randomized trial of laparoscopic repair versus open-mesh inguinal hernia repair conducted in the United States indicate that both types of herniorrhaphy are cost-effective (Hynes and others 2006). In this study, investigators used the generally accepted threshold of cost-effectiveness in the United States of US$50,000 per quality-adjusted life year (QALY).

In an analysis of inguinal hernia repair using nationally collected, patient-reported outcome measures from the National Health Service (NHS) in the United Kingdom, Coronini-Cronberg and others (2013) calculated the cost per QALY of open and laparoscopic inguinal herniorrhaphy to be £1,746 ($2,970) and £1,540 ($2,620), respectively. The United Kingdom's National Institute for Health and Clinical Excellence committee routinely uses a cutoff of £20,000 to £30,000 ($34,000 to $51,000) per QALY to determine treatment cost-effectiveness and define the scope of NHS therapies. These findings suggest that inguinal hernia repair is especially cost-effective in the United Kingdom.

In Sweden, Nordin and others (2007) found that inguinal hernia repair performed under local anesthesia has significant cost advantages when compared with the use of spinal and general anesthesia techniques. This result has important implications for inguinal herniorrhaphy in LMICs, where the use of local anesthesia may be an important cost-saving strategy for hernia repair.

Inguinal hernia repair with mosquito-net mesh has been demonstrated to be cost-effective in LMICs even when compared with more traditional public health interventions. In a study using Operation Hernia data from Ghana, Shillcutt, Clarke, and Kingsnorth (2010) found that inguinal hernia repair with mosquito-net mesh costs approximately US$12.88 per DALY averted. This figure means that inguinal hernia repair with low-cost mesh in Ghana is as cost-effective as a vaccine and 10 times as cost-effective as HIV treatment (Ozgidez and Riviello 2008). Of note, approximately 70 percent of hernias in the Shillcutt, Clarke, and Kingsnorth (2010) study were repaired under local anesthesia, a technique that likely increased the cost-effectiveness of hernia repair in this patient cohort.

In India, low-cost polyethylene mesh has been shown not only to be safe and effective for use in inguinal hernia repair but also 2,808 times cheaper than commercially available polypropylene mesh (Gundre, Iyer, and Subramaniyan 2012). Mosquito-net mesh is the ultimate in surgical cost savings: one polyester mosquito net can repair approximately 3,000 hernias (Shillcutt, Clarke, and Kingsnorth 2010), and all symptomatic hernias in Ghana could be repaired today using an estimated US$15,000 worth of mesh (Beard, Oresanya, Ohene-Yeboa, and others 2013).

Shillcutt and others (2013) also demonstrated the cost-effectiveness of mosquito-net mesh hernia repair in Ecuador, a middle-income country. The mean cost-effectiveness for herniorrhaphy in this study is US$78.18 per DALY, a good buy considering Ecuador's gross national income of US$3,850. These data are strong evidence of the cost-effectiveness of hernia repair with low-cost mesh in LMIC contexts and of the need to prioritize surgery for inguinal hernia when allocating scarce resources.

The findings of Shillcutt's Ghana and Ecuador studies should be interpreted with some caution because the DALYs averted per hernia repair were based on expert opinion and may be overestimated (Shillcutt, Clarke, and Kingsnorth 2010; Shillcutt and others 2013). In addition, both studies included hernias repaired on Operation Hernia missions, which may not represent the typical scenario in a low-resource setting. Further research is needed to characterize the cost-effectiveness of inguinal hernia repair performed by local practitioners using both low-cost mesh and traditional tissue techniques to get a clearer picture of herniorrhaphy cost-effectiveness in LMICs.

HYDROCELE

Definitions of Hydrocele

A hydrocele is an abnormal accumulation of fluid most commonly occurring in the scrotum in men or the labia majora in women:

- A *communicating hydrocele* is similar to a hernia except that the sac connecting the abdomen to the scrotum or labia majora contains only fluid rather than abdominal contents.

- A *noncommunicating hydrocele* is a collection of scrotal fluid that is isolated from the abdomen. This type of hydrocele is caused by an imbalance between secretion, absorption, and drainage of fluid in the scrotal sac. Increased scrotal fluid secretion may be caused by local inflammation from bacteria or viruses, whereas poor absorption commonly results from thickening of the sac or lymphatic malfunction. Noncommunicating hydroceles are the most common type of hydrocele globally, affecting more than 30 million men and boys (WHO 2013a).

Risk Factors for Hydrocele in Adults

Obstruction of the testicular venous or lymphatic vessels is associated with acute hydrocele development. Venous or lymphatic obstruction can be caused by torsion of the testicle, lymphoma, or the death of parasitic filarial worms. In the temperate climates of Europe, North and South America, and China, most primary hydroceles in adult males are idiopathic. In tropical regions, mainly in LMICs, lymphatic filariasis (LF) is the most significant risk factor for the development of noncommunicating hydrocele. LF is caused by infection with the mosquito-borne worm *Wuchereria bancrofti* (Michael, Bundy, and Grenfell 1996; WHO 2005).

LF is a complex disease affecting several parts of the male genital anatomy. The biological predilection of adult filarial worms to live and reproduce in the lymphatic channels of the scrotum means that more than 50 percent of infected men will, with age, develop chronic hydrocele (Addiss and others 1995; Eigege and others 2002; Mathieu and others 2008). Hydroceles caused by LF are sometimes called filariceles.

In tropical or subtropical zones, the *Culex, Aedes,* and *Anopheles* mosquitoes carry the filarial parasite. The cycle of infection requires that mosquitoes deposit larvae on the host skin; the larvae migrate through the puncture site to the venous system and lymphatics, where they mature into adults. Nests of the male and female adults are most commonly identified in the male scrotal lymphatics, where they produce the first-stage larvae (microfilariae) that are subsequently consumed by mosquitoes.

Clinical Features of Filarial Hydrocele

Studies have identified living adult worms within the scrotal lymphatics in a large cohort of patients with hydrocele in northern Brazil (Dreyer and others 2002; Norões and others 1996; Norões and others 2003). Filarial parasites can be identified by ultrasound (the filarial dance sign) or by visual examination during surgery. In practice, clinical demonstration of the living adult parasite confirms the filarial origin of the hydrocele and can be useful in distinguishing actively evolving disease from residual scrotal disease after medical treatment.

Filarial hydroceles can be either acute or chronic. Acute hydroceles are associated with painful, inflammatory nodules caused by the death of adult worms (Dreyer and others 2002; Figueredo-Silva and others 2002). They are often seen after medical treatment for LF but can also be unrelated to treatment. In these cases, they are a response to acute lymphatic inflammation or infection known as acute adenolymphangitis (ADLA).

Chronic hydroceles are thought to correlate with chronic dysfunction of the lymphatic drainage system of the testicular cord, the sac, or both, and this pathology may be a result of intermittent attacks of ADLA over a number of years. Hydrocele patients suffer two episodes of ADLA per year, on average, resulting in scrotal nodules (Chu and others 2010); Dreyer and others 2002; Norões and Dreyer 2010). Chronic filarial hydroceles are associated with dilation and malfunction of the lymphatics (known as lymphangiectasia), rather than chronic lymphatic obstruction; lymphangiectasia can be identified by ultrasound and direct observation. The ultrasound may have a similar appearance to a varicocele. Hydrocele fluid in these patients contains lymphatic fluid leaked from damaged lymphatic vessels (Dreyer and others 2000; Pani and Dhanda 1994).

Epidemiology and Burden of Disease of Lymphatic Filariasis and Hydrocele

In many LMICs, including India and countries in Africa, LF accounts for a significant portion of the total burden of disease. Approximately 1.3 billion people—more than one-seventh of the world's population—are at risk for LF in 83 countries (Chu and others 2010; Michael, Bundy, and Grenfell 1996; WHO 2013a). The Southeast Asia region is home to 65 percent of LF cases, and 30 percent of patients live in Sub-Saharan Africa.

Some 40 million people are estimated to have symptomatic manifestations of filariasis; one-third of these people live in India. In tropical regions, an estimated 25 million to 27 million men have filarial hydroceles (Pani, Kumaraswami and Das 2005; WHO 2013a). In many communities, the majority of men with LF eventually develop symptomatic hydroceles (Addiss 2013; Babu, Mishra, and Nayak 2009; Dreyer, Norões, and Addiss 1997; Wijers 1977; Zeldenryk and others 2011). In a summary by Haddix and Kestler (2000), a high prevalence of hydrocele was demonstrated in several LMICs. On the coasts of Tanzania and Kenya, 90 percent and 60 percent of men, respectively, were found to have hydrocele at age 70. In Pondicherry, India, 45 percent of men have hydroceles by age 60 (Haddix and Kestler 2000). Hydrocele is also common in young men and has been identified in a large number of military recruits in northern Brazil (Norões and others 1996).

Studies indicate that population-based and household surveys consistently underestimate the true prevalence of hydrocele and disability from the disease (Eigege and others 2002; Mathieu and others 2008). Personal modesty often impedes accurate reporting of hydroceles in household surveys. Clinical mapping by patient examination is the only precise method of hydrocele prevalence measurement (Eigege and others 2002; Mathieu and others 2008; Pani, Kumaraswami, and Das 2005). Spot mapping of children for LF may produce imprecise estimates of hydrocele disease burden; spot maps of men with hydrocele generally correlate highly with local LF prevalence.

Global Burden of Lymphatic Filariasis and Hydrocele. Map 9.1 illustrates that the global DALYs attributable to LF in 2004 were concentrated in tropical regions in Sub-Saharan Africa and Southeast Asia, some of the poorest areas in the world. GBD 2010 ranks disability from LF at 105.2; in men, the disease has a slightly higher disability ranking of 87. According to GBD 2010, the number of DALYs attributable to LF (2.8 million) is

approximately one-half the estimate in the WHO Global Burden of Disease study of 2004, which found a total of 5.9 million DALYs associated with the disease (Murray and others 2012; Vos and others 2012; WHO 2005). Clearly these estimates are significantly different, though the reasons for this variation in disease burden are not yet understood.

Although GBD 2010 acknowledged that the world's population is aging, and therefore years lived with disability is increasing, it did not consider that the burden of filarial hydrocele may actually increase in many regions, or that other diseases such as depression may be directly attributable to hydrocele (Vos and others 2012). In addition, the previous edition of *Disease Control Priorities in Developing Countries* (Jamison and others 2006) did not consider the burden of filarial hydroceles in its calculation of global surgical DALYs (Debas and others 2006).

Economic Burden of Lymphatic Filariasis and Hydrocele in LMICs. A number of studies have attempted to estimate the economic burden of LF. It is clear that the disease not only predominantly affects the world's poor, but it also perpetuates poverty (Haddix and Kestler 2000). The burden can be measured as direct disease-related costs to individuals and households, lost

Map 9.1 Global Disability-Adjusted Life Years Attributable to Lymphatic Filariasis (per 100,000 population), 2004

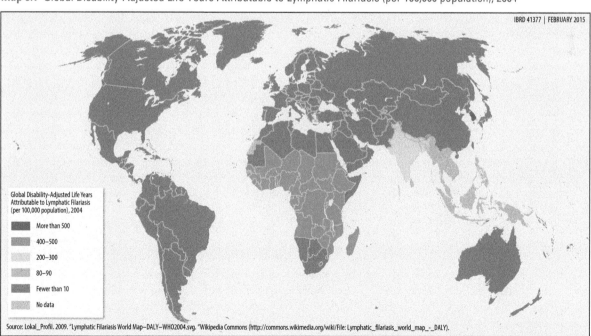

Source: Lokal_Profil. 2009. "Lymphatic Filariasis World Map–DALY–WHO2004.svg. "Wikipedia Commons (http://commons.wikimedia.org/wiki/File: Lymphatic_filariasis_world_map_-_DALY).

productivity of individuals, reduced productivity due to changes in the economies of affected communities, and costs to government-funded health care systems.

In 2000, more than 10 million people in India sought medical care for symptoms associated with LF (Haddix and Kestler 2000; Ramaiah and others 2000). However, the number of people who seek treatment varies from community to community, depending on availability of care and other factors. The economic loss due to disability from LF in India alone is estimated to be US$1 billion to US$1.5 billion per year, with another US$1 billion attributable to LF in Sub-Saharan Africa. In Sub-Saharan Africa, 83 percent of this economic loss is due to hydrocele (Gyapong and others 1996; Haddix and Kestler 2000; Pani, Kumaraswami, and Das 2005). Entire communities have had to adapt their economic structure from fishing to agriculture on the eastern coast of Sub-Saharan Africa because of the high prevalence of LF in this region (Muhondwa 1983).

Industry both suffers from, and in some cases is responsible for, the perpetuation of conditions conducive to LF. For example, workers in large irrigation projects in Ghana and in coco fiber processing in Sri Lanka are at increased risk of LF because of environmental exposure to mosquitoes carrying the filarial parasite. Migration of infected individuals and crowded living arrangements complicate disease eradication efforts.

Social Burden of Filarial Hydrocele in LMICs. The social burden of filarial hydroceles has been explored in Orissa, India, by Babu, Mishra, and Nayak (2009). In their ethnographic study, the authors interviewed hydrocele patients, their wives, and the general public to understand how hydroceles impact sexual and married life. A high rate of depression accompanied the loss of a satisfactory sexual life in these patients and their spouses. An unmarried man with a hydrocele seeking a wife was seen as a last-choice marriage prospect. Because of the severity of the psychological impact on patients, Addiss (2013) has argued for an "uprising of compassion" for people disabled with LF. He noted that the 1997 World Health Assembly resolution charged the GPELF with two missions: the elimination of filarial transmission and the alleviation of infection-related disability.

Stories of suffering due to the consequences of LF, including hydrocele, from Brazil, the Dominican Republic, Ghana, Haiti, and India highlight the very human cost of these disabilities. These disabilities have largely not received international attention to the extent that some other disabilities, yet they affect at least 15 times as many people (Addiss 2013; Addiss and others 1995; Zeldenryk and others 2011). The impact of hydroceles on communities also has been grossly underestimated, especially when the psychosocial impacts of disfiguring hydroceles are considered; the preventive role of hydrocele surgery for the human and monetary costs of DALYs attributable to depression is potentially huge (Wynd and others 2007).

Global Efforts to Combat Lymphatic Filariasis and Hydrocele

LF is categorized as a neglected tropical disease. In 1997, the WHO listed it among the six communicable diseases that could potentially be eliminated worldwide. Recognizing this, World Health Assembly Resolution 50.29 identified LF as a significant source of global disease burden and called for its elimination. In 2000, the GPELF launched a program for LF elimination by 2020 (Ottesen 2000). The GPELF set the parallel goals of alleviating disability from LF, including hydrocele, lymphedema, and ADLA, and interrupting transmission of the disease with mass drug administration (MDA).

Although MDA, mosquito control, and bednets have effectively eliminated LF in some countries, MDA has been less successful in others, for social, economic, and geographic reasons (WHO 2011). Moreover, even when transmission has been effectively prevented at a population level, large numbers of people will still suffer disability from filarial hydrocele because of cumulative damage to scrotal lymphatics.

Economic Effects of Global Elimination Efforts. In the first eight years of MDA supported by the GPELF, more than 570 million at-risk individuals were treated for four to six years. More than 1.9 billion treatments were given in 48 of the 83 endemic countries (map 9.2). Economic benefits have been measurable. This effort has rendered an estimated US$21.8 billion of economic benefit for affected individuals and US$2.2 billion in health systems savings. Approximately 6.6 million newborns have been protected from 1.4 million symptomatic hydroceles. Among those already affected with LF and subclinical disease, MDA is expected to prevent its progression (Chu and others 2010).

In individual terms, the cost of preventing one case of hydrocele, ADLA, or lymphedema in India has been calculated to be US$8.41, which would save 58.35 working days per year and improve wages by US$39.39. The cost-benefit ratio has been calculated to be 52.6, which is among the most cost-effective of any disease control program (Remme and others 2006).

The potential economic benefit of hydrocelectomy has not yet been calculated but may be similar to that of hernia surgery, scaled to the known number of cases of

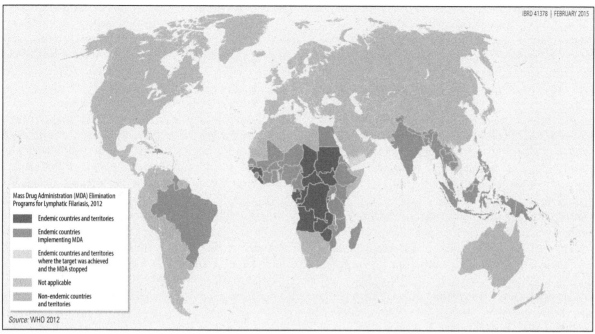

Mass Drug Administration (MDA) Elimination
Programs for Lymphatic Filariasis, 2012

- Endemic countries and territories
- Endemic countries
  implementing MDA
- Endemic countries and territories
  where the target was achieved
  and the MDA stopped
- Not applicable
- Non-endemic countries
  and territories

Source: WHO 2012

existing disease. Unfortunately, access to hydrocelectomy in LMICs is limited. The waitlists for hydrocele repair in government-sponsored health programs annually exceed 2,000 to 5,000 in endemic Sub-Saharan African countries. The need for hydrocelectomy in these areas clearly exceeds the surgical capacity (Odoom, personal communication, 2013).

Surgical Management of Hydrocele

Idiopathic Hydrocele. The surgical management of benign idiopathic hydroceles can be complex. Although the technical drainage of hydrocele via a scrotal incision appears to be straightforward, the complexity of vascular and lymphatic anatomy is often underappreciated (Gottesman 1976; Ku and others 2001; Rodriguez, Rodriguez, and Fortuño 1981). Complication rates after hydrocelectomy are high, even in HICs. In a retrospective series during the period 1998–2004 in the United States, a posthydrocelectomy complication rate of 20 percent was found (Swartz, Morgan, and Krieger 2007), including recurrences of hydrocele, hematoma, infection, and testicular infarction. The surgical techniques used in this series included sac partial excision and eversion (47 percent), sac eversion alone (22 percent), and excision alone (18 percent). The authors

concluded that subtotal excision of the sac is superior to complete excision. However, the generalizability of this study is limited because there was no standardization of perioperative care or surgical technique.

Filarial Hydrocele. Surgical management of filarial hydrocele is especially critical. In LMICs, patients may present with massive, disfiguring hydroceles requiring more specialized care. Scrotal skin and lymphatics are damaged by the parasitic infection, leading to increased inflammation in the operative field and poor wound healing. Given this situation, complications after repair of filarial hydroceles, including infection, recurrence, and hematoma, have been shown to be even higher than those after surgical repair of benign idiopathic hydroceles (deVries 2002; Fasana 1982; Thambugala 1971; Thomas and others 2009; WHO 2002).

In Brazil, postoperative infection rates after filarial hydrocelectomy have been reported to be as high as 30 percent; recurrence was as high as 19 percent in a large series of patients who underwent sac-sparing surgery for LF (Norões and Dreyer 2010). In this series, a total of 1,128 surgical patients with hydroceles received complete excision of the hydrocele sac. Postoperative outcomes in these patients were compared with those of a group of 218 patients with "sac-sparing" subtotal excision of the sac, done elsewhere. With a mean follow-up of 8.6 years, recurrence rates for complete excision were 0.3 percent compared with 19 percent in sac-sparing surgery. Although resection of the sac is more challenging and requires special care for hemostasis, it has become the standard of care in Brazil, Haiti, and the West African Filariasis Program (Mante 2012; Mante and Seim 2007).

Particular care must be taken when the skin of the scrotum is thickened, especially when dripping with lymphatic fluid—a condition known as "lymph scrotum." These cases require reconstructive surgery. Simple hydrocelectomy is contraindicated. Successful lymphovenous shunts for hydroceles and lymphedema secondary to LF have also been reported in the Indian literature (Manokaran 2005).

The surgical management of filarial hydroceles in LMICs is largely not standardized. In our experience, protocols for LF hydrocelectomy appear to improve outcomes by standardizing the use of antibiotics, surgical techniques, dressings, and perioperative management, although little published data on this topic are available.

CONCLUSIONS

The global burden of groin hernia and hydrocele is significant. We estimate that 223 million people in the world, equivalent to about two-thirds of the population of the United States, have inguinal hernia, while nearly 30 million men suffer from filarial hydrocele. Elective hernia repair and hydrocelectomy are curative public health interventions. Herniorrhaphy prevents life-threatening complications from hernia accidents, and both procedures improve quality of life. Hernia repair is also cost-effective, even when compared with more traditional public health interventions.

Many people in the world do not have access to safe groin hernia surgery or hydrocelectomy. This disparity results in higher levels of morbidity and mortality from hernia in LMICs. Limited access to hydrocelectomy in LMICs perpetuates the continuing suffering of the world's poorest people from disfiguring filarial hydroceles. Although tension-free mesh repair is the standard of care for groin hernia in HICs, it is unavailable to most patients in LMICs. Mosquito-net mesh may be a safe and cost-effective way to correct this disparity. However, pending widespread availability of a proven safe option for mesh, increased access to well-established tissue techniques of groin hernia repair should be promoted.

Task-shifting of herniorrhaphy to NPCs and non-surgeon physicians is occurring throughout Africa.

Programs to expand the capacity for inguinal hernia repair and hydrocelectomy at first-level hospitals should use existing human resources and focus on skills training for surgeons, physicians, and NPCs already performing these repairs. Local organizations such as the Ghana Hernia Society could be instrumental in spearheading training efforts. Infrastructure investment to build hospital capacity for essential surgeries like herniorrhaphy and hydrocelectomy is needed to ensure access to these procedures.

Addressing inguinal hernia and filarial hydrocele should be a high priority on any global surgery agenda. Basic surgical care, specifically, essential procedures like groin herniorrhaphy and hydrocelectomy, is a crucial part of health care services that should be available at first-level hospitals. Working toward equitable provision of hernia repair and hydrocelectomy in LMICs has the potential to strengthen health systems and ultimately increase much-needed hospital capacity.

NOTES

The World Bank classifies countries according to four income groupings. Income is measured using gross national income (GNI) per capita, in U.S. dollars, converted from local currency using the *World Bank Atlas* method. Classifications as of July 2014 are as follows:

- Low-income countries (LICs) = US$1,045 or less in 2013
- Middle-income countries (MICs) are subdivided:
  - Lower-middle-income = US$1,046 to US$4,125
  - Upper-middle-income (UMICs) = US$4,126 to US$12,745
- High-income countries (HICs) = US$12,746 or more

1. International Database, 2013, United States Census Bureau, Washington, DC. http://www.census.gov/population /international/data/idb/region.php.

REFERENCES

Abramson, J. H., J. Gofin, C. Hopp, A. Makler, and L. M. Epstein. 1978. "The Epidemiology of Inguinal Hernia: A Survey in Western Jerusalem." *Journal of Epidemiology & Community Health* 32 (1): 59–67.

Addiss, D. G. 2013. "Global Elimination of Lymphatic Filariasis: A 'Mass Uprising of Compassion.'" *PLoS Neglected Tropical Diseases* 7 (8): e2264. doi:10.1371/journal.pntd.0002264.

Addiss, D. G., K. A. Dimock, M. L. Eberhard, and P. J. Lammie. 1995. "Clinical, Parasitologic and Immunologic Observations of Patients with Hydrocele and Elephantiasis in an Area with Endemic Lymphatic Filariasis." *Journal of Infectious Diseases* 171 (3): 755–58.

Arowolo, O. A., E. A. Agbakwuru, A. O. Adisa, O. O. Lawal, M. H. Ibrahim, and others. 2011. "Evaluation of Tension-Free Mesh Inguinal Hernia Repair in Nigeria: A Preliminary Report." *West African Journal of Medicine* 30 (2): 110–13.

Babu, B. V., S. Mishra, and A. N. Nayak. 2009. "Marriage, Sex, and Hydrocele: An Ethnographic Study on the Effect of Filarial Hydrocele on Conjugal Life and Marriageability from Orissa, India." *PLoS Neglected Tropical Diseases* 3 (4): e414.

Bainbridge, D., J. Martin, M. Arango, and D. Cheng. 2012. "Perioperative and Anaesthetic-Related Mortality in Developed and Developing Countries: A Systematic Review and Meta-Analysis." *The Lancet* 380 (9847): 1075–81.

Bay-Nielsen, M., and H. Kehlet. 2008. "Anesthesia and Postoperative Morbidity after Elective Groin Hernia Repair: A Nationwide Study." *Acta Anaesthesiologica Scandinavica* 52 (2): 169–74.

Bay-Nielsen, M., L. Strand, J. Malmstrom, F. H. Anderson, and others. 2001. "Quality Assessment of 26,304 Herniorrhaphies in Denmark: A Prospective Nationwide Study." *The Lancet* 358 (9288): 1124–28.

Beard, J. H., L. B. Oresanya, L. Akoko, A. Mwanga, R. A. Dicker, and H. W. Harris. 2013. "An Estimation of Inguinal Hernia Epidemiology Adjusted for Population Age Structure in Tanzania." *Hernia* 18 (2): 289–95. doi:10.1007/s10029-013-1177-5.

Beard, J. H., L. B. Oresanya, L. Akoko, A. Mwanga, C. A. Mkony, and R. A. Dicker. 2014. "Surgical Task-Shifting in a Low-Resource Setting: Outcomes after Major Surgery Performed by Non-physician Clinicians in Tanzania." *World Journal of Surgery* 38 (6): 1398–404.

———. Not dated. "Hernia Repair Capacity in Pwanu Region, Tanzania, 2014." Unpublished.

Beard, J. H., L. B. Oresanya, M. Ohene-Yeboah, R. A. Dicker, and H. W. Harris. 2013. "Characterizing the Global Burden of Surgical Disease: A Method to Estimate Inguinal Hernia Epidemiology in Ghana." *World Journal of Surgery* 37 (3): 498–503.

Belcher, D. W., P. K. Nyame, and F. K. Wurapa. 1978. "The Prevalence of Inguinal Hernia in Adult Ghanaian Males." *Tropical Geographical Medicine* 30 (1): 39–43.

Carbonell, J. F., J. L. Sanchez, R. T. Peris, J. C. Ivorra, M. J. Del Baño, and others. 1993. "Risk Factors Associated with Inguinal Hernias: A Case Control Study." *European Journal of Surgery* 159 (9): 481–86.

Chu, B. K., P. J. Hooper, M. H. Bradley, D. A. McFarland, and E. A. Ottesen. 2010. "The Economic Benefits Resulting from the First 8 Years of the Global Programme to Eliminate Lymphatic Filariasis (2000–2007)." *PLoS Neglected Tropical Diseases* 4 (6): e708.

Clarke, M. G., C. Oppong, R. Simmermacher, K. Park, M. Kurzer, and others. 2009. "The Use of Sterilised Polyester Mosquito Net Mesh for Inguinal Hernia Repair in Ghana." *Hernia* 13 (2): 155–59.

Coronini-Cronberg, S., J. Appleby, and J. Thompson. 2013. "Application of Patient-Reported Outcome Measures (PROMs) Data to Estimate Cost-Effectiveness of Hernia Surgery in England." *Journal of the Royal Society of Medicine* 106 (7): 278–87. doi:10.1177/0141076813489679.

Debas, H. T., R. Gosselin, C. McCord, and A. Thind. 2006. "Surgery." In *Disease Control Priorities in Developing Countries*, edited by D. T. Jamison, J. G. Breman, A. R. Measham, G. Alleyne, M. Claeson, D. B. Evans, P. Jha, A. Mills, and P. Musgrove, 2nd ed., 1245–60. Washington, DC: World Bank and Oxford University Press.

deVries, C. R. 2002. "The Role of the Urologist in the Treatment and Elimination of Lymphatic Filariasis Worldwide." *BJU International* 89 (suppl 1): 37–43.

Dreyer, G., D. Addiss, J. Roberts, and J. Norões. 2002. "Progression of Lymphatic Vessel Dilatation in the Presence of Living Adult *Wuchereria bancrofti*." *Transactions of the Royal Society of Tropical Medicine and Hygiene* 96 (2): 157–61.

Dreyer, G., J. Norões, and D. Addiss. 1997. "The Silent Burden of Sexual Disability Associated with Lymphatic Filariasis." *Acta Tropica* 63 (1): 57–60.

Dreyer, G., J. Norões, J. Figueredo-Silva, and W. F. Piessens. 2000. "Pathogenesis of Lymphatic Disease in Bancroftian Filariasis: A Clinical Perspective." *Parasitology Today* 16 (12): 544–48.

Eigege, A., F. O. Richards, D. D. Blaney, E. S. Miri, I. Gontor, and others. 2002. "Rapid Assessment for Lymphatic Filariasis in Central Nigeria: A Comparison of the Immunochromaticographic Card Test and Hydrocele Rates in an Area of High Endemicity." *American Journal of Tropical Medicine and Hygiene* 68 (6): 643–46.

Everhart, J. E. 1994. "Abdominal Wall Hernia." In *Digestive Diseases in the United States: Epidemiology and Impact*, edited by J. E. Everhart, 471–507. Bethesda, MD: National Institute of Diabetes and Digestive and Kidney Diseases.

Fall, B., M. E. Betel, O. Diarra, M. Ba, A. Dia, and A. Diop. 2005. "Complications of Treatment of Adult's Groin Hernia: A Report of 100 Cases Comparative Study between Bassini and McVay's Techniques." *Dakar Médical* 50 (1): 37–40.

Fasana, F. 1982. "Treatment of Tropical Hydrocele: A Study of 273 Cases." *Medicom* 4 (3): 73–75.

Figueredo-Silva, J., J. Norões, A. Cedenho, and G. Dreyer. 2002. "The Histopathology of Bancroftian Filariasis Revisited: The Role of the Adult Worm in the Lymphatic-Vessel Disease." *Annals of Tropical Medicine and Parasitology* 96 (6): 531–41.

Fitzgibbons, R. J., Jr., A. Giobbie-Hurder, J. O. Gibbs, D. D. Dunlop, D. J. Reda, and others. 2006. "Watchful Waiting vs. Repair of Inguinal Hernia in Minimally Symptomatic Men: A Randomized Clinical Trial." *Journal of the American Medical Association* 295 (3): 285–92.

Flich, J., J. L. Alfonso, F. Delgado, M. J. Prado, and P. Cortina. 1992. "Inguinal Hernia and Certain Risk Factors." *European Journal of Epidemiology* 8 (2): 277–82.

Freudenberg, S., D. Sano, E. Ouangre, C. Weiss, and T. J. Wilhelm. 2006. "Commercial Mesh versus Nylon Mosquito Net for Hernia Repair: A Randomized

Double-Blind Study in Burkina Faso." *World Journal of Surgery* 30 (10): 1784–89.

Gallegos, N. C., J. Dawson, M. Jarvis, and M. Hibsely. 1991. "Risk of Strangulation in Groin Hernias." *British Journal of Surgery* 78 (10): 1171–73.

Galukande, M., J. von Schreeb, A. Wladis, N. Mbembati, H. de Miranda, and others. 2010. "Essential Surgery at the District Hospital: A Retrospective Descriptive Analysis in Three African Countries." *PLoS Medicine* 7 (3): e1000243. doi:10.1371/journal.pmed.1000243.

Gessessew, A., G. A. Barnabas, N. Prata, and K. Weidert. 2011. "Task Shifting and Sharing in Tigray, Ethiopia, to Achieve Comprehensive Emergency Obstetric Care." *International Journal of Gynaecology and Obstetrics* 113 (1): 28–31.

Gottesman, J. E. 1976. "Hydrocelectomy: Evaluation of Technique." *Urology* 7 (4): 386–87.

Grimes, C. E., R. S. Law, E. S. Borgstein, N. C. Mkandawire, C. B. Lavy, and others. 2012. "Systematic Review of Met and Unmet Need of Surgical Disease in Rural Sub-Saharan Africa." *World Journal of Surgery* 36 (1): 8–23.

Gundre, N. P., S. P. Iyer, and P. Subramaniyan. 2012. "Prospective Randomized Controlled Study Using Polyethylene Mesh for Inguinal Hernia Meshplasty as a Safe and Cost-Effective Alternative to Polypropylene Mesh." *Updates in Surgery* 64 (1): 37–42.

Gyapong, J. O., M. Gyapong, D. B. Evans, M. K. Aikins, and S. Adjei. 1996. "The Economic Burden of Lymphatic Filariasis in Northern Ghana." *Annals of Tropical Medicine and Parasitology* 90 (1): 39–48.

Haddix, A. C., and A. Kestler. 2000. "Lymphatic Filariasis: Economic Aspects of the Disease and Programmes for Its Elimination." *Transactions of the Royal Society of Tropical Medicine and Hygiene* 94 (6): 592–93.

Hair, A., C. Paterson, D. Wright, J. N. Baxter, and P. J. O'Dwyer. 2001. "What Effect Does the Duration of an Inguinal Hernia Have on Patient Symptoms?" *Journal of the American College of Surgeons* 193 (2): 125–29.

Hakeem, A., and V. Shanmugam. 2011. "Inguinodynia Following Lichtenstein Tension-Free Hernia Repair: A Review." *World Journal of Gastroenterology* 17 (14): 1791–96.

Harouna, Y., H. Yaya, I. Abdou, and L. Bazira. 2000. "Prognosis of Strangulated Hernia in Adult with Necrosis of Small Bowel: A 34 Cases Report." *Bulletin de la Société de Pathologie Exotique* 93: 317–20.

Heikkinen, T., K. Haukipuro, J. Leppälä, and A. Hulkko. 1997. "Total Costs of Laparoscopic and Lichtenstein Inguinal Hernia Repairs: A Prospective Study." *Surgical Laparoscopy, Endoscopy, and Percutaneous Techniques* 7 (1): 1.

Herszage, L. 2004. "Hernia Surgery in the South American Woodlands: A Surgical Adventure in Argentina." *Hernia* 8 (4): 306–10.

Hynes, D. M., K. T. Stroupe, P. Luo, A. Giobbie-Hurder, D. Reda, and others. 2006. "Cost Effectiveness of Laparoscopic versus Open Mesh Hernia Operation: Results of a Department of Veterans Affairs Randomized Clinical Trial." *Journal of the American College of Surgeons* 203 (4): 447–57.

Jamison, D. T., J. G. Brennan, A. R. Measham, G. Alleyne, M. Claesen, and others, eds. 2006. *Disease Control Priorities in Developing Countries*, 2nd ed. New York: Oxford University Press.

Kingsnorth, A. N., C. Oppong, J. Akoh, B. Stephenson, and R. Simmermacher. 2006. "Operation Hernia to Ghana." *Hernia* 10 (5): 376–79.

Koch, A., A. Edwards, S. Haapaniemi, P. Nordin, and A. Kald. 2005. "Prospective Evaluation of 6895 Groin Hernia Repairs in Women." *British Journal of Surgery* 92 (12): 1553–58.

Krishna, A., M. C. Misra, V. K. Bansal, S. Kumar, S. Rajeshwari, and others. 2012. "Laparoscopic Inguinal Hernia Repair: Transabdominal Preperitoneal (TAPP) versus Totally Extraperitoneal (TEP) Approach: A Prospective Randomized Controlled Trial." *Surgical Endoscopy* 26 (3): 639–49.

Kruk, M. E., A. Wladis, N. Mbembati, S. K. Ndao-Brumblay, R. Y. Hsia, and others. 2010. "Human Resource and Funding Constraints for Essential Surgery in District Hospitals in Africa: A Retrospective Cross-Sectional Survey." *PLoS Medicine* 7 (3): e1000242.

Ku, J. H., M. E. Kim, N. K. Lee, and Y. H. Park. 2001. "The Excisional, Plication and Internal Drainage Techniques: A Comparison of the Results for Idiopathic Hydrocele." *BJU International* 87 (1): 82–84.

Lau, H., C. Fang, W. K. Yuen, and N. G. Patil. 2007. "Risk Factors for Inguinal Hernia in Adult Males: A Case-Control Study." *Surgery* 141 (2): 262–66.

Linden, A. F., F. S. Sekidde, M. Galukande, L. M. Knowlton, S. Chackungal, and K. A. McQueen. 2012. "Challenges of Surgery in Developing Countries: A Survey of Surgical and Anesthesia Capacity in Uganda's Public Hospitals." *World Journal of Surgery* 36 (5): 1056–65.

Löfgren, J., F. Makumbi, E. Galliwango, P. Nordin, C. Ibingira, and others. 2014. "Prevalence of Treated and Untreated Groin Hernia in Eastern Uganda." *British Journal of Surgery* 101 (6): 728–34.

Mabula, J. B., and P. L. Chalya. 2012. "Surgical Management of Inguinal Hernias at Bugando Medical Center in Northwestern Tanzania: Our Experiences in a Resource-Limited Setting." *BMC Research Notes* 5: 585.

Manokaran, G. 2005. "Management of Genitourinary Manifestations of Lymphatic Filariasis." *Indian Journal of Urology* 21 (1): 39–43.

Mante, S. D. 2012. "The African Filariasis Morbidity Project: The Past, the Present, and the Future." http://filariasis.org /documents/4.TheAfricanMorbidityProject.pdf.

Mante, S. D., and A. R. Seim. 2007. *West African Lymphatic Filariasis Morbidity Project Surgical Handbook: An Aid to District Hospital Surgeons*. 2nd ed. Fjellstrand, Norway: Health and Development International. http://hdi.no/pdfs /LF/lymphatic-filariasis-guide.pdf.

Manyilirah, W., S. Kijambu, A. Upoki, and J. Kiryabwire. 2012. "Comparison of Non-mesh (Desarda) and Mesh (Lichtenstein) Methods for Inguinal Hernia Repair among Black African Patients: A Short-Term Double-Blind RCT." *Hernia* 16 (2): 134–44.

Mathieu, E., J. Amann, A. Eigege, F. Richards, and Y. Sodahhlon. 2008. "Collecting Baseline Information for National Morbidity Alleviation Programs: Different Methods to Estimate Lymphatic Filariasis Morbidity Prevalence." *American Journal of Tropical Medicine and Hygiene* 78: (1): 153–58.

Mbah, N. 2007. "Morbidity and Mortality Associated with Inguinal Hernia in Northwestern Nigeria." *West African Journal of Medicine* 26 (4): 288–92.

McCord, C., G. Mbaruku, C. Pereira, C. Nzabuhakwa, and S. Bergstrom. 2009. "The Quality of Emergency Obstetrical Surgery by Assistant Medical Officers in Tanzanian District Hospitals." *Health Affairs* 28 (5): w876–85.

McCormack, K., N. W. Scott, P. M. Go, S. Ross, A. M. Grant, and others. 2003. "Laparoscopic Techniques versus Open Techniques for Inguinal Hernia Repair." *Cochrane Database of Systematic Reviews* 1: Cd001785. doi:10.1002/14651858. CD001785.

Michael, E., D. A. Bundy, and B. T. Grenfell. 1996. "Re-Assessing the Global Prevalence and Distribution of Lymphatic Filariasis." *Parasitology* 112 (4): 409–28.

Mock, C., M. Cherian, C. Julliard, P. Donkor, S. Bickler, and others. 2010. "Developing Priorities for Addressing Surgical Conditions Globally: Furthering the Link between Surgery and Public Health Policy." *World Journal of Surgery* 34 (3): 381–85.

Muhondwa, E. P. Y. 1983. "Community Participation in Filariasis Control: The Tanzania Experiment." *TDR/SER /SWG (4)/WP/83.13*, WHO, Geneva.

Murray, C. J. L., T. Vos, R. Lozano, M. Naghavi, A. D. Flaxman, and others. 2012. "Disability-Adjusted Life Years (DALYs) for 291 Diseases and Injuries in 21 Regions, 1990–2010: A Systematic Analysis for the Global Burden of Disease Study 2010." *The Lancet* 380 (9859): 2197–223.

National Bureau of Statistics and Coast Regional Commissioners Office. 2007. "United Republic of Tanzania Coast Region Socioeconomic Profile."

Neuhauser, D. 1977. "Elective Inguinal Herniorrhaphy versus Truss in the Elderly." In *Costs, Risks, and Benefits of Surgery*, edited by J. P. Bunker, B. A. Barnes, and F. Mosteller, 223–39. New York: Oxford University Press.

Neumayer, L., A. Giobbie-Hurder, O. Jonasson, R. Fitzgibbons, Jr., D. Dunlop, and others. 2004. "Open Mesh versus Laparoscopic Mesh Repair of Inguinal Hernia." *New England Journal of Medicine* 350: 1819.

Nilsson, H., G. Stylianidis, M. Haapamaki, E. Nilsson, and P. Nordin. 2007. "Mortality after Groin Hernia Surgery." *Annals of Surgery* 245 (4): 656–60.

Nordberg, E. 1984. "Incidence and Estimated Need of Cesarean Section, Inguinal Hernia Repair, and Operation for Strangulated Hernia in Rural Africa." *British Medical Journal* (Clinical Research Edition) 289 (6437): 92–93.

Nordin, P., H. Zetterstrom, P. Carlsson, and E. Nilsson. 2007. "Cost-Effectiveness Analysis of Local, Regional and General Anaesthesia for Inguinal Hernia Repair Using Data from a Randomized Controlled Trial." *British Journal of Surgery* 94 (4): 500–05.

Norões, J., D. Addiss, F. Amaral, A. Coutinho, Z. Medeiros, and others. 1996. "Occurrence of Living Adult *Wuchereria bancrofti* in the Scrotal Area of Men with Microfilaraemia." *Transactions of the Royal Society of Tropical Medicine and Hygiene* 90 (1): 55–56.

Norões, J., D. Addiss, A. Cedenho, J. Figueredo-Silva, G. Lima, and G. Dreyer. 2003. "Pathogenesis of Filarial Hydrocele: Risk Associated with Intrascrotal Nodules Caused by Death of Adult *Wuchereria bancrofti*." *Transactions of the Royal Society of Tropical Medicine and Hygiene* 97 (5): 561–66.

Norões, J., D. Addiss, A. Santos, Z. Medeiros, A. Coutinho, and G. Dreyer. 1996. "Ultrasonographic Evidence of Abnormal Lymphatic Vessels in Young Men with Adult *Wuchereria bancrofti* Infection in the Scrotal Area." *Journal of Urology* 156 (2 Pt 1): 409–12.

Norões, J., and G. Dreyer. 2010. "A Mechanism for Chronic Filarial Hydrocele with Implications for Its Surgical Repair." *PLoS Neglected Tropical Diseases* 4 (6): e695.

Ohene-Yeboah, M., and F. A. Abantanga. 2011. "Inguinal Hernia Disease in Africa: A Common but Neglected Surgical Problem." *West African Journal of Medicine* 30 (2): 77–83.

Ohene-Yeboah, M., J. Oppong, B. Togbe, B. Nimako, and others. 2009. "Some Aspects of the Epidemiology of External Hernia in Kumasi, Ghana." *Hernia* 13 (5): 529–32.

Ottesen, E. A. 2000. "The Global Programme to Eliminate Lymphatic Filariasis." *Tropical Medicine and International Health* 5 (9): 591–94.

Ozgediz, D., and R. Riviello. 2008. "The 'Other' Neglected Diseases in Global Public Health: Surgical Conditions in Sub-Saharan Africa." *PLoS Medicine* 5 (6): 850–54.

Pani, S. P., and V. Dhanda. 1994. "Natural History and Dynamics of Progression of Clinical Manifestations of Filariasis." In *Tropical Disease: Molecular Biology and Control Strategies*, edited by Sushil Kumar, A. K. Sen, G. P. Dutta, and R. N. Sharma. New Delhi: Publications and Information Directorate.

Pani, S. P., V. Kumaraswami, and L. K. Das. 2005. "Epidemiology of Lymphatic Filariasis with Special Reference to Urogenital-Manifestations." *Indian Journal of Urology* 21 (1): 44–49.

Pereira, C., A. Bugalho, S. Bergstrom, F. Vaz, and M. Cotiro. 1996. "A Comparative Study of Cesarean Deliveries by Assistant Medical Officers and Obstetricians in Mozambique." *British Journal of Obstetrics and Gynaecology* 103 (6): 508–12.

Poobalan, A. S., J. Bruce, W. C. Smith, P. M. King, Z. H. Krukowski, and others. 2003. "A Review of Chronic Pain after Inguinal Herniorrhaphy." *Clinical Journal of Pain* 19 (1): 48.

Primatesta, P., and M. J. Goldacre. 1996. "Inguinal Hernia Repair: Incidence of Elective and Emergency Surgery, Readmission and Mortality." *International Journal of Epidemiology* 25 (4): 835–39.

Ramaiah, K. D., P. K. Das, E. Michael, and H. Guyatt. 2000. "The Economic Burden of Lymphatic Filariasis in India." *Parasitology Today* 16 (6): 251–23.

Ramyil, V. M., D. Iya, B. C. Ogbonna, and M. K. Dakum. 2000. "Safety of Daycare Hernia Repair in Jos, Nigeria." *East African Medical Journal* 77 (6): 326–28.

RAND Corporation. 1983. *Conceptualization and Measurement of Physiologic Health of Adults.* Santa Monica, CA: RAND Corporation.

Remme, J. H. F., P. Feenstra, P. R. Lever, A. C. Medici, C. M. Morel, and others. 2006. "Tropical Diseases Targeted for Elimination: Chagas Disease, Lymphatic Filariasis, Onchocerciasis, and Leprosy." In *Disease Control Priorities in Developing Countries*, edited by D. T. Jamison, J. G. Brennan, A. R. Measham, G. Alleyne, S. Claesen, and others, 2nd ed., 433–44. New York: Oxford University Press.

Rodriguez, W. C., D. D. Rodriguez, and R. F. Fortuño. 1981. "The Operative Treatment of Hydrocele: A Comparison of 4 Basic Techniques." *Journal of Urology* 125 (6): 804–05.

Ruhl, C. E., and J. E. Everhart. 2007. "Risk Factors for Inguinal Hernia among Adults in the US Population." *American Journal of Epidemiology* 165 (10): 1154–61.

Sanders, D. L., A. N. Kingsnorth, R. Moate, and J. A. Steer. 2013. "An In Vitro Study Assessing the Infection Risk of Low-Cost Polyethylene Mosquito Net Compared with Commercial Hernia Prosthetics." *Journal of Surgical Research* 183 (2): e31–37.

Sanders, D. L., A. N. Kingsnorth, and B. M. Stephenson. 2013. "Mosquito Net Mesh for Abdominal Wall Hernioplasty: A Comparison of Material Characteristics with Commercial Prosthetics." *World Journal of Surgery* 37 (4): 737–45.

Sanders, D. L., C. S. Porter, C. D. Mitchell, and A. N. Kingsnorth. 2008. "A Prospective Cohort Study Comparing the African and European Hernia." *Hernia* 12 (5): 527–29.

Sani, R., B Nameoua, A. Yahaya, I. Hassane, R. Adamou, and others. 2009. "The Impact of Launching Surgery at the District Level in Niger." *World Journal of Surgery* 33 (10): 2063–68.

Schneider, B. E., J. M. Castillo, L. Villegas, D. J. Scott, and D. B. Jones. 2003. "Laparoscopic Totally Extraperitoneal versus Lichtenstein Herniorrhaphy: Cost Comparison at Teaching Hospitals." *Surgical Laparoscopy, Endoscopy, and Percutaneous Techniques* 13 (4): 261–67.

Shillcutt, S. D., M. G. Clarke, and A. N. Kingsnorth. 2010. "Cost-Effectiveness of Groin Hernia Surgery in the Western Region of Ghana." *Archives of Surgery* 145 (10): 954–61.

Shillcutt, S. D., D. L. Sanders, M. T. Butron-Vila, and A. N. Kingsnorth. 2013. "Cost-Effectiveness of Inguinal Hernia Surgery in Northwestern Ecuador." *World Journal of Surgery* 37 (1): 32–41.

Stephenson, B. M., and A. N. Kingsnorth. 2011. "Safety and Sterilization of Mosquito Net Mesh for Humanitarian Inguinal Hernioplasty." *World Journal of Surgery* 35 (9): 1957–60.

Swadia, N. D. 2011. "Laparoscopic Totally Extra-Peritoneal Inguinal Hernia Repair: 9 Year's Experience." *Hernia* 15 (3): 273–79.

Swartz, M., T. M. Morgan, and J. N. Krieger. 2007. "Complications of Scrotal Surgery for Benign Conditions." *Urology* 69 (4): 616–19.

Szopinski, J., S. Dabrowiecki, S. Pierscinski, M. Jackowski, M. Jaworski, and Z. Szuflet. 2012. "Desarda versus Lichtenstein Technique for Primary Inguinal Hernia Treatment: 3-Year Results of a Randomized Clinical Trial." *World Journal of Surgery* 36 (5): 984–92.

Thambugala, R. L. 1971. "The Radical Cure of Hydrocele of the Tunica Vaginalis: The Technique of Excision of the Sac." *British Journal of Surgery* 58 (7): 517–51.

Thomas, G., F. O. Richards, Jr., A. Eigege, N. K. Dakum, M. P. Azzuwut, and others. 2009. "A Pilot Program of Mass Surgery Weeks for Treatment of Hydrocele Due to Lymphatic Filariasis in Central Nigeria." *American Journal of Tropical Medicine and Hygiene* 80 (3): 447–51.

Tongaonkar, R. R., B. V. Reddy, V. K. Mehta, N. S. Singh, and S. Shivade. 2003. "Preliminary Multicentric Trial of Cheap Indigenous Mosquito-Net Cloth for Tension-Free Hernia Repair." *Indian Journal of Surgery* 65 (1): 89–95.

Turaga, K., R. J. Fitzgibbons, and V. Puri. 2008. "Inguinal Hernias: Should We Repair?" *Surgical Clinics of North America* 88 (1): 127–38.

Vos, T., A. D. Flaxman, M. Naghavi, R. Lozano, C. Michaud, and others. 2012. "Years Lived with Disability (YLDs) for 1,160 Sequelae of 289 Diseases and Injuries, 1990–2010: A Systematic Analysis for the Global Burden of Disease Study 2010." *The Lancet* 380 (9859): 2163–96.

Walker, I. A., and I. H. Wilson. 2008. "Anaesthesia in Developing Countries—A Risk for Patients." *The Lancet* 371 (9617): 968–69.

WHO (World Health Organization). 2002. Surgical Approaches to the Urogenital Manifestations of Lymphatic Filariasis. Geneva: WHO. http://whqlibdoc.who.int/hq/2002/WHO _CDS_CPE_CEE_2002.33.pdf.

———. 2005. "Global Programme to Eliminate Lymphatic Filariasis: Progress Report for 2004." *Weekly Epidemiological Record* 80: 202–12. http://www.who.int/wer/2005/wer8023 .pdf.

———. 2011. Accelerating Work to Overcome the Global Impact of Neglected Tropical Diseases: A Roadmap for Implementation. Geneva: WHO. http://www.who.int /neglected_diseases/NTD_RoadMap_2012_Fullversion.pdf.

———. 2012. "Global Programme to Eliminate Lymphatic Filariasis: Progress Report, 2011." *Weekly Epidemiological Record* 87: 345–56. http://www.who.int/wer/2012/REH _37.pdf.

———. 2013a. "Lymphatic Filariasis." Factsheet No. 102, WHO, Geneva. http://www.who.int/mediacentre/factsheets /fs102/en/.

———. 2013b. "World Health Organization Media Center: Maternal Mortality." Factsheet No. 348, WHO, Geneva. http://www.who.int/mediacentre/factsheets/fs348/en/.

Wijers, D. J. B. 1977. "Bancroftian Filariasis in Kenya I. Prevalence Survey among Adult Males in the Coast Province." *Annals of Tropical Medicine and Parasitology* 71 (3): 313–33.

Wilhelm, T. J., S. Freudenberg, E. Jonas, R. Gobholz, S. Post, and P. Kyamanywa. 2007. "Sterilized Mosquito Net versus Commercial Mesh for Hernia Repair: An Experimental Study in Goats in Mbarara/Uganda." *European Surgical Research* 39 (5): 312–17.

Wilhelm, T. J., I. Thawe, B. Mwatabu, H. Mothes, and S. Post. 2011. "Efficacy of Major General Surgery Performed by Non-physician Clinicians at a Central Hospital in Malawi." *Tropical Doctor* 41 (2): 71–75.

Wynd, S., W. D. Melrose, D. N. Durrheim, J. Carron, and M. Gyapong. 2007. "Understanding the Community Impact of Lymphatic Filariasis: A Review of the Sociocultural Literature." *Bulletin of the World Health Organization* 85 (6): 493–98.

Yang, J., D. Papandria, D. Rhee, H. Perry, and F. Abdullah. 2011. "Low-Cost Mesh for Inguinal Hernia Repair in Resource-Limited Settings." *Hernia* 15 (5): 485–89.

Yardov, Y. S., and S. K. Stoyanov. 1969. "The Incidence of Hernia on the Island of Pemba." *East African Medical Journal* 46 (12): 687–91.

Zeldenryk, L. M., M. Gray, R. Speare, S. Gordon, and W. Melrose. 2011. "The Emerging Story of Disability Associated with Lymphatic Filariasis: A Critical Review." *PLoS Neglected Tropical Diseases* 5 (12): e1366.

Zendejas, B., T. Ramirez, T. Jones, A. Kuchena, S. M. Ali, and others. 2013. "Incidence of Inguinal Hernia Repairs in Olmsted County, MN: A Population-Based Study." *Annals of Surgery* 257 (3): 520–26.

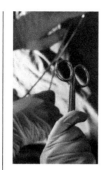

Chapter 10

Dentistry

Richard Niederman, Magda Feres,
and Eyitope Ogunbodede

INTRODUCTION

The oral health chapter in *Disease Control Priorities in Developing Countries*, second edition, focused on noncommunicable disease models for health systems (Bratthall and others 2006). The current chapter provides a complementary approach based on the definition of health care delivery as the "effective provision of services to people with diseases for which proven therapies exist" (Kim, Farmer, and Porter 2013, 1060–61). These complementary approaches—top down and bottom up, respectively—are both necessary; neither alone is sufficient to improve oral health. More specifically, we focus on the effective provision of preventive services and the implications of this goal for global policy changes, and the upstream value and economic choices that must be made to effect these positive changes.

Oral health maladies can be divided into four categories:

- Largely preventable bacterial or viral infections, for example, caries, periodontitis, noma, as well as oral manifestations of HIV/AIDS
- Largely preventable cellular transformations, for example, oral cancer
- Congenital defects, for example, cleft lip and cleft palate
- Trauma.

This chapter addresses the first category—the largely preventable bacterial infections of caries, periodontitis, and noma. It does not specifically address oral-systemic interactions or associations. The other maladies in the remaining three categories are addressed in other chapters and volumes in this series.

We identify evidence-based, cost-effective, preventive interventions that community health care workers can deliver at the community level. These same workers provide better sanitation and clean water, as well as treat a range of diseases, such as diabetes, helminthiasis, HIV/AIDS, malaria, malnutrition, and tuberculosis. These community-based preventive interventions for oral health will increase access to care, improve health, and reduce the burden of disease and the costs of care, compared with traditional surgical approaches to care.

However, in low- and middle-income countries (LMICs), access to the identified services, as well as the financial resources and infrastructure to deliver them, vary. Accordingly, in the initial stages, stakeholders need to be very selective in the starting points.

We specifically selected caries and periodontitis for the following reasons (Marcenes and others 2013):

- They are the first and sixth most prevalent global diseases.
- They are increasing in prevalence because of population growth and aging.

Corresponding author: Richard Niederman, DMD, New York University, rniederman@nyu.edu.

- They are largely preventable bacterial infections of epidemic proportions.

Additional considerations include the following:

- Preventing and controlling these maladies will address the goals of the World Health Organization's (WHO's) Basic Package of Oral Care (Frencken and others 2002).
- Cost-effective preventive measures can be implemented globally (Benzian and others 2012).
- Multiple effective training, workforce, and care models are available to support global implementation (Mathu-Muju, Friedman, and Nash 2013; Nash and others 2012). However, cross-cultural applications will need to be validated.

Like caries and periodontitis, noma is a preventable infection. Unlike caries and periodontitis, which have high prevalence but low morbidity and low mortality, noma has a low prevalence (approximately 0.0005 percent; 0.5 per 100,000), but very high morbidity and mortality (approximately 80 percent) (Marck 2003).

We focus on the critical few preventive measures with demonstrated benefit based on the following:

- Multiple systematic reviews of human trials (caries and periodontitis)
- Multiple human trials exhibiting similar quantitative and qualitative directionality (caries, periodontitis, and noma).

For clarity of purpose, we do not address the other prevention and treatment modalities for which there are no systematic reviews or for which results from human trials differ from one another.

Although we address specific effective preventive measures for oral maladies, these maladies are but one reflection of social determinants of health and disease (Lee and Divaris 2014; Watt 2012; Watt and Sheiham 2012). Other factors include the following:

- Tobacco use (Benedetti and others 2013; Fiorini and others 2014; Walter and others 2012)
- Nutrition (Moynihan and Kelly 2014; Palacios, Joshipura, and Willett 2009; Ritchie and others 2002; Touger-Decker, Mobley, and American Dietetic Association 2007)
- Bidirectional impacts of oral and systemic health (Cullinan and Seymour 2013; Friedewald and others 2009a; Linden, Lyons, and Scannapieco 2013; Lockhart and others 2012).

EPIDEMIOLOGY OF CARIES, PERIODONTITIS, AND NOMA

According to assessments of the WHO and World Bank's Global Burden of Disease (Marcenes and others 2013), untreated caries, or tooth decay, is the most common of all 291 diseases and injuries assessed, affecting 35 percent of the global population. If periodontitis is added to caries, untreated oral maladies affect almost 50 percent of the global population, or 4 billion people. When people with untreated oral maladies are added to those with a history of treatment, oral diseases affect nearly 100 percent of the global population (Marcenes and others 2013).

Caries and periodontitis have the highest prevalence among oral diseases, but other oral diseases add significant morbidity and mortality, including noma, oral manifestations of HIV/AIDs, oral cancer, genetic defects, and orofacial trauma.

Of particular concern is the 11 percent increase of oral diseases between 2000 and 2011, despite the 4 percent decrease in the global burden of other diseases in this period (table 10.1). Quantitatively, and as measured by disability-adjusted life years (DALYs), 15,152,000 years of

Table 10.1 Changes in All Global Burden of Disease Causes and Oral Health, 2000–11

	2011 DALYs (thousands)	Percent change, 2000–11	2011 DALYs (per 100,000 population)	Percent change, 2000–11
All GBD causes	2,744,322	–4	39,553	–16
All oral conditions	15,152	11	218	–3
Untreated caries in primary teeth	5,031	15	73	1
Periodontitis	5,501	27	79	11
Tooth loss	4,620	–7	67	–19

Source: WHO 2013.
Note: DALYs = disability-adjusted life year (years of life lost + years lived with disability); GBD = Global Burden of Disease.

healthy life were lost because of oral conditions in 2011. This loss was almost evenly divided between untreated caries, severe periodontitis, and severe tooth loss.

The largest increases in oral disease occurred in Sub-Saharan Africa (24 percent) and South Asia (19 percent) (table 10.2). Although thought to be due primarily to population growth and aging, increases in caries and periodontitis occurred in almost all LMICs and high-income countries (HICs). Tables 10.3 through 10.5 provide details by region for untreated caries (table 10.3), periodontitis (table 10.4), and tooth loss (table 10.5) (Marcenes and others 2013).

Figure 10.1 illustrates the burden of disease for caries by income level, demonstrating the substantial differences in needs. These differences, in turn, suggest that different approaches to care are required by income level and need, both among and within countries.

MICROBIOLOGY OF CARIES, PERIODONTITIS, AND NOMA

Caries, periodontitis, and noma are largely preventable, mixed, bacterial infections. The specific causative agents for each disease are as follows:

- Caries is a microaerophilic Gram-positive mixture of *Lactobacillus* and several *Streptococci* including *mutans, sanguis, mitis, and salivarius* (Gibbons and van Houte 1975).
- Periodontitis is an anaerobic Gram-negative mixture of *Actinobacillus actinomycetemcomitans, Porphyromonas gingivalis, Campylobacter rectus, Prevotella intermedia, Prevotella nigrescens, and Fusobacterium nucleatum* (Haffajee and Socransky 1994; Socransky and Haffajee 1994), and the more

Table 10.2 Changes in Oral Health, by Region, 2000–11

	2011 DALYs (thousands)	Percent change, 2000–11	2011 DALYs (per 100,000 population)	Percent change, 2000–11
World	15,152	11	218	−3
High income	2,467	−2	225	−9
East Asia and Pacific	4,308	14	217	5
Europe and Central Asia	1,242	−6	305	−7
Latin America and the Caribbean	1,502	11	255	−3
Middle East and North Africa	627	14	189	−6
South Asia	3,614	19	219	0
Sub-Saharan Africa	1,392	24	159	−5

Source: WHO 2013.
Note: DALYs = disability-adjusted life years (years of life lost + years lived with disability); GBD = Global Burden of Disease.

Table 10.3 Untreated Caries, 2000–11

	2011 DALYs (thousands)	Percent change, 2000–11	2011 DALYs (per 100,000 population)	Percent change, 2000–11
World	5,031	15	73	1
High income	338	9	31	1
East Asia and Pacific	1,561	10	79	1
Europe and Central Asia	362	1	89	−1
Latin America and Caribbean	349	16	59	2
Middle East and North Africa	245	24	74	2
South Asia	1,581	20	96	1
Sub-Saharan Africa	594	33	68	1

Source: WHO 2013.
Note: DALY = disability-adjusted life year; GBD = Global Burden of Disease.

Table 10.4 Periodontitis, 2000–11

	2011 DALYs (thousands)	Percent change, 2000–11	2011 DALYs (per 100,000 population)	Percent change, 2000–11
World	5,501	27	79	11
High income	915	14	84	6
East Asia and Pacific	1,817	29	91	19
Europe and Central Asia	449	10	110	8
Latin America and Caribbean	635	31	108	14
Middle East and North Africa	177	42	53	17
South Asia	990	34	60	13
Sub-Saharan Africa	518	37	59	5

Source: WHO 2013.
Note: DALY = disability-adjusted life year; GBD = Global Burden of Disease.

Table 10.5 Tooth Loss, 2000–11

	2011 DALYs (thousands)	Percent change, 2000–11	2011 DALYs (per 100,000 population)	Percent change, 2000–11
World	4,620	−7	67	−19
High income	1,214	−13	111	−20
East Asia and Pacific	930	−4	47	−11
Europe and Central Asia	432	−22	106	−23
Latin America and the Caribbean	518	−8	88	−20
Middle East and North Africa	205	−10	62	−25
South Asia	1,043	6	63	−10
Sub-Saharan Africa	279	−7	32	−29

Source: WHO 2013.
Note: DALY = disability-adjusted life year; GBD = Global Burden of Disease.

recently identified or renamed *Aggregatibacter actinomycetemcomitans*, *Tannerella forsythia*, and *Treponema denticola*.

- Noma exhibits an altered oral microbiota with an increase in *Prevotella* and *Peptostreptococcus* genus exacerbated by poor nutrition, poverty, and prior infections (Huyghe and others 2013; Paster and others 2002).

CARIES

Traditional Surgical Treatment

For more than 100 years, dentists have successfully treated dental cavities with surgery, consisting of local anesthesia, followed by surgical excision of the decay, followed by filling. To ensure success, surgical excision normally extended beyond the lesion itself as a preventive measure against further decay. This approach is termed extension for prevention, or comprehensive treatment (Webster 1908). The clinical principle was that, to ensure success, all decay and all areas of potential decay had to be removed. Once this was done, additional tooth structure was removed to provide undercuts that mechanically hold the "permanent" fillings (usually silver amalgam) in place. These permanent fillings, however, have a limited life span of approximately 10 years and then require replacement (Burke and Lucarotti 2009; Chadwick and others 2001; Downer and others 1999).

The traditional surgical approach to care is office based; patients travel to dental offices multiple times for comprehensive care. Additionally, systematic reviews demonstrate that traditional fillings, with extensive excision of tooth structure, lead to a significant increase in risk of adverse events, when compared with sealing early caries lesions or providing atraumatic restorations (Ricketts and others 2013; Schwendicke, Dörfer, and Paris 2013).

There exist little or no data to demonstrate that traditional surgical care followed by fillings reduces or prevents the underlying causative infection from instigating further tooth destruction. Accordingly, the identification of causative bacterial agents, together with the identification of a number of preventive and treatment agents, led to the twenty-first-century concept, and first clinical demonstration, of minimal intervention dentistry (Frencken and others 1994).

Finally, this chapter's focus on prevention precludes discussion of surgical care (such as fillings and extractions). We recognize that fillings for treating cavities have an established history (Webster 1908); extractions for acute problems are essential components of the WHO's Basic Package of Oral Care (Frencken and others 2002), and extractions are an integral part of emergency and trauma care. However, work on both the longevity and the cost of fillings, compared with prevention, indicates that investments in prevention outweigh investments in fillings (Mickenautsch and Yengopal 2012; Mickenautsch, Yengopal, and Banerjee 2010; Ricketts and others 2013; Schwendicke and others 2013).

Preventive Approaches

Multiple systematic reviews of human randomized controlled trials from multiple LMICs and HICs have identified a number of effective caries prevention agents (table 10.6). In all cases, preventive care can be community based, in addition to office or clinic based, allowing care to be brought to patients rather than patients brought to care. Furthermore, because the biology of caries is identical globally and across the life span, the mode of action and efficacy of these agents are also similar. However, because of training deficiencies, tariffs, local regulations, and social infrastructure, the delivery of these evidence-based, cost-effective preventive therapeutics varies substantially among countries and within countries.

Systematic reviews with formal comparative comprehensive economic evaluations of all caries prevention methods are modest in both number and quality (Källestål and others 2003; Mariño, Khan, and Morgan 2013). The available work indicates that for specific countries, and for specific populations, prevention is cost-effective. However, many of these evaluations fall short of current economic evaluation standards. Accordingly, only estimated efficacy and costs are provided in table 10.6 to facilitate local assessments.

Water Fluoridation. High-quality economic evaluations of water fluoridation conducted in Australia and the United States for the general and aging populations

Figure 10.1 Proportion of Decayed, Missing, and Filled Teeth in Children, by Income Level, 1990–2004

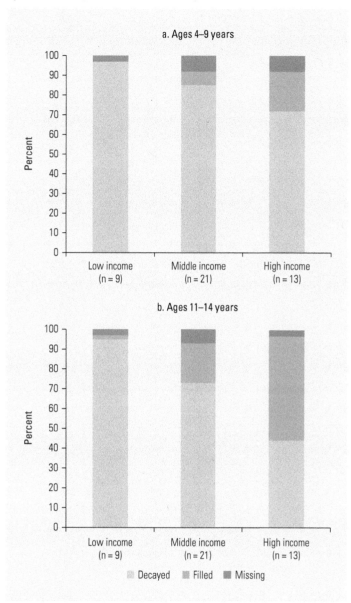

Source: Yee 2008.

indicate reductions in caries greater than 20 percent to 50 percent for approximately US$0.50 per year per person (Campain and others 2010; Doessel 1979; Griffin, Jones, and Tomar 2001; Johnson and others 2014). A caution is warranted because these studies use differing methodologies and may not relate to LMICs (Mariño, Khan, and Morgan 2013).

Studies of water fluoridation have been carried out in LMICs. Two examples of import provide object lessons on its benefits. In Brazil, a 25-year longitudinal assessment of caries demonstrates a significant

Table 10.6 Summary of Current Systematic Reviews: Identifying Effective Caries Preventive and Therapeutic Agents

Agent	Frequency	Estimated efficacy (percent)	Material cost[a] US$	Material cost[a] US$ per year	Delivery agent
Water fluoridation	Continuous	20–40[1]		$0.50[2]	Piped water
Salt fluoride	Daily	20[3]		$0.03[4]	Cooked food
Fluoride toothpaste[b]	Twice a day	25[5]	< $0.05 per dose	$0.50–36.50[6]	Individual or school
Fluoride milk	More than twice a day	>20[7]	n.a.	n.a.[8]	Individual
Silver fluoride	Twice a year	80[9]	$0.10 per dose	$0.20	Community health care worker
Fluoride varnish	More than twice a year	40[10]	$3.00 per dose	$6.00[11]	Community health care worker
Sealant	Once for posterior tooth	80[12]	$3.00 per application on multiple teeth		Community health care worker
Atraumatic restoration (therapeutic sealant)	As needed	80[13]	$3.00 per application on multiple teeth[14]		Community health care worker
Filling	As needed	80[13]	$2.00 per anesthesia and filling per tooth		Community health care worker or dentist
Extraction	As needed	100	$1.00 per tooth for anesthesia		Community health care worker or dentist

Sources:
1. Griffin and others 2007; Johnson and others 2014; McDonagh and others 2000; Parnell, Whelton, and O'Mullane 2009.
2. Kroon and van Wyk 2012b; Mariño, Fajardo, and Morgan 2012; van Wyk, Kroon, and Holtshousen 2001.
3. Yengopal and others 2010.
4. Gillespie and Marthaler 2005; Mariño, Fajardo, and Morgan 2012; Marino and others 2011.
5. Dos Santos, Nadanovsky, and de Oliveira 2012; Wong and others 2011.
6. Benzian 2012; Davies and others 2003; Splieth and Flessa 2008; Yee, McDonald, and Walker 2004.
7. Cagetti and others 2013; Espelid 2009.
8. Mariño, Fajardo, and Morgan 2012.
9. Liu and others 2012; Rosenblatt, Stamford, and Niederman 2009; Zhi, Lo, and Lin 2012.
10. Marinho and others 2013.
11. Hendrix and others 2013; Quiñonez and others 2006; Sköld and others 2008.
12. Ahovuo-Saloranta and others 2013; Mickenautsch and Yengopal 2011; Yengopal and others 2009.
13. de Amorim, Leal, and Frencken 2012; Mickenautsch and Yengopal 2011; Ricketts and others 2013; Schwendicke, Dörfer, and Paris 2013.
14. da Mata and others 2014; Schwendicke and others 2013.
Note: n.a. = not available.
a. Only includes actual material cost for active agent, not ancillary material costs (for example, toothbrush, applicators, sterile instruments, gloves, and barriers to deliver active agents), or indirect costs (for example, transportation and rent).
b. Systematic reviews support an international standard level of 1,000 parts per million fluoride for younger children and up to 1,500 parts per million for older children and adults (Wong and others 2011).

25 percent reduction in caries over five years following water fluoridation (Lauris, da Silva Bastos, and de Magalhaes Bastos 2012) at a cost of approximately US$0.03 per year per person (Frias and others 2006). Routine assessments of water fluoride levels were needed to ensure success (Buzalaf and others 2013; Moimaz and others 2012; Moimaz and others 2013). In South Africa, a Commission of Inquiry recommended community water fluoridation with regulations compelling water fluoridation. However, the water remains unfluoridated, despite multiple economic analyses demonstrating that water fluoridation can reduce caries by approximately 15 percent at a cost of approximately US$0.36 per year per person and is cost-effective (Kroon and van Wyk 2012a, 2012b; van Wyk, Kroon, and Holtshousen 2001).

Water fluoridation depends on the availability of potable piped water. However, even when fluoridated water is available, it is not 100 percent effective. Implementation of complementary effective fluoride delivery systems and preventive measures need to be considered to control and prevent caries. Efficacy studies have been carried out in LMICs for all of these fluoride delivery systems and preventive interventions (table 10.6); they are likely to be effective at local levels if affordable high-quality products are available.

Modeling and subsequent testing of the projected economic costs to achieve these health benefits need to be locally determined. Some examples from LMICs, UMICs, and HICs are relevant (Mariño, Khan, and Morgan 2013; Morgan and others 2012). Focused studies of salt fluoridation in Peru (Marino and others 2011), toothpaste in Nepal and Brazil (Frazao 2012; Yee, McDonald, and Helderman 2006; Yee, McDonald, and Walker 2004), and comparative studies in Chile (Mariño, Fajardo, and Morgan 2012) differ in methodology; however, all demonstrate the tangible clinical and economic benefits of salt, water, toothpaste, and milk fluoridation.

PERIODONTITIS

Periodontitis is an inflammatory reaction to an overgrowth of a mixed, anaerobic bacterial infection colonizing the subgingival crevices around the teeth. If untreated, this infection leads to bleeding gingiva, loose teeth, and ultimately, tooth loss. In addition, this inflammatory reaction is associated with adverse effects on systemic health (Han and others 2014). These include, for example, cardiovascular disease (Friedewald and others 2009b; Tonetti, van Dyke, and Working Group 1 2013), diabetic control (Borgnakke and others 2013), and adverse pregnancy outcomes (Ide and Papapanou 2013; Sanz, Kornman, and Working Group 3 2013).

Paradoxically, most of the bacterial species present in the oral biofilm are host-compatible or beneficial (Socransky and others 1988; Socransky and others 1998). These bacteria not only inhabit the subgingival crevice; they are also found on the supragingival tissue, tongue, cheek, and palate (Faveri and others 2006; Mager and others 2003). Thus, health or disease is a result of the balance or imbalance in the oral microbiome (Socransky and Haffajee 2002; Teles, Haffajee, and Socransky 2006).

Current data support the concept that clinical improvement is attained when there is a change from a disease-related to a health-related oral ecology (Feres 2008; Socransky and Haffajee 2002; Teles, Haffajee, and Socransky 2006). To achieve this shift, effective therapy needs to address all the oral ecological environments.

Similar to dental caries, periodontitis has been successfully treated with mechanical therapy for more than 100 years, including scaling and root planing with or without subsequent surgery. Furthermore, successful therapy requires quarterly maintenance therapy. It is of interest to note that we were unable to identify studies demonstrating beneficial long-term impact on the oral microbiome following mechanical therapy.

Two levels of care are potentially effective in the treatment of gingivitis: patient-applied toothpastes and mouthwashes, and professionally prescribed antimicrobials (Teles and Teles 2009). Gingivitis is generally considered to be a precursor to periodontitis, and patient-applied oral use of specific mouthwashes and toothpaste can potentially reduce risk of subsequent periodontitis. The agents that provide a clinically significant benefit in reducing gingivitis are triclosan copolymer toothpaste and chlorhexidine mouthwash (Gunsolley 2006; Osso and Kanani 2013; Riley and Lamont 2013; Van Strydonck and others 2012).

Seminal Clinical Trials

Three seminal trials provide key turning points and offer an alternate approach to periodontal mechanical therapy—the use of combination therapy with metronidazole and amoxicillin (250–500 milligrams of each agent, three times a day, for seven days). The first trial was a case series of 118 patients who, having failed all forms of traditional mechanical therapy, received metronidazole and amoxicillin and scaling (van Winkelhoff, Tijhof, and de Graaff 1992). The second trial was a masked randomized controlled trial of 46 patients that compared metronidazole and amoxicillin to placebo (López and Gamonal 1998). Perhaps the most surprising of all the studies, but with multiple threats to validity, was the paradigm-breaking solitary study comparing a seven-day regimen of metronidazole plus amoxicillin alone to scaling or root planing alone (López and others 2006). At 12 months, the clinical and microbial outcomes of care for patients receiving antimicrobial therapy alone were similar to those of patients receiving only mechanical therapy. In sum, in all three cases, seven days of metronidazole and amoxicillin shifted the oral ecology from disease-related to health-related and improved clinical health, compared with prior or concurrent mechanical therapy.

Systematic Reviews

Three systematic reviews of human randomized controlled trials examined combined short-term metronidazole plus amoxicillin for treating periodontitis. The results of all three reviews found significant statistical and clinical benefit of short-term (7–14 days) 250–500 milligram metronidazole and amoxicillin three times a day (Sgolastra, Gatto, and others 2012; Sgolastra, Petrucci, and others 2012; Zandbergen and others 2013).

Recent Clinical Trials

Human randomized clinical trials, published after the inclusion dates of these systematic reviews, support the use of short-term metronidazole and amoxicillin (Feres and others 2012; Goodson and others 2012; Mestnik and others 2010). Although these studies differed from each other in important ways, they reached similar conclusions: antibiotic therapy shifts the oral microbiome from disease related to health related, with substantial clinical improvement. Feres and others (2012) treated high-risk patients, Mestnik and others (2010) treated patients with aggressive disease, and Goodson and others (2012) treated patients with moderate to high disease levels. These trials demonstrate that short-term treatment with metronidazole and amoxicillin achieved the following outcomes:

- The combination therapy moved 66 percent of patients from high-risk levels to low-risk levels one year after therapy; in contrast, mechanical therapy only moved 22 percent of patients from high-risk levels to low-risk levels (Feres and others 2012).
- The combination therapy was more clinically effective than mechanical therapy in patients with aggressive periodontitis (Mestnik and others 2010).
- The combination therapy resulted in better microbial and clinical outcomes two years after therapy, compared with other treatments, for example, scaling and root planing, surgery, scaling and root planing plus surgery, and local antibiotic delivery (Goodson and others 2012).

Concerns with Antimicrobial Use

The studies described all support the demonstrated sustained clinical and statistical improvements in periodontal health in subjects receiving short-term metronidazole in combination with amoxicillin. However, antibiotic use in a public health context raises concerns about several issues: the quality, affordability, and availability of the antibiotics; resistance to the antibiotics as well as the emergence of resistant-strains of bacteria; and changes or reequilibration of the oral (and gastrointestinal) microbiome.

Multiple perspectives merit consideration:

- *Risks versus benefits.* The benefits need to clearly offset the risks. The benefits of short-term metronidazole plus amoxicillin in treating periodontitis must secure benefits that would be much more difficult, costly, inaccessible, or risky by other means, such as surgery with quarterly cleaning.
- *Recolonization.* Treating periodontitis with metronidazole plus amoxicillin facilitates oral recolonization by a health-compatible oral microbiome (Matarazzo and others 2008; Silva and others 2011).

- *Acquired resistance.* Resistance to metronidazole has rarely been reported (Soares and others 2012).
- *Allergic reactions.* Assessments vary, but current data suggest a prevalence of approximately 37 percent for nonsteroidal anti-inflammatory drugs and 5 percent to 29.4 percent for beta-lactam antibiotics (Bigby and others 1986; Dona and others 2012). Clindamycin and azithromycin are alternatives (Herrera and others 2008).
- *Global increase in antibiotic resistance.* The dramatic and effective use of metronidazole plus amoxicillin for treating *Helicobacter pylori* and the global increase in resistance provides a useful object lesson. In Latin America, amoxicillin resistance is approximately 4 percent, and metronidazole resistance is approximately 53 percent (Camargo and others 2014). Early short courses of combination therapy with the two antibiotics prevent the emergence of resistant strains (D'Agata and others 2008).
- *Relative balance (known and unknown) of direct benefits and risks.* Preliminary data suggest that antimicrobial use changes the human microbiome in the direction of increasing the risk of obesity, type 1 diabetes, inflammatory bowel disease, allergies, and asthma (Blaser 2011). Conversely, data also indicate that treating periodontitis with metronidazole plus amoxicillin facilitates oral recolonization by the health-compatible oral microbiome (Matarazzo and others 2008; Silva and others 2011). The potential benefits of effectively treating periodontal infections include reductions in the negative impacts that the inflammatory response has on cardiovascular disease, diabetes, and pregnancy outcomes (Borgnakke and others 2013; Friedewald and others 2009b; Ide and Papapanou 2013; Sanz, Kornman, and Working Group 3 2013; Tonetti, van Dyke, and Working Group 1 2013).

In sum, the most effective approach to controlling and preventing periodontitis appears to be short-term metronidazole and amoxicillin, with or without concordant mechanical therapy. However, in countries without access to professional treatment, metronidazole and amoxicillin alone may be the only effective and efficient option. This assumption will need rigorous testing under local conditions for widespread validation. The additional potential benefits of local testing will be the secondary benefits of improved systemic health. The alternative to testing is the absence of care or the implementation of mechanical therapy, which is more expensive and less effective.

Additional Considerations

Two additional points relevant to systemic health are noteworthy with respect to the available data.

First, we were unable to identify any human trials supporting the concept that a single round of mechanical therapy alone (for example, scaling and root planing, with or without surgery) will prevent or control periodontal infections or improve oral health in the long term (Loesche and Grossman 2001; Sampaio, Araújo, and Oliveira 2011; Worthington and others 2013). This lack of support was not unexpected. Mechanical therapy targets specific tooth surfaces but does not comprehensively address other areas of microbial residence, such as tongue and oral mucosal; nor is mechanical therapy capable of removing residual disease-related microbial colonies from the treated tooth surfaces.

Second, only a few studies address the economics of mechanical periodontal therapy, and these indicate that scaling and root planing do not confer an economic benefit (Braegger 2005; Gaunt and others 2008). In light of the enhanced clinical benefit of antimicrobial intervention (with or without scaling and root planing), the wider opportunity for intervention and access to care provided by nondental personnel, the broader potential beneficial impact of antimicrobials on systemic disease, and the broader potential negative impact on antimicrobial resistance, we await demonstration programs examining the clinical and economic impact of antimicrobial therapy.

NOMA

Noma (cancrum oris, necrotizing ulcerative gingivitis, stomatitis gangrenosa) is a destructive ulceration of the gingival-oral mucosa that spreads extraorally, degrading the tissues of the face and bone (Ogbureke and Ogbureke 2010). The disease leads to severe destruction of the midface—the lips, cheek, maxilla, mandible, nose, and orbital floor—with unsightly facial disfigurement, impaired self-nutrition, impaired speech, trismus, and social alienation (Marck 2003; Ogbureke and Ogbureke 2010).

Prevalence and Incidence

Noma is most commonly found in Sub-Saharan Africa, where extreme poverty, malnutrition, and childhood infections are common (Feller and others 2014). Noma is commonly described as the "face of poverty" because of its facial location and prevalence among children ages one to four years in LMICs (Marck 2003). Estimates suggest a global prevalence of 500,000 people; an annual incidence of 140,000; and a mortality rate of 80 percent to 90 percent (Bourgeois and Leclercq 1999). In local

regions of Nigeria, the incidence is estimated to reach 6.4 per 1,000 children, which extrapolates to a global incidence of 30,000 to 40,000 (Fieger and others 2003). However, these estimates are based on cases and projections and may overestimate or underestimate the prevalence and incidence.

Contributing Factors

The precipitating events are unclear. The most recent and best studies are a matched and powered case control and a parallel microbial analysis. They indicate three contributing factors:

- An altered oral flora, specifically an increase in the percentage of *Prevotella* and *Peptostreptococcus* genus, and a decrease in the percentage of *Fusobacterium*, *Capnocytophaga*, *Neisseria*, and *Spirochaeta*
- Malnutrition
- Recent illness of respiratory or intestinal origin or compromised immune response, for example, the presence of HIV/AIDS (Baratti-Mayer, Pittet, and Montandon 2004; Bolivar and others 2012; Feller and others 2014).

Treatment

When detected early, noma responds to antibiotic treatment with metronidazole plus amoxicillin. Recommended doses vary with age and body weight; they range from 100 milligrams to 500 milligrams of each agent three times per day for seven days. When antibiotics are used in conjunction with nutritional rehabilitation, the mortality rate drops from more than 80 percent to less than 10 percent (Baratti-Mayer, Pittet, and Montandon 2004; Bolivar and others 2012; Tempest 1966). These findings support a bacterial and nutritional etiology.

For survivors, postinfection surgical reconstruction, when available, is extensive. No standardized approach can be advocated because of the variety of anatomical manifestations (Marck and others 2010). The current consensus is that surgical techniques will largely depend on the extent and location of the lesions, the availability of technical facilities, the competence of the surgical teams, and the timing of surgery (Ogbureke and Ogbureke 2010).

Treatment normally consists of excising all scar tissue, correcting the trismus, raising and transposing local and distant soft tissue flaps, and bone grafting in cases of considerable loss of facial bone or jawbone. Multiple flap, transposition, and closure designs have been implemented, often paralleling oncologic reconstruction.

Reconstruction for noma, however, differs from oncologic reconstruction in several ways (Huijing and others 2011):

- Compound tissue losses are common.
- The bony defect and soft-tissue scar affect facial skeleton and dental development, producing gross asymmetry, with loss of normal anatomical reference points.
- Patients usually suffer nutritional deficiencies and extreme deprivation.
- Postoperative complications, such as poor healing and infection, are common.

Even in the most advanced medical environments, however, the results of surgical repair are less than perfect (Bisseling and others 2010; Bouman and others 2010), but preoperative planning, multiple staged surgeries, and a multidisciplinary team approach have been found to be useful in reducing postoperative complications (Huijing and others 2011; Marck and others 2010). These include the following precautions:

- Postponement of surgical treatment until the acute phase has abated
- Routine presurgical clinical workup, including dental care, hyperalimentation, multivitamin and anthelminthic treatment, and general hygiene measures
- Multidisciplinary team approach of plastic and maxillofacial surgeons, orthodontists, pedodontists, prosthodontists, physical therapists, and psychologists.

Additional studies demonstrate the benefits of anesthesiologists who can provide special airway and ventilation techniques needed for the limited openings (Coupe and others 2013), as well as psychiatric support and societal reintegration (Yunusa and Obembe 2012).

Economic analysis of this care is unavailable, possibly because of the low prevalence, high morbidity, and variability and complexity of care.

IMPLICATIONS FOR GLOBAL HEALTH POLICY

The oral diseases discussed in this chapter are preventable global epidemics that affect more than 50 percent of the population and have increasing prevalence (Marcenes and others 2013). The systematic reviews and clinical studies cited indicate that effective preventive measures are available. However, effective dissemination and implementation that improve oral health depend on two complementary approaches: a top-down noncommunicable disease model (Bratthall and others 2006), and a bottom-up health care delivery model (Kim, Farmer, and Porter 2013). In marked contrast to the traditional surgical model of oral care, these preventive measures can be delivered outside of clinical settings by community health workers (Benzian and others 2012; Monse and others 2010; Nash and others 2012).

Delivery Models for Prevention

The widespread incidence and increasing prevalence; the attendant long-term detrimental educational, medical, and social effects; the absolute and relative inequalities in care for HICs as well as LMICs (and within countries); and the collocation of these diseases with other noncommunicable diseases combine to suggest that it is appropriate to consider alternative approaches to traditional surgical care delivered by dentists.

Prevention Choices. Nationally, regionally, and locally, the preventive choices and modes of delivery will vary. These variations will depend on local needs, values, circumstances, and infrastructure, as well as on product availability and cost (box 10.1). Furthermore, if the goal is sustainable, long-term improvements in oral health, then systemic changes will be required at all stakeholder levels: patients, care providers, organizations, and governments. These evidence-based, effective, preventive methods will need to be culturally integrated into the social systems of personal care, care-provider training, and workforce models, as well as into community-based care delivery, compensation, and incentive systems.

Elements of a High-Value Program. An effective population- and patient-centered delivery framework is hypothesized to have four elements essential to delivering and optimizing value (Kim, Farmer, and Porter 2013; Porter 2010; Porter, Pabo, and Lee 2013):

- Integration of care for every individual condition over the cycle of care
- Shared delivery infrastructure across medical conditions
- Implemented knowledge of local patient and community constraints
- Maximized equitable economic and community development to improve value.

Delivery Choices. Oral prevention could be delivered in three ways, depending on local values, circumstances, infrastructure, and product availability:

- By patients themselves, for example, by the use of *affordable* fluoridated toothpaste and fluoride salt

Box 10.1

Guidelines for Selecting and Implementing the Basic Package of Oral Care

Guidelines for selecting and implementing the Basic Package of Oral Care (BPOC) in LMICs follow. The selection of interventions will be determined locally, regionally, and nationally.

Examples of partial implementation of the BPOC:

- **Cambodia:** Training of rural nurses to provide simple extractions, draining of abscess under local anesthesia, and atraumatic restorative treatment (Chher and others 2009).
- **Nepal:** Implementation of affordable toothpaste resulted in 27 percent decrease in caries prevalence and 10 percent decrease in oral pain (Yee, McDonald, and Helderman 2006).
- **The Philippines:** Training of teachers and education staff members to implement hand washing, fluoride tooth brushing, and school deworming programs (Monse and others 2013).
- **Tanzania:** Training of primary health care workers in the provision of simple extractions and atraumatic restorative treatment, resulting in improved oral health and quality of life (Kikwilu, Frencken, and Mulder 2009; Mashoto and others 2010).

Barriers to Implementing the BPOC:

- An absence of knowledge of the BPOC among government entities, nongovernmental organizations, and clinicians collaborating to improve oral health
- Knowledge of the BPOC, but failure to accept its utility based on the perceived absence of evidence, advantage, simplicity, compatibility with values, and trust in concept
- Acceptance of BPOC, but an absence of methodological knowledge of implementation and improvement, or determination of how BPOC might be integrated into existing health or educational structures
- A reluctance on the part of the dental profession to accept oral care provision by ancillary personnel.

Implementation precepts:

- **Safe:** Care should be as safe for patients in health care facilities as in their homes.
- **Effective:** The science and evidence behind health care should serve as the standard in the delivery of care and be applied.
- **Efficient:** Both process and outcomes of care should achieve maximum outcome with minimal time, effort, or expense.
- **Timely:** Patients should not experience excessive delays in receiving care and service.
- **Patient centered:** The system of care should be patient centered, respect patient preferences, and put patients in control.
- **Equitable:** Disparities in care should be eliminated.
- **Feasible:** The initiating clinical, organizational, or governmental stakeholders should have the financial, organizational, technical, capacity, and collaborative commitments to implement the programs.
- **Sustainable:** The delivery system must be financially, organizationally, and technically sustainable.
- **Improvement:** Process and outcome measures should be systematically implemented and the results evaluated to reduce waste and variation.
- **Regulatory compliance:** Compliance with all local and national regulations should be ensured.
- **Communicated outcomes:** Outcomes must be disseminated to overcome implementation barriers.

Implementation Steps

Step 1. Ask three questions:

- What is to be improved at the local, regional, or national level?
- What change will be made?
- How will we know that the change effected improvement?

box continues next page

Box 10.1 (continued)

Step 2. Determine local, regional, or national needs and capacities:

- Oral health needs (to see if implementation is needed)
- Costs and availability of funding
- Availability of necessary supplies, personnel, and collaborating health groups
- Quality of supplies

Step 3. Develop improvement plan to accomplish the following:

- A pilot program manual of procedures
- Carrying out of pilot

- Evaluation of impact (for example, Reach multiplied by Effectiveness for patient-centered outcomes)
- Identification and reduction of waste and variations

Step 4. Develop improvement plan to accomplish the following:

- Scale up effective pilot programs
- Evaluate wider impact validity
- Evaluate fidelity of adoption and maintenance

Sources: Chher and others 2009; Glasgow and others 2005; Greenhalgh and others 2004; IHI 2014; IOM 2001; Kikwilu, Frencken, and Mulder 2009; Langley and others 2009; Mashoto and others 2010; Monse and others 2013; Rogers 2002; Yee, McDonald, and Helderman 2006.

- By nondentist community health workers and school systems, for example, by the provision of fluoride toothpaste, silver fluoride, fluoride varnish, sealants, atraumatic restorations, antibiotics, and improved nutrition
- By community-wide programs and capacities, for example, the provision of water fluoridation and fluoride salt.

Of the three ways, the modest training of community health workers and school system staff, and the expansion of their current services, may provide the most immediate opportunity for oral health care improvement. Community water fluoridation is perhaps the most cost-effective preventive measure for caries, but it requires the most significant prior systematic infrastructure—piped potable water. Until such infrastructure exists, mobile clinics that bring dental services to rural communities may be cost-effective solutions for secondary prevention, such as restorative care, as demonstrated in South Africa and Thailand (Holtshousen and Smit 2007; Tianviwat, Chongsuvivatwong, and Birch 2009). For individual community-based care, affordable fluoridated toothpaste needs to be locally available for home use.

At least two narrative and two systematic reviews support the community-based delivery of preventive oral health care by nondentists (Calache and Hopcraft 2012; Mathu-Muju, Friedman, and Nash 2013; Nash and others 2012; Wright and others 2013). These studies indicate that community health care workers can increase access to care, improve health, and reduce costs by eliminating the proximal need for dentists. Much of the data in table 10.6 come from studies employing community health workers. Local values and circumstances will guide decisions, and local pilot and scaling programs will be required to quantitatively validate local process and outcome effectiveness.

One example of the beneficial and significant impact of an integrated community-based care program using a noncommunicable disease model is the award-winning Fit for School program in the Philippines. This program marries once-a-year school-based deworming with school-based tooth brushing with fluoridated toothpaste (box 10.2) (Benzian 2012; Benzian and others 2012; Monse and others 2010).

Fit for School parallels numerous improvement initiatives in LMICs (see box 10.1 for oral health examples). These initiatives include agriculture, education, environment, finance, governance, labor, and health. Many of these effective programs are chronicled in Banerjee and Duflo (2011). This work ranges from evaluating effectiveness, building capacity, and changing policies for deworming, bed nets, and chlorine in Kenya; to water disinfectants in Zambia; to hand washing with soap in India and Pakistan.[1]

Fees. Among the key counterintuitive policy findings is that the evidence does not support the practice of charging small fees to poor people for health products and

The Fit for School Approach

The Philippine Department of Education, supported by the German Enterprise for International Cooperation, the Philippine *Fit for School Inc.,* and other partners, initiated the Essential Health Care Program (EHCP) in public elementary schools. The program is based on the Fit for School Approach and integrates three evidence-based prevention measures for the most prevalent childhood diseases: soil-transmitted intestinal worm infections, hygiene-related diseases such as diarrhea and respiratory infections, and rampant tooth decay.

The program implements the following activities run by teachers:

- Daily group hand washing with soap
- Daily group tooth brushing with fluoride toothpaste

- Biannual deworming according to the WHO guidelines

These evidence-based interventions are complemented by the construction of facilities for group hand washing and sanitation and the provision of clean water to schools without access to it. The EHCP currently reaches more than 2.5 million Filipino children and is also implemented in Cambodia, Indonesia, and the Lao People's Democratic Republic. Material costs average US$0.50 per child per year. Affordability increases the probability that this program can be integrated into the regular government budgets, even in resource-poor countries, thereby ensuring sustainability beyond the initial start-up costs.

Sources: Benzian 2012; Monse and others 2013.

services, a policy promoted to help reduce waste. Even small fees for prevention services substantially reduce use. This finding suggests that prevention programs should be provided at no charge to patients and should be sustained by governmental funding.[2]

Examples, Principles, and Guidelines. Box 10.1 provides examples of programs implementing the Basic Package of Oral Care, as well as the principles and guidelines for selecting and implementing prevention programs.

Lessons Learned from Current Care Delivery Models in High-Income Countries

The unchanging high oral health needs in the United Kingdom and the United States provide the counterfactual to focusing on traditional surgical rather than preventive care.

In the United Kingdom, 33 percent of children age five years have active decay, and 2.3 percent have sepsis (NHS 2007). The need for care extends to adults: 31 percent have untreated cavities, 22 percent have urgent conditions, and 9 percent have dental pain (NHS 2009). The reviews of National Health Service dental care during the past 30 years repeatedly call for increases in both prevention and access to care, and for reductions in both the inequality of service distribution and waste through

overuse, underuse, and misuse of services (NHS 2005; Steele 2009).

In the United States, the Healthy People initiative reports that, from 1990 to 2010, the percentage of studied children with untreated decay remained virtually unchanged at almost 30 percent.[3] For underserved, rural, and minority populations, the percentage is significantly higher, reaching almost 50 percent (Dye and Thornton-Evans 2010). During the same period, yearly governmental dental expenditures for children increased from US$1 billion to US$7 billion. Spending is expected to reach US$15 billion by 2020 (CMS 2011b). In parallel, national spending for oral health care reached US$105 billion in 2010 (CMS 2011b). This level is second only to that of cardiac care (AHRQ 2007) and is expected to be US$170 billion by 2020 (CMS 2011b). Yet, data from the national Healthy People initiative indicate that oral health is not improving in concert with spending.[4] As a result, the need for a change to prevention-focused care is chronicled in multiple government and foundation publications (CMS 2011a; HHS 2010; IOM 2011a, 2011b).

Dental Workforce

The immediate need for considering alternatives to the current surgical-mechanical model of care is also clear when the current dental workforce is taken into account.

The 188 countries for which there are data have, on average, 0.3 (plus or minus 0.4 standard deviation) dentists per 1,000 residents (WHO 2006). The United States, which has five times the global average, has not been able to improve oral health during the past 20 years.[4]

These findings suggest that new education, training, and workforce models are needed (Bhutta and others 2010; Frenk and others 2010; Mathu-Muju, Friedman, and Nash 2013; Nash and others 2012). The current surgical-mechanical care model will not solve the global oral health problem. Countries need two complementary prevention frameworks for improving oral health care:

- A community-based health care provider model for providing services to people with diseases for which proven therapies exist (Kim, Farmer, and Porter 2013)
- A noncommunicable disease model (Bratthall and others 2006).

To succeed, the community-based health care worker model will need to consider the following:

- Preventive care delivered by nondentists
- Triage prevention, extractions, and complex surgical care
- Innovative methods to increase access to care at all levels, such as focused prevention integrated with other health initiatives, and focused mobile extraction service, to overcome the many barriers to access to safe oral health care.

Quality of Care

The Institute of Medicine's report *Crossing the Quality Chasm* identified six quality aims for clinical care (IOM 2001). From this perspective, using surgery rather than prevention as the primary mode of dental care seems to violate five of the six quality aims. This is not to say that surgery is unsafe or unwarranted; clearly, it is critical for treatment of acute abscesses, extractions, and noma.

However, for the most common infections—caries and periodontitis—surgical care appears to have the following limitations:

- It is not effective in treating the underlying causative infection.
- It is not patient centered in that clinicians are well compensated to intervene surgically but patients are better served by prevention.

- It is not timely in that multiple appointments, travel, and missed work or school are required to treat multiple teeth.
- It is not efficient in that surgical care requires a dental office, and preventive care can be delivered in locations where people learn, work, play, or pray.
- It is not equitable in that care is available only to people who are geographically near clinics, have a means of transportation, and can pay for care.

The surgical approach provides an example of the overuse of ineffective treatment and the underuse of effective prevention (Kohn, Corrigan, and Donaldson 2000).

INCREASING CLINICAL VALUE WITH COMMUNITY-BASED PREVENTION

A conceptual strategic starting point for thinking about alternative care models is value-based oral health care. *Value for global health care delivery* is defined as the aggregate health outcomes per aggregate costs (value = outcomes divided by costs) (Kim, Farmer, and Porter 2013; Porter 2010; Porter, Pabo, and Lee 2013). Outcomes depend on patient results rather than process measures such as numbers of patients seen and procedures completed.

Work from multiple groups (IOM 2013; Kaplan and Porter 2011; Porter 2010; Schoen and others 2013), an international comparison of 12 countries (Soderlund and others 2012), and assessments of oral health care (Glassman 2011) all indicate that focusing on values can be a key driver for health improvement. The goal is to simultaneously address a set of interrelated patient circumstances for a distinct population with distinct prevention and care challenges using an integrated and shared delivery infrastructure to improve health and reduce costs.

Value can be increased in two ways: by continually implementing the current best evidence to improve outcomes, and by reducing the costs accruing from waste and variation. In short, value can be improved by implementing safe, effective, patient-centered, timely, efficient, and equitable care (Kohn, Corrigan, and Donaldson 2000).

Outcomes

With the exception of noma, for which only case series are available, the data cited all derive primarily from systematic reviews of studies done in LMICs; the reviews indicate that the success rates for prevention are equivalent to or exceed those for surgery. For noma, the available data indicate that population-based and immediate prevention is more effective than surgery.

These comments are independent of the geographic location, the patient age, and the longevity of the study. The findings for caries and periodontitis contradict the conventional clinical thinking and training, which tend to focus on the individual clinical techniques of comprehensive surgical treatment and overlook community-based comprehensive prevention.

Short-Term Costs

In the traditional clinical setting, short-term costs accrue directly and indirectly. Surgically related direct costs for personnel, equipment, and supplies are all substantially higher than those associated with preventive care delivered by community health workers, plus prevention supplies, and antibiotics. Similarly, the indirect costs for surgery (for example, office space rent; utilities; patients' travel to dental offices or hospitals; and time away from work, school, and family, and for multiple visits) are all substantially higher than prevention delivered in community locations. Although the absolute costs may vary among LMICs, we suspect that the relative cost differentials are similar. This assumption calls for local validation.

Long-Term Costs

The impact of long-term costs may be even more substantial than short-term costs because of surgical longevity. Caries, periodontitis, and noma typically require cycles of surgical treatment and retreatment.

In the case of filling for the treatment of dental caries, the standard of care—excavating potential carious lesions and placing undercuts to mechanically secure the fillings (Webster 1908)—undermines the long-term structural integrity of the tooth. Consequently, the "permanent" fillings have an average lifespan of about 10 years (Burke and Lucarotti 2009; Chadwick and others 2001; Downer and others 1999); the net result is the initiation of a rerestoration cycle. Estimates indicate that 70 percent of the replacement restorations are larger than the original fillings (Brantley and others 1995; Elderton 1990). With sequential restorations, the ultimate outcome in some cases is tooth loss and the need for bridges or implants. The attendant cost implications are significant (Shugars and Bader 1996). Therefore, in marked contrast to

traditional thought regarding the efficacy of fillings (Mickenautsch and Yengopal 2012), complete caries removal is contraindicated for effective comprehensive prevention (Frencken and others 2012; Ricketts and others 2013).

The data for periodontitis and noma are less extensive but nonetheless informative. For periodontal health, current thinking recommends quarterly mechanical scaling. In marked contrast, clinical trials indicate that one round of a week-long regimen of metronidazole and amoxicillin shifts the oral ecology from disease related to health related, improves clinical health, and remains stable for up to five years without further intervention. For noma, the week-long costs for a regimen of metronidazole and amoxicillin and hyperalimentation are significantly less than extensive, repetitive, hospital-based surgeries. Further, with preventive care the patient is left with far fewer functional, esthetic, and emotional challenges.

In sum, the following approaches increase health care value:

- Effectively providing preventive services to people with diseases for which proven therapies exist
- Implementing integrated care delivery across multiple disease conditions
- Implementing local knowledge to ensure quality and equity.

Benefits of Focus on Prevention

The efficacy trials distilled in the multiple systematic reviews cited here indicate that prevention offers several theoretical and actual benefits:

- Moving oral health toward achieving health care's triple aim of increasing access, improving health, and reducing costs
- Facilitating the prevention and treatment of disease earlier in life and earlier in the disease progress, obviating the multitude of negative biological and social downstream consequences
- Improving health for both the well served and underserved, reducing one aspect of the social gradients.

The indicated benefits require vigorous testing in country- and region-specific effectiveness trials to demonstrate the universality of the findings (Banerjee and Duflo 2011; Glasgow and others 2005). These trials need to be supported by a noncommunicable disease system infrastructure to ensure care delivery across multiple systems.

Barriers and Challenges to Prevention Programs

Significant challenges to comprehensive prevention can be expected from governments, organizations, professional schools, clinicians, and regulatory agencies (Benzian and others 2011) (box 10.1). The reasons are relatively simple. First, these evidence-based, effective, preventive measures violate many of the oral health profession's closely held assumptions and clinical principles that focus on surgical treatment of dental diseases. Second, the current predominant stakeholders support an infrastructure, value system, and economy of training, licensing, boarding, and compensation that was created more than 100 years ago. This established social architecture will be difficult to change.

CONCLUSIONS

The challenge to achieving Alma-Ata's promise of "health care for all" (WHO 1978) and health care's triple aim will be to coordinate and integrate a top-down, noncommunicable disease policy change and a pragmatic bottom-up innovation approach (Christensen and others 2009; Frenk 2009). It seems unlikely that a top-down policy change will occur rapidly (Benzian and others 2011). It is much more likely that a bottom-up, pragmatic innovation approach to oral health care improvement will be successful in the short- and long-terms. Data-driven measures of bottom-up success will demonstrate the plausibility of and necessity for policy change.

Functionally, the challenge for pragmatic innovative programs will be to quantitatively improve health and document value, using methods of health improvement (IHI 2014; Langley and others 2009). Successful examples using local improvement initiatives with accompanying data are emerging (Banerjee and Duflo 2011; Monse and others 2013), but more are needed. Additionally, the incremental cost for delivering comprehensive prevention is likely to provide significantly greater benefit and value than incremental prevention. However, this economic assumption will require local validation. The effective preventive interventions identified in this chapter provide starting points.

If the multiple local and regional pilot oral health improvement initiatives simultaneously implement the multiple preventive interventions identified here, use community health workers to deliver care, and quantitatively assess outcomes and value, they are more likely to organically change policy and ensure sustainability than approaches that start with policy change. Finally, to effect this sea change, stakeholder advocates will need to consider actively providing evidence that is more easily understood by policy makers, specifically, advantage, simplicity, values, trust, and choice (Backer and Rogers 1998; Rogers 2002). These will be significant undertakings (Sheiham and others 2011; Williams 2011).

NOTES

The World Bank classifies countries according to four income groupings. Income is measured using gross national income (GNI) per capita, in U.S. dollars, converted from local currency using the *World Bank Atlas* method. Classifications as of July 2014 are as follows:

- Low-income countries (LICs) = US$1,045 or less in 2013
- Middle-income countries (MICs) are subdivided:
  - Lower-middle-income = US$1,046 to US$4,125
  - Upper-middle-income (UMICs) = US$4,126 to US$12,745
- High-income countries (HICs) = US$12,746 or more

1. Abdul Latif Jameel Poverty Action Lab (http://www.povertyactionlab.org/).
2. Abdul Latif Jameel Poverty Action Lab (http://www.povertyactionlab.org/health).
3. "2020 Topics and Objectives Oral Health." http://www.healthypeople.gov/2020/topicsobjectives2020/ebr.aspx?topicId=32.
4. "2020 Topics and Objectives Oral Health." http://www.healthypeople.gov/2020/topicsobjectives2020/ebr.aspx?topicId=32.

REFERENCES

Ahovuo-Saloranta, A., H. Forss, T. Walsh, A. Hiiri, A. Nordblad, and others. 2013. "Sealants for Preventing Dental Decay in the Permanent Teeth." *Cochrane Database of Systematic Reviews* 3: CD001830.

AHRQ (Agency for Healthcare Research and Quality). 2007. "Medical Expenditure Panel Survey 2007." Rockville, MD: Agency for Healthcare Research and Quality.

Backer, T. E., and E. M. Rogers. 1998. "Diffusion of Innovations Theory and Work-Site AIDS Programs." *Journal of Health Communication* 3 (1): 17–28.

Banerjee, A. V., and E. Duflo. 2011. *Poor Economics: A Radical Rethinking of the Way to Fight Global Poverty*. 1st edition. New York: Public Affairs.

Baratti-Mayer, D., B. Pittet, and D. Montandon. 2004. "[GESNOMA (Geneva Study Group on Noma): State-of-the-Art Medical Research for Humanitarian Purposes]." *Annales de chirurgie plastique et esthétique* 49 (3): 302–05. doi:10.1016/j.anplas.2004.04.005.

Benedetti, G., G. Campus, L. Strohmenger, and P. Lingstrom. 2013. "Tobacco and Dental Caries: A Systematic Review." *Acta Odontologica Scandinavica* 71 (3–4): 363–71. doi:10.3109/00016357.2012.734409.

Benzian, H. 2012. *Keeping Children 'Fit for School': Simple, Scalable and Sustainable School Health in the Philippines.* German Health Practice Collection. Bonn: Deutsche Gesellschaft für Internationale Zusammenarbeit (GIZ).

———, M. Hobdell, C. Holmgren, R. Yee, B. Monse, and others. 2011. "Political Priority of Global Oral Health: An Analysis of Reasons for International Neglect." *International Dental Journal* 61 (3): 124–30.

Benzian, H., B. Monse, V. Belizario, A. Schratz, M. Sahin, and W. van Palenstein Helderman. 2012. "Public Health in Action: Effective School Health Needs Renewed International Attention." *Global Health Action* 5: 14870.

Bhutta, Z. A., L. Chen, J. Cohen, N. Crisp, T. Evans, and others. 2010. "Education of Health Professionals for the 21st Century: A Global Independent Commission." *The Lancet* 375 (9721): 1137–38. doi:10.1016/S0140-6736(10)60450-3.

Bigby, M., S. Jick, H. Jick, and K. Arndt. 1986. "Drug-Induced Cutaneous Reactions: A Report from the Boston Collaborative Drug Surveillance Program on 15,438 Consecutive Inpatients, 1975 to 1982." *Journal of the American Medical Association* 256 (24): 3358–63.

Bisseling, P., J. Bruhn, T. Erdsach, A. M. Ettema, R. Sautter, and others. 2010. "Long-Term Results of Trismus Release in Noma Patients." *International Journal of Oral and Maxillofacial Surgery* 39 (9): 873–77.

Blaser, M. 2011. "Antibiotic Overuse: Stop the Killing of Beneficial Bacteria." *Nature* 476 (7361): 393–94. doi:10.1038/476393a.

Bolivar, I., K. Whiteson, B. Stadelmann, D. Baratti-Mayer, Y. Gizard, and others. 2012. "Bacterial Diversity in Oral Samples of Children in Niger with Acute Noma, Acute Necrotizing Gingivitis, and Healthy Controls." *PLoS Neglected Tropical Diseases* 6 (3): e1556.

Borgnakke, W. S., P. V. Ylostalo, G. W. Taylor, and R. J. Genco. 2013. "Effect of Periodontal Disease on Diabetes: Systematic Review of Epidemiologic Observational Evidence." *Journal of Periodontology* 84 (Suppl 4): S135–52. doi:10.1902/jop.2013.1340013.

Bouman, M. A., K. W. Marck, J. E. M. Griep, R. E. Marck, M. A. Huijing, and others. 2010. "Early Outcome of Noma Surgery." *Journal of Plastic, Reconstructive and Aesthetic Surgery: JPRAS* 63 (12): 2052–56.

Bourgeois, D. M., and M. H. Leclercq. 1999. "The World Health Organization Initiative on Noma." *Oral Diseases* 5 (2): 172–74.

Braegger, U. J. 2005. "Cost-Benefit, Cost-Effectiveness and Cost-Utility Analyses of Periodontitis Prevention." *Periodontology* 32 (Suppl.6): 301–13.

Brantley, C. F., J. D. Bader, D. A. Shugars, and S. P. Nesbit. 1995. "Does the Cycle of Rerestoration Lead to Larger Restorations?" *Journal of the American Dental Association* (1939) 126 (10): 1407–13.

Bratthall, D., P. E. Petersen, J. R. Stjernsward, and L. J. Brown. 2006. "Oral and Craniofacial Diseases and Disorders." In *Disease Control Priorities in Developing Countries*, edited by D. T. Jamison, J. G. Breman, A. R. Measham, G. Alleyne, M. Claeson, D. B. Evans, P. Jha, A. Mills, and P. Musgrove 723–36. 2nd ed. Washington, DC: World Bank.

Burke, F. J. T., and P. S. K. Lucarotti. 2009. "How Long Do Direct Restorations Placed within the General Dental Services in England and Wales Survive?" *British Dental Journal* 206 (1): E2; discussion 26–7.

Buzalaf, M. A., C. M. Moraes, K. P. Olympio, J. P. Pessan, L. T. Grizzo, and others. 2013. "Seven Years of External Control of Fluoride Levels in the Public Water Supply in Bauru, São Paulo, Brazil." *Journal of Applied Oral Science* 21 (1): 92–98.

Cagetti, M. G., G. Campus, E. Milia, and P. Lingström. 2013. "A Systematic Review on Fluoridated Food in Caries Prevention." *Acta Odontologica Scandinavica* 71 (3–4): 381–87.

Calache, H., and M. Hopcraft. 2012. "The Role of the Oral Health Therapist in the Provision of Oral Health Care to Patients of All Ages." In *Oral Health Care: Prosthodontics, Periodontology, Biology, Research and Systemic Conditions*, edited by M. Virdi, 249–68. Rijeka, Croatia: InTech Europe.

Camargo, M. C., A. Garcia, A. Riquelme, W. Otero, C. A. Camargo, and others. 2014. "The Problem of *Helicobacter pylori* Resistance to Antibiotics: A Systematic Review in Latin America." *American Journal of Gastroenterology* 109 (4): 485–95. doi:10.1038/ajg.2014.24.

Campain, A. C., R. J. Marino, F. A. Wright, D. Harrison, D. L. Bailey, and others. 2010. "The Impact of Changing Dental Needs on Cost Savings from Fluoridation." *Australian Dental Journal* 55 (1): 37–44. doi:10.1111/j.1834-7819.2010.01173.x.

Chadwick, B., E. Treasure, P. Dummer, F. Dunstan, A. Gilmour, and others. 2001. "Challenges with Studies Investigating Longevity of Dental Restorations: A Critique of a Systematic Review." *Journal of Dentistry* 29 (3): 155–61.

Chher, T., S. Hak, F. Courtel, and C. Durward. 2009. "Improving the Provision of the Basic Package of Oral Care (BPOC) in Cambodia." *International Dental Journal* 59 (1): 47–52.

Christensen, C. M., J. H. Grossman, J. Hwang, and N. Y. York. 2009. *The Innovator's Prescription: A Disruptive Solution for Health Care.* New York: McGraw-Hill.

CMS (Centers for Medicare and Medicaid Services). 2011a. "Improving Access to and Utilization of Oral Health Services for Children in Medicaid and CHIP Programs." CMS, Washington, DC.

———. 2011b. "National Health Expenditure Projections 2011–2021." U.S. Department of Health and Human Services, Washington, DC.

Coupe, M. H., D. Johnson, P. Seigne, and B. Hamlin. 2013. "Special Article: Airway Management in Reconstructive Surgery for Noma (Cancrum Oris)." *Anesthesia and Analgesia* 117 (1): 211–18.

Cullinan, M. P., and G. J. Seymour. 2013. "Periodontal Disease and Systemic Illness: Will the Evidence Ever Be Enough?" *Periodontology 2000* 62 (1): 271–86. doi:10.1111/prd.12007.

D'Agata, E. M., M. Dupont-Rouzeyrol, P. Magal, D. Olivier, and S. Ruan. 2008. "The Impact of Different Antibiotic Regimens on the Emergence of Antimicrobial-Resistant Bacteria." *PLoS One* 3 (12): e4036. doi:10.1371/journal.pone.0004036.

da Mata, C., P. F. Allen, M. Cronin, D. O'Mahony, G. McKenna, and others. 2014. "Cost-Effectiveness of ART Restorations in Elderly Adults: A Randomized Clinical Trial." *Community Dentistry and Oral Epidemiology* 42 (1): 79–87.

Davies, G. M., H. V. Worthington, R. P. Ellwood, A. S. Blinkhorn, G. O. Taylor, and others. 2003. "An Assessment of the Cost Effectiveness of a Postal Toothpaste Programme to Prevent Caries among Five-Year-Old Children in the North West of England." *Community Dental Health* 20 (4): 207–10.

de Amorim, R. G., S. C. Leal, and J. E. Frencken. 2012. "Survival of Atraumatic Restorative Treatment (ART) Sealants and Restorations: A Meta-Analysis." *Clinical Oral Investigations* 16 (2): 429–41.

Doessel, D. P. 1979. *Cost-Benefit Analysis and Water Fluoridation: An Australian Study.* Canberra: Australian National University Press.

Dona, I., N. Blanca-Lopez, M. J. Torres, J. Garcia-Campos, I. Garcia-Nunez, and others. 2012. "Drug Hypersensitivity Reactions: Response Patterns, Drug Involved, and Temporal Variations in a Large Series of Patients." *Journal of Investigative Allergology and Clinical Immunology* 22 (5): 363–71.

Dos Santos, A. P., P. Nadanovsky, and B. H. de Oliveira. 2012. "A Systematic Review and Meta-Analysis of the Effects of Fluoride Toothpastes on the Prevention of Dental Caries in the Primary Dentition of Preschool Children." *Community Dentistry and Oral Epidemiology* 41 (1): 1–12. doi:10.1111/j.1600-0528.2012.00708.x.

Downer, M. C., N. A. Azli, R. Bedi, D. R. Moles, and D. J. Setchell. 1999. "How Long Do Routine Dental Restorations Last? A Systematic Review." *British Dental Journal* 187 (8): 432–39.

Dye, B. A., and G. Thornton-Evans. 2010. "Trends in Oral Health by Poverty Status as Measured by Healthy People 2010 Objectives." *Public Health* 125 (6): 817–30.

Elderton, R. J. 1990. "Clinical Studies Concerning Re-restoration of Teeth." *Advances in Dental Research* 4: 4–9.

Espelid, I. 2009. "Caries Preventive Effect of Fluoride in Milk, Salt and Tablets: A Literature Review." *European Archives of Paediatric Dentistry* 10 (3): 149–56.

Faveri, M., M. Feres, J. A. Shibli, R. F. Hayacibara, M. M. Hayacibara, and others. 2006. "Microbiota of the Dorsum of the Tongue after Plaque Accumulation: An Experimental Study in Humans." *Journal of Periodontology* 77 (9): 1539–46.

Feller, L., M. Altini, R. Chandran, R. A. Khammissa, J. N. Masipa, and others. 2014. "Noma (Cancrum Oris) in the South African Context." *Journal of Oral Pathology and Medicine* 43 (1): 1–6. doi:10.1111/jop.12079.

Feres, M. 2008. "Antibiotics in the Treatment of Periodontal Diseases: Microbiological Basis and Clinical Applications." *Annals of the Royal Australasian College of Dental Surgeons* 19: 37–44.

Feres, M., G. M. S. Soares, J. A. V. Mendes, M. P. Silva, M. Faveri, and others. 2012. "Metronidazole Alone or with Amoxicillin as Adjuncts to Non-surgical Treatment of Chronic Periodontitis: A 1-Year Double-Blinded, Placebo-Controlled, Randomized Clinical Trial." *Journal of Clinical Periodontology* 39 (12): 1149–58.

Fieger, A., K. W. Marck, R. Busch, and A. Schmidt. 2003. "An Estimation of the Incidence of Noma in North-West Nigeria." *Tropical Medicine and International Health* 8 (5): 402–07.

Fiorini, T., M. L. Musskopf, R. V. Oppermann, and C. Susin. 2014. "Is There a Positive Effect of Smoking Cessation on Periodontal Health? A Systematic Review." *Journal of Periodontology* 85 (1): 83–91. doi:10.1902/jop.2013.130047.

Frazao, P. 2012. "[Cost-Effectiveness of Conventional and Modified Supervised Toothbrushing in Preventing Caries in Permanent Molars among 5-Year-Old Children]." *Cadernos de Saúde Pública* 28 (2): 281–90.

Frencken, J. E., C. Holmgren, W. Helderman, and WHO. 2002. "Van Palenstein Basic Package of Oral Care (BPOC)." Centre for Oral Health Care Planning and Future Scenarios, University of Nijmegen, Nijmegen, Netherlands.

Frencken, J. E., M. C. Peters, D. J. Manton, S. C. Leal, V. V. Gordan, and E. Eden. 2012. "Minimal Intervention Dentistry for Managing Dental Caries: A Review: Report of a FDI Task Group." *International Dental Journal* 62 (5): 223–43.

Frencken, J. E., Y. Songpaisan, P. Phantumvanit, and T. Pilot. 1994. "An Atraumatic Restorative Treatment (ART) Technique: Evaluation after One Year." *International Dental Journal* 44 (5): 460–64.

Frenk, J. 2009. "Reinventing Primary Health Care: The Need for Systems Integration." *The Lancet* 374 (9684): 170–73. doi:10.1016/S0140-6736(09)60693-0.

Frenk, J., L. Chen, Z. A. Bhutta, J. Cohen, N. Crisp, and others. 2010. "Health Professionals for a New Century: Transforming Education to Strengthen Health Systems in an Interdependent World." *The Lancet* 376 (9756): 1923–58. doi:10.1016/S0140-6736(10)61854-5.

Frias, A. C., P. C. Narvai, M. E. Araujo, C. Zilbovicius, and J. L. Antunes. 2006. "[Cost of Fluoridating the Public Water Supply: A Study Case in the City of São Paulo, Brazil, 1985–2003]." *Cadernos de Saude Publica* 22 (6): 1237–46. doi:S0102-311X2006000600013.

Friedewald, V. E., K. S. Kornman, J. D. Beck, R. Genco, A. Goldfine, and others. 2009a. "The American Journal of Cardiology and Journal of Periodontology Editors' Consensus: Periodontitis and Atherosclerotic Cardiovascular Disease." *American Journal of Cardiology* 104 (1): 59–68. doi:10.1016/j.amjcard.2009.05.002.

———. 2009b. "The American Journal of Cardiology and Journal of Periodontology Editors' Consensus: Periodontitis and Atherosclerotic Cardiovascular Disease." *Journal of Periodontology* 80 (7): 1021–32. doi:10.1902 /jop.2009.097001.

Gaunt, F., M. Devine, M. Pennington, C. Vernazza, E. Gwynnett, and others. 2008. "The Cost-Effectiveness of Supportive Periodontal Care for Patients with Chronic Periodontitis." *Journal of Clinical Periodontology* 35 (8 Suppl): 67–82.

Gibbons, R. J., and J. van Houte. 1975. "Dental Caries." *Annual Review of Medicine* 26: 121–36.

Gillespie, G. M., and T. M. Marthaler. 2005. "Cost Aspects of Salt Fluoridation." *Schweizer Monatsschrift* fur Zahnmedizin=Revue mensuelle suisse d'odonto-stomatologie=Rivista mensile svizzera di odontologia e stomatologia. SSO 115 (9): 778–84.

Glasgow, R. E., D. J. Magid, A. Beck, D. Ritzwoller, and P. A. Estabrooks. 2005. "Practical Clinical Trials for Translating Research to Practice: Design and Measurement Recommendations." *Medical Care* 43 (6): 551–57.

Glassman, P. 2011. *Oral Health Quality Improvement in the Era of Accountability*. Report prepared for the W. K. Kellogg Foundation, Battle Creek, MI. https://www.dentaquestinstitute.org/sites/default/files/reports/2011/12/Pacific_Center_for_Special_Care_Report.pdf.

Goodson, J. M., A. D. Haffajee, S. S. Socransky, R. Kent, R. Teles, and others. 2012. "Control of Periodontal Infections: A Randomized Controlled Trial I. The Primary Outcome Attachment Gain and Pocket Depth Reduction at Treated Sites." *Journal of Clinical Periodontology* 39 (6): 526–36. doi:10.1111/j.1600-051X.2012.01870.x.

Greenhalgh, T., G. Robert, F. Macfarlane, P. Bate, and O. Kyriakidou. 2004. "Diffusion of Innovations in Service Organizations: Systematic Review and Recommendations." *Milbank Quarterly* 82 (4): 581–629. doi:10.1111/j.0887-378X.2004.00325.x.

Griffin, S. O., K. Jones, and S. L. Tomar. 2001. "An Economic Evaluation of Community Water Fluoridation." *Journal of Public Health Dentistry* 61 (2): 78–86.

Griffin, S. O., E. Regnier, P. M. Griffin, and V. Huntley. 2007. "Effectiveness of Fluoride in Preventing Caries in Adults." *Journal of Dental Research* 86 (5): 410–15.

Gunsolley, J. C. 2006. "A Meta-Analysis of Six-Month Studies of Antiplaque and Antigingivitis Agents." *Journal of the American Dental Association* 137 (12): 1649–57.

Haffajee, A. D., and S. S. Socransky. 1994. "Microbial Etiological Agents of Destructive Periodontal Diseases." *Periodontology 2000* 5: 78–111.

Han, Y. W., W. Houcken, B. G. Loos, H. A. Schenkein, and M. Tezal. 2014. "Periodontal Disease, Atherosclerosis, Adverse Pregnancy Outcomes, and Head-and-Neck Cancer." *Advances in Dental Research* 26 (1): 47–55. doi:10.1177/0022034514528334.

Hendrix, K. S., S. M. Downs, G. Brophy, C. C. Doebbeling, and N. L. Swigonski. 2013. "Threshold Analysis of Reimbursing Physicians for the Application of Fluoride Varnish in Young Children." *Journal of Public Health Dentistry* 73 (4): 297–303.

Herrera, D., B. Alonso, R. Leon, S. Roldan, and M. Sanz. 2008. "Antimicrobial Therapy in Periodontitis: The Use of Systemic Antimicrobials against the Subgingival Biofilm." *Journal of Clinical Periodontology* 35 (Suppl. 8): 45–66. doi:10.1111/j.1600-051X.2008.01260.x.

HHS (Health and Human Services). 2010. "Promoting and Enhancing the Oral Health of the Public." HHS, Washington, DC. http://www.hrsa.gov/publichealth/clinical/oralhealth/hhsinitiative.pdf.

Holtshousen, W. S., and A. Smit. 2007. "A Cost-Efficiency Analysis of a Mobile Dental Clinic in the Public Services." *SADJ [Journal of the South African Dental Association]* 62 (8): 334, 336–38, 340.

Huijing, M. A., K. W. Marck, J. Combes, K. D. Mizen, L. Fourie, and others. 2011. "Facial Reconstruction in the Developing World: A Complicated Matter." *British Journal of Oral and Maxillofacial Surgery* 49 (4): 292–96.

Huyghe, A., P. François, A. Mombelli, M. Tangomo, M. Girard, and others. 2013. "Microarray Analysis of Microbiota of Gingival Lesions in Noma Patients." *PLoS Neglected Tropical Diseases* 7 (9): e2453.

Ide, M., and P. N. Papapanou. 2013. "Epidemiology of Association between Maternal Periodontal Disease and Adverse Pregnancy Outcomes: Systematic Review." *Journal of Periodontology* 84 (Suppl. 4): S181–94. doi:10.1902/jop.2013.134009.

IHI (Institute for Healthcare Improvement). 2014. "How to Improve." IHI, Cambridge, MA. http://www.ihi.org/resources/Pages/HowtoImprove/default.aspx.

IOM (Institute of Medicine). 2001. *Crossing the Quality Chasm: A New Health System for the 21st Century*. Washington, DC: National Academies Press.

———. 2011a. *Advancing Oral Health in America*. Washington, DC: National Academies Press.

———. 2011b. Children and Adolescent Health and Health Care Quality: Measuring What Matters. Washington, DC: National Academies Press.

———. 2013. "Roundtable on Value & Science-Driven Health Care." Institute of Medicine, Washington, DC. http://www.iom.edu/~/media/Files/Activity%20Files/Quality/VSRT/Core%20Documents/Background.pdf.

Johnson, N., R. Lalloo, J. Kroon, S. Fernando, and O. Tut. 2014. "Effectiveness of Water Fluoridation in Caries Reduction in a Remote Indigenous Community in Far North Queensland." *Australian Dental Journal*. Online in advance of print. doi:10.1111/adj.12190.

Källestål, C., A. Norlund, B. Söder, G. Nordenram, H. Dahlgren, and others. 2003. "Economic Evaluation of Dental Caries Prevention: A Systematic Review." *Acta Odontologica Scandinavica* 61 (6): 341–46.

Kaplan, R. S., and M. E. Porter. 2011. "How to Solve the Cost Crisis in Health Care." *Harvard Business Review* 89 (9): 46–52, 54, 56.

Kikwilu, E. N., J. Frencken, and J. Mulder. 2009. "Impact of Atraumatic Restorative Treatment (ART) on the Treatment Profile in Pilot Government Dental Clinics in Tanzania." *BMC Oral Health* 9: 14. doi:10.1186/1472-6831-9-14.

Kim, J. Y., P. Farmer, and M. E. Porter. 2013. "Redefining Global Health-Care Delivery." *The Lancet* 382 (9897): 1060–69. doi:10.1016/S0140-6736(13)61047-8.

Kohn, L. T., J. Corrigan, and M. S. Donaldson. 2000. *To Err Is Human: Building a Safer Health System*. Washington, DC: National Academies Press.

Kroon, J., and P. J. van Wyk. 2012a. "A Retrospective View on the Viability of Water Fluoridation in South Africa to Prevent Dental Caries." *Community Dentistry and Oral Epidemiology* 40 (5): 441–50. doi:10.1111/j.1600-0528.2012.00681.x.

———. 2012b. "A Model to Determine the Economic Viability of Water Fluoridation." *Journal of Public Health Dentistry* 72 (4): 327–33.

Langley, G. L., R. Moen, K. M. Nolan, T. W. Nolan, C. L. Norman, and others. 2009. *The Improvement Guide: A Practical Approach to Enhancing Organizational Performance.* 2nd edition. San Francisco, CA: Jossey-Bass.

Lauris, J. R., R. da Silva Bastos, and J. R. de Magalhaes Bastos. 2012. "Decline in Dental Caries among 12-Year-Old Children in Brazil, 1980–2005." *International Dental Journal* 62 (6): 308–14. doi:10.1111/j.1875-595x.2012.00124.x.

Lee, J. Y., and K. Divaris. 2014. "The Ethical Imperative of Addressing Oral Health Disparities: A Unifying Framework." *Journal of Dental Research* 93 (3): 224–30. doi:10.1177/0022034513511821.

Linden, G. J., A. Lyons, and F. A. Scannapieco. 2013. "Periodontal Systemic Associations: Review of the Evidence." *Journal of Periodontology* 84 (Suppl. 4): S8–19. doi:10.1902/jop.2013.1340010.

Liu, B. Y., E. C. M. Lo, C. H. Chu, and H. C. Lin. 2012. "Randomized Trial on Fluorides and Sealants for Fissure Caries Prevention." *Journal of Dental Research* 91 (8): 753–58.

Lockhart, P. B., A. F. Bolger, P. N. Papapanou, O. Osinbowale, M. Trevisan, and others. 2012. "Periodontal Disease and Atherosclerotic Vascular Disease: Does the Evidence Support an Independent Association? A Scientific Statement from the American Heart Association." *Circulation* 125 (20): 2520–44. doi:10.1161/CIR.0b013e31825719f3.

Loesche, W. J., and N. S. Grossman. 2001. "Periodontal Disease as a Specific, Albeit Chronic, Infection: Diagnosis and Treatment." *Clinical Microbiology Reviews* 14 (4): 727–52.

López, N. J., and J. A. Gamonal. 1998. "Effects of Metronidazole Plus Amoxicillin in Progressive Untreated Adult Periodontitis: Results of a Single 1-Week Course after 2 and 4 Months." *Journal of Periodontology* 69 (11): 1291–98.

López, N. J., S. S. Socransky, I. Da Silva, M. R. Japlit, and A. D. Haffajee. 2006. "Effects of Metronidazole Plus Amoxicillin as the Only Therapy on the Microbiological and Clinical Parameters of Untreated Chronic Periodontitis." *Journal of Clinical Periodontology* 33 (9): 648–60.

Mager, D. L., L. A. Ximenez-Fyvie, A. D. Haffajee, and S. S. Socransky. 2003. "Distribution of Selected Bacterial Species on Intraoral Surfaces." *Journal of Clinical Periodontology* 30 (7): 644–54.

Marcenes, W., N. J. Kassebaum, E. Bernabé, A. Flaxman, M. Naghavi, and others. 2013. "Global Burden of Oral Conditions in 1990–2010: A Systematic Analysis." *Journal of Dental Research* 92 (7): 592–97.

Marck, K. W. 2003. *Noma, the Face of Poverty.* Hannover, Germany: MIT-Verlag GmbH.

Marck, R., M. Huijing, D. Vest, M. Eshete, K. Marck, and others. 2010. "Early Outcome of Facial Reconstructive Surgery Abroad: A Comparative Study." *European Journal of Plastic Surgery* 33 (4): 193–97.

Marinho, V. C. C., H. V. Worthington, T. Walsh, and J. E. Clarkson. 2013. "Fluoride Varnishes for Preventing Dental Caries in Children and Adolescents." *Cochrane Database of Systematic Reviews* 7: CD002279.

Marino, R. J., J. Fajardo, A. Arana, C. Garcia, and F. Pachas. 2011. "Modeling an Economic Evaluation of a Salt Fluoridation Program in Peru." *Journal of Public Health Dentistry* 71 (2): 125–30.

Mariño, R., J. Fajardo, and M. Morgan. 2012. "Cost-Effectiveness Models for Dental Caries Prevention Programmes among Chilean Schoolchildren." *Community Dental Health* 29 (4): 302–08.

Mariño, R. J., A. R. Khan, and M. Morgan. 2013. "Systematic Review of Publications on Economic Evaluations of Caries Prevention Programs." *Caries Research* 47 (4): 265–72.

Mashoto, K. O., A. N. Astrom, M. S. Skeie, and J. R. Masalu. 2010. "Changes in the Quality of Life of Tanzanian School Children after Treatment Interventions Using the Child-OIDP." *European Journal of Oral Sciences* 118 (6): 626–34. doi:10.1111/j.1600-0722.2010.00776.x.

Matarazzo, F., L. C. Figueiredo, S. E. B. Cruz, M. Faveri, and M. Feres. 2008. "Clinical and Microbiological Benefits of Systemic Metronidazole and Amoxicillin in the Treatment of Smokers with Chronic Periodontitis: A Randomized Placebo-Controlled Study." *Journal of Clinical Periodontology* 35 (10): 885–96.

Mathu-Muju, K. R., J. W. Friedman, and D. A. Nash. 2013. "Oral Health Care for Children in Countries Using Dental Therapists in Public, School-Based Programs, Contrasted with That of the United States, Using Dentists in a Private Practice Model." *American Journal of Public Health* 103 (9): e7–e13. doi:10.2105/AJPH.2013.301251.

McDonagh, M. S., P. F. Whiting, P. M. Wilson, A. J. Sutton, I. Chestnutt, and others. 2000. "Systematic Review of Water Fluoridation." *BMJ (Clinical research ed.)* 321 (7265): 855–59.

Mestnik, M. J., M. Feres, L. C. Figueiredo, P. M. Duarte, E. A. G. Lira, and others. 2010. "Short-Term Benefits of the Adjunctive Use of Metronidazole Plus Amoxicillin in the Microbial Profile and in the Clinical Parameters of Subjects with Generalized Aggressive Periodontitis." *Journal of Clinical Periodontology* 37 (4): 353–65.

Mickenautsch, S., and V. Yengopal. 2011. "Caries-Preventive Effect of Glass Ionomer and Resin-Based Fissure Sealants on Permanent Teeth: An Update of Systematic Review Evidence." *BMC Research Notes* 4: 22.

———. 2012. "Failure Rate of High-Viscosity GIC Based ART Compared with That of Conventional Amalgam Restorations: Evidence from an Update of a Systematic Review." *SADJ [Journal of the South African Dental Association]* 67 (7): 329–31.

Mickenautsch, S., V. Yengopal, and A. Banerjee. 2010. "Atraumatic Restorative Treatment versus Amalgam Restoration Longevity: A Systematic Review." *Clinical Oral Investigations* 14 (3): 233–40.

Moimaz, S. A., O. Saliba, F. Y. Chiba, and N. A. Saliba. 2012. "External Control of the Public Water Supply in 29 Brazilian Cities." *Brazilian Oral Research* 26 (1): 12–18.

Moimaz, S. A., N. A. Saliba, O. Saliba, D. H. Sumida, N. P. Souza, F. Y. Chiba, and C. A. Garbin. 2013. "Water Fluoridation in 40 Brazilian cities: 7 Year Analysis." *Journal of Applied Oral Science* 21 (1): 92–98.

Monse, B., H. Benzian, E. Naliponguit, V. Belizario, A. Schratz, and W. van Palenstein Helderman. 2013. "The Fit for School Health Outcome Study: A Longitudinal Survey to Assess Health Impacts of an Integrated School Health Programme in the Philippines." *BMC Public Health* 13: 256. doi:10.1186/1471-2458-13-256.

Monse, B., E. Naliponguit, V. Belizario, H. Benzian, and W. Palenstein van Helderman. 2010. "Essential Health Care Package for Children: The 'Fit for School' Program in the Philippines." *International Dental Journal* 60 (2): 85–93.

Morgan, M., R. Marino, C. Wright, D. Bailey, and M. Hopcraft. 2012. "Economic Evaluation of Preventive Dental Programs: What Can They Tell Us?" *Community Dentistry and Oral Epidemiology* 40 (Suppl 2): 117–21. doi:10.1111/j.1600-0528.2012.00730.x.

Moynihan, P. J., and S. A. Kelly. 2014. "Effect on Caries of Restricting Sugars Intake: Systematic Review to Inform WHO Guidelines." *Journal of Dental Research* 93 (1): 8–18. doi:10.1177/0022034513508954.

Nash, D. A., J. W. Friedman, K. R. Mathu-Muju, P. G. Robinson, J. Satur, and others. 2012. *A Review of the Global Literature on Dental Therapists*. Battle Creek, MI: W. K. Kellogg Foundation.

NHS (National Health Service). 2005. *Choosing Better Oral Health: An Oral Health Plan for England*. Edited by Department of Health: Dental and Ophthalmic Services Division, London. http://webarchive.nationalarchives.gov .uk/20130107105354/http://www.dh.gov.uk/prod_consum _dh/groups/dh_digitalassets/@dh/@en/documents /digitalasset/dh_4123253.pdf.

———. 2007. "Oral Health Survey of 5 Year Old Children 2007/2008." London. http://www.nwph.net/dentalhealth /reports/NHS_DEP_for_England_OH_Survey_5yr_2007 -08_Report.pdf.

———. 2009. "Adult Dental Health Survey 2009." London. http://www.hscic.gov.uk/pubs/dentalsurveyfullreport09.

Ogbureke, K. U. E., and E. I. Ogbureke. 2010. "Noma: A Preventable 'Scourge' of African Children." *Open Dentistry Journal* 4: 201–06.

Osso, D., and N. Kanani. 2013. "Antiseptic Mouth Rinses: An Update on Comparative Effectiveness, Risks and Recommendations." *Journal of Dental Hygiene* 87 (1): 10–18.

Palacios, C., K. Joshipura, and W. Willett. 2009. "Nutrition and Health: Guidelines for Dental Practitioners." *Oral Diseases* 15 (6): 369–81. doi:10.1111/j.1601-0825.2009.01571.x.

Parnell, C., H. Whelton, and D. O'Mullane. 2009. "Water Fluoridation." *European Archives of Paediatric Dentistry* 10 (3): 141–48.

Paster, B. J., W. A. Falkler Jr., C. O. Enwonwu, E. O. Idigbe, K. O. Savage, and others. 2002. "Prevalent Bacterial Species and Novel Phylotypes in Advanced Noma Lesions." *Journal of Clinical Microbiology* 40 (6): 2187–91.

Porter, M. E. 2010. "What Is Value in Health Care?" *New England Journal of Medicine* 363 (26): 2477–81.

Porter, M. E., E. A. Pabo, and T. H. Lee. 2013. "Redesigning Primary Care: A Strategic Vision to Improve Value by Organizing around Patients' Needs." *Health Affairs (Millwood)* 32 (3): 516–25. doi:10.1377/hlthaff.2012.0961.

Quiñonez, R. B., S. C. Stearns, B. S. Talekar, R. G. Rozier, and S. M. Downs. 2006. "Simulating Cost-Effectiveness of Fluoride Varnish during Well-Child Visits for Medicaid-Enrolled Children." *Archives of Pediatrics and Adolescent Medicine* 160 (2): 164–70.

Ricketts, D., T. Lamont, N. P. T. Innes, E. Kidd, and J. E. Clarkson. 2013. "Operative Caries Management in Adults and Children." *Cochrane Database of Systematic Reviews* 3: CD003808.

Riley, P., and T. Lamont. 2013. "Triclosan/Copolymer Containing Toothpastes for Oral Health." *Cochrane Database of Systematic Reviews* 12: CD010514. doi:10.1002/14651858 .CD010514.pub2.

Ritchie, C. S., K. Joshipura, H. C. Hung, and C. W. Douglass. 2002. "Nutrition as a Mediator in the Relation between Oral and Systemic Disease: Associations between Specific Measures of Adult Oral Health and Nutrition Outcomes." *Critical Reviews in Oral Biology and Medicine* 13 (3): 291–300.

Rogers, E. M. 2002. "Diffusion of Preventive Innovations." *Addictive Behaviors* 27 (6): 989–93.

Rosenblatt, A., T. C. M. Stamford, and R. Niederman. 2009. "Silver Diamine Fluoride: A Caries 'Silver-Fluoride Bullet.'" *Journal of Dental Research* 88 (2): 116–25.

Sampaio, A. L. L., M. F. S. Araújo, and C. A. C. P. Oliveira. 2011. "New Criteria of Indication and Selection of Patients to Cochlear Implant." *International Journal of Otolaryngology* 2011: 573968.

Sanz, M., K. Kornman, and EFP/AAP Workshop Working Group 3. 2013. "Periodontitis and Adverse Pregnancy Outcomes: Consensus Report of the Joint EFP/AAP (European Federation of Periodontology and American Academy of Peridontology) Workshop on Periodontitis and Systemic Diseases." *Journal of Periodontology* 84 (Suppl. 4): S164–69. doi:10.1902/jop.2013.1340016.

Schoen, C., S. Guterman, M. Zezza, and M. Abrams. 2013. "Confronting Costs: Stabilizing U.S. Health Spending While Moving toward a High Performance Health Care System." Publication 1653, The Commonwealth Fund Commission on a High Performance Health System, Washington, DC.

Schwendicke, F., C. E. Dörfer, and S. Paris. 2013. "Incomplete Caries Removal: A Systematic Review and Meta-Analysis." *Journal of Dental Research* 92 (4): 306–14.

Schwendicke, F., M. Stolpe, H. Meyer-Lueckel, S. Paris, and C. E. Dörfer. 2013. "Cost-Effectiveness of One- and Two-Step Incomplete and Complete Excavations." *Journal of Dental Research* 92 (10): 880–87.

Sgolastra, F., R. Gatto, A. Petrucci, and A. Monaco. 2012. "Effectiveness of Systemic Amoxicillin/Metronidazole as Adjunctive Therapy to Scaling and Root Planing in the Treatment of Chronic Periodontitis: A Systematic Review and Meta-Analysis." *Journal of Periodontology* 83 (10): 1257–69.

Sgolastra, F., A. Petrucci, R. Gatto, and A. Monaco. 2012. "Effectiveness of Systemic Amoxicillin/Metronidazole as an Adjunctive Therapy to Full-Mouth Scaling and Root Planing in the Treatment of Aggressive Periodontitis: A Systematic Review and Meta-Analysis." *Journal of Periodontology* 83 (6): 731–43.

Sheiham, A., D. Alexander, L. Cohen, V. Marinho, S. Moysés, and others. 2011. "Global Oral Health Inequalities: Task Group: Implementation and Delivery of Oral Health Strategies." *Advances in Dental Research* 23 (2): 259–67.

Shugars, D. A., and J. D. Bader. 1996. "Cost Implications of Differences in Dentists' Restorative Treatment Decisions." *Journal of Public Health Dentistry* 56 (4): 219–22.

Silva, M. P., M. Feres, T. A. Sirotto, G. M. Soares, J. A. Mendes, and others. 2011. "Clinical and Microbiological Benefits of Metronidazole Alone or with Amoxicillin as Adjuncts in the Treatment of Chronic Periodontitis: A Randomized Placebo-Controlled Clinical Trial." *Journal of Clinical Periodontology* 38 (9): 828–37. doi:10.1111/j.1600-051X.2011.01763.x.

Sköld, U. M., L. G. Petersson, D. Birkhed, and A. Norlund. 2008. "Cost-Analysis of School-Based Fluoride Varnish and Fluoride Rinsing Programs." *Acta Odontologica Scandinavica* 66 (5): 286–92.

Soares, G. M., L. C. Figueiredo, M. Faveri, S. C. Cortelli, P. M. Duarte, and M. Feres. 2012. "Mechanisms of Action of Systemic Antibiotics Used in Periodontal Treatment and Mechanisms of Bacterial Resistance to These Drugs." *Journal of Applied Oral Science* 20 (3): 295–309.

Socransky, S. S., and A. D. Haffajee. 1994. "Evidence of Bacterial Etiology: A Historical Perspective." *Periodontology 2000* 5: 7–25.

———. 2002. "Dental Biofilms: Difficult Therapeutic Targets." *Periodontology 2000* 28: 12–55.

———, M. A. Cugini, C. Smith, and R. L. Kent. 1998. "Microbial Complexes in Subgingival Plaque." *Journal of Clinical Periodontology* 25 (2): 134–44.

Socransky, S. S., A. D. Haffajee, J. L. Dzink, and J. D. Hillman. 1988. "Associations between Microbial Species in Subgingival Plaque Samples." *Oral Microbiology and Immunology* 3 (1): 1–7.

Soderlund, N., J. Kent, P. Lawyer, and S. Larsson. 2012. "Progress toward Value-Based Health Care: Lessons Learned from 12 Countries." Boston Consulting Group.

Splieth, C. H., and S. Flessa. 2008. "Modelling Lifelong Costs of Caries with and without Fluoride Use." *European Journal of Oral Sciences* 116 (2): 164–69.

Steele, J. 2009. "NHS Dental Services in England: An Independent Review Led by Professor Jimmy Steele." NHS Department of Health, London. http://www.sigwales.org/wp-content/uploads/dh_101180.pdf.

Teles, R. P., A. D. Haffajee, and S. S. Socransky. 2006. "Microbiological Goals of Periodontal Therapy." *Periodontology 2000* 42: 180–218.

Teles, R. P., and F. R. Teles. 2009. "Antimicrobial Agents Used in the Control of Periodontal Biofilms: Effective Adjuncts to Mechanical Plaque Control?" *Brazilian Oral Research* 23 (Suppl. 1): 39–48.

Tempest, M. N. 1966. "Cancrum Oris." *British Journal of Surgery* 53 (11): 949–69.

Tianviwat, S., V. Chongsuvivatwong, and S. Birch. 2009. "Estimating Unit Costs for Dental Service Delivery in

Institutional and Community-Based Settings in Southern Thailand." *Asia Pacific Journal of Public Health* 21 (1): 84–93. doi:10.1177/ 1010539508327246.

Tonetti, M. S., T. E. Van Dyke, and EFP/AAP (European Federation of Periodontology and American Academy of Peridontology) Working Group 1. 2013. "Periodontitis and Atherosclerotic Cardiovascular Disease: Consensus Report of the Joint EFP/AAP Workshop on Periodontitis and Systemic Diseases." *Journal of Periodontology* 84 (Suppl. 4): S24–9. doi:10.1902/jop.2013.1340019.

Touger-Decker, R., C. C. Mobley, and American Dietetic Association. 2007. "Position of the American Dietetic Association: Oral Health and Nutrition." *Journal of the American Dietetic Association* 107 (8): 1418–28.

Van Strydonck, D. A., D. E. Slot, U. van der Velden, and F. Van der Weijden. 2012. "Effect of a Chlorhexidine Mouthrinse on Plaque, Gingival Inflammation and Staining in Gingivitis Patients: A Systematic Review." *Journal of Clinical Periodontology* 39 (11): 1042–55. doi:10.1111/j.1600-051X.2012.01883.x.

van Winkelhoff, A. J., C. J. Tijhof, and J. de Graaff. 1992. "Microbiological and Clinical Results of Metronidazole Plus Amoxicillin Therapy in *Actinobacillus actinomycetemcomitans*–Associated Periodontitis." *Journal of Periodontology* 63 (1): 52–57.

van Wyk, P. J., J. Kroon, and W. S. Holtshousen. 2001. "Cost Evaluation for the Implementation of Water Fluoridation in Gauteng." *SADJ [Journal of the South African Dental Association]* 56 (2): 71–76.

Walter, C., F. R. Rodriguez, B. Taner, H. Hecker, and R. Weiger. 2012. "Association of Tobacco Use and Periapical Pathosis: A Systematic Review." *International Endodontic Journal* 45 (12): 1065–73. doi:10.1111/j.1365-2591.2012.02072.x.

Watt, R. G. 2012. "Social Determinants of Oral Health Inequalities: Implications for Action." *Community Dental and Oral Epidemiology* 40 (Suppl 2): 44–48. doi:10.1111/j.1600-0528.2012.00719.x.

Watt, R. G., and A. Sheiham. 2012. "Integrating the Common Risk Factor Approach into a Social Determinants Framework." *Community Dental and Oral Epidemiology* 40 (4): 289–96. doi:10.1111/j.1600-0528.2012.00680.x.

Webster, A. E. 1908. "Preparation of Cavities for Fillings." In *A Textbook of Operative Dentistry*, edited by C. N. Johnson, 161–214. Philadelphia, PA: P. Blakiston's Son & Co.

WHO (World Health Organization). 1978. "Declaration of Alma-Ata." International Conference on Primary Health Care, Alma-Ata, Kazakhstan, September 6–12.

———. 2006. *The World Health Report 2006: Working Together for Health.* Geneva: WHO. http://www.who.int/whr/2006/whr06_en.pdf.

———. 2013. "Global Health Estimates for Deaths by Cause, Age, and Sex for Years 2000–2011." WHO, Geneva. http://www.who.int/healthinfo/global_health_estimates/en/.

Williams, D. M. 2011. "Global Oral Health Inequalities: The Research Agenda." *Journal of Dental Research* 90 (5): 549–51. doi:10.1177/0022034511402210.

Wong, M. C. M., J. Clarkson, A. M. Glenny, E. C. M. Lo, V. C. C. Marinho, and others. 2011. "Cochrane Reviews on the Benefits/Risks of Fluoride Toothpastes." *Journal of Dental Research* 90 (5): 573–79.

Worthington, H. V., J. E. Clarkson, G. Bryan, and P. V. Beirne. 2013. "Routine Scale and Polish for Periodontal Health in Adults." *Cochrane Database of Systematic Reviews* 11: CD004625.

Wright, J. Timothy, F. Graham, C. Hayes, A. I. Ismail, K. W. Noraian, and others. 2013. "A Systematic Review of Oral Health Outcomes Produced by Dental Teams Incorporating Midlevel Providers." *Journal of the American Dental Association (1939)* 144 (1): 75–91.

Yee, R. 2008. "Healthy Choices, Healthy Smiles: Appropriate and Affordable Fluorides in Nepal." Dissertation. Radboud University of Nijmegen.

———, N. McDonald, and W. H. Helderman. 2006. "Gains in Oral Health and Improved Quality of Life of 12-13-Year-Old Nepali Schoolchildren: Outcomes of an Advocacy Project to Fluoridate Toothpaste." *International Dental Journal* 56 (4): 196–202.

Yee, R., N. McDonald, and D. Walker. 2004. "A Cost-Benefit Analysis of an Advocacy Project to Fluoridate Toothpastes in Nepal." *Community Dental Health* 21 (4): 265–70.

Yengopal, V., U. M. E. Chikte, S. Mickenautsch, L. B. Oliveira, and A. Bhayat. 2010. "Salt Fluoridation: A Meta-analysis of Its Efficacy for Caries Prevention." *SADJ [Journal of the South African Dental Association]* 65 (2): 60–4, 66.

Yengopal, V., S. Mickenautsch, A. C. Bezerra, and S. C. Leal. 2009. "Caries-Preventive Effect of Glass Ionomer and Resin-Based Fissure Sealants on Permanent Teeth: A Meta Analysis." *Journal of Oral Science* 51 (3): 373–82.

Yunusa, M., and A. Obembe. 2012. "Prevalence of Psychiatric Morbidity and Its Associated Factors among Patients Facially Disfigured by Cancrum Oris in Nigeria: A Controlled Study." *Nigerian Journal of Medicine: Journal of the National Association of Resident Doctors of Nigeria* 21 (3): 277–81.

Zandbergen, D., D. E. Slot, C. M. Cobb, and F. A. Van der Weijden. 2013. "The Clinical Effect of Scaling and Root Planing and the Concomitant Administration of Systemic Amoxicillin and Metronidazole: A Systematic Review." *Journal of Periodontology* 84 (3): 332–51.

Zhi, Q. H., E. C. Lo, and H. C. Lin. 2012. "Randomized Clinical Trial on Effectiveness of Silver Diamine Fluoride and Glass Ionomer in Arresting Dentine Caries in Preschool Children." *Journal of Dentistry* 40 (11): 962–67.

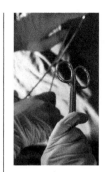

11

Cataract Surgery

N. Venkatesh Prajna, Thulasiraj D. Ravilla,
and Sathish Srinivasan

THE GLOBAL CHALLENGE OF BLINDNESS

Prevalence

The worldwide estimate of blindness (defined as best corrected visual acuity [BCVA] of 3/60 [recognizing at 3 meters what a person with normal acuity can recognize at 60 meters] and less in the better eye) is 39 million people (Pascolini and Mariotti 2012). This figure is just the tip of the iceberg; a significantly larger proportion of people suffer from low vision (defined as BCVA in the range of 6/18 to 3/60), which reduces their levels of independence, safety, and productivity (Thylefors and others 1995). The World Health Organization (WHO) has expanded the scope of the definition of blindness by using presenting visual acuity instead of BCVA. Table 11.1 provides a classification of severity of visual impairment as recommended by the International Council of Ophthalmology (2002) and the recommendations of the WHO (2003).

Risk Factors

The distribution of the burden of disease is disparate; 90 percent of all blind and visually impaired people live in low- and middle-income countries (LMICs) (Cunningham 2001; Thylefors 1998). A study performed in 2010 indicates that visual impairment is unequally distributed among the WHO regions (Stevens and others 2013). The bulk of the blind population resides in Asia and Sub-Saharan Africa (Pascolini and Mariotti 2012). Even in high-income countries (HICs), the prevalence is more common among the economically poorer segments of the population.

Other major risk factors for blindness include advancing age, illiteracy, and rural residence (Abdull and others 2009; Huang and others 2009; Li and others 2008; Li and others 2009; Murthy and others 2010; Salomão and others 2008; Woldeyes and Adamu 2008). Conflicting data have been reported with respect to potential gender-based risks. Although some studies conducted in Sub-Saharan Africa (Komolafe and others 2010; Lewallen and others 2009; Rabiu and Muhammed 2008), China (Li and others 2008; Li and others 2009), and India (Neena and others 2008) report that the prevalence of blindness is more common in women, other studies conducted in Brazil (Salomão and others 2008), China (Huang and others 2009), India (Murthy and others 2010), and Nepal (Sherchan and others 2010) have not established an association.

Costs

The estimation of the cost of blindness has been a subject of considerable interest. One 1996 study estimates the annual worldwide productivity cost of blindness to be US$168 billion, using the data on prevalence rates, GDP, and populations (Smith and Smith 1996). This estimate is based on an assumption that all blind

Corresponding author: N. Venkatesh Prajna, DNB, FRCOphth, Aravind Eye Hospital, prajna@aravind.org

Table 11.1 Visual Acuity Scale

Presenting visual acuity Category	Worse than	Equal to or better than
Mild or no visual impairment	n.a.	6/18
0		3/10 (0.3)
		20/70
Moderate visual impairment	6/18	6/60
1	3/10 (0.3)	1/10 (0.1)
	20/70	20/200
Severe visual impairment	6/60	3/60
2	1/10 (0.1)	1/20 (0.05)
	20/200	20/400
Blindness	3/60	1/60[a]
3	1/20 (0.05)	1/50 (0.02)
	20/400	5/300 (20/1200)
Blindness	1/60[a]	Light perception
4	1/50 (0.02)	
	5/300 (20/1200)	
Blindness	No light perception	
5		
9	Undetermined or unspecified	

Source: WHO 2008.
Note: Three visual acuity measurements are included for each category because countries express visual acuity in different ways. The first notation is given in metric form and is expressed as meters. The second notation is expressed in decimal form. The third notation is given in imperial form and expressed as feet.
Note: n.a. = not applicable.
a. Or counts fingers at 1 meter.

individuals are completely unproductive, while all other adults and children are assumed to be productive. A subsequent study, using data from 2000 and based on a more conservative estimate of personal productivity losses associated with blindness, estimates the economic productivity loss to be US$19 billion (Frick and Foster 2003). Another study estimates the direct investment required to treat the backlog of avoidable blindness and visual impairment over 10 years, to 2020, to be US$23.1 billion (PwC 2012).

CATARACT DISEASE

Description and Prevalence

Cataract is defined as a significant opacity in the crystalline lens that obstructs or distorts light entering the eye. The WHO in 2004 estimated that cataract was responsible for blindness in 17.7 million people, or 47.8 percent of all blindness (Resnikoff and others 2004). A more recent estimate from Pascolini and Mariotti (2012) finds cataract the leading cause of avoidable blindness, responsible for 51 percent of cases (figure 11.1). The prevalence of cataract as a proportion of the blind population shows large variations across countries. The figure is as low as 5 percent in developed countries such as Australia, the United Kingdom, and the United States; it is more than 55 percent in countries such as Peru and some parts of Sub-Saharan Africa (Resnikoff and others 2004). An estimate based on the number of cataract surgery procedures

Figure 11.1 Global Burden of Cataract
Percent

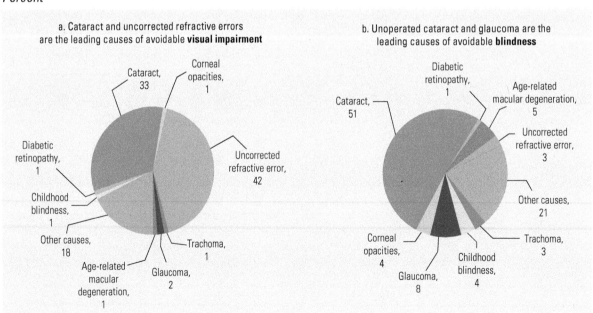

a. Cataract and uncorrected refractive errors are the leading causes of avoidable **visual impairment**

Cataract, 33
Corneal opacities, 1
Uncorrected refractive error, 42
Diabetic retinopathy, 1
Childhood blindness, 1
Other causes, 18
Age-related macular degeneration, 1
Glaucoma, 2
Trachoma, 1

b. Unoperated cataract and glaucoma are the leading causes of avoidable **blindness**

Diabetic retinopathy, 1
Cataract, 51
Age-related macular degeneration, 5
Uncorrected refractive error, 3
Other causes, 21
Trachoma, 3
Childhood blindness, 4
Glaucoma, 8
Corneal opacities, 4

Source: Pascolini and Mariotti 2012.

per million population shows interesting variations. Even among high-income countries (HICs), annual cataract surgical rates per million population vary dramatically; for example, there are 1,200 in the United Arab Emirates versus 8,000 in Australia (WHO 2010).

The burden of visual loss due to cataract can markedly reduce the quality of life (QOL) of the affected elderly population because routine activities like reading, driving, walking, and remaining independent are severely affected (Salive and others 1994; Stuck and others 1999; West and others 1997). Impaired vision may be associated with an increased risk of falls, which can cause broken hips and associated increased morbidity (Patino and others 2010). Studies have suggested that this visual disability may pose an increased risk for mental depression and suicide (Lam and others 2008; Zheng and others 2012).

Cataract has no proven preventive or medical therapy. Surgery, the only option, consists of removing the cloudy natural lens and replacing it with an artificial, transparent intraocular lens (IOL). Studies have clearly established that this surgery with the implantation of IOL significantly improves vision-related QOL (Fletcher and others 1998). Although economic conditions play a significant role, the availability of adequate and appropriate surgical resources and patients' perceptions of the benefits could be significant factors in increasing the utility of cataract surgery.

A visual acuity measurement can serve as a guiding factor, but the timing of surgery should be based on the visual needs of individual patients. In general, patients in developed countries are more likely to seek and obtain cataract surgery early in the course of the disease because of the widespread availability and easy accessibility of quality eye care services and probably because of government-provided or -subsidized health care, to an extent. Anecdotal experiences in India suggest that this phenomenon of early cataract surgery intervention has increased in recent years, probably due to the country's improving economy and access to affordable quality interventions. Early surgery also helps the individual make informed decisions before loss of social independence.

Preoperative Evaluation

A comprehensive ocular examination evaluates the cornea, anterior chamber, pupil, lens status, retina, and optic nerve; this examination is the first step in determining the need for a surgical procedure. This examination is useful for identifying associated comorbidities, such as glaucoma or retinal and optic nerve disorders, given that their presence may contribute to a poor final visual outcome. Räsänen and others (2006) highlight the

importance of this examination; 33 percent of patients surveyed had a secondary ophthalmic diagnosis, indicating that they may receive a reduced benefit from the surgery. Systemic conditions such as diabetes mellitus, hypertension, and compromised cardiac status should be evaluated before the decision is made to subject patients to surgery.

The power of the IOL to be placed inside the eye should be customized for each individual. Ultrasonography is performed to estimate the axial length of the eye; this estimate is used to determine the power of the IOL. It might be argued that the vast majority of patients may benefit from receiving a standard 20-diopter IOL, which would eliminate the high cost of obtaining an ultrasound, but the advantage of having a customized power IOL is far greater.

The amount of preoperative testing performed for healthy patients undergoing cataract surgery may vary significantly, which might influence the ultimate cost of the intervention. A national survey in the United States assessed variations in preoperative medical tests ordered by physicians (Bass and others 1995). Results indicate that 50 percent of ophthalmologists, 40 percent of internists, and 33 percent of anesthesiologists frequently or always obtained chest x-rays; in contrast, 20 percent of ophthalmologists, 27 percent of internists, and 37 percent of anesthesiologists never obtained x-rays. Similar significant differences were also seen with respect to the ordering of routine blood tests. Many respondents (32 percent to 80 percent) believed that these tests may be unnecessary, but they cited medico-legal reasons or institutional requirements for ordering them (Bass and others 1995).

SURGICAL INTERVENTIONS

Surgery is the only treatment choice for visually disabling cataract. If surgery is delayed, the following sequelae may occur:

1. Cataract may become denser (hard or brunescent, which implies a browner color) or whiter (mature cataract).
2. If still untreated, it may proceed to the following stages:
   - Phacolytic glaucoma: A hypermature cataract can leak, causing increased intraocular pressure.
   - Phacomorphic glaucoma: A mature cataract can sometimes cause crowding of the anterior chamber, leading to increased intraocular pressure. Surgery at these stages has to be undertaken as an emergency to prevent irreversible blindness.

Surgical Types and Procedures

There are three basic types of cataract surgery:

Phacoemulsification (PE)
Manual small-incision cataract surgery (MSICS)
Extracapsular cataract extraction (ECCE)

The basic steps in all three surgical procedures are the following: making an entry wound into the eye, removing the cloudy natural lens, and replacing the lens with an artificial IOL.

Incision. In PE, a small incision of approximately 2.5 millimeters (mm) is made, either in the sclera or the cornea. This wound is triplanar, which provides a self-sealing trapdoor incision. The configuration of the incision is more important than the size, with respect to the maintenance of the self-sealing property. In most cases, no sutures are used that could distort the corneal edge, any resultant induced astigmatism is negligible, and the visual rehabilitation is very quick.

In MSICS, a triplanar incision, similar in configuration to that in PE but considerably wider (8 to 9 mm), is made in the sclera. This incision is large enough to let the lens be delivered through it, but it is self-sealing because of the triplanar configuration. Hence, the entry wounds for PE and MSICS are superior to those of ECCE in ensuring quick visual rehabilitation.

In ECCE, the entry wound is biplanar, placed at the limbus, and is 10 to 12 mm in length. Because this incision is biplanar, it requires meticulous suturing. These sutures may have many inherent problems, the most important of which is suture-induced astigmatism, which prolongs visual rehabilitation. Occasionally, the sutures may cause significant irritation and may serve as a locus for potential intraocular infection.

Removal of the Cloudy Natural Lens. In PE, the nucleus is fragmented and emulsified using ultrasound within the eye. Hence, this surgery requires a smaller incision, only wide enough to allow the ultrasound probe to enter the eye and access the lens. In ECCE and MSICS, the nuclear and corneal material is manually delivered, which requires a wide incision to allow the lens to be retrieved.

Replacement with an Artificial Lens. Following the cataract extraction, an IOL of a customized dioptric power is placed in the posterior chamber of the eye. The power is determined preoperatively using a formula based on keratometry and the axial length measurement. These posterior chamber IOLs are manufactured from one of two types of material: PE uses an acrylic lens (which is foldable), and MSICS and ECCE use a rigid lens of polymethylmethacrylate (PMMA) (which is rigid).

PE is the most commonly performed cataract surgery in HICs. However, in LMICs, most surgeries are done using the MSICS and ECCE techniques. There are valid reasons for these different approaches. Patients seek cataract surgery much later than in developed countries. The surgery is often postponed until the disease progresses, by which time the cataract may have become advanced and mature. It is not uncommon to see phacolytic and phacomorphic glaucoma, the sequelae of longstanding cataract. Even though PE can be performed for hard cataract, MSICS is easier and more cost-effective in this situation. MSICS has been reported to be safer in situations such as brunescent cataract (Gogate and others 2003; Venkatesh and others 2009), white mature cataract (Venkatesh, Das, and others 2005; Venkatesh and others 2010), and cataract causing phacolytic and phacomorphic glaucomas (Ramakrishanan and others 2010; Venkatesh and others 2007), which are more prevalent in LMICs.

Another deterrent for large-scale adoption of the PE procedure in LMICs is the high cost of the instruments and the consumables, which include tubings, cassettes, and the surgical tips of the machine, and the need for trained technical personnel to maintain these sophisticated instruments. In contrast, MSICS does not require sophisticated equipment, except for an operating microscope, which is an essential requirement for all intraocular procedures.

The scarcest resource for an effective intervention is the availability of a trained ophthalmic surgeon; this can be an important rate-limiting step in eye care service delivery in LMICs. Effective use of surgeons' time by using well-organized and efficient supporting teams is a prerequisite to improving cost-effectiveness. Surgeries that take less time mean that more surgeries can be performed in a given period. In general, PE takes significantly more time than MSICS; Ruit and others (2007) and Gogate and others (2005) report mean surgical time of 15.5 minutes for PE and 9 minutes for MSICS. In high-volume settings, the mean surgical time can be reduced to as low as 4.5 minutes for MSICS, making it an extremely fast procedure (Balent and others 2001; Venkatesh and others 2005).

COMPARATIVE SAFETY OF SURGICAL INTERVENTIONS

Many studies have compared the incidence of intraoperative and postoperative complications of these procedures (Ruit and others 2007; Venkatesh and others 2010).

Posterior Capsular Rupture

During cataract surgery, the anterior capsule, the nucleus, and the cortex of the cataractous lens are removed, while the posterior capsule is retained. The integrity of the posterior capsule acts as a scaffold for keeping the artificial IOL in place. Posterior capsular rupture (PCR) with or without vitreous loss is one of the important intraoperative complications during cataract surgery and may lead to suboptimal visual outcomes.

The occurrence of PCR is often used as a surrogate for estimation of safety in cataract surgeries. Ruit and others (2007) report a 1.85 percent PCR rate in the PE group, versus none in the MSICS group. Venkatesh and others (2010) report that PCR occurred in 2.2 percent of PE cases, compared with 1.4 percent in MSICS cases. Gogate and others (2005) report a higher incidence of PCR in both groups: 6 percent in the MSICS group versus 3.5 percent in the PE group. These studies show that the incidence of PCR is comparable between the groups; anecdotal experience among high-volume surgeons suggests that the incidence of PCR declines with increasing surgical experience.

Endophthalmitis

Endophthalmitis is a serious postoperative complication that can cause significant ocular morbidity. Infection within the eye is more difficult to treat because antibiotics are not able to cross the blood-ocular barrier with ease. Hence, the results are very often devastating and all efforts should be made to prevent this complication. A retrospective observational study reported the comparative incidence for PE and MSICS (Ravindran and others 2009). This study was performed at Aravind Eye Hospital, a large eye care facility in India that offers services to two distinct subsets of patients: private patients who come from comparatively good economic backgrounds; and poor patients who come from distant areas, where outreach screening eye examinations are conducted. This study reports lower incidence of endophthalmitis in private patients, who had a better standard of living, than in patients from eye camps.

Posterior Capsule Opacification

Posterior capsule opacification (PCO) is one of the significant postoperative occurrences following cataract surgery, and the incidence increases over longer follow-up periods. Although a minimal PCO does not warrant any treatment, a significant PCO may cause a substantial reduction in visual acuity and requires an additional surgical intervention called yttrium-aluminum garnet laser capsulotomy. Ruit and others (2007) report an incidence of grade-one PCO (defined as a non-vision-threatening, mild peripheral PCO) of 26.1 percent of MSICS patients, compared with 14.6 percent in PE patients. The incidence of grade-two PCO was 17.4 percent in the MSICS group, and none in the PE group. However, in this study, IOLs made of different materials were used for these two interventions. The design of the IOL also matters. Square-edged IOLs are known to cause less PCO than round-edged IOLs.

COMPARATIVE EFFICACY OF SURGICAL INTERVENTIONS

Visual Acuity

The visual outcomes following cataract surgery are often reported either as uncorrected visual acuity (UCVA) or BCVA. UCVA, which is the visual acuity of the operated eye without the aid of additional refractive tools like spectacles, often reflects the real-life situation in LMICs, in which patients often do not have easy access to spectacles. BCVA represents the best possible visual potential of the operated eye, usually with the aid of spectacles. The WHO recommends that 88 percent of surgically operated patients should have a UCVA of 6/18 and better (WHO 1998).

The three randomized trials mentioned compare the visual outcomes between PE and MSICS. Venkatesh and others (2010) randomize 270 consecutive patients, who presented with white mature cataract (a common occurrence in many LMICs), to receive either PE or MSICS. At six weeks' follow-up, 87.6 percent of the eyes in the PE group and 82.0 percent in the MSICS group had a UCVA of 6/18 and better. The BCVA comparison revealed that 99.0 percent of the eyes in the PE group and 98.2 percent of the eyes in the MSICS group had vision of 6/18 and better. Gogate and others (2005), who compare PE with MSICS in a prospective randomized trial of 400 eyes, report that UCVA of 6/18 or better was achieved by 81.1 percent of the PE eyes, versus 71.1 percent of the MSICS eyes, at six weeks. The BCVA was 6/18 or better in 98.4 percent of the PE group and 98.4 percent of the MSICS group at six weeks. Ruit and others (2007) report longer-term visual outcomes in a prospective trial of 108 eyes in Nepal. The patients were randomized to PE or MSICS, with each type of surgery performed by an acknowledged expert in that technique. They report comparable rates of 98 percent achieving BCVA of 6/18 or better at six months.

Surgically Induced Astigmatism

The main determinant in the difference between UCVA and BCVA is the amount of surgically induced astigmatism (SIA). SIA is the most important reason for patients to have a suboptimal UCVA, while their BCVA may be normal. The lower the SIA created, the closer UCVA and BCVA will be to each other, an ideal situation. Hence, one of the main strategies for optimizing the visual acuity of the patient is to keep the incidence of SIA as low as possible.

The size and location of the incision play key roles in the occurrence of SIA; larger incisions cause more SIA. A prospective Japanese study compares the SIA between two sizes of surgical incision in MSICS, 3.2 mm and 5.5 mm, and finds a reduction of SIA by 0.3 diopter when the smaller incision size is used (Kimura and others 1999). Surgical incisions created in the temporal side of the corneo-scleral junction are known to cause less SIA than the traditional superior incisions (Gokhale and Sawhney 2005; Reddy, Raj, and Singh 2007).

Studies have also looked at the SIA created by PE and MSICS. At six months' follow-up, Ruit and others (2007) report a mean astigmatism of 0.7 diopter for the PE group and 0.88 for the MSICS group. This difference of astigmatism was not statistically significant. At six weeks postoperatively, Gogate and others (2005) report mean astigmatism of 1.1 diopters for PE and 1.2 diopters for MSICS, which were also comparable. Other authors, however, report that PE causes significantly less SIA than MSICS at six weeks postoperatively (George and others 2005; Venkatesh and others 2010). Astigmatism caused by MSICS is greater when a superior incision is used; accordingly, it can be lessened to a great extent by using a temporal incision, thereby improving the UCVA of MSICS (Gokhale and Sawhney 2005; Kimura and others 1999).

FACTORS AFFECTING THE EFFICACY OF SURGICAL INTERVENTIONS

Advantages of Interventions

Cataract surgery has several advantages over other ophthalmic conditions, including the following:

- Because cataract causes visual disability early in the disease course, patients become symptomatic and seek medical care, which is in contrast to other ocular morbidities, such as diabetic retinopathy and glaucoma, in which patients may be asymptomatic and may not seek care until the disease is more advanced.

- The treatment is often a one-time surgical intervention with excellent visual rehabilitation. This is one of the few age-related conditions for which surgical intervention will result in near-normal functional levels. Because there is no need for routine systemic antibiotics, the cost of postoperative medications is lower.

- Visual acuity becomes normal after the initial convalescent period of one month, and patients are able to resume their occupations with near-normal productivity.

Despite these factors and the availability of time-tested surgical options, cataract continues to constitute a major global health care burden, not because of the lack of a clinical solution, but because of the challenging issues in effective program implementation. These challenges include identifying patients in need, making services available, creating supportive infrastructures, ensuring quality, and developing sustainable service delivery systems.

Identifying Patients in Need

The first strategy for a successful cataract surgery program is to ensure a high throughput of patients into an efficient, quality-conscious, and cost-effective service delivery system. Emerging evidence indicates that the incidence of blinding cataract varies among regions. Studies have suggested that the burden of cataract disease may be lower in Sub-Saharan Africa than in India (Mathenge and others 2007; Neena and others 2008; Oye and Kuper 2007; Oye and others 2006). The proportion of people in India who are older than age 50 years is about 16 percent of the total population, which is twice that of some Sub-Saharan African countries (Lewallen and Thulasiraj 2010). Given that advancing age is a significant risk factor for the development of cataract, it may be prudent to assume that the incidence in these Sub-Saharan African countries may be lower than that in India. In addition, physical access to patients in remote locations such as the mountainous regions of Nepal and in some Sub-Saharan African countries with low population density may be considerably more difficult than in a country such as India, which has high population density.

Increasing Access to Care

It is often difficult to provide continuous ophthalmic services to sparsely populated areas. However, evidence exists that even when such services are provided, they are underutilized (Brilliant and Brilliant 1985;

Brilliant and others 1991; Courtright, Kanjaloti, and Lewallen 1995; Gupta and Murthy 1995; Venkataswamy and Brilliant 1981). In India, screening eye camps have been available for decades to identify and advise surgery to people affected by cataract. A study conducted by the Aravind Eye Hospital investigated service uptake in rural Indian populations served by regular outreach camps and tried to identify the barriers (Fletcher and others 1999). The authors found that, of the people with eye problems, only 7 percent attended the eye camps. The major barriers were lack of resources such as money, transportation, and attendants.

The cost of getting cataract patients to hospitals can also vary significantly between geographic settings. Whereas it costs about US$4.50 to transport one patient for cataract surgery to Aravind Eye Hospital in southern India, the same effort is estimated to cost US$40 to US$60 in the much less densely populated areas of eastern Africa (Lewallen, Eliah, and Gilbert 2006). Innovative programs, such as the creation of low-cost permanent facilities staffed by ophthalmic assistants connected with an ophthalmologist in a central location through telemedicine connectivity, may positively influence eye care–seeking behavior.

Optimizing Productivity

The lack of availability of ophthalmologists and their disproportional distribution is a major issue. There are approximately 200,000 ophthalmologists worldwide. Although this number is growing annually by 1.2 percent, the population older than age 60 years, which is more at risk of developing cataract, is growing by 2.9 percent. Sub-Saharan Africa has three ophthalmologists per 1 million population in contrast to 79 ophthalmologists per 1 million population in HICs (Resnikoff and others 2012).

Although the presence of skilled ophthalmologists is a key factor, this alone may not solve the issue of optimal productivity. Good infrastructure with optimal paramedical support is crucial for the productivity of ophthalmologists. In a study in Sub-Saharan Africa, Courtright and others (2007) show that the creation of an enabling environment improves the productivity of a cataract surgeon by four- to five-fold, from a low of 100 to a high of nearly 500 surgeries per year.

The establishment of such a system has produced a successful high-volume, high-quality eye care service model in India (Natchiar and others 1994). Maximizing operating room efficiency is extremely important in achieving high-volume productivity. Venkatesh, Muralikrishnan, and others (2005) describe how the

Aravind Eye Hospital operating room staff supports a single surgeon; the staff includes three scrub nurses, one orderly, one circulating nurse, and one nurse to clean and sterilize instruments. To minimize the surgical turnaround time, the ophthalmologist alternates between two adjacent operating tables. A centrally placed operating microscope can rotate between the two tables. While the surgeon is operating on one patient, the paramedical team positions and prepares the next patient on an adjacent table. The average surgical time is about 3.5 minutes, with 16 to 18 surgeries performed by a single surgeon per hour. The complication rate and the visual results are comparable to the best global standards (Venkatesh, Muralikrishnan, and others 2005).

Ensuring Quality

The WHO recommends that 80 percent of eyes should have presenting visual acuity better than 6/18 after surgery, and fewer than 5 percent should be worse than 6/60 (Lewallen and Thulasiraj 2010). However, several population-based studies have reported poor visual outcome of less than 6/60, which would be defined as blind in most countries (Courtright and others 2004; Habiyakire and others 2010; Kimani and others 2008; Oye and Kuper 2007; Oye and others 2006). These population-based studies may have encompassed patients operated over a large time span; hence, the results may reflect services offered both in the past and in the present. Nevertheless, these data clearly indicate significant room for improvement. Poor outcomes start a vicious cycle that will result in lower demand and lower patient volumes.

Building Sustainable Service Delivery Systems

Excellent programs are not able to continue without sustainable strategies. Although philanthropy can be an initial source of support, programs need to devise ways to become self-sustaining to continue to be efficient. Eye care service providers can allow patients to choose the type of surgical procedure and the IOL from a menu of options. For example, Aravind Eye Hospitals have developed a tiered service system. Using this system, it offers free surgery to patients from eye camps, subsidized by fees paid by wealthier patients who choose to pay for special services such as PE procedures with costlier IOLs or for private rooms. Paying customers also have high standards for quality care, and these standards are used as the benchmark for nonpaying customers as well (Rangan and Thulasiraj 2007).

MEASURING COSTS OF SURGICAL PROGRAMS

There are different ways of analyzing the economic implications of cataract surgical procedures.

Cost-Minimization Analysis

Cost-minimization analysis compares events that have similar outcomes and determines which procedures are less costly (Brown and others 2003). The results are expressed in units of currency expended for each outcome. Various studies report the cost of providing PE and MSICS services (table 11.2).

The data in table 11.2 show, in the three studies, that provider costs for MSICS are consistently less than those for PE. Provider costs for PE show a wide variation, ranging from US$25.50 to US$70 even though these studies were in similar geographic locations with comparable socioeconomic dynamics. The cost difference was mainly attributable to the different types of IOLs used. For example, in the Nepal study (Ruit and others 2007), the provider cost was US$70, of which US$52 was due to the more expensive, imported, foldable acrylic IOL. In comparison, the cost of an indigenous IOL made of PMMA would be US$3. If a PMMA lens had been used instead of a foldable acrylic IOL, the provider cost would have been reduced dramatically and would have been similar to the costs reported in the other studies (Gogate and others 2005; Muralikrishnan and others 2004). Muralikrishnan and others (2004) study the societal costs (obtained by summing the provider costs and the patient costs) of the two procedures and arrive at US$29.40 for MSICS and US$37.92 for PE. Even though rigid PMMA IOLs were used in both arms of this study, PE procedures were more expensive because of the capital costs of the machine and the costs of the consumables. Compared with PE, MSICS clearly reduces the costs for the health care delivery system (Gogate, Deshpande, and Nirmalan 2007).

Table 11.2 Providers' Cost of PE and MSICS
US$ per procedure

Study	PE	MSICS
Muralikrishnan and others 2004	25.55	17.03
Gogate and others 2005	42.10	15.34
Ruit and others 2007	70	15

Source: Venkatesh and others 2012.

Note: MSICS = manual small-incision cataract surgery; PE = phacoemulsification.

Cost-Effectiveness Analysis

Cost-effectiveness analysis looks beyond the concepts of cost minimization and cost-benefit analysis to measure the costs expended upon an intervention and compares them for a single outcome (Brown and others 2003). These outcomes can be analyzed as measured by life-years gained, vision-years gained, or disability-adjusted life years (DALYs) averted, and expressed in cost per output unit (Lansingh, Carter, and Martens 2007). The first Global Burden of Disease study quantified health effects by employing DALYs (Murray and Lopez 1996). This metric integrates parameters such as morbidity, mortality, and disability information, and arrives at a single unit. In essence, this unit aims to measure the difference between the current health status of individuals and ideal situations in which people would live to old age without disease or disability.

Data from the WHO's Global Health Estimates study indicate that the global burden of eye disease was an estimated 25 million DALYs, accounting for 1 percent of total DALYs (WHO 2013). The highest number of DALYs was found in South Asia (including India), and East Asia and the Pacific (including China), followed by Sub-Saharan Africa and the other LMICs. Among the ocular noncommunicable diseases, cataract was most unevenly distributed across the globe, with increased presence in LMICs, and contributed to 7 million DALYs. In HICs such as Australia and the United States, cataract surgery is offered to people with early lens changes and not delayed until cases are severe, probably because of market demand (Ono, Hiratsuka, and Murakami 2010).

Cost-effectiveness can vary among countries and also among providers in the same country. Singh, Garner, and Floyd (2000) compare the cost-effectiveness of cataract surgery in southern India in three types of facilities: government camps, a nongovernment hospital, and a state medical college functioning as a first-level hospital. This study reports that even though camps were a low-cost option, the poor outcomes experienced there reduced their cost-effectiveness to US$97 per patient. The state medical college hospital was least cost-effective at US$176 per patient; the nongovernmental hospital was the most cost-effective at US$54 per patient. A study from Nepal reports that under a best-estimate scenario, cataract surgery had a cost of US$5.06 per DALY, which places it among the most cost-effective public health interventions (Marseille 1996).

Cost Utility Analysis

Cost utility analysis is more exhaustive than simple cost-effectiveness in that it includes evaluation of both QOL as perceived by the patient and longevity (Brown and Brown 2005; Brown, Brown, and Sharma 2004; Lansingh, Carter, and Martens 2007). Improvement in visual outcome following an intervention is often used as the indicator of success after the procedure. However, this result does not effectively illuminate the intrinsic value of the intervention from patients' perspectives.

Utility value is a quantifiable measure of data derived from patient-preference-based value, clinician, and community (Groot 2000). The time tradeoff (TTO) method is a major tool for measuring utility value; subjects are asked what proportion of their lives they would be willing to trade in return for guaranteed perfect vision in each eye (Brown, Brown, Sharma, Busbee, and Brown 2001; Brown, Brown, Sharma, and Garrett 1999; Brown, Brown, Sharma, and Shah 1999; Brown, Sharma, Brown, and Garrett 1999; Wakker and Stiggelbout 1995). TTO utility values were significantly higher in patients with ocular disease and good bilateral visual acuity than in those with good unilateral visual acuity (Brown, Brown, Sharma, Busbee, and Brown 2001). Patients who had undergone cataract surgery in both eyes had a better QOL than those who had surgery in only one eye (Castells and others 1999; Desai and others 1996; Javitt, Brenner, and others 1993; Javitt, Steinberg, and others 1995). A 2012 cataract surgery cost utility study finds that cataract surgery yielded a remarkable 36.2 percent gain in QOL for surgery in both eyes. Additionally, it was highly cost-effective, being 34.4 percent less expensive than in 2000 and 85 percent less expensive than in 1985. Initial cataract surgery was estimated to yield an extraordinary 4.57 percent financial return

on investment to society over 13 years (Brown and others 2013).

Surgery on the First Eye. The results of the cost utility analysis are expressed using cost per quality-adjusted life year ($/QALY) gained. Vision improvement after cataract surgery has been shown to positively affect utility values and, in most instances, to correlate positively with health-related QOL instruments or utility measuring methods (Brown, Brown, Sharma, Busbee, and Brown 2001; Gafni 1994; Lee and others 2000; Rosen, Kaplan, and David 2005). Studies have been performed on cost utility following cataract surgery; the results have been depicted in the form of QALY per unit of currency (table 11.3).

A Swedish study that analyzes the cost utility of cataract surgery based on cost data and vision and disability scores estimates the cost utility in 2006 to be US$4,800 per QALY, using the common benefit discount of 3 percent (Kobelt, Lundström, and Stenevi 2002). In HICs such as the United States, interventions costing less than US$100,000 per QALY gained have been considered cost-effective (Laupacis and others 1992). Cost-effectiveness is accentuated when the cost is less than US$20,000.

The benefit of any surgery is increased if the duration of the benefit is extended. One study tries to determine the duration of the visual improvement following cataract surgery (Lundstrom and Wendel 2005). This study, performed in Sweden on 615 patients, assesses the patients preoperatively, at one year, and at eight years after the surgery, using clinical data and the Catquest questionnaire. The results indicate that 80 percent of patients reported improved visual function at the

Table 11.3 Studies Reporting Cost Utility of Cataract Surgery Using Intraocular Implants for the First Eye, Unless Otherwise Stated

Study	Year published	Country	Cost utility (US$/QALY)	Method used to measure utility	Remarks
Aribaba	2004	Nigeria	1,928–2,875	TTO	Cost utility for four scenarios
Busbee and others	2002	United States	2,020	TTO	Cost/QALYs discounted 3 percent over 12 years (life expectancy)
Busbee and others	2003	United States	2,727	TTO	Cost utility of surgery for second eye
Kobelt, Lundström, and Stenevi	2002	Sweden	4,900	EQ-5D and Catquest*	Undiscounted costs; QALYs discounted 3 percent over 5 years (life expectancy); correlation of Catquest and EQ-5D
Räsänen and others	2006	Finland	13,018	15D	QALYs discounted 3 percent; costs not discounted; life expectancy unknown

Source: Lansingh, Carter, and Martens 2007.

Note: EQ-5D = Euro quality of life measure on five dimensions; QALY = quality-adjusted life year; TTO = time tradeoff; 15D = 15 dimensions of the health-related quality of life.

*Catquest = a disease-specific, health-related quality-of-life instrument measuring the benefit of surgery as a function of a patient's specifics at baseline.

latest follow-up, implying that the cost utility benefit of cataract surgery may continue throughout individuals' life spans. As life expectancy increases, higher numbers of QALYs can be expected. The costs will also be discounted over the longer period. Brown and others (2013) find that cataract surgery is very effective at $2,222 per QALY, from the third-party insurer cost perspective.

Surgery on the Second Eye. Cost utility studies have demonstrated the benefit of surgery on the second eye in cases of bilateral cataract. Busbee and others (2003) analyze the cost utility of cataract surgery in the second eye of the same patient in the outcomes research team study cohort; they find that patients gained 0.92 QALYs. This figure is similar to the cost utility for the first eye reported by the same authors (Busbee and others 2002). These studies indicate that the cost utilities for surgeries on both eyes are similar when calculated using the same methodology.

Utility values can also be used to compare the cost-effectiveness analyses of medical interventions across different specialties. One study compares the cost-effectiveness of cataract surgery and other surgical options; results indicate that cataract surgery is more cost-effective than knee arthroplasty, epileptic surgery, or implantation of a defibrillator, but it may be less cost-effective than hip arthroplasty (Lansingh, Carter, and Martens 2007). Another study states that when total benefits are compared with total costs (estimated to eliminate avoidable blindness and visual impairment), the result shows a 2:1 benefit-to-cost ratio (PwC 2012).

CONCLUSIONS

Rising Costs

Health care expenditures are rising throughout the world and hence must be considered in any health care delivery intervention. In 1970, total health care expenditure in the United States was US$73.1 billion, which was 7 percent of GDP. By 2001, this figure had risen to US$1,425 billion or 14.1 percent of GDP (Brown and others 2003).

In 2000, the WHO published a health system performance assessment of its 191 member states that measured how efficiently health systems translate expenditures into health care (Brown and others 2003; WHO 2000). The United States, which incurred the highest health care expenditures per capita, adjusted for cost of living differences in 1997, achieved a ranking of 72, between Argentina and Bhutan. Clearly, increasing the

amount of per capita spending on health alone does not translate into an efficient health system. It is imperative to find more effective, sustainable, and equitable solutions to meet the needs of the world's population.

Changing Demographics

Demographic projections suggest that there will be a significant increase in the general population and in the proportion of the population that is older (Lutz, Sanderson, and Scherbov 1997). Without new interventions, the global number of blind individuals is likely to increase from 44 million in 2000 to 76 million in 2020 (Frick and Foster 2003). Providing quality eye care, with its projected increase in costs, is going to be an increasing challenge for both LMICs and HICs. The government of the United Kingdom had to increase its eye care budget by £730 million between 2003 and 2009, a 60 percent increase (figure 11.2) (Malik and others 2013). In this era of financial austerity, such increased expenditures cannot be sustained.

Current Scenario

Realizing the need for an increasing thrust to combat avoidable blindness, the WHO, in partnership with the International Agency for the Prevention of Blindness, launched the VISION 2020 Right to Sight initiative in 1999. At that time, it was envisaged that if successfully implemented, this initiative would lower the projected number of people who are blind to 24 million in 2020 and lead to 429 million blind person-years avoided.

Recent studies done across the world have shown encouraging trends in the reduction of vision loss. In Southeast Asia, blindness decreased significantly from

Figure 11.2 Gross Expenditure on Vision Program, 2003–09

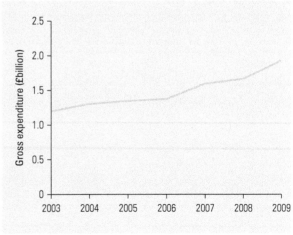

Source: Malik and others 2013.

1.4 percent in 1990 to 0.8 percent in 2010, a 43 percent decrease (Keeffe and others 2014). Similarly, in Central Asia, the estimated age-standardized prevalence of blindness decreased from 0.4 percent in 1990 to 0.2 percent in 2010, while in South Asia, blindness has decreased from 1.7 percent to 1.1 percent in the same period (Jonas and others 2014). East Asia was no different, and the blindness prevalence dropped from 0.7 percent in 1990 to 0.4 percent in 2010 (Wong and others 2014). The change in these figures can be linked to major cataract programs that have been conducted in the most populous countries, such as India, which now has a cataract surgery rate of 4,000 per 1 million population (Keeffe and others 2014). However, in absolute numbers, the number of blind people remains constant because of the rapid increase in the older adult population (Stevens and others 2013).

Demand and Supply Strategies

In an early study, cataract surgery was identified by the World Bank as one of the most cost-effective interventions that can be offered in LMICs (Javitt, Venkataswamy, and Somme 1983). Programs need to put effective teams and processes in place to create an environment that can address both the demand and the supply sides of the equation. Strategies on demand creation would ensure that all those who can benefit from cataract surgery will actively seek it; such strategies also need to facilitate the efficient delivery of cataract services with good visual outcomes. The scenario of increasing backlogs of patients, low surgical productivity, and poor visual outcomes indicates that this demand-supply equation needs to be refined, evaluated, and monitored. Although the resource bases such as infrastructure, equipment, ophthalmologists, and paramedical staff should be strengthened, an equal emphasis is needed on management aspects and competencies (Lewallen and Thulasiraj 2010) to build the effective processes and organizational capabilities to use resources optimally.

LMICs have to use their economic resources even more judiciously in light of competing and compelling health care needs, such as maternal and child health programs and immunizations. Resources are neither infinite nor indefinite. The law of diminishing returns states that for a certain period, the benefits to patients increase when health care resources are increased. After a certain point, however, additional resources may lead to a reduction in net benefits to patients (Malik and others 2013). Supporting literature indicates that PE and MSICS procedures are comparable with respect to safety and efficacy, and MSICS is more cost-effective and more appropriate in these settings.

NOTE

The World Bank classifies countries according to four income groupings. Income is measured using gross national income (GNI) per capita, in U.S. dollars, converted from local currency using the *World Bank Atlas* method. Classifications as of July 2014 are as follows:

- Low-income countries (LICs) = US$1,045 or less in 2013
- Middle-income countries (MICs) are subdivided:
  - Lower-middle-income = US$1,046 to US$4,125
  - Upper-middle-income (UMICs) = US$4,126 to US$12,745
- High-income countries (HICs) = US$12,746 or more

REFERENCES

Abdull, M. M., S. Sivasubramaniam, G. V. S. Murthy, C. Gilbert, T. Abubakar, and others. 2009. "Causes of Blindness and Visual Impairment in Nigeria: The Nigeria National Blindness and Visual Impairment Survey." *Investigative Ophthalmology and Visual Science* 50 (4): 4114–20.

Aribaba, O. T. "Cost Effectiveness Analysis of Cataract Services in Lagos University Teaching Hospital [LUTH], Lagos, Nigeria." Master's thesis summary. http://www.iceh.org.uk/alumni/more/aribaba04.htm.

Balent, L. C., K. Narendran, S. Patel, S. Kar, and D. A. Patterson. 2001. "High Volume Sutureless Intraocular Lens Surgery in a Rural Eye Camp in India." *Ophthalmic Surgery, Lasers, and Imaging* 32 (6): 446–55.

Bass, E. B., E. P. Steinberg, R. Luthra, O. D. Schein, J. M. Tielsch, and others. 1995. "Do Ophthalmologists, Anesthesiologists, and Internists Agree about Preoperative Testing in Healthy Patients Undergoing Cataract Surgery?" *Archives of Ophthalmology* 113 (10): 1248–56.

Brilliant, G. E., and L. B. Brilliant. 1985. "Using Social Epidemiology to Understand Who Stays Blind and Who Gets Operated for Cataract in a Rural Setting." *Social Science and Medicine* 21 (5): 553–58.

Brilliant, G. E., J. M. Lepkowski, B. Zurita, and R. D. Thulasiraj. 1991. "Social Determinants of Cataract Surgery Utilization in South India: The Operations Research Group." *Archives of Ophthalmology* 109 (4): 584–89.

Brown, M. M., and G. C. Brown. 2005. "How to Interpret a Healthcare Economic Analysis." *Current Opinion in Ophthalmology* 16 (3): 191–94.

Brown, G. C., M. M. Brown, A. Menezes, B. G. Busbee, H. B. Lieske, and P. A. Lieske. 2013. "Cataract Surgery Cost Utility Revisited in 2012: A New Economic Paradigm." *Ophthalmology* 120 (12): 2367–76.

Brown, G. C., M. M. Brown, and S. Sharma. 2004. "Health Care Economic Analyses." *Retina* 24 (1): 139–46.

Brown, M. M., G. C. Brown, S. Sharma, B. Busbee, and H. Brown. 2001. "Quality of Life Associated with Unilateral and Bilateral Good Vision." *Ophthalmology* 108 (4): 643–47; discussion 647–48.

Brown, M. M., G. C. Brown, S. Sharma, and S. Garrett. 1999. "Evidence-Based Medicine, Utilities, and Quality of Life." *Current Opinion in Ophthalmology* 10 (3): 221–26.

Brown, M. M., G. C. Brown, S. Sharma, H. Hollands, and A. F. Smith. 2001. "Physician Manpower and Health Care Expenditures in the United States: A Thirty-Year Perspective." *Journal of Health Care Finance* 27 (4): 55–64.

Brown, M. M., G. C. Brown, S. Sharma, and J. Landy. 2003. "Health Care Economic Analyses and Value-Based Medicine." *Survey of Ophthalmology* 48 (2): 204–23.

Brown, M. M., G. C. Brown, S. Sharma, and G. Shah. 1999. "Utility Values and Diabetic Retinopathy." *American Journal of Ophthalmology* 128 (3): 324–30.

Brown, G. C., S. Sharma, M. M. Brown, and S. Garrett. 1999. "Evidence-Based Medicine and Cost-Effectiveness." *Journal of Health Care Finance* 26 (2): 14–23.

Busbee, B. G., M. M. Brown, G. C. Brown, and S. Sharma. 2002. "Incremental Cost-Effectiveness of Initial Cataract Surgery." *Ophthalmology* 109 (3): 606–12; discussion 612–13.

———. 2003. "Cost-Utility Analysis of Cataract Surgery in the Second Eye." *Ophthalmology* 110 (12): 2310–17.

Castells, X., J. Alonso, C. Ribó, A. Casado, J. A. Buil, and others. 1999. "Comparison of the Results of First and Second Cataract Eye Surgery." *Ophthalmology* 106 (4): 676–82.

Courtright, P., S. Kanjaloti, and S. Lewallen. 1995. "Barriers to Acceptance of Cataract Surgery among Patients Presenting to District Hospitals in Rural Malawi." *Tropical Geographical Medicine* 47 (1): 15–18.

Courtright, P., N. Metcalfe, A. Hoechsmann, M. Chirambo, S. Lewallen, and others. 2004. "Cataract Surgical Coverage and Outcome of Cataract Surgery in a Rural District in Malawi." *Canadian Journal of Ophthalmology* 39 (1): 25–30.

Courtright, P., L. Ndegwa, J. Msosa, and J. Banzi. 2007. "Use of Our Existing Eye Care Human Resources: Assessment of the Productivity of Cataract Surgeons Trained in Eastern Africa." *Archives of Ophthalmology* 125 (5): 684–87.

Cunningham, E. T., Jr. 2001. "World Blindness—No End in Sight." *British Journal of Ophthalmology* 85 (3): 253.

Desai, P., A. Reidy, D. C. Minassian, G. Vafidis, and J. Bolger. 1996. "Gains from Cataract Surgery: Visual Function and Quality of Life." *British Journal of Ophthalmology* 80 (10): 868–73.

Fletcher, A., M. Donoghue, J. Devavaram, R. D. Thulasiraj, S. Scott, and others. 1999. "Low Uptake of Eye Services in Rural India: A Challenge for Programs of Blindness Prevention." *Archives of Ophthalmology* 117 (10): 1393–99.

Fletcher, A., V. Vijaykumar, S. Selvaraj, R. D. Thulasiraj, and L. B. Ellwein. 1998. "The Madurai Intraocular Lens Study. III: Visual Functioning and Quality of Life Outcomes." *American Journal of Ophthalmology* 125 (1): 26–35.

Frick, K. D., and A. Foster. 2003. "The Magnitude and Cost of Global Blindness: An Increasing Problem That Can Be Alleviated." *American Journal of Ophthalmology* 135 (4): 471–76.

Gafni, A. 1994. "The Standard Gamble Method: What Is Being Measured and How It Is Interpreted." *Health Services Research* 29 (2): 207–24.

George, R., P. Rupauliha, A. V. Sripriya, P. S. Rajesh, P. V. Vahan, and S. Praveen. 2005. "Comparison of Endothelial Cell Loss and Surgically Induced Astigmatism Following Conventional Extracapsular Cataract Surgery, Manual Small-Incision Surgery and Phacoemulsification." *Ophthalmic Epidemiology* 12 (5): 293–97.

Gogate, P., M. Deshpande, and P. K. Nirmalan. 2007. "Why Do Phacoemulsification? Manual Small-Incision Cataract Surgery Is Almost as Effective, but Less Expensive." *Ophthalmology* 114 (5): 965–68.

Gogate, P. M., M. Deshpande, R. P. Wormald, R. Deshpande, and S. R. Kulkarni. 2003. "Extracapsular Cataract Surgery Compared with Manual Small Incision Cataract Surgery in Community Eye Care Setting in Western India: A Randomised Controlled Trial." *British Journal of Ophthalmology* 87 (6): 667–72.

Gogate, P. M., S. R. Kulkarni, S. Krishnaiah, R. D. Deshpande, S. A. Joshi, and others. 2005. "Safety and Efficacy of Phacoemulsification Compared with Manual Small-Incision Cataract Surgery by a Randomized Controlled Clinical Trial: Six-Week Results." *Ophthalmology* 112 (5): 869–74.

Gokhale, N. S., and S. Sawhney. 2005. "Reduction in Astigmatism in Manual Small Incision Cataract Surgery through Change of Incision Site." *Indian Journal of Ophthalmology* 53 (3): 201–03.

Groot, W. 2000. "Adaptation and Scale of Reference Bias in Self-Assessments of Quality of Life." *Journal of Health Economics* 19 (3): 403–20.

Gupta, S. K., and G. V. Murthy. 1995. "Where Do Persons with Blindness Caused by Cataracts in Rural Areas of India Seek Treatment and Why?" *Archives of Ophthalmology* 113 (10): 1337–40.

Habiyakire, C., G. Kabona, P. Courtright, and S. Lewallen. 2010. "Rapid Assessment of Avoidable Blindness and Cataract Surgical Services in Kilimanjaro Region, Tanzania." *Ophthalmic Epidemiology* 17 (2): 90–94.

Huang, S., Y. Zheng, P. J. Foster, W. Huang, and M. He. 2009. "Prevalence and Causes of Visual Impairment in Chinese Adults in Urban Southern China." *Archives of Ophthalmology* 127 (10): 1362–67.

International Council of Ophthalmology. 2002. "Visual Standards—Aspects and Range of Vision Loss, with Emphasis on Population Surveys." A report at the 29th International Congress of Ophthalmology, Sydney, Australia.

Javitt, J. C., M. H. Brenner, B. Curbow, M. W. Legro, and D. A. Street. 1993. "Outcomes of Cataract Surgery: Improvement in Visual Acuity and Subjective Visual Function after Surgery in the First, Second, and Both Eyes." *Archives of Ophthalmology* 111 (5): 686–91.

Javitt, J. C., E. P. Steinberg, P. Sharkey, O. D. Schein, J. M. Tielsch, and others. 1995. "Cataract Surgery in One Eye or Both: A Billion Dollar per Year Issue." *Ophthalmology* 102 (11): 1583–92; discussion 1592–93.

Javitt, J., G. Venkataswamy, and A. Somme. 1983. "The Economic and Social Aspects of Restoring Sight." In *ACTA: 24th International Congress of Ophthalmology*, edited by P. Henkind, 1308–12. New York: J. B. Lippincott.

Jonas, J. B., R. George, R. Asokan, S. R. Flaxman, J. Keeffe, and others. 2014. "Prevalence and Causes of Vision Loss in Central and South Asia: 1990–2010." *British Journal of Ophthalmology* 98 (5): 592–98.

Keeffe, J., H. R. Taylor, K. Fotis, K. Pesudovs, S. R. Fkaxnab, and others. 2014. "Prevalence and Causes of Vision Loss in Southeast Asia and Oceania: 1990–2010." *British Journal of Ophthalmology* 98 (5): 586–91.

Kimani, K., W. Mathenge, M. Sheila, O. Oscar, W. Wachira, and others. 2008. "Cataract Surgical Services, Outcomes and Barriers in Kericho, Bureti and Bomet Districts, Kenya." *East African Journal of Ophthalmology* 13: 36–41.

Kimura, H., S. Kuroda, N. Mizoguchi, H. Terauchi, M. Matsumura, and M. Nagata. 1999. "Extracapsular Cataract Extraction with a Sutureless Incision for Dense Cataracts." *Journal of Cataract and Refractive Surgery* 25 (9): 1275–79.

Kobelt, G., M. Lundström, and U. Stenevi. 2002. "Cost-Effectiveness of Cataract Surgery: Method to Assess Cost-Effectiveness Using Registry Data." *Journal of Cataract and Refractive Surgery* 28 (10): 1742–49.

Komolafe, O. O., A. O. Ashaye, B. G. K. Ajayi, and C. O. Bekibele. 2010. "Visual Impairment from Age-Related Cataract among an Indigenous African Population." *Eye* 24 (1): 53–58.

Lam, B. L., S. L. Christ, D. J. Lee, D. D. Zheng, and K. L. Arheart. 2008. "Reported Visual Impairment and Risk of Suicide: The 1986–1996 National Health Interview Surveys." *Archives of Ophthalmology* 126 (7): 975–80.

Lansingh, V. C., M. J. Carter, and M. Martens. 2007. "Global Cost-Effectiveness of Cataract Surgery." *Ophthalmology* 114 (9): 1670–78.

Laupacis, A., D. Feeny, A. S. Detsky, and P. X. Tugwell. 1992. "How Attractive Does a New Technology Have to Be to Warrant Adoption and Utilization? Tentative Guidelines for Using Clinical and Economic Evaluations." *Canadian Medical Association Journal* 146 (4): 473–81.

Lee, J. E., P. J. Fos, M. A. Zuniga, P. R. Kastl, and J. H. Sung. 2000. "Assessing Health-Related Quality of Life in Cataract Patients: The Relationship between Utility and Health-Related Quality of Life Measurement." *Quality of Life Research* 9 (10): 1127–35.

Lewallen, S., E. Eliah, and S. Gilbert. 2006. "The Cost of Outreach Services in Eastern Africa." *IAPB (International Agency for the Prevention of Blindness) News* 50: 16–17.

Lewallen, S., A. Mousa, K. Bassett, and P. Courtright. 2009. "Cataract Surgical Coverage Remains Lower in Women." *British Journal of Ophthalmology* 93 (3): 295–98.

Lewallen, S., and R. D. Thulasiraj. 2010. "Eliminating Cataract Blindness: How Do We Apply Lessons from Asia to Sub-Saharan Africa"? *Global Public Health* 5 (6): 639–48.

Li, L., H. Guan, P. Xun, J. Zhou, and H. Gu. 2008. "Prevalence and Causes of Visual Impairment among the Elderly in Nantong, China." *Eye* 22 (8): 1069–75.

Li, Z., H. Cui, L. Zhang, P. Liu, and H. Yang. 2009. "Cataract Blindness and Surgery among the Elderly in Rural Southern Harbin, China." *Ophthalmic Epidemiology* 16 (2): 78–83.

Lundstrom, M., and E. Wendel. 2005. "Duration of Self Assessed Benefit of Cataract Extraction: A Long Term Study." *British Journal of Ophthalmology* 89 (8): 1017–20.

Lutz, W., W. Sanderson, and S. Scherbov. 1997. "Doubling of World Population Unlikely." *Nature* 387 (6635): 803–05.

Malik, A. N. J., A. Cassels-Brown, R. Wormald, and J. A. M. Gray. 2013. "Better Value Eye Care for the 21st Century: The Population Approach." *British Journal of Ophthalmology* 97 (5): 553–57.

Marseille, E. 1996. "Cost-Effectiveness of Cataract Surgery in a Public Health Eye Care Programme in Nepal." *Bulletin of the World Health Organization* 74 (3): 319–24.

Mathenge, W., J. Nkurikiye, H. Limburg, and H. Kuper. 2007. "Rapid Assessment of Avoidable Blindness in Western Rwanda: Blindness in a Postconflict Setting." *PLoS Medicine* 4: e217.

Muralikrishnan, R., R. Venkatesh, N. V. Prajna, and K. J. D. Frick. 2004. "Economic Cost of Cataract Surgery Procedures in an Established Eye Care Centre in Southern India." *Ophthalmic Epidemiology* 11 (5): 369–80.

Murray, C. J. L., and A. D. Lopez, eds. 1996. *The Global Burden of Disease: A Comprehensive Assessment of Mortality and Disability from Diseases, Injuries, and Risk Factors in 1990 and Projected to 2020*. Cambridge, MA: Harvard University Press.

Murthy, G. V. S., P. Vashist, N. John, G. Pokharel, and L. B. Ellwein. 2010. "Prevalence and Causes of Visual Impairment and Blindness in Older Adults in an Area of India with a High Cataract Surgical Rate." *Ophthalmic Epidemiology* 17 (4): 185–95.

Natchiar, G., A. L. Robin, R. D. Thulasiraj, and S. Krishnaswamy. 1994. "Attacking the Backlog of India's Curable Blind: The Aravind Eye Hospital Model." *Archives of Ophthalmology* 112 (7): 987–93.

Neena, J., J. Rachel, V. Praveen, and G. V. S. Murthy. 2008. "Rapid Assessment of Avoidable Blindness in India." *PLoS One* 3: e2867.

Ono, K., Y. Hiratsuka, and A. Murakami. 2010. "Global Inequality in Eye Health: Country-Level Analysis from the Global Burden of Disease Study." *American Journal of Public Health* 100 (9): 1784–88.

Oye, J. E., B. Dineen, R. Befidi-Mengue, and A. Foster. 2006. "Prevalence and Causes of Blindness and Visual Impairment in Muyuka: A Rural Health District in South West Province, Cameroon." *British Journal of Ophthalmology* 90 (5): 538–42.

Oye, J. E., and H. Kuper. 2007. "Prevalence and Causes of Blindness and Visual Impairment in Limbe Urban Area, South West Province, Cameroon." *British Journal of Ophthalmology* 91 (11): 1435–39.

Pascolini, D., and S. P. Mariotti. 2012. "Global Estimates of Visual Impairment: 2010." *British Journal of Ophthalmology* 96 (5): 614–18.

Patino, C. M., R. McKean-Cowdin, S. P. Azen, J. C. Allison, F. Choudhury, and R. Varma. 2010. "Central and Peripheral Visual Impairment and the Risk of Falls and Falls with Injury." *Ophthalmology* 117 (2): 199–206.e1.

PwC (PricewaterhouseCoopers). 2012. *The Price of Sight: The Global Cost of Eliminating Avoidable Blindness*. Final report for the Fred Hollows Foundation. Melbourne, Australia: PricewaterhouseCoopers.

Rabiu, M. M., and N. Muhammed. 2008. "Rapid Assessment of Cataract Surgical Services in Birnin-Kebbi Local Government Area of Kebbi State, Nigeria." *Ophthalmic Epidemiology* 15 (6): 359–65.

Ramakrishanan, R., D. Maheshwari, M. A. Kader, R. Singh, N. Pawar, and M. J. Bharathi. 2010. "Visual Prognosis, Intraocular Pressure Control and Complications in Phacomorphic Glaucoma Following Manual Small Incision Cataract Surgery." *Indian Journal of Ophthalmology* 58 (4): 303–6.

Rangan, V. K., and R. D. Thulasiraj. 2007. "Making Sight Affordable." *Innovations* 2 (4): 35–49.

Räsänen, P., K. Krootila, H. Sintonen, T. Leivo, A.-M. Koivisto, and others. 2006. "Cost-Utility of Routine Cataract Surgery." *Health Quality of Life Outcomes* 4: 74.

Ravindran, R. D., R. Venkatesh, D. F. Chang, S. Sengupta, J. Gyatsho, and B. Talwar. 2009. "Incidence of Post-cataract Endophthalmitis at Aravind Eye Hospital: Outcomes of More than 42,000 Consecutive Cases Using Standardized Sterilization and Prophylaxis Protocols." *Journal of Cataract and Refractive Surgery* 35 (4): 629–36.

Reddy, B., A. Raj, and V. P. Singh. 2007. "Site of Incision and Corneal Astigmatism in Conventional SICS versus Phacoemulsification." *Annals of Ophthalmology* (Skokie) 39 (3): 209–16.

Resnikoff, S., W. Felch, T. M. Gauthier, and B. Spivey. 2012. "The Number of Ophthalmologists in Practice and Training Worldwide: A Growing Gap Despite More than 200,000 Practitioners." *British Journal of Ophthalmology* 96 (6): 783–87.

Resnikoff, S., D. Pascolini, D. Etya'ale, I. Kocur, R. Pararajasegaram, and others. 2004. "Global Data on Visual Impairment in the Year 2002." *Bulletin of the World Health Organization* 82 (11): 844–51.

Rosen, P. N., R. M. Kaplan, and K. David. 2005. "Measuring Outcomes of Cataract Surgery Using the Quality of Well-Being Scale and VF-14 Visual Function Index." *Journal of Cataract and Refractive Surgery* 31 (2): 369–78.

Rubin, G. S., S. K. West, B. Muñoz, K. Bandeen-Roche, S. Zeger, and others. 1997. "A Comprehensive Assessment of Visual Impairment in a Population of Older Americans. The SEE Study. Salisbury Eye Evaluation Project." *Investigative Ophthalmology and Visual Science* 38 (3): 557–68.

Ruit, S., G. Tabin, D. Chang, L. Bajracharya, D. C. Kline, and others. 2007. "A Prospective Randomized Clinical Trial of Phacoemulsification vs Manual Sutureless Small-Incision Extracapsular Cataract Surgery in Nepal." *American Journal of Ophthalmology* 143 (1): 32–38.

Salive, M. E., J. Guralnik, R. J. Glynn, W. Christen, R. B. Wallace, and A. M. Ostfeld. 1994. "Association of Visual Impairment with Mobility and Physical Function." *Journal of the American Geriatric Society* 42 (3): 287–92.

Salomão, S. R., R. W. Cinoto, A. Berezovsky, A. Araújo-Filho, M. R. Mitsuhiro, and others. 2008. "Prevalence and Causes of Vision Impairment and Blindness in Older Adults in Brazil: The São Paulo Eye Study." *Ophthalmic Epidemiology* 15 (3): 167–75.

Sherchan, A., R. P. Kandel, M. K. Sharma, Y. D. Sapkota, J. Aghajanian, and K. L. Bassett. 2010. "Blindness Prevalence and Cataract Surgical Coverage in Lumbini Zone and Chetwan District of Nepal." *British Journal of Ophthalmology* 94 (2): 161–66.

Singh, A. J., P. Garner, and K. Floyd. 2000. "Cost-Effectiveness of Public-Funded Options for Cataract Surgery in Mysore, India." *The Lancet* 355 (9199): 180–84.

Smith, A. F., and J. G. Smith. 1996. "The Economic Burden of Global Blindness: A Price Too High." *British Journal of Ophthalmology* 80 (4): 276–77.

Stevens, G. A., R. A. White, S. R. Flaxman, H. Price, J. B. Jonas, and others, for the Vision Loss Expert Group. 2013. "Global Prevalence of Vision Impairment and Blindness: Magnitude and Temporal Trends, 1990–2010." *Ophthalmology* 120 (12): 2377–84.

Stuck, A. E., J. M. Walthert, T. Nikolaus, C. J. Büla, C. Hohmann, and J. C. Beck. 1999. "Risk Factors for Functional Status Decline in Community-Living Elderly People: A Systematic Literature Review." *Social Science and Medicine* 48 (4): 445–69.

Thylefors, B. 1998. "A Global Initiative for the Elimination of Avoidable Blindness." *American Journal of Ophthalmology* 125 (1): 90–93.

Thylefors, B., A. D. Négrel, R. Pararajasegaram, and K. Y. Dadzie. 1995. "Global Data on Blindness." *Bulletin of the World Health Organization* 73 (1): 115–21.

Venkataswamy, G., and G. Brilliant. 1981. "Social and Economic Barriers to Cataract Surgery in Rural South India: A Preliminary Report." *Journal of Visual Impairment and Blindness* 405–08.

Venkatesh, R., D. F. Chang, R. Muralikrishnan, K. Hemal, P. Gogate, and S. Sengupta. 2012. "Manual Small Incision Cataract Surgery: A Review." *Asia Pacific Journal of Ophthalmology* 1 (2): 113–19.

Venkatesh, R., M. Das, S. Prashanth, and R. Muralikrishnan. 2005. "Manual Small Incision Cataract Surgery in Eyes with White Cataracts." *Indian Journal of Ophthalmology* 53: 173–76.

Venkatesh, R., R. Muralikrishnan, L. C. Balent, S. K. Prakash, and N. V. Prajna. 2005. "Outcomes of High Volume Cataract Surgeries in a Developing Country." *British Journal of Ophthalmology* 89 (9): 1079–83.

Venkatesh, R., C. S. H. Tan, T. T. Kumar, and R. D. Ravindran. 2007. "Safety and Efficacy of Manual Small Incision Cataract Surgery for Phacolytic Glaucoma." *British Journal of Ophthalmology* 91 (3): 279–81.

Venkatesh, R., C. S. H. Tan, S. Sengupta, R. D. Ravindran, K. T. Krishnan, and D. F. Chang. 2010. "Phacoemulsification versus Manual Small-Incision Cataract Surgery for White Cataract." *Journal of Cataract and Refractive Surgery* 36 (11): 1849–54.

Venkatesh, R., C. S. H. Tan, G. P. Singh, K. Veena, K. T. Krishnan, and R. D. Ravindran. 2009. "Safety and Efficacy of Manual

Small Incision Cataract Surgery for Brunescent and Black Cataracts." *Eye* 23 (5): 1155–57.

Wakker, P., and A. Stiggelbout. 1995. "Explaining Distortions in Utility Elicitation through the Rank-Dependent Model for Risky Choices." *Medical Decision Making* 15 (2): 180–86.

West, S. K., B. Munoz, G. S. Rubin, O. D. Schein, K. Bandeen-Roche, and others. 1997. "Function and Visual Impairment in a Population-Based Study of Older Adults: The SEE Project. Salisbury Eye Evaluation." *Investigative Ophthalmology and Visual Science* 38 (1): 72–82.

WHO (World Health Organization). 1998. "Informal Consultation on Analysis of Blindness Prevention Outcomes." WHO/PBL/98.68, Geneva, WHO.

———. 2000. *World Health Report 2000—Health Systems: Improving Performance.* Geneva: WHO.

———. 2003. "Consultation on Development of Standards for Characterization of Vision Loss and Visual Functioning." WHO/PUBL/03.91, WHO, Geneva.

———. 2010. "Prevention of Blindness and Visual Impairment." WHO/NMH/PBD/12.01. WHO, Geneva. http://www.who .int/blindness/GLOBALDATAFINALforweb.pdf

———. 2008. "Change the Definition of Blindness." WHO, Geneva. http://www.who.int/blindness/Change%20the%20 Definition%20of%20Blindness.pdf.

———. 2013. "Global Health Estimates for Deaths by Cause, Age, and Sex for Years 2000–2011." WHO, Geneva. http:// www.who.int/healthinfo/global_health_estimates/en/.

Woldeyes, A., and Y. Adamu. 2008. "Gender Differences in Adult Blindness and Low Vision, Central Ethiopia." *Ethiopian Medical Journal* 46 (3): 211–18.

Wong, T. Y., Y. Zheng, J. B. Jonas, S. R. Flaxman, J. Keeffe, and others. 2014. "Prevalence and Causes of Vision Loss in East Asia: 1990–2010." *British Journal of Ophthalmology* 98 (5): 599–604.

World Bank. 2001. *World Development Indicators 2001.* CD-ROM. Washington, DC: World Bank.

———. 2009. "World Bank List of Economies." World Bank, Washington, DC. http://siteresources.worldbank.org /DATASTATISTICS/Resources/CIASS.xls.

Zheng, D. D., S. L. Christ, B. L. Lam, K. L. Arheart, A. Galor, and D. J. Lee. 2012. "Increased Mortality Risk among the Visually Impaired: The Roles of Mental Well-Being and Preventive Care Practices." *Investigative Ophthalmology and Visual Science* 53 (6): 2685–92.

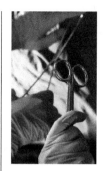

Organization of Essential Services and the Role of First-Level Hospitals

Colin McCord, Margaret E. Kruk, Charles N. Mock, Meena Cherian, Johan von Schreeb, Sarah Russell, and Mike English

INTRODUCTION

Every country has some sort of system to provide surgical and other health services at various levels, with a progressive increase in the capacity to treat more complicated problems. Reliable evidence indicates that properly functioning small hospitals and health centers can deliver effective basic surgical services at very low cost; these surgical services can be one of the most cost-effective components of the public health system in low- and middle-income countries (LMICs) (Alkire and others 2012; Debas and others 2006; Gosselin, Maldonado, and Elder 2010; Gosselin, Thind, and Bellardinelli 2006; McCord and Chowdhury 2003). *Properly functioning* is a key phrase; a hospital lacking personnel trained in surgery and in the administration of anesthesia cannot provide major surgical procedures. Even minor surgery requires trained personnel. More than 50 percent of the disability-adjusted life years (DALYs) averted in a small hospital can derive from surgical treatment, (McCord and Chowdhury 2003) so the cost-effectiveness of these units is drastically reduced if this treatment is not available. Box 12.1 defines the three levels of hospital care.

Recommended Skills and Services

The World Health Organization (WHO) and others have provided descriptions of what services would be available at properly functioning first-, second-, and third-level

facilities, and how such systems could function (Debas and others 2006; WHO 1992, 2003, 2010). The WHO has assisted countries in analyzing their current systems and asked them to make realistic plans to get from where they are to a point closer to the ideal. Chapter 67 in *Disease Control Priorities in Developing Countries*, second edition (DCP2), presents a detailed outline of what skills, services, and infrastructure would be available in an ideal district hospital and calculates the cost in 2004 U.S. dollars (Debas and others 2006).

This chapter considers, and generally follows, the recommendations of DCP2 and the WHO, discusses what is actually available in LMICs, and considers how to move from the current situation to an achievable improvement. The emphasis is on first-level hospitals—the lowest level hospital that provides major surgery—and the systems to support them.

Referral Systems

Referrals of surgical patients from lower levels such as clinics to first-level hospitals, as well as from first-level facilities to second- and third-level facilities, is an essential part of any system; however, in LMICs, the transport of referred patients is a major problem for families with low incomes. If surgical care is not available at an accessible first-level hospital, it is effectively beyond the reach of at least 1 billion people (Weiser and others 2008). This group includes 80 percent of the population

Corresponding author: Colin McCord, MD, Columbia University (retired), cwm1@columbia.edu

Box 12.1

Levels of Hospital Care in Low- and Middle-Income Countries

Crucial treatment for surgical conditions can be available in clinics and dispensaries, especially treatment for surgical infections and simple trauma. However, the lack of trained staff, limited supplies, and unavailability of anesthesia seriously restrict the services that can be offered in these facilities, so most patients with important problems need to find hospitals (table B12.1.1).

The principal function of second- and third-level hospitals is to provide more complex clinical care to patients referred from lower levels; however, no agreed-on international definition determines which specific services should be provided at hospitals at the three levels in these settings. The range of services offered tends to vary substantially, even between third-level hospitals within the same country, as much because of historical accident as deliberate design. Also, almost all second- and third-level hospitals provide emergency services for local areas and thereby function as first-level hospitals to varying degrees.

Important differences exist among regions:

- In Sub-Saharan Africa, first-level hospitals are usually small facilities, serving populations of fewer than 500,000. They rarely have specialized physicians on staff. Surgical services are provided by general practitioners, often recent medical school graduates. In some countries (notably Malawi, Mozambique, Tanzania, and Zambia), nonphysician clinicians (NPCs) have been trained to do major surgery.
- In South Asia, first-level hospitals are larger and commonly serve much larger populations of 1 million to 2 million or more. They usually have several specialists on staff. Nonphysicians rarely perform major surgery.
- In Latin America and the Caribbean, small hospitals often provide first-level surgical services to populations of fewer than 100,000. They usually have a surgeon and an obstetrician, and nonphysicians do not perform major surgery.

Table B12.1.1 Definitions of Levels of Hospital Care

Level of care	Alternative terms commonly found in the literature
First-level hospitals: Few specialties—mainly internal medicine, obstetrics and gynecology, pediatrics, and general surgery; often only one general practice physician or a nonphysician practitioner; limited laboratory services available for general but not specialized pathological analysis; from 50 to 250 beds.	Primary-level hospital
	District hospital
	Rural hospital
	Community hospital
	General hospital
Second-level hospitals: More differentiated by function with as many as 5 to 10 clinical specialties; from 200 to 800 beds.	Regional hospital
	Provincial hospital (or equivalent administrative area such as county)
	General hospital
Third-level hospitals: Highly specialized staff and technical equipment—for example, cardiology, intensive care unit, and specialized imaging units; clinical services highly differentiated by function; could have teaching activities; from 300 to 1,500 beds.	National hospital
	Central hospital
	Academic or teaching or university hospital

Source: Adapted from Mulligan and others 2003.

of Sub-Saharan Africa and 60 percent of the population of South Asia, as well as large parts of the populations of Latin America and the Caribbean and middle-income countries (MICs) in other regions.

Distance and lack of transportation restrict patient travel outside of local areas, but the real barrier is cost.

Transportation can generally be found, but the cost usually falls on the patient. Additional high costs include transportation of and accommodations for family members to accompany patients, the opportunity costs of family members taken away from work, medical supplies not provided by hospitals, and often "informal payments" to hospital staff. Moreover, many patients are not in any condition to withstand a long trip, even if they can afford it.

The need for first-level hospitals is not limited to rural areas. In cities, population growth can overwhelm the third-level central hospitals; smaller urban hospitals are too often unable to provide 24-hour emergency services, except in private facilities that are too costly for most urban residents in LMICs.

Capacity Constraints

These issues place first-level hospitals at the center of any system to provide surgery in LMICs (Kushner and others 2010). Major constraints limit their capacity. These constraints reflect the extremely low budgets within which these hospitals must function—usually less than US$30 per day per patient in Sub-Saharan Africa (Kruk and others 2010)—and include the following:

- Lack of trained staff
- Inadequate supplies
- Inadequate maintenance of basic equipment
- Poor condition of buildings and intermittent or absent water and electricity
- Transportation challenges that restrict the effectiveness of a functioning referral system

FIRST-LEVEL HOSPITALS: POTENTIAL VERSUS REALITY

The Ideal

Although most health systems are organized as a pyramid, with primary care facilities at the base and national third-level hospitals at the apex, the specifics vary among countries (Chatterjee, Levin, and Laxminarayan 2013; Galukande and others 2010; Lebrun and others 2013; Zafar and McQueen 2011). In most of Sub-Saharan Africa, dispensaries and health centers provide primary care, deliver newborns, and usually perform minor surgery. When patients need major surgery, they are meant to be referred to a district (first-level) hospital, usually with 100 to 200 beds, serving a population of 100,000 to 500,000 (Galukande and others 2010). In Bangladesh, India, and Pakistan, the smallest unit regularly providing major surgery is also called a *district hospital*, but the districts are much bigger, usually with a population of 2 million or more (Chatterjee, Levin, and Laxminarayan 2013; Lebrun and others 2013; Zafar and McQueen 2011). In Latin America and the Caribbean, many quite small "basic hospitals" provide first-level surgical functions for populations of fewer than 100,000, and

refer patients to a fairly extensive network of second- and third-level hospitals (Lebrun and others 2012; Solis and others 2013).

However the pyramid is structured, the constraints listed previously seriously limit the way it can function. The two most important and difficult of these constraints are the shortage of trained staff, which limits the services that can be provided, especially in first-level hospitals, and the weakness of the referral system, which often makes it impossible to send patients to a higher level, where more highly trained staff may be available. Clearly, the two problems work against each other. If trained staff are not available, patients should be referred. If they cannot be referred, they often do not receive appropriate treatment, which can lead to death or serious disability. Although the emphasis today needs to be on initiatives to increase the capacity of peripheral first-level hospitals, access to transportation and referral can reduce the need for this expansion of capacity and lead to a more efficient system.

In DCP2, Debas and others (2006) list the resource requirements for surgical services in ideal LMIC clinics and hospitals, based on their own estimates and those of the WHO (table 12.1).

The Reality

Table 12.2 presents the actual situation in 3 first-level hospitals in Tanzania, as well as the averages for 11 hospitals in Bolivia and 7 in Bangladesh.

- The Kasulu District Hospital is typical of the second-level hospitals in Tanzania and most other Sub-Saharan African countries, except that the population served is more than twice the national average. The one physician also serves as the district medical officer, an administrative job that occupies most of the physician's time. No specialists and no one fully qualified in surgery or obstetrics is on staff. Assistant medical officers (NPCs with six months of formal surgical and obstetrical training) perform the surgery.
- The Maweni Regional Hospital serves as the first-level hospital for two districts and receives few patients as referrals for higher-level care, a common situation in Tanzania. There are six physicians, including one academically qualified pediatrician, but no qualified surgeon or obstetrician. NPCs perform all of the surgery.
- The St. Francis Designated District Hospital is a large, faith-based hospital that serves as a designated first-level hospital for two districts. Although it has been named a regional referral hospital, it still serves a first-level function because a new first-level hospital has not yet been created. The six qualified specialists

Table 12.1 Resource Requirements for Surgical Services by Level of Care: The Ideal

Category of requirement	Community clinic	100-bed district (second-level) hospital	Third-level hospital
Infrastructure	Weatherproof building (100 square meters) Storage space Clean water supply Power supply	Inpatient facility of 100 beds, including several wards and an isolation ward Outpatient facility including an emergency room; operating rooms (at least two: one clean, one contaminated) Labor and delivery rooms Recovery room or intensive care unit Blood bank Pharmacy Clinical laboratory Radiology and ultrasonography suite	A major facility providing • Full emergency services with advanced diagnostic services • Inpatient wards for complex general medical and surgical care • Various types of specialty services • Several delivery rooms and operating rooms • One or more recovery rooms and intensive care units • Rehabilitation and occupational therapy facilities
Equipment and supplies	Furniture Refrigerator Blood pressure machine Minor surgical trays Sterile and burn dressings Autoclave Intravenous sets and solutions Bandages and splints Drugs: local anesthetics, nonsteroidal anti-inflammatory drugs, antibiotics, tetanus toxoid, silver nitrate ointment, oxytocin, magnesium sulfate Wireless communication equipment Materials for recordkeeping	Anesthetic machines and inhalation gases Monitors (electrocardiogram, blood pressure, pulse oximetry) Fully equipped operating room Fully equipped delivery room Fully equipped recovery room or intensive care unit Respirators and oxygen supply Blood products and intravenous fluids Basic microbiology equipment Pharmaceuticals, (anesthetics, analgesics, antibiotics) Surgical materials (drapes, gowns, dressings, gloves), and other consumables (disposable equipment and devices)	Equipment and supplies as for the 100-bed (first-level) hospital, plus all required equipment and supplies to undertake the range of routine and complex services provided
Human resources[a]	Nurse or nurse equivalent Skilled birth attendant Orderly	Nurses (50+) Midwives (5+) Anesthetists (2–3) Anesthesiologist (1)[b] Primary care physicians (4)[c] Obstetrician/gynecologist (1 or 2) General surgeons (2) Pharmacy assistants (2) Pharmacist (1)[b] Radiology technician (1) Radiologist (1) Physiotherapist (1)	Nurses (100+) Midwives (20+) Anesthetists (5) Anesthesiologists (3) Primary care physicians (10) Obstetricians and gynecologists (5) General surgeons (5) Orthopedic surgeon (1) Pharmacy assistants (2) Pharmacist (1) Radiology technicians (5)

table continues next page

Table 12.1 Resource Requirements for Surgical Services by Level of Care: The Ideal **(continued)**

Category of requirement	Community clinic	100-bed district (second-level) hospital	Third-level hospital
			Radiologists (2)
			Physiotherapists (5)
			Neurosurgeon (1)[b]
			Cardiac surgeon[b]
			Reconstructive surgeon[b]

Source: Debas and others 2006.

a. The variability in the size and the complexity of services provided by third-level hospitals makes it difficult to describe a standard third-level hospital; the human resource needs given in the table represent what is thought to be minimally adequate.

b. Desirable but not absolutely necessary.

c. May be a general internist, general practitioner, or general pediatrician.

Table 12.2 Human Resources and Infrastructure at Selected First-Level Hospitals in Three Regions: The Reality

	Kasulu District Hospital, Tanzania, 2010	Maweni Regional Hospital, Tanzania, 2013	St. Francis Designated District Hospital, Tanzania, 2013	11 "basic" (first-level) hospitals Bolivia,[a] 2012	7 district (first-level) hospitals, Bangladesh,[a] 2013
Population served	677,000	850,000	500,000+	134,000	1,879,000
Beds	200	256	372	54	140
Admissions per year	12,900	25,800	18,140	3,644	20,000
Operating rooms	3	3	3	2.1	2.4
Physicians	1	6	14	29.4	29.3
General surgeons	0	0	2	3.4	1.6
Obstetricians and gynecologists	0	0	3	3.5	1.4
Orthopedic surgeons	0	0	1	1.4	1.1
Anesthesiologists	0	0	2	3	1
Nurses	61	57	126	24.5	50.5
Beds per nurse	3.3	4.5	3.0	2.2	2.8
Nonphysician clinicians	23	29	8	0	0
Physicians and nonphysician clinicians per 100 beds	12	14	6	54	21

Sources: Kruk and others 2010; Lebrun and others 2012, 2013.

a. Average for all hospitals reviewed.

provide approximately 50 percent of the surgery, and NPCs provide the remainder.

- Bolivia, a lower-middle-income country with a large, very poor population, has trained enough physicians to be able to staff its first-level hospitals with qualified specialists.
- In Bangladesh, as in India, Pakistan, and Sri Lanka, districts are much larger (usually 2 million people or more); first-level surgery is rarely available below the level of the district hospital. Qualified surgeons, obstetricians, and orthopedists are usually present.

Data are not available from these hospitals to permit a calculation of nursing hours per patient-day. One staff nurse per bed is normally required to achieve the usually recommended five to six hours per patient per day for an average hospital (Coffman, Seago, and Spetz 2002; McHugh, Berez, and Small 2013; Needleman and others 2011). The number of beds per nurse far exceeds this level in all of these hospitals.

Surgical and obstetrical specialists are rarely available in Sub-Saharan African first-level hospitals, which typically have one or two general practitioners (often a recently graduated doctor) for whom surgery is one of many clinical and administrative responsibilities. Tanzania is one of several Sub-Saharan African countries that have trained NPCs to provide basic surgery at this level, especially for obstetrical emergencies. In Mozambique, this training is a three-year program focused on all types of basic emergency surgery; but in most countries with these cadres, surgery and obstetrics are part of a course designed to produce general practitioners (see chapter 17).

Virtually every country has a private health sector, which is often divided into charitable facilities (usually faith based) and for-profit facilities. In much of Latin America and the Caribbean, multiple systems work in parallel: a public system for the poorest; a system serving those with insurance usually derived from salaried employment; and a private sector for the more affluent segment of the population (Lebrun and others 2012; Solis and others 2013).

In India, where the private sector accounts for 78 percent of health expenditure (Kumar and others 2011), the supply of medical school graduates is large, and in some places, excessive. In Sub-Saharan Africa the private health sector is much smaller but is growing rapidly, as is the supply of graduate doctors. In both South Asia and Sub-Saharan Africa, no matter how large the supply of doctors, persuading physicians, especially specialists, to work in rural areas or to serve the poor majority in the cities has been difficult. In Latin America and the Caribbean, the number of physicians is much higher, and many first-level hospitals, even

in lower-middle-income countries such as Bolivia and Nicaragua, have specialists (Lebrun and others 2012; Solis and others 2013).

In many Sub-Saharan African countries, mission hospitals (faith-based) can offer to serve as the district (first-level) hospital for a specified area. In Tanzania, for example, if accepted as a "designated district hospital," these faith-based hospitals receive government support for salaries and supplies, and the government does not provide another first-level hospital for that area.

Everywhere, almost all of the second- and third-level hospitals act as first-level hospitals for local emergencies.

Table 12.3 presents the surgical volume and procedures in the same hospitals described in table 12.2. The detailed information presented in these tables is not available on a national scale for any of these countries, but the selected hospitals are probably typical for Latin America and the Caribbean, South Asia, and Sub-Saharan Africa. In Tanzania, private (usually faith-based) hospitals that have become designated district hospitals often have several surgical specialists on staff, and some of them have a larger number of nurses. Second-level hospitals are meant to be referral hospitals, but many in Sub-Saharan Africa have few or no surgical specialists and primarily function as larger first-level hospitals (Sanders and others 1998; Siddiqi and others 2001). South Asia has more physicians and specialists for a given population than Sub-Saharan Africa and Latin America and the Caribbean countries usually have many more than other LMIC regions. In Latin America and the Caribbean, this larger professional force is reflected

Table 12.3 Current Surgical Volume and Major Procedures Performed at Selected First-Level Hospitals in Three Regions

	Kasula District Hospital, Tanzania, 2010	Maweni Regional Hospital, Tanzania, 2013	St. Francis Designated District Hospital, Tanzania, 2013	11 "basic" (first-level) hospitals, Bolivia,[a] 2012	7 "district" (first-level) hospitals, Bangladesh,[a] 2013
Total operations per year	893	915	2,034[c]	730	3,215
General surgery	99 (11%)	119 (13%)	252 (12%)	284 (39%)	845 (26%)
Obstetrics and gynecology	635 (71%)	499 (55%)	1,386 (68%)	311 (43%)[b]	1,077 (33%)
Other	159 (18%)	297 (32%)	396 (19%)	135 (18%)	1,293 (40%)[c]
Population served	677,000	850,000	500,000	134,000	1,879,000
Operations per specialist	n.a.	n.a.	339	88	784
Operations per 100,000 population	132	108	407	545	171

Sources: Kruk and others 2010; Lebrun and others 2012, 2013.

Note: % = percentage of total annual operations that fall within a category; n.a. = not applicable (no specialist surgeons).

a. Average for all hospitals reviewed.

b. Average for hospitals in towns with no maternity hospital.

c. Includes 717 orthopedic operations; 349 ocular operations; and 199 ear, nose, and throat operations.

in adequate (even excessive) numbers of physicians and specialists in small first-level hospitals (Lebrun and others 2012; Solis and others 2013).

In Bangladesh as well as Pakistan, Sri Lanka, and much of India, most major surgery is provided at the district level or above. District hospitals in these countries serve populations of 1 million to 2 million people. These hospitals have specialists available, but the populations served are so large that the numbers of major operations per 100,000 people is comparable to those in Sub-Saharan Africa (Chatterjee, Levin, and Laxminarayan 2013; Lebrun and others 2013; Zafar and McQueen 2011).

The "population served" by these five hospital groups is an approximation given that patients often move in and out of an area to seek hospital care. In some places, such as Kasulu in tables 12.2 and 12.3, transportation is so difficult that practically no movement of patients to other districts occurs, so the population cited is the true catchment area.

In all three regions, operations for obstetrical emergencies are the largest single component of surgical activity; in Tanzania they are by far the most common kind of surgery. All over the world women are aware that these operations can prevent maternal, fetal, and newborn death. The demand for emergency obstetrical surgery is limited primarily by persistent restricted access to hospitals that can provide surgical care. Because the operations are common, relatively safe, and uncomplicated, general practitioners and NPCs have been trained to perform them with considerable success (McCord and others 2009; Pereira and others 1996). Still, met need for obstetrical surgery is 25 percent or less in most of Sub-Saharan Africa and much of South Asia (Paxton, Bailey, and Lobis 2006; Pearson and Shoo 2005). Latin America and the Caribbean have a much larger supply of obstetrical specialists working in first-level hospitals and a correspondingly higher met need and lower maternal mortality, even in very poor countries (Bailey 2005; Hogan and others 2010).

More general surgical operations (including trauma, acute abdomen, and other surgical emergencies) are performed in hospitals that have specialists available, but estimates indicate that in all regions, the met need for these emergencies is even lower than the met need for obstetrical care (chapters 5 and 6). The list of operations actually performed in one year in eight first-level hospitals in Sub-Saharan Africa (table 12.4) shows

Table 12.4 Annual Major Operations at Eight First-Level Hospitals in Sub-Saharan Africa
Percent, except as noted

Procedure	Tanzania, 2007		Mozambique, 2007		Uganda, 2006			
	Bagamoyo	Kasulu	Chokwe	Catandica	Mityana	Kiryandongo	Buluba	Iganga
Major nonobstetric (number)	428	242	171	133	456	80	125	711
Amputation	0	3	2	8	0	1	10	1
Appendectomy	11	2	6	2	2	0	1	4
Circumcision	0	1	13	18	1	68	1	0
Excision	0	10	0	5	0	0	0	0
Herniorrhaphy	22	24	17	20	41	16	24	29
Hydrocelectomy	13	8	4	20	2	1	4	0
Hysterectomy (elective)	6	2	9	0	5	1	2	17
Laparotomy	6	26	20	10	3	5	10	43
Open fracture reduction	3	0	2	0	31	0	0	0
Other	9	24	29	17	15	8	48	5
Obstetric (number)	431	883	377	110	754	35	100	915
Tubal ligation	6	11	7	4	10	14	0	0
Cesarean	61	62	80	73	63	74	88	88
Evacuation of uterus	30	22	0	1	19	0	0	0
Other	3	5	13	23	8	11	12	12

Source: Galukande and others 2010.
Note: Data are based on annual aggregate hospital statistics extracted from hospital information systems.

Table 12.5 Surgical Procedures That Could Be Managed at First- and Second-Level Hospitals

First-level hospitals with general practitioner surgeon or nonphysician clinician surgeon	Second-level hospitals with qualified specialist available (all first-level operations, as well as the following)
Emergency obstetrical surgery (including repair of ruptured uterus and emergency hysterectomy)	Elective major gynecological surgery
Salpingectomy for ruptured ectopic pregnancy	
Evacuation of the uterus	
Appendectomy	Gall bladder and biliary tract
Herniorrhaphy (elective repair and emergency)	Intestinal resection and repair
Intestinal obstruction	
Suture of intestinal perforation	
Plication of perforated ulcer	Operation for bleeding peptic ulcer
Colostomy	
Tube thoracostomy	
Cricothyroidotomy	
Closed fracture reduction and stabilization	
Open fracture management	
Amputation	
Minor burn care	Major burn care
Conservative management of head injury	Drainage of epidural and subdural hematoma
Wound care and repair	
Surgical infections	

that many of the problems in table 12.5 that could be addressed in these facilities were not treated at all. Wide variations exist among hospitals; in some cases, there was complete omission of operations that are urgently needed, not complicated, and within the competence of general practitioners with brief surgical training (for example, open reduction of compound fractures). Such omissions can lead to a major loss of cost-effectiveness in these hospitals.

Closed fracture treatment and some uterine evacuations may not have been recorded in the operating room logbooks (the source of data for this study) because they are not always carried out in the main operating rooms. Trauma is not listed separately, but the very small number of open fracture reductions (with the exception of Kiryandongo) indicates that major trauma either is not being seen or is being referred elsewhere.

If general anesthesia and a qualified surgeon are available in a first-level hospital, all of the procedures in table 12.5 can be done at this level, which would be ideal, since referral often is not possible or practical. If all of the procedures in the first-level hospitals column

could be mastered by the staff available at this level, few patients would need to be referred. The ideal will be to put fully qualified surgeons and obstetricians in all hospitals, but better training of the general practitioners and NPCs now serving as the only surgeons in many first-level hospitals could bring these facilities closer to the ideal.

HEALTH CENTERS AS A SURGICAL PLATFORM

Health centers (clinics, usually without inpatient beds except for normal deliveries) deliver babies, suture small lacerations, and drain small abscesses, but very few provide more comprehensive services. The primary reason for the limited range of services is the limited training available to health care personnel; another reason is the shortage of medical personnel of all kinds, which results in heavy workloads and makes additional responsibilities and skill acquisition a problem.

As these issues are resolved, it will be important to ensure that basic surgical training is provided. The list of services that could be provided at the health center level is substantial and includes the following:

- Treatment of simple fractures, burns, and other injuries
- Resuscitation of major trauma patients: control of bleeding, airway maintenance, fluid replacement, and shock prevention and treatment
- Tubectomy, intrauterine device insertion, and other contraceptive procedures
- Early management of postpartum bleeding, eclampsia, and prolonged labor; suture of perineal lacerations; extraction of retained placentas
- Uterine curettage for incomplete abortion
- Circumcision
- Removal of foreign bodies in eyes, ears, and noses

A functioning referral system with patient access to transportation will increase the efficiency and the effectiveness of these services.

BURDEN OF SURGICALLY TREATABLE DISEASE AND THE UNMET NEED

This volume has shown that universal provision of a package of essential surgical services would avert an estimated 1.5 million deaths per year, or 6–7 percent of all avertable deaths in LMICs (Debas and others 2006; Mock and others 2015). For many of the conditions treated by this package, surgical care is the only option. There are no preventive strategies for many pregnancy-related complications or for most general surgical emergencies. Similarly, road traffic crashes and other injuries are increasing in LMICs, and there is a substantial and growing burden of chronic, congenital, and acquired conditions that can be treated surgically.

Surgery for Obstetrical Emergencies

The need for emergency obstetrical surgery is relatively easy to calculate because the birth rate is almost always known, and it is generally accepted that 10 percent to 15 percent of births are likely to have complications, most of them requiring surgical treatment, that threaten the lives of the mothers or newborns. There are important exceptions: El Salvador, Honduras, and Sri Lanka, for example, have reduced the unmet obstetrical need to 25 percent or lower, with a corresponding drop in the maternal mortality ratio to well below 100 per 100,000 births (AMDD Working Group 2003; Paxton and others 2005).

Surgery for Trauma and General Surgical Emergencies

The surgical burdens due to trauma and general surgical emergencies are harder to estimate, but the burdens are unquestionably high; for trauma, the estimated burden is much higher than that due to obstetrical emergencies, even though trauma has been found to be a relatively small part of surgical activities in hospitals in LMICs (Canoodt and others 2012; Mock and others 2012; Mock and others 1998). The reason for this discrepancy in met need between traumatic and obstetrical emergencies seems clear: childbirth is a predictable event; when emergencies occur, there is usually enough time to bring patients to hospitals, even distant ones. That the unmet need for emergency obstetrical care is still greater than 80 percent in most of Sub-Saharan Africa is a measure of the very serious deficiencies in the health systems in the region. That the unmet need has been less than 25 percent in Sri Lanka for more than 20 years shows that these deficiencies can be corrected, even in LMICs.

Most of the causes of the unmet need for trauma care lie outside of the hospitals. Immediate emergency assistance and prompt transfer for definitive care are often needed and rarely available in LMICs; 21 percent of serious vehicle accident victims die before reaching a hospital in the United States compared with 51 percent in Ghana (Henry and Reingold 2012; Mock and others 1998). Emergency resuscitation is usually not well organized in LMICs, neither before nor after arrival at hospitals. Furthermore, the general practitioners or NPCs available for emergencies at most first-level hospitals are not well trained for trauma care after resuscitation.

Surgery for Disabling Conditions

Most LMICs have a high burden of surgically treatable disabling conditions (Beard and others 2013; Petroze and others 2013; Wu, Poenaru, and Poley 2013). Specialists visiting first-level hospitals can effectively treat cataracts, complicated fractures, burn contractures, congenital anomalies, vesico-vaginal fistulas, and many other conditions that are beyond the capacity and skills of the permanent staff of first-level hospitals; during the same visit, the specialists can provide in-service training and supervision. Many successful programs bring specialists to these hospitals, but too often the visits are sporadic and uncoordinated. Regular visits to provide continuity and follow-up can greatly increase the effectiveness of these programs (see chapter 13).

SURGICAL OUTCOMES AT FIRST-LEVEL HOSPITALS

Of the surgical patients seen in first-level hospitals, 50 percent to 80 percent present with emergencies. Problems with transportation to a higher-level facility and the attendant costs of families' travel place a very high premium on managing these cases at first-level facilities. Fortunately, the surgical treatment needed for these emergencies is usually straightforward, relatively simple, and well standardized. Outcomes are remarkably good, given reasonable training to manage a relatively short list of problems, even when a fully qualified surgeon is not available.

Surgery for Obstetrical Emergencies

Obstetrical emergency surgery is the most common surgical problem presenting in first-level hospitals. The standard established in the United Nations process indicators (Paxton, Bailey, and Lobis 2006) calls for case fatality rates of 1 percent or less for mothers with obstetrical complications requiring hospital treatment. Many hospitals in LMICs, including those in which this work is usually done by NPCs, come close to this target, with mortality rates less than 2 percent (McCord and others 2009; Pereira and others 1996).

Surgery for General Emergencies

General surgical emergencies, including acute abdominal conditions, surgical infections, thoracic emergencies, and airway obstruction, can almost always be managed at first-level hospitals, with overall mortality rates of less than 5 percent (see chapter 4).

Surgery for Trauma Emergencies

Trauma can lead to very serious and complicated problems. Unfortunately, most seriously injured patients die before arrival, leaving first-level hospitals with patients who usually have treatable problems and a smaller group that can be stabilized and transferred. Because the number of accident victims is so high, caring for patients with manageable problems and treating them with straightforward procedures to prevent death and disability should be the most important surgical activity in first-level surgical systems. This potential is not realized in most LMICs, primarily because transportation systems to bring injured patients to hospitals safely are so poorly developed.

Postsurgical Treatment Needs

Successful operations will cure most patients requiring emergency surgery at first-level hospitals, and these patients usually will not need further treatment. A few exceptions exist: patients with peptic ulcers will need medical treatment for ulcer disease; many fractures will not have a positive outcome without follow-up basic physiotherapy; and patients with emergency relief of sigmoid volvulus will need resection of the sigmoid intestine to prevent recurrence, which is common.

Serious operative complications are also relatively rare. Infections are usually minor, and the proper use of anesthetics for these short operations is safe and effective. This surgical capacity relies on medical personnel, usually nurses, who have been trained to administer anesthesia, and surgeons who know when to take simple measures to prevent major infections, such as leaving the skin open with subsequent secondary closure in heavily contaminated operations, and using antibiotics appropriately.

SURGICAL COST AND COST-EFFECTIVENESS

When DALYs averted were calculated for all patients discharged from a first-level nongovernmental hospital in Bangladesh, surgical and obstetrical patients contributed the largest share by far: 80 percent of 3,309 DALYs averted in three months. The cost per DALY averted for the whole hospital was US\$11, which was comparable to the cost per DALY of many public health interventions at that time (McCord and Chowdhury 2003).

Debas and others (2006) estimate a cost per DALY averted of the surgical services in the ideal first-level hospital described in table 12.1 at US\$33 in Sub-Saharan Africa, US\$38 in South Asia, and US\$95 in Latin America and the Caribbean. Gosselin, Thind, and Bellardinelli (2006); Gosselin and Heitto (2008); and Gosselin, Maldonado, and Elder (2010) calculate US\$32.78 per DALY averted for surgical services in a nongovernmental hospital in Sierra Leone, and US\$172, US\$223, and US\$77 in nongovernmental trauma centers in Cambodia, Haiti, and Nigeria, respectively. These directly observed cost-per-DALY averted estimates, all of them in nongovernmental facilities (and three of the four were hospitals that did not provide obstetrical care), need to be supplemented by other studies in LMICs, with a focus on government hospitals, local private hospitals, and hospitals unable to provide major surgical services. It is likely that small, Sub-Saharan African government hospitals with active surgical services will have costs per DALY averted comparable to the Bangladesh hospital, given that hospital costs in these government hospitals are comparable (table 12.6). Government third-level hospitals and private hospitals are more costly and probably will be less cost-effective (Barnum and Kutzin 1993; Chatterjee, Levin, and Laxminarayan 2013).

Conducting cost analysis in hospitals in LMICs, especially in public hospitals, is difficult, and not many

Table 12.6 Hospital Costs and Surgical Services Costs at Hospitals in Sub-Saharan Africa (2010) and India (2012)

U.S. dollars

	Bagamoyo District Hospital, Tanzania	Kasulu District Hospital, Tanzania	Chokwe District Hospital, Mozambique	Hospital Catandica, Mozambique	Mityana Hospital, Uganda	Kiryandongo Hospital, Uganda	Private Hospital, India	District Hospital, India	Private Teaching hospital, India	Third-level Hospital, India
Total annual expenditures	329,716	800,662	286,593	155,908	251,448	369,419	13,758,650	2,315,165	4,606,788	10,152,380
Surgery annual expenditures	31,700	84,492	19,358	11,376	33,980	33,470	1,158,319	181,468	915,350	517,657
	(9.6%)	(10.6%)	(6.7%)	(7.3%)	(13.5%)	(9.1%)	(8.4%)	(7.8%)	(19.9%)	(5.1%)
Beds	125	135	214	91	100	100	200	400	655	778
Admissions	6,545	10,296	8,089	3,861	9,106	5,713	5,925	25,871	19,139	205,949
Expenditure per bed	2,640	5,933	1,341	1,714	2,510	3,690	68,795	5,788	7,034	13,049
Expenditure per admission	53.02	85.24	43.33	42.11	39.96	68.81	134.54	7.58	6.63	11.81
Expenditure per day	17.70	26.84	10.79	18.16	11.22	22.05	n.a.	n.a.	n.a.	n.a.
Operations	980	2,045	601	256	1,484	248	2,508	3,623	2,788	3,219
Expenditure per operation	56.41	98.82	41.54	49.03	55.34	304.28	461.85	50.10	330.69	160.81

Source: Chatterjee, Levin, and Laxminarayan 2013; Galukande and others 2010; Kruk and others 2010.
Note: % = annual surgical expenditure as a percentage of total annual expenditure; n.a. = data not available.

comprehensive cost reports dealing with LMIC hospitals are available. Government funds come from different sources; there are nongovernmental gifts, grants, and programs; supplies and equipment may be provided in kind; the contribution of "cost recovery" (patient payments to the hospital) is often not well documented; and "informal payments" are usually not documented at all. Table 12.6 summarizes some of the findings in three analyses of annual recurrent cost, including depreciation of buildings and equipment, for several hospitals in India and Sub-Saharan Africa. No estimates of DALYs averted were available. Cost per surgical operation for most of the second-level hospitals in both regions was low and comparable. In the one Sub-Saharan African second-level hospital with high cost per operation, surgical activity was very low. The cost per operation in the single Indian third-level hospital was three times higher than the average for the six low-cost second-level hospitals; in the Indian private hospitals, it was seven times higher. There are some inconsistencies in these reports; the very high number of admissions to the Indian third-level hospital probably includes both inpatient admissions and outpatient visits.

In all public hospitals, personnel costs were considerably higher than those of any other cost centers within the hospital. Salaries were low, and staff shortages were pervasive, so relatively high personnel costs probably reflect inadequate funding for supplies, maintenance, and transportation, and certainly not large numbers of staff or excessive salaries. More analysis of this kind is urgently needed and could be combined with estimates of DALYs averted to better define the true cost and cost effectiveness of properly functioning hospital systems in LMICs.

Reasons for the Cost-Effectiveness of First-Level Hospitals

The high cost-effectiveness of surgery in a small first-level hospital is due to three factors: self-selection, effective and inexpensive technology, and efficient use of limited resources. Furthermore, the most common operations performed in first-level hospitals are very effective and low-cost procedures, including cesarean sections, acute abdominal emergencies, and herniorrhaphies.

- *Self-selection*: Few people want to be in a hospital, but the resource-starved hospitals in LMICs can be especially unpleasant places. People quickly come to know what services a hospital can and cannot provide, and they generally make intelligent choices with respect to the places where service provided is

worth the cost in time, money, and discomfort. Very few patients with cancer select first-level hospitals for treatment in LMICs, but many women experiencing pregnancy-related complications will seek competent obstetrical care, if available. If the outcomes are suboptimal at a particular facility, patients will find better ones (Kruk and others 2009). The end result is a patient population that has self-selected itself so that individuals who seek treatment can be effectively treated.

- *Effective, inexpensive technology*: Operating rooms are not expensive; affordable antibiotics, anesthesia, and other supplies are usually effective. Training and mobilizing staff members is the largest expense. The total hospital cost in a first-level hospital is usually less than US$30 per patient-day (Kruk and others 2010), compared with US$1,000 per day or more in high-income countries (HICs), and surgical services cost is a fraction of total hospital costs (table 12.6).

- *Resource-limited hospitals*: Hospital budgets, even though they are a major part of total health budgets in LMICs, are low by any international standard. Despite this limitation, these hospitals are able to achieve good results in patient care. Undoubtedly, they could do better with more resources, but this relative starvation keeps costs down. One of the most important reasons for further analysis of the cost-effectiveness of different levels of hospitals in different places is to determine the most efficient ways to improve and expand services delivery with minimum increases in cost.

OBSTACLES TO LOW COST AND HIGH COST-EFFECTIVENESS

Not every hospital is cost-effective. The third-level hospitals and the private hospitals in table 12.6 are much more expensive than the smaller, first- and second-level government or nongovernmental facilities. Anything that diverts patients from low-cost hospitals to higher-cost, third-level ones increases the costs of the whole system and lowers the effectiveness of the first- and second-level hospitals.

Fixed expenses, notably for personnel, are the major component of hospital costs, so the cost per unit of service delivery rises when utilization is low.

Training

Less-than-optimal training may be the most important contributor to a reduction in cost-effectiveness. First-level hospitals in LMICs usually do not have a fully qualified surgeon, obstetrician, or orthopedist on staff. General practitioners or NPCs generally learn to treat obstetric emergencies, but they often refer serious trauma and acute abdominal emergencies to higher-level facilities. If patient transfer could be made efficient and inexpensive, this process might work well. However, in many places, most transferred patients never arrive at the referral hospitals (Urassa and others 2005); death en route is common. Moreover, the receiving hospitals may be no better able to provide care than the hospitals from which the patients were sent (Grimes and others 2011; Siddiqi and others 2001). Patients bypass hospitals known to refer often, reducing surgical volume to inefficient levels. The operations and surgical conditions listed for first-level hospitals in table 12.5 are all within the competence of general practitioners or NPCs, given appropriate training. A six-month program in a busy second-level facility could provide substantial benefits. If this training could be combined with follow-up in-service training and supervision, the capacity and outcomes could be further improved.

Anesthesia

Major surgery usually requires general or spinal anesthesia. Doctors, nurses, and NPCs are not routinely trained to administer anesthesia. Many first-level hospitals do not perform surgery or perform very limited surgery simply because they lack trained staff to administer anesthesia. This relatively simple staff deficiency can be readily addressed. A one- or two-year course for nurses or NPCs can produce a sufficient level of competence for the safe administration of general and spinal anesthesia; a six-month course can be enough for hospitals to make spinal and Ketamine anesthesia available.[1] The same short course can produce competency in the resuscitation of patients with severe trauma, blood loss, or respiratory insufficiency.

Poor Quality of Service and Low Utilization

Poor quality of patient care reduces the number of positive outcomes and is a common reason for low utilization. Low utilization, in turn, reduces the experience of hospital staff and can lead to even poorer outcomes.

Informal Payments

The issue of informal payments has two components. The first is that hospitals with inadequate inventories ask patients to purchase medicine and other needed supplies, which adds considerably to patients' costs.

The second component is outright corruption in the form of payments to staff for presumably better service; in some areas this abuse can more than double the costs to patients (Lewis 2007). Increased costs plus the associated loss of confidence in hospital staff can lead to further reductions in utilization and increase the cost per unit of service.

Epidemiological Transition

The epidemiological transition (from infectious to noninfectious, degenerative disease) is in full swing in MICs and among the upper classes in many low-income countries, with consequent increases in the incidence of cancer, diabetes, and complications from arteriosclerosis. Surgery for these conditions is generally more complicated and often will not be curative; the underlying disease remains and complications of the disease can recur. Costs are higher and cost-effectiveness is lower. Universal health coverage is increasing, and treatment for degenerative diseases certainly cannot be excluded, but health budgets in LMICs will not support, for example, the universal availability of cardiac surgery for coronary artery disease. Fortunately, diabetes, arteriosclerosis, and many cancers are preventable. Energetic efforts at primary and secondary prevention will pay off in lower hospital costs. The elimination of tobacco use and better management of hypertension could be the most important activities.

New Technology

New diagnostic and therapeutic technologies are usually expensive and have the further disadvantage of imposing an additional training burden to teach staff to use and maintain equipment. There are exceptions:

- Replacement lenses for cataract operations are made in India and Nepal at very low cost.
- The mesh for hernia repair greatly improves long-term results; mosquito netting seems to work well, but factories in LMICs could produce a standardized, sterile product at low cost.
- The pulse oximeter is a simple, sturdy, and relatively inexpensive electronic instrument that can greatly improve the safety of anesthesia and the control of respiration and circulation during resuscitation of severely injured patients.
- Flexible gastroscopes are expensive, but they can control bleeding from stomach and duodenal ulcers so well as to virtually eliminate the need for surgery for bleeding ulcers.

Careful evaluation, including cost analysis, of each example of new technology should be able to control a technological cost spiral, at least in the public sector. However, little is being done to make this increasingly important evaluation. The National Institute for Health and Care Excellence of the British National Health Service provides a model of how such an evaluation can be conducted (http://www.nice.org.uk).

FINANCING SURGICAL CARE

Financial support for surgical services delivery is discussed in chapter 18. The reality is that no matter how cost-effective it is, most people in low-income countries (LICS) and many in lower-middle-income countries, cannot afford surgery unless it is available without charge at the point of care. Although El Salvador, Honduras, and Sri Lanka, for example, have shown that free service can be made available within very low budget public health systems, most lower-middle-income countries, and many upper-middle-income countries, have hospital systems that reach only a fraction of the population, largely because of the cost barrier. Economic growth and increased government budgets for health are reducing this disparity, but progress is slow. In many LMICs, availability of trained staff and other resources has not improved at all in the past 20 years, especially in the first-level hospital network. Efforts to mobilize nongovernmental funds to support health care have had limited success.

- Although the private health sector is growing rapidly everywhere, it reaches only a fraction of the population. In India, 78 percent of health expenditures occur in the private sector, but in most Indian states, only a fraction of the population has access to private hospital care (Kumar and others 2011).
- Cost-sharing (fees for service) in public hospitals has been shown to reduce utilization, but it contributes very little to covering hospital costs (Lagarde and Palmer 2011; Robert and Ridde 2013).
- Government-run insurance systems that provide direct government financing of essential services have been shown to be possible on a large scale (Kruk 2013; Kumar and others 2011). The most common example is free emergency obstetrical care. If such plans can be successfully implemented, they will have a double benefit: they reduce the financial barrier to the use of clinical services, and they give purchasing power to patients, thereby directing income to the hospitals and clinics that provide the most popular, and it is to be hoped the best, services. The key is to direct the benefits to those who need them most

and to those services that can give the greatest public health outcome, for example, obstetrics, trauma, emergency surgery, and neonatal care. However, equitable utilization of "free surgery" is by no means guaranteed; poor people continue to face high costs for transportation, supplies, food, and informal charges (El-Khoury, Hatt, and Gandaho 2012).

Financing of surgical care is further complicated by the large number of first-level surgical procedures that are emergencies. The need for out-of-pocket user fees (especially fees required before treatment can be provided) has been found to be a major barrier to the provision of emergency care in many places (Canoodt, Mock, and Bucagu 2012).

STRENGTHENING FIRST-LEVEL SURGICAL FACILITIES

The first-level hospitals and the clinics below them described in table 12.1 are an ideal, achieved in a few LMICs but far from a reality in most. Although existing first-level hospitals are cost-effective, and their surgical services seem to be especially so, they could be doing much more, especially for trauma, general surgical emergencies, and the backlog of treatable disabling conditions. The successful development more than 20 years ago of effective hospital systems in countries such as Sri Lanka has shown that this is possible even with low budgets for health. The number of available trained health personnel is increasing rapidly in almost all countries, and health budgets are rising, so that it should be possible for all LMICs to achieve a much better level of care in the next 20 years. The question is how to accomplish this rapidly and efficiently, so that the poor majorities in these countries are not left behind.

Removing Roadblocks

The following are three major roadblocks to better care:

- *Access to well-functioning health centers and first-level hospitals is critical*: These clinics and hospitals must have better patient transport available, and the financial barriers to travel should be removed to the extent possible. All of the financial barriers for families cannot be eliminated, but the cost of transport and the cost of the hospital's or clinic's services are the two most important. Not enough is known about how much free transport would cost, but it would probably not be an unbearable burden. The creation and analysis of real-life models will facilitate the raising of funds for this purpose. Hospitals with limited budgets will not be able to pay for all of this, so outside funding sources will need to be found.

- *Staffing is inadequate, both in numbers and in training.* Many years will pass before fully trained staff can be available at all levels; therefore, it is important to identify intermediate solutions. These solutions include training general physicians and NPCs to perform basic surgery; training nurses to administer anesthesia; and providing in-service training of staff at all levels in such skills as better management of nonsurgical obstetric emergencies, patient resuscitation on arrival at the clinic or hospital, and appropriate care during transport for referral. Functioning models with cost analysis are needed.
- *Logistical systems to provide supplies and maintain equipment are usually underfunded and inadequate.* Closer consideration of areas in which such systems seem to be working better, such as Sri Lanka, will help solutions for widespread implementation to be developed.

Expanding Capacity

If the roadblocks are removed, utilization will increase and it will be necessary to expand facilities, eliminate the gross inadequacies in such fundamentals as water and electricity supply, and, in some cases, create new clinics and hospitals. Upgrading health centers to provide more surgical services will help ease the burden for hospitals.

As the medical workload increases, paying attention to staff morale in health centers and hospitals will be essential. Adequate pay, decent housing, sufficient staff numbers, and professional satisfaction from supportive supervision and recognition are all important.

FUTURE DIRECTIONS FOR SURGICAL SERVICES

Research and Training

Better determination of the burden of surgical disease is needed, but retrospective population surveys produce incomplete and imprecise information, and prospective surveys are expensive. Prospective studies in places with ongoing demographic surveillance could produce more useful information.

However, enough is known to begin the implementation of programs to improve services and increase access to services. Monitoring and evaluating the effectiveness and cost of these improvements as they are implemented will be important. Monitoring can provide ongoing evidence of the effect on utilization and outcomes.

Evaluation can include the evaluation of the population impact as well as of the costs and benefits. Training, especially to increase the availability of surgical skills in first-level hospitals, will be an essential element of these programs. National professional societies could play a crucial role in this process, and qualified surgeons from HICs could provide important assistance, improving the availability of trained staff in the first- and second-level hospitals that will be the principal venues for this training.

Finance

Hospitals and the systems to support them are terribly underfunded in most LMICs, as are all of the health services for the poor segments of the population in these places. For most people in these countries, a generation or more will pass before incomes rise sufficiently to provide purchasing power for basic surgical services. LMICs are increasingly embracing universal health coverage, primarily funded through taxes, as a means of improving access to services and ensuring that medical bills do not force families into poverty. Essential and life-saving surgeries are likely to be core components of these insurance programs.

Epidemiological Transition

Controlling the inevitable increase in cost and decrease in effectiveness associated with surgery for complications of arteriosclerosis, cancer, and diabetes is an important issue. The best approach is probably through primary and secondary prevention. Investments to control tobacco use and improve the medical management of hypertension could produce significant benefits to individual health, as well as reduce inefficient hospital use. Nevertheless, surgeons still need to be prepared to address the sequelae of chronic diseases.

Technological Advances

Although new technology can improve treatment and, in some cases, reduce costs, it initially increases costs for equipment, materials, and training. The demand for video-assisted surgery, computerized tomography scanning, and coronary artery stenting is likely to increase. These advances should be carefully evaluated before they are incorporated into public programs.

Referral Systems

Patient transportation is generally available, but paying for it is difficult. The most practical approach may be to provide ambulances to hospitals and health centers, with adequate budgets for fuel and maintenance. A realistic evaluation of the cost for provision of adequate transport is needed; the costs may be less than expected if corruption and misuse can be controlled. Monitoring by community and district government councils could help. For example, second-level health teams in Uganda have established local transport committees to manage dispatch, communications, and repair and maintenance of donated vehicles.

There should be a tradeoff between more referral and less need for surgical facilities, but how important this tradeoff will be remains unknown. It is likely that the combination of more and better trained staff in first-level units, with better transport between units, will improve service, as well as pay for itself by reducing the need for multiple hospitals delivering service.

Supervision Systems

First-level hospital surgeons and other surgeons in LMICs generally work without effective supervision, oversight, and in-service training. These shortcomings can only be corrected if enough qualified specialists can be made available to provide training and supervision, as well as direct service. In the long term, most countries will have adequate numbers of specialists, but ways need to be found to make service provision in first-level hospitals and clinics an important part of their work.

Logistical Systems

Logistical systems need to be decentralized, adequately funded, simplified, and controlled. At all hospital levels in the public system, the cost of personnel is the largest budgetary component. It makes no sense to pay for trained staff and deny them the relatively small funds needed for basic supplies that make it possible to do what they are trained to do.

Health Policy and National Health Plans

Service delivery in almost all LMIC public hospitals is a government responsibility, but delivery of emergency and essential surgical services is usually not mentioned in health plans at either the central or the local level. Attention to surgical services in these plans would help focus attention on its importance (Hedges, Mock, and Cherian 2010).

Professional Societies

National professional societies need to play a more active role in the development of robust first-level surgical care in their countries; they have taken too little interest in first-level hospitals to date. Professional societies could take responsibility for equitable delivery of services; work with communities and government to develop the needed political will; and provide guidance in the development of programs for training, supervision, and logistical support.

Traditionally, advancement and recognition within the surgical community and within surgical organizations are based on factors such as the skills of individual surgeons; training of residents to become fully trained surgeons, and especially subspecialists; and research on basic science or operative surgical issues. Surgeons who develop and master the most difficult, complicated procedures are usually those who are most highly regarded. However, most of the burden of surgical disease could be lowered by improved access to fairly simple procedures that are both very cost-effective and very suitable to being performed in first-level hospitals. The surgical community and surgical organizations need to develop a focus on the wider population. Surgeons who choose to devote themselves to improving access to the most-needed procedures (whether through their own labor or through the training and research activities they conduct) need to be better recognized for these contributions. Professional organizations need to develop their own mechanisms for supporting and encouraging such work.

NOTES

One of the authors of this chapter is a WHO staff member. The authors alone are responsible for the views expressed in this publication and they do not necessarily represent the decisions or policies of the World Health Organization.

The World Bank classifies countries according to four income groupings. Income is measured using gross national income (GNI) per capita, in U.S. dollars, converted from local currency using the *World Bank Atlas* method. Classifications as of July 2014 are as follows:

- Low-income countries (LICs) = US$1,045 or less in 2013
- Middle-income countries (MICs) are subdivided:
  - Lower-middle-income = US$1,046 to US$4,125
  - Upper-middle-income (UMICs) = US$4,126 to US$12,745
- High-income countries (HICs) = US$12,746 or more

1. Ketamine is a relatively new and safe anesthetic agent that can induce general anesthesia without paralysis of respiration and the need for artificial respiration or a tracheal tube.

REFERENCES

Alkire, B. C., J. R. Vincent, C. T. Burns, I. S. Metzler, P. E. Farmer, and others. 2012. "Obstructed Labor and Caesarean Delivery: The Cost and Benefit of Surgical Intervention." *PLoS One* 7 (4): e34595. doi:10.1371/journal.pone.0034595.

AMDD Working Group (Averting Maternal Death and Disability Working Group). 2003. "Using UN Process Indicators to Assess Needs in Emergency Obstetric Services: Morocco, Nicaragua and Sri Lanka." Program note. *International Journal of Gynaecology and Obstetrics* 80 (2): 222–30.

Bailey, P. 2005. "Using UN Process Indicators to Assess Needs in Emergency Obstetric Services: Bolivia, El Salvador and Honduras." Program note. *International Journal of Gynaecology and Obstetrics* 89 (2): 221–30. doi:10.1016 /j.ijgo.2004.12.045.

Barnum, B., and B. H. Kutzin. 1993. *Public Hospitals in Developing Countries*. Baltimore, MD: Johns Hopkins University Press.

Beard, J. H., L. B. Oresanya, M. Ohene-Yeboah, R. A. Dicker, and H. W. Harris. 2013. "Characterizing the Global Burden of Surgical Disease: A Method to Estimate Inguinal Hernia Epidemiology in Ghana." *World Journal of Surgery* 37 (3): 498–503. doi:10.1007/s00268-012-1864-x.

Cannoodt, L., C. Mock, and M. Bucagu. 2012. "Identifying Barriers to Emergency Care Services." *International Journal of Health Planning and Management* 27 (2): e104–20. doi:10.1002/hpm.1098.

Chatterjee, S., and R. Laxminarayan. 2013. "Costs of Surgical Procedures in Indian Hospitals." *British Medical Journal Open* 3 (6). doi:10.1136/bmjopen-2013-002844.

Chatterjee, S., C. Levin, and R. Laxminarayan. 2013. "Unit Cost of Medical Services at Different Hospitals in India." *PLoS One* 8 (7): e69728. doi:10.1371/journal.pone.0069728.

Coffman, J. M., J. S. Seago, and J. Spetz. 2002. "Minimum Nurse-to-Patient Ratios in Acute Care Hospitals in California." *Health Affairs (Millwood)* 21 (5): 53–64.

Debas, H. T., R. Gosselin, C. McCord, and A. Thind. 2006. "Surgery." In *Disease Control Priorities in Developing Countries*, 2nd ed. edited by D. T. Jamison, J. G. Breman, A. R. Measham, G. Alleyne, M. Claeson, D. B. Evans, P. Jha, A. Mills, and P. Musgrove, 1245–60. Washington, DC: World Bank and Oxford University Press.

El-Khoury, M., L. Hatt, and T. Gandaho. 2012. "User Fee Exemptions and Equity in Access to Caesarean Sections: An Analysis of Patient Survey Data in Mali." *International Journal of Equity in Health* 11 (49). doi:10.1186/1475-9276-11-49.

Galukande, M., J. von Schreeb, A. Wladis, N. Mbembati, H. de Miranda, and others. 2010. "Essential Surgery at the District Hospital: A Retrospective Descriptive Analysis in Three African Countries." *PLoS Medicine* 7 (3): e1000243. doi:10.1371/journal.pmed.1000243.

Gosselin, R. A., and M. Heitto. 2008. "Cost-Effectiveness of a District Trauma Hospital in Battambang, Cambodia." *World Journal of Surgery* 32 (11): 2450–53. doi:10.1007 /s00268-008-9708-4.

Gosselin, R. A., A. Maldonado, and G. Elder. 2010. "Comparative Cost-Effectiveness Analysis of Two MSF Surgical Trauma Centers." *World Journal of Surgery* 34 (3): 415–19. doi:10.1007/s00268-009-0230-0.

Gosselin, R. A., A. Thind, and A. Bellardinelli. 2006. "Cost/ DALY Averted in a Small Hospital in Sierra Leone: What Is the Relative Contribution of Different Services?" *World Journal of Surgery* 30 (4): 505–11. doi:10.1007 /s00268-005-0609-5.

Grimes, C. E., K. G. Bowman, C. M. Dodgion, and C. B. Lavy. 2011. "Systematic Review of Barriers to Surgical Care in Low-Income and Middle-Income Countries." *World Journal of Surgery* 35 (5): 941–50. doi:10.1007/s00268-011-1010-1.

Hedges, J. P., C. Mock, and M. N. Cherian. 2010. "The Political Economy of Emergency and Essential Surgery in Global Health." *World Journal of Surgery* 34 (9): 2003–06.

Henry, J. A., and A. L. Reingold. 2012. "Prehospital Trauma Systems Reduce Mortality in Developing Countries: A Systematic Review and Meta-Analysis." *Journal of Trauma and Acute Care Surgery* 73 (1): 261–68. doi:10.1097 /TA.0b013e31824bde1e.

Hogan, M. C., K. J. Foreman, M. Naghavi, S. Y. Ahn, M. Wan, and others. 2010. "Maternal Mortality for 181 Countries, 1980–2008: A Systematic Analysis of Progress towards Millennium Development Goal 5." *The Lancet* 375 (9726): 1609–23. doi:10.1016/s0140-6736(10)60518-1.

Kruk, M. E. 2013. "Universal Health Coverage: A Policy Whose Time Has Come." *British Medical Journal* 347: f6360. doi:10.1136/bmj.f6360.

Kruk, M. E., G. Mbaruku, C. W. McCord, M. Moran, P. C. Rockers, and others. 2009. "Bypassing Primary Care Facilities for Childbirth: A Population-Based Study in Rural Tanzania." *Health Policy and Planning* 24 (4): 279–88. doi:10.1093/heapol/czp011.

Kruk, M. E., A. Wladis, N. Mbembati, S. K. Ndao-Brumblay, R. Y. Hsia, and others. 2010. "Human Resource and Funding Constraints for Essential Surgery in District Hospitals in Africa: A Retrospective Cross-Sectional Survey." *PLoS Medicine* 7 (3): e1000242. doi:10.1371/ journal.pmed.1000242.

Kumar, A. K., L. C. Chen, M. Choudhury, S. Ganju, V. Mahajan, and others. 2011. "Financing Health Care for All: Challenges and Opportunities." *The Lancet* 377 (9766): 668–79. doi:10.1016/s0140-6736(10)61884-3.

Kushner, A. L., M. N. Cherian, L. Noel, D. A. Spiegel, S. Groth, and others. 2010. "Addressing the Millennium Development Goals from a Surgical Perspective: Essential Surgery and Anesthesia in 8 Low- and Middle-Income Countries." *Archives of Surgery* 145 (2): 154–59. doi:10.1001/ archsurg.2009.263.

Lagarde, M., and N. Palmer. 2011. "The Impact of User Fees on Access to Health Services in Low- and Middle-Income Countries." *Cochrane Database of Systematic Reviews* (4): Cd009094. doi:10.1002/14651858.cd009094.

Lebrun, D. G., D. Dhar, M. I. Sarkar, T. M. Imran, S. N. Kazi, and others. 2013. "Measuring Global Surgical Disparities: A Survey of Surgical and Anesthesia Infrastructure in Bangladesh." *World Journal of Surgery* 37 (1): 24–31. doi:10.1007/s00268-012-1806-7.

Lebrun, D. G., I. Saavedra-Pozo, F. Agreda-Flores, M. L. Burdic, M. R. Notrica, and others. 2012. "Surgical and Anesthesia Capacity in Bolivian Public Hospitals: Results from a National Hospital Survey." *World Journal of Surgery* 36 (11): 2559–66. doi:10.1007/s00268-012-1722-x.

Lewis, M. 2007. "Informal Payments and the Financing of Health Care in Developing and Transition Countries." *Health Affairs (Millwood)* 26 (4): 984–97. doi:10.1377/hlthaff.26.4.984.

McCord, C., and Q. Chowdhury. 2003. "A Cost Effective Small Hospital in Bangladesh: What It Can Mean for Emergency Obstetric Care." *International Journal of Gynaecology and Obstetrics* 81 (1): 83–92.

McCord, C., G. Mbaruku, C. Pereira, C. Nzabuhakwa, and S. Bergstrom. 2009. "The Quality of Emergency Obstetrical Surgery by Assistant Medical Officers in Tanzanian District Hospitals." *Health Affairs (Millwood)* 28 (5): w876–85. doi:10.1377/hlthaff.28.5.w876.

McHugh, M. D., J. Berez, and D. S. Small. 2013. "Hospitals with Higher Nurse Staffing Had Lower Odds of Readmissions Penalties than Hospitals with Lower Staffing." *Health Affairs (Millwood)* 32 (10): 1740–47. doi:10.1377/hlthaff.2013.0613.

Mock, C. N., P. Donkor, A. Gawande, D. T. Jamison, M. E. Kruk, and H. T. Debas. 2015. "Essential Surgery: Key Messages of This Volume." In *Disease Control Priorities* (third edition): Volume 1, *Essential Surgery*, edited by H. T. Debas, P. Donkor, A. Gawande, D. T. Jamison, M. E. Kruk, and C. N. Mock. Washington, DC: World Bank.

Mock, C. N., M. Joshipura, C. Arreola-Risa, and R. Quansah. 2012. "An Estimate of the Number of Lives That Could Be Saved through Improvements in Trauma Care Globally." *World Journal of Surgery* 36 (5): 959–63. doi:10.1007/s00268-012-1459-6.

Mock, C. N., G. J. Jurkovich, D. nii-Amon-Kotei, C. Arreola-Risa, and R. V. Maier. 1998. "Trauma Mortality Patterns in Three Nations at Different Economic Levels: Implications for Global Trauma System Development." *Journal of Trauma* 44 (5): 804–12; discussion 812–04.

Mulligan, J., J. Fox-Rushby, T. Adams, B. Johns, and A. Mills. 2003. "Unit Costs of Health Care Inputs in Low and Middle Income Regions." Working Paper 9, Disease Control Priorities Project, Fogarty International Center, National Institutes of Health, Bethesda, MD.

Needleman, J., P. Buerhaus, V. S. Pankratz, C. L. Leibson, S. R. Stevens, and others. 2011. "Nurse Staffing and Inpatient Hospital Mortality." *New England Journal of Medicine* 364 (11): 1037–45. doi:10.1056/NEJMsa1001025.

Paxton, A., P. Bailey, and S. Lobis. 2006. "The United Nations Process Indicators for Emergency Obstetric Care: Reflections Based on a Decade of Experience." *International Journal of Gynaecology and Obstetrics* 95 (2): 192–208. doi:10.1016/j.ijgo.2006.08.009.

Paxton, A., D. Maine, L. Freedman, D. Fry, and S. Lobis. 2005. "The Evidence for Emergency Obstetric Care." *International Journal of Gynaecology and Obstetrics* 88 (2): 181–93. doi:10.1016/j.ijgo.2004.11.026.

Pearson, L., and R. Shoo. 2005. "Availability and Use of Emergency Obstetric Services: Kenya, Rwanda, Southern Sudan, and Uganda." *International Journal of Gynaecology and Obstetrics* 88 (2): 208–15. doi:10.1016/j.ijgo.2004.09.027.

Pereira, C., A. Bugalho, S. Bergstrom, F. Vaz, and M. Cotiro. 1996. "A Comparative Study of Caesarean Deliveries by Assistant Medical Officers and Obstetricians in Mozambique." *British Journal of Obstetrics and Gynaecology* 103 (6): 508–12.

Petroze, R. T., R. S. Groen, F. Niyonkuru, M. Mallory, E. Ntaganda, and others. 2013. "Estimating Operative Disease Prevalence in a Low-Income Country: Results of a Nationwide Population Survey in Rwanda." *Surgery* 153 (4): 457–64. doi:10.1016/j.surg.2012.10.001.

Robert, E., and V. Ridde. 2013. "Global Health Actors No Longer in Favor of User Fees: A Documentary Study." *Global Health* 9 (1): 29. doi:10.1186/1744-8603-9-29.

Sanders, D., J. Kravitz, S. Lewin, and M. McKee. 1998. "Zimbabwe's Hospital Referral System: Does It Work?" *Health Policy and Planning* 13 (4): 359–70.

Siddiqi, S., A. Kielmann, M. Khan, N. Ali, A. Ghaffar, and others. 2001. "The Effectiveness of Patient Referral in Pakistan." *Health Policy and Planning* 16 (2): 193–98.

Solis, C., P. Leon, N. Sanchez, M. Burdic, L. Johnson, and others. 2013. "Nicaraguan Surgical and Anesthesia Infrastructure: Survey of Ministry of Health Hospitals." *World Journal of Surgery* 37 (9): 2109–21. doi:10.1007/s00268-013-2112-8.

Urassa, D. P., A. Carlstedt, L. Nystrom, S. N. Massawe, and G. Lindmark. 2005. "Are Process Indicators Adequate to Assess Essential Obstetric Care at District Level? A Case Study from Rufiji District, Tanzania." *African Journal of Reproductive Health* 9 (3): 100–11.

Weiser, T. G., S. E. Regenbogen, K. D. Thompson, A. B. Haynes, S. R. Lipsitz, and others. 2008. "An Estimation of the Global Volume of Surgery: A Modeling Strategy Based on Available Data." *The Lancet* 372 (9633): 139–44. doi:10.1016/s0140-6736(08)60878-8.

WHO (World Health Organization). 1992. "The Hospital in Rural and Urban Districts. Report of a WHO Study Group on the Functions of Hospitals at the First Referral Level." World Health Organization Technical Report 819, WHO, Geneva.

———. 2003. *Surgical Care at the District Hospital.* Geneva: WHO.

———. 2010. "Planning Tool for Emergency and Essential Care Surgical Services." WHO, Geneva. http://www.who.int/surgery/publications/Planning_toolEESC.pdf.

Wu, V. K., D. Poenaru, and M. J. Poley. 2013. "Burden of Surgical Congenital Anomalies in Kenya: A Population-Based Study." *Journal of Tropical Pediatrics* 59 (3): 195–202. doi:10.1093/tropej/fmt001.

Zafar, S. N., and K. A. McQueen. 2011. "Surgery, Public Health, and Pakistan." *World Journal of Surgery* 35 (12): 2625–34. doi:10.1007/s00268-011-1304-3.

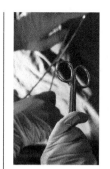

Chapter 13

Specialized Surgical Platforms

Mark G. Shrime, Ambereen Sleemi,
and Thulasiraj D. Ravilla

INTRODUCTION

A large fraction of the burden of disease comprises conditions that are potentially amenable to surgical intervention (chapters 1 and 2) (Bickler and others 2015; Mock and others 2015). The proportion is higher in low- and middle-income countries (LMICs) (Shrime, Sleemi, and Ravilla 2014). Because of difficulties in access to surgical care—often due to issues of cost, transportation, infrastructure, and a lack of providers (Chao and others 2012; Ilbawi, Einterz, and Nkusu 2013; Knowlton and others 2013; Linden and others 2012)—this surgical burden is sometimes borne by the international charitable sector.

Historically, first-level hospitals in LMICs have tended primarily to treat conditions associated with a low disability-adjusted life year (DALY) burden. These hospitals have done so with a high loss to follow-up; patients scheduled for surgeries often do not return for their operations (Ilbawi, Einterz, and Nkusu 2013), especially as the complexity and up-front costs of the surgeries increase. Meanwhile, charitable sector involvement has grown rapidly: the charitable sector in the United States, which includes many international charitable surgical organizations, has grown at a pace exceeding the growth of gross domestic product by 20 percent and is currently larger than its counterpart agriculture, construction, transportation, and utilities sectors (Casey 2007). Médecins Sans Frontières (also known as Doctors Without Borders) alone has an annual budget of more than US$700 million, much of which comes from private funders (McCoy, Chand, and Sridhar 2010). This review focuses specifically on the charitable sector's role in the delivery of surgical care in LMICs.

This chapter uses the World Health Organization's (WHO's) six geographical regions: African Region, Region of the Americas, South-East Asia Region, European Region, Eastern Mediterranean Region, and Western Pacific Region.

Challenges to Defining Platforms for Service Delivery

Any attempt to examine the specialized platforms that nongovernmental organizations (NGOs) establish for surgical delivery must necessarily define these platforms. This is a daunting task—an entire galaxy of NGOs provide surgical care, few of which easily fit into any single category, and many of which overlap. Fully 50 percent of international surgical organizations operate in Southeast Asia, with another 46 percent each in Central and South America and 43 percent in Sub-Saharan Africa. Only 20 percent of the organizations provide services in East Asia and the Pacific, the Middle East and North Africa, Europe, or North America (McQueen and others 2010). Organizations vary broadly in surgical scope: 70 percent provide general surgery, 60 percent provide plastic and reconstructive surgery or gynecologic surgery, 50 percent provide ophthalmology services. A minority of surveyed organizations provide other services, including orthopedics; ear, nose, and throat; burns; cardiac; and transplant surgeries (McQueen and others 2010).

Corresponding author: Mark G. Shrime, MD, MPH, FACS, Harvard University, shrime@mail.harvard.edu

Most of the literature evaluating these organizations focuses on breaking down NGOs by the conditions that each treats. This approach is not, however, informative; it masks salient similarities and differences between platforms, and, in doing so, may actually promote fragmentation in delivery.

New Classification by Delivery Platform

This chapter proposes a novel classification scheme by delivery *platform*. Focusing on the platform of care, rather than on disease-specific organizations themselves, allows for a discussion of the costs and effectiveness of the platforms and for benefit patterns common to the respective platforms to emerge, distinct from the diseases treated and the organizations providing treatment. Using this new framework, nongovernmental surgical platforms are compared along metrics of effectiveness, cost-effectiveness, sustainability, and training.

It should be noted that although the vast majority of providers of specialized surgical care in low- and middle-income countries are NGOs, not all are, and that the concentration of NGOs varies by region. At least one of the organizations discussed—Babbar Ruga Fistula Teaching Hospital—is better described as a public-private (or public-charitable) partnership. Other organizations, such as Médecins Sans Frontières and the International Committee of the Red Cross, provide primarily humanitarian emergency services, although both have been involved in training and capacity building (Chu, Ford, and Trelles 2010, 2011; Chu, Trelles, and Ford 2011). Therefore, although the focus of this chapter is the charitable sector, it is not the only model for delivering surgical care; when other platforms are discussed, they are highlighted as such.

Other methods of delivering surgery by external organizations are not discussed:

- Telemedicine (Bai and others 2007), in which surgeons from high-income countries (HICs) diagnose conditions or guide surgeons in LMICs, is not considered a platform for the actual delivery of surgery.
- Cancer screening (Bailie 1996), despite the surgical nature of many cancers, is not included for similar reasons.

METHODOLOGY

A systematic review of the literature was performed to assess the cost, effectiveness, sustainability, and training role of various surgical platforms. The following search strategy was used to query the MEDLINE database, with similar strategies for EMBASE and Google Scholar:

(Surgical Procedures, Operative[MeSH Terms] OR surgery[tiab] OR surgeries[tiab] OR surgical[tiab] OR operative[tiab] OR operating room[tiab] OR operation[tiab] OR cleft lip[tiab] OR cleft palate[tiab] OR eye[tiab] OR congenital[tiab] OR heart[tiab] OR cardiac[tiab] OR vesicovaginal[tiab] OR obstetric fistula[tiab] OR genital fistula[tiab] OR trauma[tiab])

AND

(Medical Missions, Official[MeSH Terms] OR Missions and Missionaries[MeSH Terms] OR Mobile Health Units[MeSH Terms] OR Relief Work[MeSH Terms] OR Voluntary Workers[MeSH Terms] OR humanitarian[tiab] OR surgical mission*[tiab] OR missionary[tiab] OR resource limited[tiab] OR low income countr*[tiab] OR middle income countr*[tiab] OR developing countr*[tiab] OR LMIC[tiab])

NOT "case reports"[publication type]

Bibliographies of the retrieved studies were searched for other relevant publications. Inclusion and exclusion criteria were determined a priori. Only published, peer-reviewed articles were included. The search was not limited to articles in English. Data were extracted using piloted forms and performed by all three authors. Because of a high risk of heterogeneity in studies across multiple disease conditions, countries, and platforms of delivery, no mathematical summary measure was calculated.

Of 8,854 records retrieved, 6,741 were screened by title and abstract; one additional article was found on bibliographic review, and the full texts of 322 were screened. From these, 104 articles were selected for inclusion. The review process, as well as the previously determined inclusion and exclusion criteria, is described in figure 13.1.

CHARITABLE SURGICAL DELIVERY PLATFORMS

Charitable surgical delivery platforms can be divided into two basic types: temporary surgical delivery platforms and specialty surgical hospitals.

Temporary Surgical Delivery Platforms

These platforms are, by definition, temporary, and do not establish hospitals in-country. Although they are almost exclusively run by NGOs, they are different enough to warrant subclassification into short-term surgical trips and self-contained mobile surgical platforms.

Short-Term Surgical Trips. Short-term surgical trips are by far the most common model for surgical delivery by the charitable sector in LMICs; these platforms send surgeons, anesthesiologists, nurses, and supporting staff—along with, at times, surgical instruments and technology—into hospitals in LMICs for short, time-limited periods. Often, these NGOs perform a restricted set of surgeries, using existing local infrastructure for surgical delivery, and relying on local physicians for follow-up. Operation Smile (Bermudez, Trost, and Ayala 2013; Bermudez and others 2010; Magee 2010; Magee, Vander Burg, and Hatcher 2010; Magee and others 2012), the Kenya Orthopedic Program (Cousins and others 2012), and many others fit this model.

Self-Contained Mobile Surgical Platforms. A significantly rarer model for surgical delivery, NGOs functioning as self-contained mobile surgical platforms spend longer periods (months to years) in-country than the short-term trips and, an important distinction, they carry their entire infrastructure with them. Contained on airplanes, ships, and other modes of transportation, these organizations tend not to leave behind any physical structure. Organizations such as Mercy Ships (Cheng, McColl, and Parker 2012; Harris 2013), CinterAndes, and, in some settings, Médecins Sans Frontières fit this model.

Specialty Surgical Hospitals

Another common model for surgical delivery by the charitable sector, specialty surgical hospitals establish an entire physical plant, either completely new or within an existing structure, dedicated to the treatment of one or a few related surgical conditions. Unlike the temporary platforms, specialized surgical hospitals tend to be a mixture of charitable organizations and government institutions. Organizations such as the Addis Ababa Fistula Hospital and the Aravind Eye Hospital fit this model.

TEMPORARY SURGICAL DELIVERY PLATFORMS

Temporary surgical platforms are legion and span the spectrum from one-week mission trips, through recurring mission trips, to mobile platforms that remain on a near-permanent basis in a region. Short-term surgical trips and self-contained mobile platforms are evaluated separately.

Short-Term Surgical Missions

Short-term, disease-specific surgical missions are myriad (McQueen and others 2010), and services rendered, lengths of surgical trips, and resultant efficacy vary.

Figure 13.1 Search Strategy Results, Inclusion Criteria, Exclusion Criteria, and Final Records Included in Qualitative Systematic Review

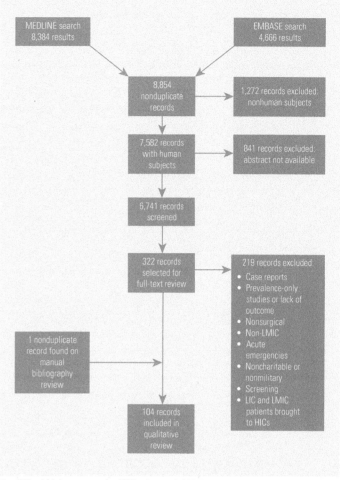

Note: HICs = high-income countries; LMICs = low- and middle-income countries.

Short-term surgical platforms have been used for the following:

- Eye camps in India (Balent and others 2001; Civerchia and others 1993, 1996; Kapoor and others 1999; van der Hoek 1997; Venkataswamy 1975)
- Ear camps in Namibia (Lehnerdt, van Delden, and Lautermann 2005)
- Surgery for facial clefts (Bermudez, Trost, and Ayala 2013; Bermudez and others 2010; Magee 2010; Magee, Vander Burg, and Hatcher 2010; Magee and others 2012)
- Surgery for hernias in Ghana (Sanders and Kingsnorth 2007)
- Cardiac surgery in Papua New Guinea (Tefuarani and others 2007)
- Surgery on endemic goiter in Burkina Faso (Rumstadt and others 2008)

Underpinning these diverse platforms, however, is a uniting model: surgeons and other specialists are flown into regions with high burdens of specific surgical diseases, where they operate for short periods, often one to two weeks (Gosselin, Gialamas, and Atkin 2011) and often in partnership with in-country physicians, to whom is left all but the most immediate follow-up care. These missions, which have alternately been called surgical safaris (Frampton 1993) or surgical blitzes (Nthumba 2010), not infrequently carry their own equipment to local hospitals in which they work (Gosselin, Gialamas, and Atkin 2011; Hodges and Hodges 2000). Often, they return to the same region in subsequent years (Cousins and others 2012; de Buys Roessingh and others 2012; Haskell and others 2002; Ruiz-Razura, Cronin, and Navarro 2000) and strive toward close partnership with local hospitals and ministries of health (Wright, Walker, and Yacoub 2007; Yeow and others 2002).

Despite the plethora of organizations that adopt the short-term surgical model, evaluations of its effectiveness and cost-effectiveness are few, in part because of the difficulty with follow-up. Of 4,100 operations for cleft lip and palate by one organization in 40 simultaneous sites, for example, only 703 patients returned for a six- to nine-month postoperative visit (Bermudez and others 2010).

Effectiveness of Short-Term Surgical Missions. In a survey of 99 international organizations providing surgeries, nearly two-thirds provided fewer than 500 operative interventions per year (McQueen and others 2010). Strong evidence indicates an association between surgical volume and outcomes in Canada and the United States (Birkmeyer and others 2002). More specifically, evidence also points to a stronger impact on outcomes by *hospital* volume than by *surgeon* volume, especially for more complex procedures (Birkmeyer and others 2003; Eskander and others 2014).

Despite myriad organizations using the short-term model, surgeries performed by these missions tend to suffer from higher mortality and complication rates and to produce mixed results, especially for more complex pathologies. In an evaluation of more than 17,000 operations performed in Sub-Saharan Africa during 114 surgical missions in two decades, overall mortality was 3.3 percent (Poilleux and Lobry 1991). The vast majority of these operations were for hernias, for which a mortality as high as 1 percent was observed—20 times higher than the observed mortality for similar procedures in HICs (Rodgers and others 2000).

Both the success of an operative mission and its complication rates, however, vary by surgical procedure.

Simpler procedures, like tonsillectomy, appear safe when performed by short-term surgical missions (Sykes and others 2012). Others are less so: Maine and others (2012) report a rate of fistulization between the mouth and the nose after cleft palate repair more than 20 times higher in surgical missions than in HICs. In this study, operations performed by experienced Ecuadorean and North American cleft surgeons on a mission in Ecuador were compared with cases performed by similar surgeons at a third-level referral hospital in the United States. Notably, all surgeons showed this 20-fold increase in complication rates, and no statistically significant difference was found between surgeries performed by U.S. surgeons on short-term surgical missions and those performed by Ecuadorean surgeons on the same mission. Although patient-level factors obviously confound this increased complication rate, the finding lends further credence to an assertion that mission volume potentially has a greater impact than surgeon experience (Maine and others 2012). De Buys Roessingh and others (2012) similarly report relatively poor functional results in the repair of cleft palates on short-term surgical missions; the lack of a multidisciplinary approach to the repair of these conditions, inherent in short-term surgical blitzes, may contribute to worse outcomes (Furr and others 2011).

Results from cataract surgeries performed in eye camps are equally variable. Some (Kapoor and others 1999) report good vision outcomes, while others (Singh, Garner, and Floyd 2000) report poor outcomes. Similar variability is also seen in studies on otologic surgery. In surgical camps in Greenland, Homøe, Siim, and Bretlau (2008) and Homøe and others (2008) find low complication rates and good results in patients with chronic ear disease; mobile surgical units in Thailand have similarly high success rates. Other authors, however, report success rates tied very strongly to either pathologic diagnosis (Horlbeck and others 2009) or the age of the surgical mission, with better results occurring a few years after the mission's establishment (Barrs and others 2000). Finally, in cardiac surgery, Adams and others (2012) find relatively acceptable results in patients operated on for rheumatic, congenital, and ischemic heart disease during two surgical missions to Peru, but these results come from a survey of very few patients.

Overall, a solid pattern emerges in a review of the effectiveness of surgical missions: the more complex the surgery, the more unsatisfactory the results. Both Marck and others (2010) and Huijing and others (2011) find this pattern in complex reconstructions, which, combined with the findings of Maine and others (2012), leads them to recommend against short-term surgical missions for all but the simplest conditions.

Cost-Effectiveness of Short-Term Surgical Missions.
With a significant caveat to be discussed below, the few cost-effectiveness analyses that have been performed on surgical missions point, in general, to a beneficial ratio of costs to effectiveness. The cost of a short-term surgical mission is difficult to calculate and very sensitive to assumptions made regarding discounting, analysis perspective, the inclusion of nonmedical patient costs, and the inclusion of opportunity costs for the volunteering staff (Corlew 2013). Cleft missions have been estimated to range from approximately US$40 per case to US$335 per case (Hodges and Hodges 2000; Moon, Perry, and Baek 2012), and up to US$65,500 per mission (Magee, Vander Burg, and Hatcher 2010). Orthopedic missions cost more than US$170,000 each (Gosselin, Gialamas, and Atkin 2011), and short-term cataract camps cost $50 per case (Singh, Garner, and Floyd 2000).

These estimates translate to cost-effectiveness ratios comparable with other global health interventions: Cleft lip and palate repair costs anywhere from US$52/DALY averted (up to US$97 per DALY averted when costs of lost income to the physician are included) (Moon, Perry, and Baek 2012) to US$1,827 per DALY averted (Magee, Vander Burg, and Hatcher 2010). Orthopedic surgeries are slightly more expensive; elective and emergency operative procedures cost between US$340 and US$360 per DALY averted in Haiti (the emergency figures, notably, come from efforts surrounding the 2010 earthquake, and their generalizability may be limited) (Gosselin, Gialamas, and Atkin 2011).

These findings, however, must be interpreted with extreme caution, especially because they do not square with the assessment that surgical results of short-term surgical missions tend toward the unsatisfactory. The apparent cost-effectiveness of surgical missions is, in fact, very likely simply an artifact of the way in which the cost-effectiveness analyses were conducted. All of the cited studies compared intervention with no intervention—as opposed, for example, to surgery by a surgical mission versus surgery by the local infrastructure. This analytic method will frequently result in a misleadingly small cost-effectiveness ratio, which must, in turn, be interpreted very narrowly: only when *no other* platform exists to deliver care for the condition treated by the mission do these results imply that a surgical mission is cost-effective. If the condition can be treated by other platforms, including first-level hospitals, these cost-effectiveness results cannot be applied.

One cost-effectiveness analysis was found that actually compares the surgical mission with other platforms for the delivery of identical surgeries. Singh, Garner, and Floyd (2000) examine the cost-effectiveness of cataract surgeries performed at specialized eye camps, at NGO hospitals, and at the state medical college. Although not the worst value—that distinction fell to the state medical college—cataract surgery performed at short-term eye camps was much less cost-effective than that performed in permanent, nongovernmental hospitals.

Sustainability and Training Role of Short-Term Surgical Missions. Many authors laud the salutary role that short-term surgical missions can have in the education of HIC surgical trainees. Alterman and Goldman (2008); Aziz, Ziccardi, and Chuang (2012); Belyansky and others (2011); Boyd and Cruz (2011); Cameron and others (2010); Campbell, Sherman, and Magee (2010); Campbell and others (2011); Haskell and others (2002); Henry and others (2013); Hughes and others (2010); Jarman, Cogbill, and Kitowski (2009); Lee and Weinstein (2009); and Matar and others (2012) are among many who have written about this beneficial impact on surgical trainees and the surgeons with whom they travel. Although this role is not to be discounted, the benefits to surgical residents in HICs clearly cannot come at the cost of delivery of unsatisfactory care in LMICs (Wall 2011).

No published evidence was found for the role that short-term missions play in training within LMICs themselves. Short-term surgical missions have, however, been put forward as a method to alleviate the disease burden—especially given that these NGOs frequently offer surgery for free. Unfortunately, with higher complication rates and unsatisfactory results in more complex operations, the sustainable role of the surgical mission is unclear. It is not altogether unlikely, for example, that these surgical missions treat the same conditions that would be treated otherwise in first-level hospitals, and that fragmentation in delivery (Butler 2010) contributes to poor coordination and often a frank inability to meet the large burden of unmet need by the short-term mission (Cam and others 2010).

The structure of the short-term medical mission itself may also be detrimental to sustainability. Patients are usually identified before the surgical team's arrival by local medical staff (Nthumba 2010). While the team is there, a large volume of cases are performed, often overwhelming the local infrastructure during and after the team's visit (Nthumba 2010).

Finally, it should also be noted that, in the communities they serve, these platforms create an awareness of a given surgical condition and the potential to address it surgically. This awareness can often have counterintuitively *detrimental* effects on health care utilization among the population. When outcomes are consistently good, increased awareness influences positive health-seeking behavior in potential patients. Even the most sporadic of bad outcomes, however, seem to discourage care-seeking outright (Fletcher and others 1999).

Despite its ubiquity, then, the short-term surgical mission appears to have a relatively limited role in the delivery of surgical care. In settings in which surgical conditions cannot otherwise be treated, the short-term mission is cost-effective and appears to have a role in the amelioration of the surgical burden. However, in settings in which other platforms exist for surgical delivery, the short-term mission is unlikely to be either the most effective or the most cost-effective method with which to alleviate the large burden of surgical disease in LMICs. Given potentially unsatisfactory results with complex surgeries, potentially detrimental effects on health-seeking behavior, and stress on the local surgical infrastructure, the short-term stand-alone surgical mission, when other options exist, is likely to be inefficient (Browning and Patel 2004).

Self-Contained Mobile Surgical Platforms

The fact that complex procedures performed by short-term missions yield unsatisfactory results, (Huijing and others 2011; Marck and others 2010), combined with the fact that most first-level hospitals are also unable to provide this care consistently (Hsia and others 2012; Ilbawi, Einterz, and Nkusu 2013; Linden and others 2012), leads to an obvious question. Many LMICs are committed to improving their surgical capacity; while they do so, how can the interim unmet need be best met, if not with short-term missions? Are specialized surgical hospitals the best way to provide adequate complex care that the local health infrastructure cannot yet provide—and to do so cost-effectively? Or can a different temporary model, better structured than the short-term mission, provide this level of care?

Few examples of such an intermediate model for surgical delivery exist, but those that do are promising. Mercy Ships, for example, maintains hospital ships that provide specialized surgical care in West Africa. They carry their entire infrastructure with them, including pathology and radiology (Harris 2013), and they are able to provide ophthalmologic, reconstructive, general, orthopedic, and obstetric fistula surgeries (Cheng, McColl, and Parker 2012; Lewis and de Bernis 2006). The limited studies on the effectiveness of surgical procedures performed using this platform indicate a complication rate that is comparable with complication rates for cases performed in centers in HICs (Cheng, McColl, and Parker 2012). No literature on similar platforms, such as Floating Doctors, was found.

Military organizations adopt a similar model. The United States Navy maintains two hospital ships that report mortality and complication rates that are equivalent to, if not better than, those found in hospitals in HICs (Troup 2007; Walk and others 2011, 2012). There have been, as yet, no cost evaluations and no cost-effectiveness evaluations of these self-contained surgical platforms.

SPECIALTY SURGICAL HOSPITALS

Demand and Supply Constraints

Specialized surgical hospitals are myriad (table 13.1). Many have evolved from temporary surgical platforms. Cataract surgeries in India, for example, were initially performed in makeshift surgical facilities, schools, or community halls, before their care made the transition to specialized hospitals. Technologies were very basic, limited essentially to surgical instruments and the skills of the surgeons. Although this sort of outreach—with improved technology—continues to be common, a population-based study estimates that those accessing these outreach eye camps represent a mere 7 percent of those in need of eye care (Fletcher and others 1998).

Similarly, current global estimates put resource utilization of eye care facilities at 25 percent of incident cases of blindness (WHO 2005). Research by

Table 13.1 Examples of Surgical Specialty Hospitals in LMICs

Cardiac
Salam Centre for Cardiac Surgery, Khartoum, Sudan
Narayana Hrudayalaya Hospitals, Bangalore, India
Innova Children's Heart Hospital, Hyderabad, India
Ophthalmic
ORBIS
Aravind Eye Hospitals, Tamilnadu, India
LRBT Eye Hospitals, Pakistan
Obstetric Fistula
Babbar Ruga Fistula Teaching Hospital, Katsina, Nigeria
Addis Ababa Fistula Hospital, Addis Ababa, Ethiopia
Danja Fistula Center, Danja, Niger
Maternity Services
Life Spring Hospitals, India
Cancer
Adayar Cancer Institute, Chennai, India
Tata Memorial Hospital, Mumbai, India

Note: LMICs = low- and middle-income countries.

Browning and Patel (2004, 321) in the obstetric fistula setting indicates that "at the world's current capacity to repair fistula, it would take at least 400 years to clear the backlog of patients, provided that there are no more new cases." At present, less than 1 percent of the surgical need for fistula repair is met (Browning and Patel 2004). In Ethiopia alone, it is estimated that of the 2.9 million women who give birth annually, almost 9,000 will develop an obstetric fistula (Hamlin, Muleta, and Kennedy 2002; Muleta, Rasmussen, and Kiserud 2010). Similar statements can be made about the unmet need for cardiac surgery, maternity services, and cancer care.

In addition to constituting a large unmet need, many surgical conditions—especially those treated by specialized hospitals—are chronic, allowing (with notable exceptions) these surgeries to be performed electively. Because at least some of these conditions (cataracts, hernias, and cardiac conditions, for example) also tend to be age related, and because these interventions can dramatically enhance activities of daily living and the quality of life (Fletcher and others 1998), an aging population will make it crucial that such services are provided in a sustainable manner.

Demand is, however, constrained by a number of factors: a large, underserved, and dispersed population; scarce capital and human resources; poor in-country logistics; and patient-level characteristics—barriers to market entry, fluctuating incomes with little disposable surplus, unfamiliarity with surgical procedures, and multiple domestic necessities (figure 13.2) (Prahalad 2009). Finally, many complex conditions cannot be treated by a single surgical procedure and require treatment of specialized preoperative and postoperative needs—including physiotherapy, economic rehabilitation, preoperative nourishment, social counseling, and physical environments that are geared toward specific surgical conditions—for which the specialized hospital may be well suited.

Effectiveness of Specialty Surgical Hospitals

The challenge for specialized surgical hospitals is not one of discovering novel clinical solutions to these conditions—time-tested surgical interventions for many of the conditions treated by long-term surgical platforms exist (Ruit and others 2007)—but of effective long-term implementation in permanent centers located in resource-limited settings. Effectiveness data for specialized surgical hospitals are, however, limited and come primarily from ophthalmologic and fistula centers. We found no evidence from specialty hospitals treating other conditions.

Figure 13.2 Demand and Supply Levers in Delivering Surgical Care in LMICs

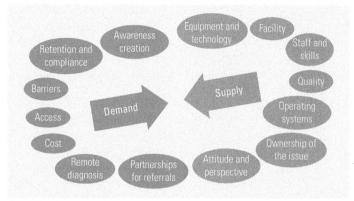

Note: LMICs = low- and middle-income countries.

Evidence for the effectiveness of ophthalmologic centers has already been presented: specialized NGO hospitals are more cost-effective than other platforms in the provision of cataract surgery (Singh, Garner, and Floyd 2000).

Repair of obstetric fistula is complex. Fistula surgeons are not considered expert until they have performed at least 300 cases (FIGO and Partners 2011); even expert surgeons deliver, on average, closure and continence to only 85 percent of patients. The volume of surgeries required to qualify as an expert and competent fistula surgeon may not be met in short-term missions, or at a first-level hospital, for years (FIGO and Partners 2011). Published studies, however, document good results for specialized fistula hospitals: the Addis Ababa Fistula Hospital (a charitable organization) and Babbar Ruga Fistula Teaching Hospital (an initiative sponsored by the Nigerian government with reliance on external funding) do well, reporting rates of successful fistula closure and return to continence of greater than 90 percent (Muleta 1997; Waaldijk 2008).

In addition to issues of volume and success rates, complex surgical conditions, such as obstetric fistula and cleft palate, place specific demands on the design of the physical facility, often not feasible on a short-term mission. For instance, Hamlin, Muleta, and Kennedy (2002) highlight needs unique to the vulnerable fistula population: traditional multistoried hospitals are not in sympathy with the poor communities from which these women come, while grassy areas can absorb leaking urine, and wide, open walkways and corridors allow the "pervasive smell of urine … to escape more readily" (Hamlin, Muleta, and Kennedy 2002, 51), both of which improve morale. Finally, specialized long-term platforms can provide physical therapy services and rehabilitation and reintegration services, all deemed to be important to an effective fistula program. Similar rehabilitative considerations—including speech and swallowing therapy—are required for the repair of cleft palate.

Temporary surgical platforms—especially those espousing a short-term model—are unlikely to be able to meet these needs; and while first-level hospitals may meet some of them, they often cannot prioritize such additional services and facilities over more life-threatening surgical conditions, further preventing the delivery of complex surgery (Wall 2007). In keeping with these findings, an expert elicitation study also concludes that outcomes for complicated obstetric fistula cases are most likely best at the high-volume, specialized surgical hospitals as opposed to first-level hospitals (Colson and others 2013).

Cost-Effectiveness of Specialty Surgical Hospitals

The single comparison of cataract care across platforms demonstrates the superior cost-effectiveness of permanent NGO hospitals (Singh, Garner, and Floyd 2000). Compared with US$50 per case at short-term cataract hospitals, NGO hospitals treat cataracts at US$46 per case, with nearly double the patient satisfaction (Singh, Garner, and Floyd 2000). No adequate data, unfortunately, exist to assess the cost-effectiveness of fistula repair centers, cardiac centers, or other specialized surgical hospitals.

Sustainability and Training Role of Specialty Surgical Hospitals

Whether a hospital is run for profit or as a nonprofit, it must be sustainable across the several dimensions of financial stability, clinical services, leadership, and community support. Financial stability is addressed by developing sustainable sources of income, as well as by ensuring high efficiency, appropriate pricing, and effective cost control measures that do not adversely affect quality or productivity. Standard protocols, processes for continuous improvement, and succession planning also contribute to stability and sustainability. The ability to continue to provide clinical services once they have departed is difficult for short-term surgical platforms—most teams take the technical skills, support, and equipment with them when they leave.

The high volume of specialized centers, however, allows for sustainable surgical training programs. The Babbar Ruga Fistula Teaching Hospital has trained more than 315 fistula surgeons and 320 nurses worldwide (Waaldijk 2008); to meet ophthalmic training needs, internal training programs at the Aravind Eye Hospital now graduate about 400 mid-level ophthalmic personnel and 33 ophthalmologists each year. Consistent with

Browning and Patel's 2004 estimates, the experience of one of this review's authors (A. Sleemi) with short-term surgical missions for obstetric fistula demonstrates the level of sustainability required for education: the training of two Eritrean fistula surgeons required at least five years before competency levels and adequate case numbers were met.

Finally, from an academic standpoint, the bulk of the literature comes from such specialized training centers: both Addis Ababa and Babbar Ruga Fistula Hospitals have provided key data and landmark papers on the management of obstetric fistula. Specialized surgical centers, because of their high volumes, may have a role in filling the void of an evidence base in global surgery.

DISCUSSION

Surgical conditions constitute up to 26 percent of the global burden of disease, and the current surgical infrastructure in many LMICs meets very little of that need. Access to surgical care is low (Brilliant and others 1985; Browning and Patel 2004; WHO 2005), and most hospitals in LMICs are themselves unable to meet the demand of high-DALY surgical conditions (Ilbawi, Einterz, and Nkusu 2013). Simultaneously, a rich, rapidly growing, and often fragmented charitable sector has stepped in to meet surgical need—a sector that, despite its growth, has not been systematically evaluated (Butler 2010). This review summarizes the known evidence on the impact of the charitable sector in delivering surgical care in LMICs.

Unfortunately, what evaluations have been done may actually promote fragmentation—examining surgical missions in isolation, as most studies have, prevents informative similarities and differences among these missions from becoming explicit. We propose, instead, to structure evaluations around *platforms* for the delivery of care, rather than around disease types or individual missions. Doing so highlights the relative effectiveness or ineffectiveness of models that underpin charitable surgical delivery.

Accordingly, we have broken down the galaxy of surgical NGOs into two types: temporary surgical platforms—including short-term, surgical missions and self-contained mobile surgical programs—and freestanding specialized surgical centers. The overall findings from this systematic review are presented in table 13.2.

Short-Term Surgical Missions

The available evidence suggests that, despite its ubiquity and benefit to HIC medical resident training, the role

Table 13.2 Summary of Results

Domain	Platform		
	Temporary, short-term mission	Temporary, self-contained[a]	Surgical specialty hospital
Effectiveness	Poor results for complex procedures; effective for simple procedures	Potentially equivalent to outcomes in HICs	Equivalent to outcomes in HICs
Cost-effectiveness	Yes if serving as the only platform for surgery; unlikely otherwise	No data available	Most cost-effective of the competing choices
Sustainability	Unlikely; may have a detrimental impact on health-seeking behavior	No data available	Platform suitable for sustainability
Training	Effective for HIC surgeons; limited data on surgeons in LMICs	Available for training	Definite role in LMICs

Note: HICs = high-income countries; LMICs = low- and middle-income countries.
a. Sparse data on this platform limit the certainty of these conclusions.

of short-term temporary surgical missions should be limited to areas and conditions for which no other surgical delivery platform is available. In these settings, this platform delivers care very cost-effectively.

In settings in which alternative delivery systems exist, the short-term mission appears to be an inefficient way to meet the global burden of high-DALY surgical disease (Cam and others 2010). These missions may not be effective at reaching the patients with unmet need, given that they treat conditions that first-level hospitals may already be treating (Browning and Patel 2004; Butler 2010) and may risk delivering unsatisfactory results, especially for complex reconstructions (Huijing and others 2011; Maine and others 2012; Marck and others 2010). Although some conditions are amenable to surgical blitzes (Sykes and others 2012), the blitzes themselves often stress the underlying local surgical infrastructure (Nthumba 2010) and may discourage health-seeking behavior (Fletcher and others 1999), which undermines this platform's sustainability.

For conditions for which cost-effectiveness evidence exists (facial clefting and orthopedic care), these surgical missions provide cost-effective service—but they do so only, again, in comparison with settings that do not provide *any* surgery (Gosselin, Gialamas, and Atkin 2011; Hodges and Hodges 2000; Magee, Vander Burg, and Hatcher 2010; Moon, Perry, and Baek 2012). In analyses in which they are compared with other platforms in delivering identical services, surgical missions become less cost-effective (Singh, Garner, and Floyd 2000).

Self-Contained Mobile Surgical Platforms

Self-contained mobile platforms are rare, but they fit in the negative space between the surgical mission and the

specialty hospital. They offer services, such as radiology, that are usually not found in the short-term mission (Harris 2013) and are able to deliver care comparable to that found in HICs (Cheng, McColl, and Parker 2012). Studies on this platform are few, and cost-effectiveness studies are nonexistent; in the interim, while surgical infrastructure develops, a scale-up of this model should be considered, given that it might meet the burden of surgical disease in a more effective and efficient way than its short-term counterpart.

Specialty Surgical Hospitals

Finally, the literature suggests that specialized surgical centers might be effective in providing a high volume of care with good outcomes (Muleta 1997; Waaldijk 2008). These long-term platforms are also able to provide for some of the unique needs faced by patients with more complex conditions (Hamlin, Muleta, and Kennedy 2002; Wall 2007; Wall and others 2006). One cost-effectiveness analysis that makes comparisons across platforms does demonstrate the superiority of these specialized surgical hospitals to short-term missions (Singh, Garner, and Floyd 2000), but further analyses are necessary.

This review is the first to attempt a broad, systematic evaluation of charitable surgical delivery in LMICs, distinct from the conditions treated and the individual organizations that treat them. As such, it has certain limitations. It should be noted, for example, that any taxonomy is leaky. Some organizations that establish hospitals also send short-term missions to other countries; some of the self-contained organizations have themselves established hospitals. That no classification system can adequately characterize any NGO does not, however, mean that research into these organizations must remain fragmented. This taxonomy, incomplete though it may be, proposes a structure for future research into a large sector of the health system.

The peer-reviewed literature in this area is small, all outcomes studies are case series, and nearly all the cost-effectiveness studies are predicated on heroic assumptions. In addition, although some studies do show less-than-optimal results, publication bias very likely exists. More important, a lack of evidence does not imply evidence of a lack. Many surgeons in LMICs, in addition to surgeons who work with these charitable organizations, have little time to devote to producing peer-reviewed publications. As such, a dearth of evidence exists as to the comparative effectiveness of NGO platforms and first-level hospitals within the same setting. This evidence void highlights the need for further investigation into the effectiveness of surgery as delivered in these settings, as well as the potential role for other research methods—such as realist synthesis—in the study of surgical delivery by charities in LMICs.

Finally, of the domains along which delivery platforms were evaluated (cost-effectiveness, effectiveness, sustainability, and training role), the first is especially controversial, especially given the various platforms used. Some organizations, for example, work entirely with volunteer staff; others pay. Therefore, cost-effectiveness claims must be interpreted with caution.

CONCLUSIONS AND RECOMMENDATIONS

Limitations in the literature highlight the clear need for more, and larger, evaluations of the effectiveness and cost-effectiveness of the charitable sector's role in the delivery of surgical care in LMICs. This sector is large and spends a significant amount of donor money (Casey 2007). Determining the most effective platform for the delivery of care stands to benefit patients, for whom this is often the only affordable avenue of care; determining the most cost-effective platform stands also to align donor interests with those of the patients they seek to help.

The available literature allows the following recommendations to be made:

- Evaluations of charitable surgery should be undertaken from the perspective of the care-delivery platform—short-term surgical trips, self-contained mobile platforms, and specialty hospitals—instead of by the disease condition addressed by individual organizations.

- Short-term surgical missions are useful when access to surgical services is nonexistent. This recommendation must, however, be made with caution because, although any surgical access is better than none, poor outcomes may have a chilling effect on health-seeking behavior.
- Consideration should be given to expansion of self-contained mobile platforms instead of short-term surgical trips to meet the unmet surgical need in countries developing their surgical infrastructure.
- Rigorous evaluations of the cost-effectiveness and sustainability of various charitable delivery platforms should be undertaken.
- Because training already occurs within the confines of some NGOs, further evaluations of the effectiveness of this training should be undertaken—with respect to the retention of surgical skills, to improvements in outcomes, and to the retention of in-country providers.

Although the paucity of data implies a measure of uncertainty in these recommendations, this literature review suggests that following them may help in decreasing the fragmentation found in the nongovernmental sector, to the ultimate benefit of surgical patients (Ilbawi, Einterz, and Nkusu 2013).

ACKNOWLEDGMENTS

The authors are indebted to Dr. Peggy Lai, Sweta Adhikari, and Vittoria Lutje for help in the literature search.

NOTES

This chapter uses the World Health Organization's (WHO's) six geographical regions: African Region, Region of the Americas, South-East Asia Region, European Region, Eastern Mediterranean Region, and Western Pacific Region.

The World Bank classifies countries according to four income groupings. Income is measured using gross national income (GNI) per capita, in U.S. dollars, converted from local currency using the *World Bank Atlas* method. Classifications as of July 2014 are as follows:

- Low-income countries (LICs) = US$1,045 or less in 2013
- Middle-income countries (MICs) are subdivided:
  - lower-middle-income = US$1,046 to US$4,125
  - upper-middle-income (UMICs) = US$4,126 to US$12,745
- High-income countries (HICs) = US$12,746 or more

REFERENCES

Adams, C., P. Kiefer, K. Ryan, D. Smith, G. McCabe, and others. 2012. "Humanitarian Cardiac Care in Arequipa, Peru: Experiences of a Multidisciplinary Canadian Cardiovascular Team." *Canadian Journal of Surgery* 55 (3): 171–76. doi:10.1503/cjs.029910.

Alterman, D. M., and M. H. Goldman. 2008. "International Volunteerism during General Surgical Residency: A Resident's Experience." *Journal of Surgical Education* 65 (5): 378–83. doi:10.1016/j.jsurg.2008.07.009.

Aziz, S. R., V. B. Ziccardi, and S. K. Chuang. 2012. "Survey of Residents Who Have Participated in Humanitarian Medical Missions." *Journal of Oral and Maxillofacial Surgery* 70 (2): e147–57. doi:10.1016/j.joms.2011.10.007.

Bai, V. T., V. Murali, R. Kim, and S. K. Srivatsa. 2007. "Teleophthalmology-Based Rural Eye Care in India." *Telemedicine Journal and e-Health* 13 (3): 313–21. doi:10.1089/tmj.2006.0048.

Bailie, R. 1996. "An Economic Appraisal of a Mobile Cervical Cytology Screening Service." *South African Medical Journal* 86 (9 Suppl): 1179–84.

Balent, L. C., K. Narendrum, S. Patel, S. Kar, and D. A. Patterson. 2001. "High Volume Sutureless Intraocular Lens Surgery in a Rural Eye Camp in India." *Ophthalmic Surgery and Lasers* 32 (6): 446–55.

Barrs, D. M., S. P. Muller, D. B. Worrndell, and E. W. Weidmann. 2000. "Results of a Humanitarian Otologic and Audiologic Project Performed outside of the United States: Lessons Learned from the Oye, Amigos! Project." *Otolaryngology—Head and Neck Surgery* 123 (6): 722–27. doi:10.1067/mhn.2000.110959.

Belyansky, I., K. B. Williams, M. Gashti, and R. F. Heitmiller. 2011. "Surgical Relief Work in Haiti: A Practical Resident Learning Experience." *Journal of Surgical Education* 68 (3): 213–17. doi:10.1016/j.jsurg.2010.12.003.

Bermudez, L., V. Carter, W. Magee, Jr., R. Sherman, and R. Ayala. 2010. "Surgical Outcomes Auditing Systems in Humanitarian Organizations." *World Journal of Surgery* 34 (3): 403–10. doi:10.1007/s00268-009-0253-6.

Bermudez, L., K. Trost, and R. Ayala. 2013. "Investing in a Surgical Outcomes Auditing System." *Plastic Surgery International* 2013: 671786. doi:10.1155/2013/671786.

Bickler, S. W., T. G. Weiser, N. Kassebaum, H. Higashi, D. C. Chang, and others. 2015. "Global Burden of Surgical Conditions." In *Disease Control Priorities* (third edition): Volume 1, *Essential Surgery*, edited by H. T. Debas, P. Donkor, A. Gawande, D. T. Jamison, M. E. Kruk, and C. N. Mock. Washington, DC: World Bank.

Birkmeyer, J. D., A. E. Siewers, E. V. Finlayson, T. A. Stukel, F. L. Lucas, and others. 2002. "Hospital Volume and Surgical Mortality in the United States." *New England Journal of Medicine* 346 (15): 1128–37.

Birkmeyer, J. D., T. A. Stukel, A. E. Siewers, P. P. Goodney, and D. E. Wennberg. 2003. "Surgeon Volume and Operative Mortality in the United States." *New England Journal of Medicine* 349 (22): 2117–27.

Boyd, N. H., and R. M. Cruz. 2011. "The Importance of International Medical Rotations in Selection of an Otolaryngology Residency." *Journal of Graduate Medical Education* 3 (3): 414–16. doi:10.4300/jgme-d-10-00185.1.

Brilliant, L. B., R. P. Pokrel, N. C. Grasset, J. M. Lepkowski, A. Kolstad, and others. 1985. "Epidemiology of Blindness in Nepal." *Bulletin of the World Health Organization* 63 (2): 375–86.

Browning, A., and T. L. Patel. 2004. "FIGO Initiative for the Prevention and Treatment of Vaginal Fistula." *International Journal of Gynecology and Obstetrics* 86 (2): 317–22.

Butler, M. W. 2010. "Fragmented International Volunteerism: Need for a Global Pediatric Surgery Network." *Journal of Pediatric Surgery* 45 (2): 303–09. doi:10.1016/j.jpedsurg.2009.10.064.

Cam, C., A. Karateke, A. Ozdemir, C. Gunes, C. Celik, and others. 2010. "Fistula Campaigns—Are They of Any Benefit?" *Taiwanese Journal of Obstetrics and Gynecology* 49 (3): 291–96. doi:10.1016/s1028-4559(10)60063-0.

Cameron, B. H., M. Rambaran, D. P. Sharma, and R. H. Taylor. 2010. "International Surgery: The Development of Postgraduate Surgical Training in Guyana." *Canadian Journal of Surgery* 53 (1): 11–16.

Campbell, A., R. Sherman, and W. P. Magee. 2010. "The Role of Humanitarian Missions in Modern Surgical Training." *Plastic and Reconstructive Surgery* 126 (1): 295–302. doi:10.1097/PRS.0b013e3181dab618.

Campbell, A., M. Sullivan, R. Sherman, and W. P. Magee. 2011. "The Medical Mission and Modern Cultural Competency Training." *Journal of the American College of Surgeons* 212 (1): 124–19. doi:10.1016/j.jamcollsurg.2010.08.019.

Casey, K. M. 2007. "The Global Impact of Surgical Volunteerism." *Surgical Clinics of North America* 87 (4): 949–60, ix. doi:10.1016/j.suc.2007.07.018.

Chao, T. E., M. Burdic, K. Ganjawalla, M. Derbew, C. Keshian, and others. 2012. "Survey of Surgery and Anesthesia Infrastructure in Ethiopia." *World Journal of Surgery* 36 (11): 2545–53. doi:10.1007/s00268-012-1729-3.

Cheng, L. H., L. McColl, and G. Parker. 2012. "Thyroid Surgery in the UK and on Board the Mercy Ships." *British Journal of Oral and Maxillofacial Surgery* 50 (7): 592–96. doi:10.1016/j.bjoms.2011.10.009.

Chu, K. M., N. Ford, and M. Trelles. 2010. "Operative Mortality in Resource-Limited Settings: The Experience of Médecins Sans Frontières in 13 Countries." *Archives of Surgery* 145 (8): 721–25.

———. 2011. "Providing Surgical Care in Somalia: A Model of Task-Shifting." *Conflict and Health* 5: 12.

Chu, K. M., M. Trelles, and N. Ford. 2011. "Quality of Care in Humanitarian Surgery." *World Journal of Surgery* 35 (6): 1169–72; discussion 1173–74.

Civerchia, L., S. W. Apoorvananda, G. Natchiar, A. Balent, R. Ramakrishnan, and others. 1993. "Intraocular Lens Implantation in Rural India." *Ophthalmic Surgery* 24 (10): 648–52; discussion 652–53.

Civerchia, L., R. D. Ravindran, S. W. Apoorvananda, R. Ramakrishnan, A. Balent, and others. 1996. "High-Volume

Intraocular Lens Surgery in a Rural Eye Camp in India." *Ophthalmic Surgery Lasers* 27 (3): 200–08.

Colson, A., S. Adhikari, A. Sleemi, and R. Laxminarayan. 2013. "Quantifying Uncertainty in Intervention Effectiveness: An Application in Obstetric Fistula." DCP3 Working Paper No. 7.

Corlew, D. S. 2013. "Economic Modeling of Surgical Disease: A Measure of Public Health Interventions." *World Journal of Surgery* 37 (7): 1478–85.

Cousins, G. R., L. Obolensky, C. McAllen, V. Acharya, and A. Beebeejaun. 2012. "The Kenya Orthopaedic Project: Surgical Outcomes of a Travelling Multidisciplinary Team." *Journal of Bone and Joint Surgery British Volume* 94 (12): 1591–94. doi:10.1302/0301-620x.94b12.29920.

de Buys Roessingh, A. S., M. Dolci, C. Zbinden-Trichet, R. Bossou, B. J. Meyrat, and others. 2012. "Success and Failure for Children Born with Facial Clefts in Africa: A 15-Year Follow-Up." *World Journal of Surgery* 36 (8): 1963–69. doi:10.1007/s00268-012-1607-z.

Eskander, A., J. Irish, P. A. Groome, J. Freeman, P. Gullane, and others. 2014. "Volume-Outcome Relationships in the Surgical Management of Head and Neck Cancer in a Universal Health Care System." *Laryngoscope.* Advance online publication. doi:10.1002/lary.24704.

FIGO (International Federation of Gynecology and Obstetrics) and Partners. 2011. "Global Competency-Based Fistula Surgery Training Manual." London: FIGO. http://www.figo.org/files/figo-corp/FIGO_Global_Competency-Based_Fistula_Surgery_Training_Manual_0.pdf.

Fletcher, A., M. Donoghue, J. Devavaram, R. D. Thulasiraj, S. Scott, and others. 1999. "Low Uptake of Eye Services in Rural India: A Challenge for Programs of Blindness Prevention." *Archives of Ophthalmology* 117 (10): 1393–99.

Fletcher, A., V. Vijaykumar, S. Selvaraj, R. D. Thulasiraj, and L. B. Ellwein. 1998. "The Madurai Intraocular Lens Study. III: Visual Functioning and Quality of Life Outcomes." *American Journal of Ophthalmology* 125 (1): 26–35.

Frampton, M. C. 1993. "Otological Relief Work in Romania." *Journal of Laryngology and Otology* 107 (12): 1185–89.

Furr, M. C., E. Larkin, R. Blakeley, T. W. Albert, L. Tsugawa, and others. 2011. "Extending Multidisciplinary Management of Cleft Palate to the Developing World." *Journal of Oral and Maxillofacial Surgery* 69 (1): 237–41. doi:10.1016/j.joms.2010.06.214.

Gosselin, R. A., G. Gialamas, and D. M. Atkin. 2011. "Comparing the Cost-Effectiveness of Short Orthopedic Missions in Elective and Relief Situations in Developing Countries." *World Journal of Surgery* 35 (5): 951–55. doi:10.1007/s00268-010-0947-9.

Hamlin, E. C., M. Muleta, and R. C. Kennedy. 2002. "Providing an Obstetric Fistula Service." *British Journal of Urology International* 89 (S1): 50–53.

Harris, R. D. 2013. "Radiology on the *Africa Mercy*, the Largest Private Floating Hospital Ship in the World." *American Journal of Roentgenology* 200 (2): W124–29. doi:10.2214/ajr.12.9087.

Haskell, A., D. Rovinsky, H. K. Brown, and R. R. Coughlin. 2002. "The University of California at San Francisco International Orthopaedic Elective." *Clinical Orthopaedics and Related Research* (396): 12–18.

Henry, J. A., R. S. Groen, R. R. Price, B. C. Nwomeh, T. P. Kingham, and others. 2013. "The Benefits of International Rotations to Resource-Limited Settings for U.S. Surgery Residents." *Surgery* 153 (4): 445–54. doi:10.1016/j.surg.2012.10.018.

Hodges, A. M., and S. C. Hodges. 2000. "A Rural Cleft Project in Uganda." *British Journal of Plastic Surgery* 53 (1): 7–11. doi:10.1054/bjps.1999.3238.

Homøe, P., G. Nikoghosyan, C. Siim, and P. Bretlau. 2008. "Hearing Outcomes after Mobile Ear Surgery for Chronic Otitis Media in Greenland." *International Journal of Circumpolar Health* 67 (5): 452–60.

Homøe, P., C. Siim, and P. Bretlau. 2008. "Outcome of Mobile Ear Surgery for Chronic Otitis Media in Remote Areas." *Otolaryngology—Head and Neck Surgery* 139 (1): 55–61. doi:10.1016/j.otohns.2008.03.014.

Horlbeck, D., M. Boston, B. Balough, B. Sierra, G. Saenz, and others. 2009. "Humanitarian Otologic Missions: Long-Term Surgical Results." *Otolaryngology—Head and Neck Surgery* 140 (4): 559–65. doi:10.1016/j.otohns.2008.12.033.

Hsia, R. Y., N. A. Mbembati, S. Macfarlane, and M. E. Kruk. 2012. "Access to Emergency and Surgical Care in Sub-Saharan Africa: The Infrastructure Gap." *Health Policy and Planning* 27 (3): 234–44. doi:10.1093/heapol/czr023.

Hughes, C., S. Zani, B. O'Connell, and I. Daoud. 2010. "International Surgery and the University of Connecticut Experience: Lessons from a Short-Term Surgical Mission." *Connecticut Medicine* 74 (3): 157–60.

Huijing, M. A., K. W. Marck, J. Combes, K. D. Mizen, L. Fourie, and others. 2011. "Facial Reconstruction in the Developing World: A Complicated Matter." *British Journal of Oral and Maxillofacial Surgery* 49 (4): 292–96. doi:10.1016/j.bjoms.2009.08.044.

Ilbawi, A. M., E. M. Einterz, and D. Nkusu. 2013. "Obstacles to Surgical Services in a Rural Cameroonian District Hospital." *World Journal of Surgery* 37 (6): 1208–15. doi:10.1007/s00268-013-1977-x.

Jarman, B. T., T. H. Cogbill, and N. J. Kitowski. 2009. "Development of an International Elective in a General Surgery Residency." *Journal of Surgical Education* 66 (4): 222–24. doi:10.1016/j.jsurg.2009.07.003.

Kapoor, H., A. Chatterjee, R. Daniel, and A. Foster. 1999. "Evaluation of Visual Outcome of Cataract Surgery in an Indian Eye Camp." *British Journal of Ophthalmology* 83 (3): 343–46.

Knowlton, L. M., S. Chackungal, B. Dahn, D. LeBrun, J. Nickerson, and others. 2013. "Liberian Surgical and Anesthesia Infrastructure: A Survey of County Hospitals." *World Journal of Surgery* 37 (4): 721–29. doi:10.1007/s00268-013-1903-2.

Lee, D. K., and S. Weinstein. 2009. "International Public Health in Third World Country Medical Missions: When Small Legs Walk, We All Stand a Little Taller." *Journal of the American Podiatric Medical Association* 99 (4): 371–76.

Lehnerdt, G., A. van Delden, and J. Lautermann. 2005. "Management of an 'Ear Camp' for Children in Namibia." *International Journal of Pediatric Otorhinolaryngology* 69 (5): 663–68. doi:10.1016/j.ijporl.2004.12.007.

Lewis, G., and L. de Bernis. 2006. *Obstetric Fistula: Guiding Principles for Clinical Management and Programme Development.* Geneva: World Health Organization. http://www.endfistula.org/webdav/site/endfistula/shared /documents/publications/who_obstetric_fistula.pdf.

Linden, A. F., F. S. Sekidde, M. Galukande, L. M. Knowlton, S. Chackungal, and others. 2012. "Challenges of Surgery in Developing Countries: A Survey of Surgical and Anesthesia Capacity in Uganda's Public Hospitals." *World Journal of Surgery* 36 (5): 1056–65. doi:10.1007/s00268-012-1482-7.

Magee, W. P., Jr. 2010. "Evolution of a Sustainable Surgical Delivery Model." *Journal of Craniofacial Surgery* 21 (5): 1321–26. doi:10.1097/SCS.0b013e3181ef2a6c.

———, H. M. Raimondi, M. Beers, and M. C. Koech. 2012. "Effectiveness of International Surgical Program Model to Build Local Sustainability." *Plastic Surgery International* 2012: 185725. doi:10.1155/2012/185725.

Magee, W. P., Jr., R. Vander Burg, and K. W. Hatcher. 2010. "Cleft Lip and Palate as a Cost-Effective Health Care Treatment in the Developing World." *World Journal of Surgery* 34 (3): 420–27. doi:10.1007/s00268-009-0333-7.

Maine, R. G., W. Y. Hoffman, J. H. Palacios-Martinez, D. S. Corlew, and G. A. Gregory. 2012. "Comparison of Fistula Rates after Palatoplasty for International and Local Surgeons on Surgical Missions in Ecuador with Rates at a Craniofacial Center in the United States." *Plastic and Reconstructive Surgery* 129 (2): 319e–26e. doi:10.1097/PRS.0b013e31823aea7e.

Marck, R., M. Huijing, D. Vest, M. Eshete, K. Marck, and others. 2010. "Early Outcome of Facial Reconstructive Surgery Abroad: A Comparative Study." *European Journal of Plastic Surgery* 33 (4): 193–97. doi:10.1007 /s00238-010-0409-5.

Matar, W. Y., D. C. Trottier, F. Balaa, R. Fairful-Smith, and P. Moroz. 2012. "Surgical Residency Training and International Volunteerism: A National Survey of Residents from 2 Surgical Specialties." *Canadian Journal of Surgery* 55 (4): S191–99. doi:10.1503/cjs.005411.

McCoy, D., S. Chand, and D. Sridhar. 2010. "Global Health Funding: How Much, Where It Comes from, and Where It Goes." *Health Policy and Planning* 24 (6): 407–17.

McQueen, K. A., J. A. Hyder, B. R. Taira, N. Semer, F. M. Burkle, Jr., and others. 2010. "The Provision of Surgical Care by International Organizations in Developing Countries: A Preliminary Report." *World Journal of Surgery* 34 (3): 397–402. doi:10.1007/s00268-009-0181-5.

Mock, C. N., P. Donkor, A. Gawande, D. T. Jamison, M. E. Kruk, and H. T. Debas. 2015. "Essential Surgery: Key Messages of This Volume." In *Disease Control Priorities* (third edition): Volume 1, *Essential Surgery*, edited by H. T. Debas, P. Donkor, A. Gawande, D. T. Jamison, M. E. Kruk, and C. N. Mock. Washington, DC: World Bank.

Moon, W., H. Perry, and R. M. Baek. 2012. "Is International Volunteer Surgery for Cleft Lip and Cleft Palate a Cost-Effective and Justifiable Intervention? A Case Study from East Asia." *World Journal of Surgery* 36 (12): 2819–30. doi:10.1007/s00268-012-1761-3.

Muleta, M. 1997. "Obstetric Fistulae: A Retrospective Study of 1210 Cases at the Addis Ababa Fistula Hospital." *Journal of Obstetrics and Gynecology* 17 (1): 68–70.

Muleta, M., S. Rasmussen, and T. Kiserud. 2010. "Obstetric Fistula in 14,928 Ethiopian Women." *Acta Obstetrica et Gynecologica Scandinavica* 89 (7): 945–51. doi:10.3109 /00016341003801698.

Nthumba, P. M. 2010. "'Blitz Surgery': Redefining Surgical Needs, Training, and Practice in Sub-Saharan Africa." *World Journal of Surgery* 34 (3): 433–37. doi:10.1007 /s00268-009-0256-3.

Poilleux, J., and P. Lobry. 1991. "Surgical Humanitarian Missions: An Experience over 18 Years." *Chirurgie* 117 (8): 602–06.

Prahalad, C. K. 2009. *The Fortune at the Bottom of the Pyramid: Eradicating Poverty through Profits.* 5th ed. Upper Saddle River, NJ: Prentice Hall.

Rodgers, A., N. Walker, S. Schug, A. McKee, H. Kehlet, and others. 2000. "Reduction of Postoperative Mortality and Morbidity with Epidural or Spinal Anaesthesia: Results from Overview of Randomised Trials." *British Medical Journal* 321 (7275): 1493.

Ruit, S., G. Tabin, D. Chang, L. Bajracharya, D. C. Kline, and others. 2007. "A Prospective Randomized Clinical Trial of Phacoemulsification vs Manual Sutureless Small-Incision Extracapsular Cataract Surgery in Nepal." *American Journal of Ophthalmology* 143 (1): 32–38.

Ruiz-Razura, A., E. D. Cronin, and C. E. Navarro. 2000. "Creating Long-Term Benefits in Cleft Lip and Palate Volunteer Missions." *Plastic and Reconstructive Surgery* 105 (1): 195–201.

Rumstadt, B., B. Klein, H. Kirr, N. Kaltenbach, W. Homenu, and others. 2008. "Thyroid Surgery in Burkina Faso, West Africa: Experience from a Surgical Help Program." *World Journal of Surgery* 32 (12): 2627–30. doi:10.1007 /s00268-008-9775-6.

Sanders, D. L., and A. N. Kingsnorth. 2007. "Operation Hernia: Humanitarian Hernia Repairs in Ghana." *Hernia* 11 (5): 389–91. doi:10.1007/s10029-007-0238-z.

Shrime, M. G., A. Sleemi, and T. D. Ravilla. 2014. "Charitable Platforms in Global Surgery: A Systematic Review of Their Effectiveness, Cost-Effectiveness, Sustainability, and Role in Training." *World Journal of Surgery*, March 29. doi: 10.1007 /s00268-014-2516-0.

Singh, A. J., P. Garner, and K. Floyd. 2000. "Cost-Effectiveness of Public-Funded Options for Cataract Surgery in Mysore, India." *The Lancet* 355 (9199): 180–84.

Sykes, K. J., P. T. Le, K. A. Sale, and P. J. Nicklaus. 2012. "A 7-Year Review of the Safety of Tonsillectomy during Short-Term Medical Mission Trips." *Otolaryngology— Head and Neck Surgery* 146 (5): 752–56. doi:10.1177 /0194599812437317.

Tefuarani, N., J. Vince, R. Hawker, G. Nunn, R. Lee, and others. 2007. "Operation Open Heart in PNG, 1993–2006." *Heart, Lung and Circulation* 16 (5): 373–77. doi:10.1016/j .hlc.2007.05.013.

Troup, L. 2007. "The USNS Mercy's Southeast Asia Humanitarian Cruise: The Perioperative Experience." *AORN Journal* 86 (5): 781–90. doi:10.1016/j.aorn.2007.10.004.

van der Hoek, J. 1997. "Three Months Follow Up of IOL Implantation in Remote Eye Camps in Nepal." *International Ophthalmology* 21 (4): 195–97.

Venkataswamy, G. 1975. "Massive Eye Relief Project in India." *American Journal of Ophthalmology* 79 (1): 135–40.

Waaldijk, K. 2008. *Obstetric Fistula Surgery: Art and Science: The Basics.* Katsina, Nigeria: Babbar Ruga Fistula Teaching Hospital.

Walk, R. M., T. F. Donahue, R. P. Sharpe, and S. D. Safford. 2011. "Three Phases of Disaster Relief in Haiti: Pediatric Surgical Care on Board the United States Naval Ship *Comfort.*" *Journal of Pediatric Surgery* 46 (10): 1978–84.

Walk, R. M., J. Glaser, L. M. Marmon, T. F. Donahue, J. Bastien, and others. 2012. "Continuing Promise 2009: Assessment of a Recent Pediatric Surgical Humanitarian Mission." *Journal of Pediatric Surgery* 47 (4): 652–57.

Wall, L. L. 2007. "Where Should Obstetric Vesico-Vaginal Fistulas Be Repaired: At the District General Hospital or a Specialized Fistula Center?" *International Journal of Gynecology and Obstetrics* 99 (S1): S28–31.

———. 2011. "Ethical Concerns Regarding Operations by Volunteer Surgeons on Vulnerable Patient Groups: The Case of Women with Obstetric Fistulas." *HEC Forum* 23 (2): 115–27. doi:10.1007/s10730-011-9153-x.

———, S. D. Arrowsmith, A. T. Lassey, and K. Danso. 2006. "Humanitarian Ventures or 'Fistula Tourism?': The Ethical Perils of Pelvic Surgery in the Developing World." *International Urogynecology Journal and Pelvic Floor Dysfunction* 17 (6): 559–62. doi:10.1007/s00192-005-0056-8.

WHO (World Health Organization). 2005. *State of the World's Sight: VISION 2020: The Right to Sight 1999–2005.* Geneva: WHO. http://apps.who.int/iris/bitstream/10665/43300/1/9241593458_eng.pdf?ua=1.

———. 2013. "Global Health Estimates for Deaths by Cause, Age, and Sex for Years 2000–2011." WHO, Geneva. http://www.who.int/healthinfo/global_health_estimates/en/.

Wright, I. G., I. A. Walker, and M. H. Yacoub. 2007. "Specialist Surgery in the Developing World: Luxury or Necessity?" *Anaesthesia* 62 (Suppl 1): 84–89. doi:10.1111/j.1365-2044.2007.05308.x.

Yeow, V. K., S. T. Lee, T. J. Lambrecht, J. Barnett, M. Gorney, and others. 2002. "International Task Force on Volunteer Cleft Missions." *Journal of Craniofacial Surgery* 13 (1): 18–25.

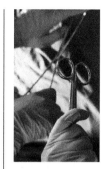

Chapter 14

Prehospital and Emergency Care

Amardeep Thind, Renee Hsia, Jackie Mabweijano,
Eduardo Romero Hicks, Ahmed Zakariah, and Charles N. Mock

INTRODUCTION

Disease or illness can strike at any time. If the condition is acute, or if the injury is life-threatening or limb-threatening, immediate care is needed. These time-dependent conditions that affect both adults and children may be due to medical, surgical, or obstetric conditions. They may result from acute injuries or illnesses or from exacerbations of chronic disease.

In low- and middle-income countries (LMICs), patients with such conditions may face delays of hours or even days before reaching the nearest medical facility or provider. Transportation may be provided by ambulance, but more often it is provided by laypersons using the handiest mode of transport available (Arellano, Mello, and Clark 2010; Khorasani-Zavareh and others 2009; Nguyen and others 2008; Ramanujam and Aschkenasy 2007). Health care before arrival at heath facilities may be provided by trained paramedics or by laypersons; quite often, however, no health care is provided (Bavonratanavech 2003; Khorasani-Zavareh and others 2009; Nguyen and others 2008; Solagberu and others 2009).

In contrast to systems in high-income countries (HICs), the prehospital and emergency medical systems of LMICs are often rudimentary. Justifiably, health systems in LMICs have focused on increasing access to health care by building facility-based health care systems. Such thinking is abetted by a perception that the provision of prehospital and emergency care is not cost-effective in LMICs (Kobusingye and others 2005), leading to policies that allocate the bulk of scarce health care resources elsewhere.

This chapter identifies the scale of the challenge by presenting data on the burden of disease that prehospital and emergency care systems in LMICs could potentially address. It then describes the common health care delivery structures in these countries and assesses the literature on costs and effectiveness of such mechanisms. It closes with a discussion of future directions in research and policy.

BURDEN OF DISEASE

The burden of disease that can potentially be addressed by prehospital and emergency care in LMICs (figure 14.1) was derived from the diseases and disease conditions used by Kobusingye and others in their chapter on emergency medical services in *Disease Control Priorities in Developing Countries*, second edition (Jamison and others 2006). The latest data for these conditions were extracted from the World Health Organization's (WHO's) Global Health Estimates (WHO 2013). Data for the diseases and conditions are clustered into three groups:

- Communicable and maternal conditions
- Chronic conditions
- Injuries

Corresponding author: Amardeep Thind, MD, PhD, University of Western Ontario, athind2@uwo.ca

Figure 14.1 Burden of Disease Potentially Addressable by Prehospital and Emergency Care in LMICs

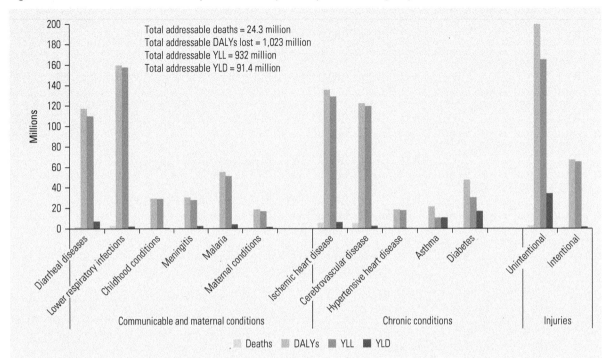

Source: Data from WHO 2013.
Note: DALYs = disability-adjusted life years; LMICs = low- and middle-income countries; YLD = years lived with disability; YLL = years of life lost.

The communicable and maternal conditions group includes the following:

- Diarrheal diseases: cholera, other salmonella infections, shigellosis, *E. coli*, campylobacter, amoebiasis, cryptosporidiosis, rotavirus, typhoid and paratyphoid fevers
- Lower respiratory infections: influenza, pneumococcal pneumonia, haemophilus influenzae pneumonia, respiratory syncytial virus pneumonia, other lower respiratory infections
- Childhood conditions: diphtheria, whooping cough, tetanus, measles
- Meningitis
- Malaria
- Maternal conditions: hemorrhage, sepsis, hypertensive disorders of pregnancy, obstructed labor, and abortion

The chronic conditions group includes the following:

- Ischemic heart disease
- Cerebrovascular disease
- Hypertensive heart disease
- Asthma
- Diabetes

The injuries group includes the following:

- Unintentional: transport and nontransport injuries, and forces of nature
- Intentional: self-harm, interpersonal violence, war, and legal intervention

Our estimates suggest that out of the approximately 45 million deaths in LMICs each year, 54 percent, or 24.3 million, are due to conditions that are potentially addressable by prehospital and emergency care. This loss translates into a staggering 1,023 million DALYs, or 932 million years of life lost (YLL) to premature mortality. From a morbidity perspective, this disease burden translates into 91.4 million years lived with disability (YLD). While ischemic heart disease and cerebrovascular disease contribute the largest number of deaths, unintentional injuries are the single largest contributor to the DALYs. The largest contributors to YLL are unintentional injuries, lower respiratory infections, and ischemic heart disease.

In this array of disease burden, maternal conditions (hemorrhage, sepsis, obstructed labor, and abortion) and injuries may require surgical intervention. Nearly 19 percent (or 4.7 million) of these 24.3 million deaths in LMICs are surgically treatable. This number corresponds to nearly 28 percent—285 million—of the DALYs, or 25 percent—286 million—of the YLL. From a morbidity perspective, surgically treatable conditions account for 38 million YLD, or 41 percent of the conditions that are potentially addressable by prehospital and emergency care.

Figures 14.2–14.5 depict the regional variations in mortality, DALYs, YLL, and YLD. By virtue of their large populations, South Asia and East Asia and the Pacific account for 56 percent of the addressable deaths (figure 14.2). South Asia and Sub-Saharan Africa account for 61 percent of the DALYs (figure 14.3), and Sub-Saharan Africa contributes 33 percent of the YLL (figure 14.4). Morbidity is the highest in East Asia and the Pacific, which accounts for 31 percent of the YLD (figure 14.5).

CURRENT DELIVERY SYSTEMS

To develop and enhance the capacity to provide effective emergency care, it is essential to view such care in the context of the overall health system rather than as a discrete and independent unit. Emergency care covers a range of services, from the care provided by laypersons at the scene to that provided in a dedicated trauma facility. Between these two phases lie the transportation systems, health centers, and first-level hospitals. Patient survival depends on how well each component functions.

The organization and operation of the prehospital care system vary by country, but should be linked to the local hospitals or facilities to which patients are to be transported. When prehospital transportation is poor or absent, deaths occur that could have been prevented by inexpensive procedures (Mock and others 1998). Most maternal deaths may fall into this category. Poor quality of care at hospitals will lead to in-hospital deaths and may eventually discourage communities that might have the capacity to promptly transfer patients to such facilities (Leigh and others 1997). Skilled and motivated personnel, appropriate supplies, pharmaceuticals, equipment, coordination, and management oriented to the needs of the critically ill all contribute to making emergency care effective in reducing death and disability.

Tiers of Care

Tier One. Prehospital care encompasses the care provided by the community—from the scene of injury, home, school, or other location—until the patient arrives at a formal health care facility. This care should comprise basic and proven strategies and the most

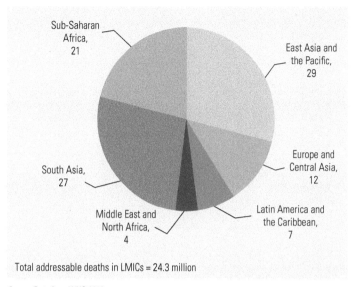

Figure 14.2 Regional Distribution of Deaths Addressable by Prehospital and Emergency Care in LMICs
Percent

Total addressable deaths in LMICs = 24.3 million

Source: Data from WHO 2013.
Note: LMICs = low- and middle-income countries.

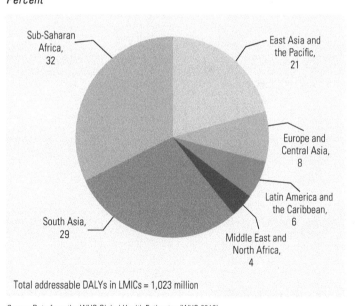

Figure 14.3 Regional Distribution of DALYs Potentially Addressable by Prehospital and Emergency Care in LMICs
Percent

Total addressable DALYs in LMICs = 1,023 million

Source: Data from the WHO Global Health Estimates (WHO 2013).
Note: DALY = disability-adjusted life year; LMICs = low- and middle-income countries.

appropriate personnel, equipment, and supplies needed to assess, prioritize, and institute interventions to minimize the probability of death or disability. The most-effective strategies are basic and inexpensive; the lack of high-technology interventions should not deter efforts

Figure 14.4 Regional Distribution of YLL Potentially Addressable by Prehospital and Emergency Care in LMICs

Percent

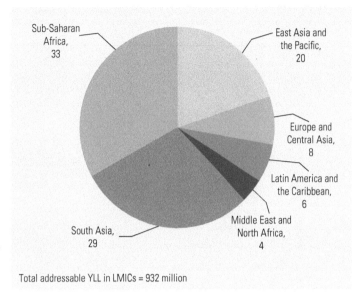

Total addressable YLL in LMICs = 932 million

Source: Data from WHO 2013.
Note: LMICs = low- and middle-income countries; YLL = years of life lost.

Figure 14.5 Regional Distribution of YLD Potentially Addressable by Prehospital and Emergency Care in LMICs

Percent

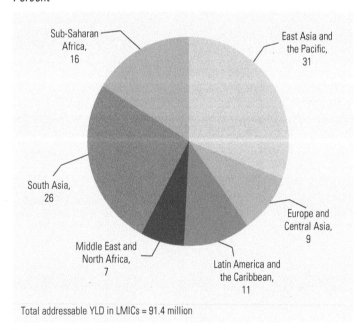

Total addressable YLD in LMICs = 91.4 million

Source: Data from WHO 2013.
Note: LMICs = low- and middle-income countries; YLD = years lived with disability.

to provide good care. Even where resources allow them, the more invasive procedures performed by physicians in some prehospital settings, such as intravenous access and fluid infusion or intubations, do not appear to

improve patient outcomes (Liberman and others 2003; Sampalis and others 1994, 1995, 1997).

Prehospital care should be simple, sustainable, and efficient. Because resource availability varies greatly across and within countries, different tiers of care are recognized. Where no formal prehospital system exists, the first tier of care may be composed of laypersons in the community who have been taught basic first aid techniques. Recruiting and training particularly motivated citizens who often confront emergencies to function as prehospital care providers can expand this resource (Geduld and Wallis 2011).

Tier Two. The second tier comprises paramedical personnel who use dedicated vehicles and equipment and are usually able to get to patients and take them to hospitals quickly. This second tier may involve the performance of advanced procedures or the administration of intravenous and other medications by physician or nonphysician providers, or both. This care is not always available in LMICs; few trained personnel and inadequate funding make around-the-clock coverage infeasible.

Although providing advanced life-saving measures in the prehospital environment may be beneficial in some cases, these benefits may be negated if such measures divert scarce resources from more basic interventions that can benefit far larger numbers of patients (Hauswald and Yeoh 1997). In most LMICs in East Asia and the Pacific, Latin America and the Caribbean, South Asia, and Sub-Saharan Africa, high maternal and child mortality are linked to inadequate emergency care, especially poor access to quality hospital care. In these settings, it is essential to integrate resources rather than to segregate systems for injuries and obstetric emergencies.

Personnel

Most of the world's population do not have access to formal prehospital care. In LMICs, personnel are not employed for the sole purpose of dealing with medical emergencies outside of hospitals, and transportation is not dedicated to the task of getting patients in need of emergency care to hospitals.

The following discussion introduces a scenario in which mortality rate reduction could be achieved in a health system in an LIC or LMIC by a small group of paramedics working together with a large group of trained lay responders. The scenario uses only emergencies caused by trauma, although it is expected that both paramedics and lay first responders would also save lives in medical or obstetric emergencies. Existing studies have not been large enough to document these effects, and they are not included in the estimates of cost-effectiveness.

Lay First Responders. The most basic tier of a pre-hospital system depends upon interested community members who serve as volunteers to learn simple, yet effective, first aid techniques. These laypersons should also ideally be able to recognize life-threatening conditions—whether obstetric, traumatic, or medical. Examples may range from traditional birth attendants or similar persons in the community who respond to obstetric emergencies to commercial taxi and minibus drivers who encounter traumatic injuries. Other examples include students or workers who receive training so that they can call for help and provide basic emergency care, such as cleansing wounds, stopping external bleeding with direct pressure, and splinting suspected fractures or necks in suspected cervical injuries. See box 14.1.

Materials to train laypersons with low rates of literacy are available, including *When Someone Is Hurt: A First Aid Guide for Lay Persons and Community Workers* (Varghese and Mohan 1998) and the British Red Cross's *Anyone Can Save a Life: Road Accidents and First Aid* (Fiander 2001). Context-specific first aid training materials have been developed, for example, in Ghana (Tiska and others 2004) and Uganda (Jayaraman and others 2009a, 2009b). These materials contain many illustrations so that learners can better understand the basic skills needed for first aid. Depending on the level of interest and availability of first responders, training can last for as little as one day or can extend to several weeks.

It is important that refresher training be incorporated into the program to allow learners to maintain and upgrade their skills; knowledge retention should be reassessed as well, as shown in previous studies of layperson training (Jayaraman and others 2009a, 2009b; Sangowawa and Owoaje 2012). An ongoing monitoring system, such as providing feedback on first aid provided, should be a major component of the system. The WHO provides a matrix of essential knowledge, skills, equipment, and supplies for prehospital providers (Kobusingye and others 2005). Emerging evidence indicates that even children as young as ages five to six years can be given basic first aid training and that their knowledge retention is good at six months (Bollig, Wahl, and Svendsen 2009; Bollig, Myklebust, and Ostringen 2011).

Husum and others (2003) and Husum, Gilbert, and Wisborg (2003) demonstrate that laypersons who are given first aid skills can effectively respond to emergencies in communities with high trauma burdens. In Ghana, it was demonstrated that taxi and minibus drivers trained in first aid could provide effective prehospital care (box 14.2) (Mock and others 2002). This experience has been replicated in other settings (Geduld and Wallis 2011; Jayaraman and others 2009a, 2009b).

Box 14.1

Critical Tasks for First Responders

The World Health Organization lists six critical tasks for first responders:

- Get involved
- Call for help
- Assess the scene for safety
- Assess the victim for life-threatening injuries
- Provide immediate assistance
- Secure essential equipment and supplies

Each of these components requires training and education—most bystanders fear getting involved, whether because of lack of knowledge or skills, or fear of exposure to body fluids, or other cultural and social barriers. Even something as simple as calling for help requires knowledge of available local resources, for example, taxi or ambulance services, private practitioners, and local police or fire departments. Scene safety includes ensuring that victims do not sustain additional injuries; this component could include managing crowds and traffic.

Source: Kobusingye and others 2005.

It is important to incorporate local needs so that the local training curricula, if they exist or are to be developed, can be adapted to address and meet specific considerations. For example, in a township outside Cape Town, South Africa, one study shows that the content of the course was adapted to specific township needs, including how to handle scene safety; penetrating injuries from violence; and medical issues, including drug overdose and alcohol abuse. This responsiveness to community needs seems to have enhanced the integration of the system into the community. This system was run by a community governing board and administered by community organizations already involved in the township (Sun, Shing, and others 2012; Sun, Twomey, and others 2012; Sun and Wallis 2011).

A study of midwives and traditional birth attendants in rural Cambodia also finds that a prehospital training course could significantly improve knowledge, compared with precourse levels, of interventions such as uterine packing to control hemorrhage and suturing tears (Chandy, Steinholt, and Husum 2007). A study from northern Iraq also shows a mortality benefit of

Box 14.2

Improving Trauma Care in the Absence of a Formal Ambulance System in Ghana

Background: The efficacy of a program that builds on the existing, although informal, system of prehospital transportation in Ghana was assessed. In Ghana, the majority of injured persons are transported to the hospital by some type of commercial vehicle, such as a taxi or bus.

Methods: A total of 335 commercial drivers were trained using a six-hour basic first aid course. The efficacy of this course was assessed by comparing the process of prehospital trauma care provided before and after the course, as determined by self-reporting from the drivers.

The course was conducted with moderate amounts of volunteer labor and gifts in kind, such as transportation to the course. The actual cost of the course amounted to US$3 per participant.

Results: Follow-up interviews were conducted on 71 of the drivers a mean of 10.6 months after the course. In the interviews, 61 percent indicated that they had provided first aid since taking the course. There was considerable improvement in the provision of the components of first aid in comparison to what was reported before the course (table B14.2.1):

Table B14.2.1 Provision of First Aid before and after Training

Percent of respondents

Component of first aid	Before	After
Crash scene management	7	35
Airway management	2	35
Bleeding control	4	42
Splint application	1	16
Triage	7	21

Conclusions: Even in the absence of a formal emergency medical system, prehospital trauma care can be improved by building on existing, although informal, prehospital transportation.

Source: Mock and others 2002.

---

first responder training (Murad and Husum 2010). Lay responders are likely to have an impact when the burden of emergencies from injuries and other causes is high. Attrition of both the responders and the skills is a concern unless they are frequently used.

Paramedical Personnel. In most middle-income countries (MICs) and some cities in low-income countries (LICs), trained paramedical personnel provide prehospital care (Mock and others 1998; Tannebaum and others 2001). These basic and advanced personnel are often paid ambulance personnel or, in some cases, specially designated cohorts of fire or police personnel who desire to acquire more medical skills. They receive professional instruction in both theory and practice, ranging from 100 to 400 hours (Sasser and others 2005). These personnel can be further categorized as follows:

- Those who are able to offer basic prehospital trauma care, including scene management, rescue, stabilization, and the transport of injured patients
- Those who can provide more advanced care, including services such as invasive airway techniques, as well as

- Systems-level developments, such as a complex regional call management center and an integrated communication network (Sasser and others 2005).

Transportation and Communication

After basic first aid has been provided and paramedical personnel have been deployed to the scene, transportation to the nearest and most appropriate health facility is critical. Efficient communication is vital to ensure that contact can be made between those who know that patients need help and the medical personnel who provide it. Although most LMICs have poor telecommunications infrastructure, cellular mobile phones are rapidly being adopted by individuals and offer an opportunity to bypass the need for traditional communications services (Kobusingye and others 2005).

In most of East Asia and the Pacific, South Asia, and Sub-Saharan Africa, where commercial ambulances may not be available, a range of options exists and can be further developed. These options include private motorized or nonmotorized vehicles (Joshipura and others 2003; Kobusingye and others 2002). In Malawi, transportation has even been achieved with bicycle ambulances (Lungu and others 2001). The establishment of rudimentary ambulance systems has been successful even in low-resource settings such as Niger, including an intervention using solar-panel-powered radios to connect health centers with the second-level hospital (Bossyns and others 2005).

When ambulance services do exist in East Asia and the Pacific, South Asia, and Sub-Saharan Africa, they are often limited to transferring patients between health facilities rather than from the scenes of injury or from homes (Joshipura and others 2003). In MICs, however, ambulance services are a major component of existing emergency care systems (Arreola-Risa and others 2000; Mock and others 2002). Their presence reduces the interval between the recognition of an emergency and the arrival of patients at the hospital (Ali and others 1993, 1997; Arreola-Risa and others 2000).

The effectiveness of well-placed dispatch sites has also been demonstrated in urban populations, where the vehicles and personnel can be optimized. Shorter prehospital times, in general, are considered an important parameter of the quality of prehospital care. These times have the following components:

- *Notification time* is the time elapsed from the occurrence of the injury or the recognition of severe illness until the prehospital or ambulance system is notified.
- *Response time* is the time elapsed from notification until arrival of an ambulance to the site of the ill or injured person.
- *Scene time* is the time elapsed from the arrival of prehospital providers on the scene until departure.
- *Transport time* is the time elapsed from departure from the scene until arrival at the hospital or other treatment facility.

Notification time is influenced by the availability of telecommunications. Response time is influenced by the capabilities of a dispatch center to handle emergency calls, and especially by the geographic distribution of sites of ambulance dispatch. The greater the number of ambulance stations and the wider their distribution, the shorter are the response times.

Geographic distribution and associated response times can be improved in some circumstances by using a tiered or layered response system. This system requires a relatively larger number of basically trained and equipped first responders with wider geographic distribution, and a smaller number of centrally located and more highly trained and equipped second responders. This approach allows the first responders to respond more rapidly and involves second responders only if needed.

With close attention to keeping costs sustainably low, paramedical personnel could be introduced in large urban areas where they do not function at present. They could be stationed at dispatch sites with dedicated vehicles, fast communications with area hospitals, and links with other emergency services, such as fire and police departments. The communities served by the system should have a well-known and rapid method of calling the paramedical teams when an emergency arises. Both lay and paramedical teams require ongoing refresher courses so that their skills do not deteriorate.

Where paramedical personnel have already been integrated into the emergency care system, their numbers and organization—location, training, deployment, and monitoring—should be enhanced to improve response times and patient outcomes, especially for cardiac and obstetric emergencies. It is essential that such systems be evaluated, not only with metrics that assess the availability of services, for example, the number of units on duty or number of sites of ambulance dispatch, but also their cost-effectiveness.

The recommended ratio of one ambulance unit for every 50,000 people suggested by McSwain (1991) results in response times as low as four to six minutes. The ratio does not distinguish between basic and advanced life-support capabilities. Traffic congestion, poor maps, and poor road signs may all increase the response time in cities with poor infrastructure. In Monterrey, Mexico, one unit per 100,000 people manages an average response time of 10 minutes. Hanoi, Vietnam, with one unit for every 3 million people, has an average response time of 30 minutes (Mock and others 1998).

Where paramedical services exist in parallel to lay responder services, the two could be integrated under the same organizational unit. The paramedical staff will be more successful in urban areas, where distances between dispatch sites, communities served, and hospitals are short. Other enabling factors are good telecommunications; rapid and dedicated transportation; and coordinating capacity among the community, hospitals, and other emergency services.

Equipment and Supplies

The provision of appropriate equipment and supplies is essential; previous studies have shown that educational interventions to paramedics are less effective if equipment availability limits the ability of these trained personnel to implement their knowledge (Arreola-Risa and others 2007; McClure and others 2007). The WHO provides a comprehensive list of equipment and supplies needed for prehospital providers, which is shown in annex 14A (Sasser and others 2005). Despite adequate provision, the utilization of appropriate equipment in LMICs is variable; a study from Malaysia finds that oxygen delivery devices were used in 45 percent of ambulance runs, the scoop stretcher in 29 percent, and wound dressings in only 23 percent (Ismail and others 2012).

HEALTH FACILITY–BASED SUBSYSTEMS

Health facility–based subsystems refer to the level within the health care system at which appropriate definitive care is delivered. Formal health facilities vary immensely across and within countries. In some countries, this subsystem may be a regional or second-level hospital with specialists; in others, a district or first-level hospital with general practitioners or nonspecialist doctors; and in still others, a health center with nonphysician clinicians. In some LMICs, some types of emergency medical care, for conditions such as acute diarrhea or severe malaria, may be effectively delivered at a health center staffed by nonphysician clinicians. However, such a facility will be inadequate for the management of severe multiple injuries or obstructed labor. The triage process in the prehospital subsystem should determine which patients receive transportation to which facility rather than merely transportation to the nearest facility. Precious time and lives may be lost when patients are taken to facilities where the desired care is not available.

The goal of an effective emergency medical system is the provision of emergency care to all who need it. This section presents guidelines on the necessary inputs. Two of the components in hospital emergency care are discussed in more detail: training, and equipment and supplies.

Training

Most in-service training for emergency care professionals working in hospitals is designed to address a particular problem, such as severe injuries, emergency pediatrics, or obstetric emergencies. Yet because of the resource constraints in LMICs, the same personnel will be confronted with all of these problems.

Few courses in emergency care have been rigorously evaluated (Black and Brocklehurst 2003). The Advanced Trauma Life Support course for physicians has resulted in improved patient outcomes in some settings, although it may be too expensive for most LMICs and inappropriate in settings in which the majority of patients are not seen by physicians. In a third-level hospital in Trinidad and Tobago, injury mortality was reduced by 50 percent following Advanced Trauma

Life Support training (Ali and others 1993). Life-saving obstetric skills training contributed to a reduction in maternal deaths. In Kebbi state in Nigeria, training led to a reduction in case-fatality rates to 5 percent from 22 percent among women with obstetric complications (Oyesola and others 1997).

Similar trends were observed in other sites at which the intervention was implemented (Oyesola and others 1997). Emergency Triage Assessment and Treatment has been used in many countries to improve pediatric emergency care (WHO and UNICEF 2000). Other examples are Primary Trauma Care, which is a trauma management course to train doctors and other health workers in first-level hospitals and remote locations (Wilkinson and Skinner 2000), and Advanced Life Support in Obstetrics (http://www.aafp.org/also). These courses have been beneficial in standardizing protocol-based emergency care, but their outcome evaluations are still awaited. Box 14.3 describes public and private initiatives to facilitate training in India.

Equipment and Supplies

A list of resources for emergency care required at different levels is available in annex 14B. This template is flexible; countries can customize it to suit local conditions such as existing facility levels and prevailing burden of emergency disease conditions. Equipment and supplies at each level should match the knowledge and skills of the personnel available to use them.

One study provides sobering evidence that one of the key barriers to the provision of emergency and surgical care in Sub-Saharan Africa is lack of basic infrastructure; in an assessment of five countries (Ghana, Kenya, Rwanda, Tanzania, and Uganda), for example, only 22 percent to 46 percent of hospitals at all levels had dependable running water and electricity. Not one surveyed hospital met the minimum WHO standards for the provision of emergency and surgical care, suggesting that these infrastructure investments must be made in conjunction with investments in the human workforce (Hsia and others 2012).

COSTS AND EFFECTIVENESS

Costs

There is a paucity of literature delineating the costs of providing prehospital and emergency care, especially in LMICs. A few studies examine the costs of specific components of this system, but none evaluates the actual cost of the entire system. Reporting on the 10-year results of the implementation and expansion of a trauma

Emergency Care Training in India

The training of personnel working in emergency medical services is crucial to the success of the efficient delivery of care. Evidence exists to support the usefulness of life-support training for emergency caregivers in low- and middle-income countries. Courses such as Advanced Trauma Life Support are available and well established in some high-income countries and middle-income countries. In most low-income countries, however, such training is not available, mainly because of prohibitive costs. The three-day Advanced Trauma Life Support course costs, on average, US$700 per trainee and is taught to 6 to 20 trainees at a time.

National Trauma Management Course
The National Trauma Management Course is a two-day course developed in India by the Academy of Traumatology with the help of international peers. The curriculum takes into account local conditions and capabilities. The cost is US$50 per trainee; local trainers teach 100 trainees at a time. Animal specimens, instead of expensive commercially produced mannequins, are used to teach life-saving procedures. More than 2,000 health professionals were trained in less than three years. The course has become a national training standard for immediate trauma care in India.

Private Initiatives
In addition, several private initiatives have increased the number of formally trained prehospital paramedics who have graduated to become Advanced Cardiac Life Support/Basic Life Support instructors. One example is the Stanford-Apollo EMT [Emergency Medical Technician]-Intermediate Training program at Apollo Hospital in Hyderabad and Chennai, in conjunction with the Stanford School of Medicine (Stanford, California). A second, also in conjunction with Stanford, is the

GVK Emergency Management and Research Institute (EMRI) in Hyderabad. The first internationally affiliated paramedic program, the Post-Graduate Program in Emergency Care, began in 2007 to develop advanced clinical educators, who are essentially paramedic-instructors, with 15 two-week modules that include simulation, interactive case-based studies, and distance learning.

Prehospital Research Center
In 2008, the Post-Graduate Program in Emergency Care also began a prehospital research center at the GVK EMRI campus in Hyderabad, India, and conducts research on obstetric emergencies, chest pain, vehicular trauma, gastrointestinal emergencies, seizures, poisoning and suicide attempts, burns, shortness of breath, and nonvehicular trauma. The program was turned over to GVK EMRI in July 2009 and continues to train Indian paramedics. In May 2013, more than 5,700 ambulances were providing prehospital care to more than 750 million Indians, including 2,121,000 medical emergencies a day, making it the largest ambulance system in the world.

Prehospital Emergency Care Protocol
Another output from the Stanford-Apollo EMT Intermediate Training has been a Prehospital Emergency Care Protocol, published in 2012, for physicians, emergency medical technicians, and educators. These protocols did not exist before March 2011. The goals of these unique protocols are to ensure countrywide uniformity and consistency of prehospital care and to espouse evidence-based practice related to ambulance systems (when this evidence is available). More than 5,000 protocol manuals have been printed and placed in ambulances and call centers throughout India.

Sources: Mahadevan and others 2009; Mantha and others 2009.

---

system (consisting of trained laypersons, paramedics, and two trauma referral centers) in north and central Iraq, Murad, Larsen, and Husum (2012) note that the per patient treatment costs—medical treatment, evacuation, data gathering, and quality control—ranged from US$130 to US$180.

Perhaps the best exercise to date in estimating system-level costs is Kobusingye and others (2006).

In their modeling exercise, they estimate system costs of establishing and running two types of prehospital and emergency care systems:

- One in which trained lay responders and paramedics provide care
- One in which staffed community ambulances provide care

For a population of 1 million, they assume that the trained laypersons and paramedics system will require 7,500 lay responders, with 2,500 trained on a rolling basis. The system would also require 50 trained paramedics annually. Training costs would include a classroom, copies of curricula, time costs, and remuneration of trainees and trainers. The training (and its costs) would be repeated every three years to maintain skill levels. Paramedics would be equipped with basic kits consisting of a stethoscope, gloves, bandages, and splint materials. Trained laypersons and paramedics would volunteer their services after training. Given these assumptions, Kobusingye and others' (2006) best estimate of cost was US$62,923 or US$0.06 per capita (ranging between US$30,254 and US$126,475).

Jayaraman and others (2009b) build on this framework to estimate the costs of scaling up their layperson first aid training pilot to cover Kampala, Uganda. They assume that 9,000 trainees (a range of 6,000 to 12,000) are required to cover the city's 1.2 million residents. Using Kobusingye and others' (2006) costs and costing assumptions, their base case scenario (of training 9,000 trainees over three years) results in an annual cost of US$47,854 or US$0.12 per capita; these costs increase to US$143,854 annually or US$0.36 per capita when the first aid kit and its restocking (US$16 each) are factored in (Jayaraman and others 2009b).

For a system that relies on staffed ambulances, Kobusingye and others (2006) assume that an ambulance unit serves 30,000 people and has a staff of seven paramedic-drivers. Accordingly, 33 such units are required for a population of 1 million; in addition, a supervisor will oversee three ambulance units per year. Ambulances can be purchased and retrofitted locally; they are assumed to have a useful life of nine years and to be driven 20,000 kilometers every year. Under these assumptions, the authors estimate the yearly cost of such a system in an urban area to be approximately US$1.27 million or US$1.27 per capita (a range of US$0.79 million to US$2.15 million), with a rural ambulance system costing three times as much.

Effectiveness

Although a prehospital and emergency care system can respond to a wide range of conditions, most studies in the literature report outcomes pertaining to trauma, with a small but growing body of literature on the effectiveness of first responders and paramedics.

Increasing evidence indicates the benefits of a well-functioning prehospital care system. Literature from high-income countries (HICs) suggests that for patients with serious injuries, preventable trauma deaths are reduced significantly after trauma system implementation (Kane and others 1992; Mullins and others 1994; Rutledge and others 1992). Similar evidence is emerging from Iraq, where the implementation and expansion of a trauma system in north and central Iraq reduced trauma mortality over a 10-year period to 4 percent from 17 percent (Murad, Larsen, and others 2012). A study from Portugal shows a reduction in mortality of approximately 50 percent in trauma patients who received some form of treatment in the prehospital phase (Gomes and others 2010). Work done in Cambodia and northern Iraq demonstrates a 9 percent reduction in mortality among trauma victims after the institution of a system comprising first-level responders and trained paramedics (Husum and others 2003); this study forms the basis of the cost-effectiveness analysis of trained laypersons and paramedics by Kobusingye and others (2006).

Experience from the northern Iraq system suggests an even greater impact of providing prehospital care to trauma patients. Murad and others (2012) report a mortality rate of 8 percent in road traffic accident patients managed onsite and evacuated by trained first responders and paramedics; the mortality rate is 40 percent in the patients admitted without any prehospital care. Similarly, a review of eight studies on prehospital care in LMICs to attempt to determine aggregate risk reduction for mortality, injury severity, and transport time found a 25 percent reduction in the risk of mortality with the implementation of a prehospital system; treatment effects were enhanced in rural settings. In addition, response times were reduced 66 minutes overall in rural settings, and 6 minutes in urban settings (Henry and Reingold 2012) (box 14.4).

An ambulance-based system can potentially save 700 lives annually: 200 from ischemic heart disease, 200 from obstetric emergencies, and 300 from trauma (Kobusingye and others 2006).

Evidence from LMICs suggests that providing basic life support (BLS) training to ambulance personnel can reduce trauma mortality, as evidenced by a decrease in mortality to 10.6 percent from 15.7 percent in Trinidad when such a system was established (Ali and others 1993). However, other LMICs are gravitating toward providing advanced life support (ALS) training to these personnel, rather than BLS training. This shift is, in part, due to evidence from HICs that attributes a reduction in trauma mortality to ALS training (Kirsch 1998; Reines and others 1988). A meta-analysis of 18 studies finds that provision of ALS care to nontraumatic cardiac arrest patients could increase their survival; it also finds no difference in survival in trauma patients who received ALS versus those receiving BLS (Bakalos and others 2011). Similarly, a Cochrane review did not find any differences in mortality among trauma victims cared for by BLS-trained versus

Training Community Paramedics and First Responders: Experiences from Iraq and Cambodia

In northern Iraq (Sulaymaniyah Governorate) and northwest Cambodia (Battambang Province), two conflict areas with extensive minefields, the estimated mortality rates for mine casualties were approximately 40 percent. Based on the concept of the Village University, laypersons recommended by their village leaders were trained by outside trainers in basic prehospital life-support and life-saving skills—for example, keeping airways open and stopping bleeding. In 1997–99, a core group of 44 trainees received 150 hours of training in basic airway, breathing, and circulation techniques; each trainee subsequently trained 50 village first helpers in two-day training sessions 6 to 12 months after the initial training.

By the end of the fifth year of the program, 135 community paramedics and 5,200 first responders had been trained. Refresher courses were also provided for the paramedics and first responders.

Care had been provided to 1,061 trauma victims, with a reduction in the mean response time from 2.9 hours (1997) to 1.8 hours (2001) from time of injury to first medical contact, although there was no change in mean prehospital transit time. Mortality for these trauma patients was reduced from a pre-intervention level of 40 percent to 8 percent postintervention at the final stage.

Further studies have shown that the time from injury to first medical help decreased even more, to 0.6 hours, and time of injury to hospital decreased to 2.8 hours from 9.6 during the period 1997–2004. These studies have shown a high retention of paramedics (72 percent) over the period.

A study has documented the benefits of the first responder program separately from the paramedic program, showing that mortality rates were 9.8 percent in those seen by first responders, and 15.6 percent in those with only paramedic contact (difference of 6 percent, 95 percent confidence interval of 2 percent to 10 percent). Of those with an injury severity score greater than 15, mortality was lower (38 percent) in those treated by first responders, compared with 51 percent in those only seen by paramedics (95 percent confidence interval on the difference of 1 percent to 24 percent). In addition, those seen by only first responders had lower mortality rates than those seen by first responders and then paramedics (4.7 percent versus 13.4 percent, 95 percent confidence interval of 3 percent to 15 percent). This is likely because shorter travel times allow for direct handoff from first responder to facility, rather than longer transit times that allow for a handoff to a paramedic who then brings the patient to a treating facility. In other words, these studies show that mortality can be lower if the injured person is treated initially by a first responder before a paramedic arrives when travel times are long.

Finally, the effect of this two-tier prehospital rural trauma system with first responders and rural paramedics has been shown to have benefits for patients in road traffic accidents with long transport times, with a mortality rate of 8 percent in the intervention areas, compared with 44 percent in the control areas.

Source: Husum and others 2003; Murad and Husum 2010; Murad and others 2012; WHO 2010; Wisborg, Murad, Edvardsen, and Brinchmann 2008; Wisborg, Murad, Edvardsen, and Husum 2008.

ALS-trained ambulance personnel (Jayaraman and Sethi 2010). On the contrary, some evidence suggests that care provided by ALS-trained personnel might have worse outcomes (Stiell and others 2008).

This evidence suggests that an advanced prehospital emergency medical system should never be developed at the expense of a broad base of basic prehospital care. ALS interventions benefit a small subset of critically ill patients who may require a large investment of resources that may be less cost-effective. Some experts recommend that the development of these more advanced systems be delayed until additional evidence demonstrates that improved outcomes can be gained by such systems. Indeed, an analysis of ALS-level interventions in Monterrey and San Pedro, Mexico, showed no significant improvements in the mortality rates of transported patients, versus a BLS training project, which did reduce mortality from 8.7 percent to 4.7 percent (Arreola-Risa and others 2004, 2007; Hauswald and Yeoh 1997). Another disadvantage of ALS training for lay personnel is that the Mexican study showed low pass rates for students in the advanced cardiac life support course; only 29 percent passed, compared with more than 80 percent who passed the BLS courses. This result could have been due to the relatively low levels of schooling for the majority of medics (Arreola-Risa and others 2007).

Cost-Effectiveness

Table 14.1 summarizes the cost-effectiveness estimates of Kobusingye and others (2006). In a population of 1 million, a system of trained laypersons and paramedics is highly cost-effective at US$170 to avert one death; an ambulance-based system in an urban area costs US$1,818 to achieve a similar result. A different metric (cost per life year gained) yields similar results; the trained layperson and paramedic system costs US$7 per year of life gained; the urban ambulance–based system costs approximately 13 times as much.

Table 14.2 is a similar synopsis of an analysis of the cost-effectiveness of scaling up a pilot layperson first aid training program to cover all of Kampala (Jayaraman and others 2009b). Mortality reductions resulting from this training program were assumed to be 15 percent (based on Husum and others 2003); the authors repeat the calculations using a more conservative 7.5 percent reduction to perform a sensitivity analysis.

However, there are caveats. The inputs in Kobusingye and others (2006) were based on 2001 data; the results are reported in 2001 U.S. dollars and may not be reflective of today's economic environment. For example, the wide availability of cellular phones has revolutionized both the availability and the cost of communications in many LMICs, decreasing the need to have dedicated communications equipment for the prehospital and emergency care system.

From a methodological perspective, certain assumptions are also important. Kobusingye and others (2006) assume that the trained laypersons and paramedics would offer their services on a volunteer basis. Both studies apply the outcome on a global basis, without taking into account regional variations. Systemic costs, or the additional burden to the health care system from additional visits, are not factored into their calculations. The ambulance system is assumed to have the same effectiveness in both rural and urban areas; the authors caution that "substantial uncertainty remains over actual effectiveness of the interventions in emergency medicine" (Kobusingye and others 2006, 1271).

FUTURE DIRECTIONS

This section summarizes considerations for LMICs as they develop their prehospital and emergency systems and highlights the gaps in evidence that hamper effective policy making.

Systems Organization

Effective emergency medical systems require careful planning, implementation, coordination, and communication

Table 14.1 Summary of Cost and Effectiveness of Interventions
U.S. dollars

	Intervention		
	Trained lay first responders and paramedic responders	Staffed community ambulance, urban	Staffed community ambulance, rural
Cost per 1 million population	62,923	1,272,705	3,827,376
Cost per death averted per 1 million population	170	1,818	5,468
Cost per life year gained per 1 million population	7	94	284

Source: Kobusingye and others 2006.
Note: Figures are unweighted averages.

Table 14.2 Cost-Effectiveness of Scaling Up Lay Person First Aid Training in Kampala
U.S. dollars

	Estimated 240 deaths averted (15 percent)		Estimated 120 deaths averted (7.5 percent)	
	Cost per death averted	Cost per life year saved	Cost per death averted	Cost per life year saved
Base case	598	25	1,196	50
Base case + US$32 supplies	1,798	75	3,596	150

Source: Jayaraman and others 2009b.

with local communities. The respective components should be linked to ensure that the entire system operates as a unit. A coordinator should be responsible for monitoring and coordinating all emergency medical care in the community or district; this coordinator should work with a central committee that reflects and represents the components.

Coordination costs are important and should not be overlooked in the development of a new emergency management system. Such costs include the salary of the coordinator, an efficient telephone or communication system, vehicle and fuel costs, and a budget to organize meetings of stakeholders at least twice a year (Bazzoli, Harmata, and Chan 1998; Nurok 2001).

Financing

To optimize outcomes, emergency care systems in LMICs should require explicit consideration of how poor people interact with these services and how barriers to acute care can be overcome. Issues of access become critical because the lack of money often keeps people from using emergency services. Direct payment of costs for transportation, medical treatment, and medications may well constitute a major barrier for poor people in every country. Emergencies frequently cripple individuals and families financially in these communities, often for many years. At the same time, evidence indicates that when services such as ambulance transport are provided, families are willing to pay (Bose and others 2012).

Financial protection for emergency health care in LMICs is a necessity that has not received adequate attention. The goal of such protection is to ensure that individuals and families do not spiral down the pathway to abject poverty as a result of obtaining needed health care. Such financial protection may be achieved by a number of different means, including community financing (Ande and others 1997; Desmet, Chowdhury, and Islam 1999; Macintyre and Hotchkiss 1999). Community loan funds to cover transportation and other requirements for emergencies, especially for obstetrics, have been explored with mixed results (Essien and others 1997; Shehu, Ikeh, and Kuna 1997). It is plausible that these approaches can help overcome barriers to accessing emergency medical services and should be considered.

Documentation and Quality Assurance

Ensuring the quality of emergency care for all people is critical. Lack of funds, lower-paying jobs, social class distinctions, ethnicity, and other affiliations make the already vulnerable poor susceptible to receiving substandard care. Systematic documentation and periodic audits or other processes to ensure quality need to be incorporated to maintain and improve patient care. The emergency medical system should include a quality management component that is simple and continuous and that allows for rapid changes.

Expensive technology and equipment and specialists should not be advocated for the urban privileged at the expense of the majority of the rural poor. The most difficult decisions concern balancing funds invested in the emergency care capacity of first-level and second-level centers against support for referral and transportation networks to feed third-level centers. These decisions are too variable and too system specific to allow uniform policy prescriptions. Two principles can help inform these difficult decisions:

- Collect data on costs, capacities, and outcomes.
- Enhance the integration of the emergency care to improve its functioning and lead to wiser investment allocations.

Legislation

The issues discussed in this chapter form the rationale for countries to enact specific legislation addressing the provision of emergency care. This area requires major cooperation between public health and the law, which together provide the legal framework for ensuring that all individuals who need emergency care can receive it, irrespective of their personal characteristics or their ability to pay. Having laws that protect trained individuals and laypersons as they provide such care is also important. Box 14.5 provides an example of how legislative action can help the coordination and creation of emergency care, from prehospital to hospital settings.

Research and Development Agenda

The research and development priorities for emergency care are challenging to define because emergency care is a neglected area of research in LMICs, and the needs are great. As a neglected topic, emergency care is part of the "10–90" gap of health research: less than 10 percent of global research investments are for problems affecting 90 percent of the world's population (GFHR and WHO 2002).

Research and Development Approach. The spectrum of research required is diverse and may be more easily understood with the help of the schematic in table 14.3.

- The rectangle is a schematic representation of the totality of the global burden of disease that can potentially be addressed by emergency care systems.

Emergency Medical Services Coordination and Legislative Efforts in Colombia

Because of the heavy burden of trauma in Colombia, numerous cities had separate emergency medical systems, with varying protocols, training, and personnel. Some cities had volunteer systems; others had publicly funded firefighters or other civil employees. This lack of centralized organizational structure made it almost impossible to coordinate mass-casualty events across cities, such as in 1985 with the eruption of the Nevado del Ruiz volcano, which was responsible for the deaths of more than 22,000 individuals.

This challenge prompted a response to standardize training. Legislation mandated additional funds for the coordination of and authority over prehospital systems. To standardize processes nationwide, the Colombian Prehospital Care Association (ACAPH, Asociación Colombiana de Atención Prehospitalaria) was constituted from stakeholders, including physicians; private and public ambulance services; hospital administrators; university researchers; and volunteer groups, such as the civil defense, Red Cross, firefighters, and volunteer rescue agencies. The ACAPH developed standardized curricula for nurse assistants, emergency technicians, and emergency technologists. In addition, the ACAPH secured increased governmental legislation. At the time, there was already a quality plan with standardized protocols for hospital-based health care staff and coordination across

hospitals; ACAPH advocated that prehospital care and training be included in the national guidelines.

These efforts ultimately resulted in the creation of the Prehospital Trauma Life Support and Basic Trauma Life Support course as well as the National Medical Prehospital Guidelines in 2005, which ACAPH developed in conjunction with the Health Sciences Institute (Instituto de Ciencias de la Salud) and the Ministry of Social Protection. Integration of prehospital and emergency medical services into national legislation continued in different resolutions to include various levels of ambulance services, which evolved into a separate decree for auditing the quality of care and accreditation of ambulance services.

The results of this national legislation have prompted six national universities to create formal prehospital career training programs, such as the National Emergency Medical Services Technologist Curriculum. In addition, coordination across emergency medical units has improved, as evidenced in the response to the 2008 Nevado del Huila volcano eruption. Although it is difficult to completely attribute the decline in mortality to these programs and legislation, injury deaths decreased from 44,000 in 2002 to 28,000 in 2007.

Source: WHO 2010.

- A portion of this potential burden is being addressed or reduced by existing interventions, defined by box A.
- If the efficiency of current interventions were enhanced and their coverage increased, then another portion of the burden defined by box B could be addressed; this increase in efficiency will require operations research, policy research, and social science research.
- If existing interventions that have not been implemented because of their high costs were made more cost-effective, then another portion of the burden defined by box C could be reduced. This process of making interventions more cost-effective will require economic analysis and clinical research in many instances.
- Finally, some portion of the burden has no existing interventions; basic and clinical research are required to develop and pilot interventions that can address other determinants of the emergency care–related burden in the future.

The schematic representation in table 14.3 is useful for demonstrating two critical needs:

- Essential research on emergency care in LMICs
- A diverse set of research studies and approaches to reduce the burden that emergency care systems can address

Priority Setting

Setting priorities for the research and development of emergency care systems needs to be a region-specific, rather than a country-specific, process. No current list exists of global research and development priorities, reflecting the need for more attention and investment in this area. This chapter does not prescribe a list of issues or topics for global research and development efforts, but rather highlights the gap in global research and development and suggests possible issues and topics

Table 14.3 Burden of Disease Potentially Addressed by Emergency Medical Services

D: No emergency care interventions currently available to address this burden		
A: Currently implemented emergency care interventions that are addressing this burden	B: Existing emergency care interventions that are able to address existing burden if efficiency enhanced	C: Potential emergency care interventions that could address this burden if they were made cost-effective

Source: Kobusingye and others 2006.

that may be broadly relevant to LMICs for these efforts in the short to medium term.

Methods for setting research priorities in the health sector are available, such as the Combined Approach Matrix promoted by the Global Forum for Health Research (GFHR and WHO 2002), and the Essential National Health Research process promoted by the Council on Health Research for Development. Countries and regions can use these approaches to help develop their individual emergency care research agendas.

The review of evidence available in the field of emergency care as applicable to LMICs reveals many gaps in global knowledge. Following from the presentation in table 14.3 is the need to better understand the epidemiology of those conditions that can be addressed by emergency care systems in LMICs and which interventions in place address them. There is little knowledge of how to enhance the efficiency of these existing interventions and reduce their costs. Most important, the lack of intervention trials in LMICs creates a major research priority for the field of emergency care. Well-designed, locally appropriate interventions that establish their effectiveness are urgently needed and should include both interventions that may be available in HICs as well as new interventions. Economic analysis is another area for major research input in the field of emergency care, where cost and cost-effectiveness information from LMICs is scant. These gaps reflect the need for a more systematic analysis of where emergency care research investments should be directed for optimal results in the future.

CONCLUSIONS: PROMISES AND PITFALLS

Emergency care is a critical and integral component of national health systems in LMICs. Governments and ministries of health in these countries need to pay specific attention to the development of emergency care and to ensure that their evolution is both evidence based and appropriate to their national needs. More important, the context and implementation of emergency care should improve health equity and not widen existing health disparities.

This chapter highlights not only the urgent need for more attention to emergency care in LMICs, but also points out an opportunity for these countries to define better emergency care systems for their needs. In promoting the systematic development of evidence-based emergency care systems, LMICs could help define more effective and more cost-effective emergency systems than currently exist in HICs. This opportunity should not be lost as a result of political inattention or lack of funds; international and national stakeholders should move forward to stem the preventable loss of life from the lack of emergency care.

Too little is known about the true extent of the need for emergency care, the design that would work well for different communities and populations, and the costs and benefits of delivering emergency care. These gaps call for more investment in the research, development, and implementation of emergency care, especially in LMICs. Universal emergency care is consistent with the right to health care; by definition, emergency care is a matter of life and death. It is essential to endeavor to ensure that prompt, appropriate care is available in critical moments when delays in care—or the delivery of inappropriate care—could mean the loss of lives.

ANNEXES

The annexes to this chapter are as follows. They are available at http://www.dcp-3.org/surgery:
- Annex 14A. Matrix of Essential Knowledge, Skills, Equipment, and Supplies for Prehospital Providers
- Annex 14B. Essential Resources for the Delivery of Emergency Care in Hospitals

NOTE

The World Bank classifies countries according to four income groupings. Income is measured using gross national income (GNI) per capita, in U.S. dollars, converted from local currency using the *World Bank Atlas* method. Classifications as of July 2014 are as follows:

- Low-income countries (LICs) = US$1,045 or less in 2013
- Middle-income countries (MICs) are subdivided:
  - Lower-middle-income = US$1,046 to US$4,125
  - Upper-middle-income (UMICs) = US$4,126 to US$12,745
- High-income countries (HICs) = US$12,746 or more

REFERENCES

Ali, J., R. Adam, A. K. Butler, H. Chang, M. Howard, and others. 1993. "Trauma Outcome Improves Following the Advanced Trauma Life Support Program in a Developing Country." *Journal of Trauma* 34 (6): 890–98; discussion 898–99.

Ali, J., R. U. Adam, T. J. Gana, and J. I. Williams. 1997. "Trauma Patient Outcome after the Prehospital Trauma Life Support Program." *Journal of Trauma* 42 (6): 1018–21; discussion 1021–12.

Ande, B., J. Chiwuzie, W. Akpala, A. Oronsaye, O. Okojie, and others. 1997. "Improving Obstetric Care at the District Hospital, Ekpoma, Nigeria: The Benin PMM Team." *International Journal of Gynaecology and Obstetrics* 59 (Suppl 2): S47–53.

Arellano, N., M. J. Mello, and M. A. Clark. 2010. "The Role of Motorcycle Taxi Drivers in the Pre-hospital Care of Road Traffic Injury Victims in Rural Dominican Republic." *Injury Prevention* 16 (4): 272–74.

Arreola-Risa, C., C. N. Mock, A. J. Herrera-Escamilla, I. Contreras, and J. Vargas. 2004. "Cost-Effectiveness and Benefit of Alternatives to Improve Training for Prehospital Trauma Care in Mexico." *Prehospital Disaster Medicine* 19 (4): 318–25.

Arreola-Risa, C., C. N. Mock, L. Lojero-Wheatly, O. de la Cruz, C. Garcia, and others. 2000. "Low-Cost Improvements in Prehospital Trauma Care in a Latin American City." *Journal of Trauma* 48 (1): 119–24.

Arreola-Risa, C., J. Vargas, I. Contreras, and C. N. Mock. 2007. "Effect of Emergency Medical Technician Certification for All Prehospital Personnel in a Latin American City." *Journal of Trauma* 63 (4): 914–19.

Bakalos, G., M. Mamali, C. Komninos, E. Koukou, A. Tsantilas, and others. 2011. "Advanced Life Support versus Basic Life Support in the Pre-hospital Setting: A Meta-Analysis." *Resuscitation* 82 (9): 1130–37.

Bavonratanavech, S. 2003. "Trauma Care Systems in Thailand." *Injury* 34 (9): 720–21.

Bazzoli, G. J., R. Harmata, and C. Chan. 1998. "Community-Based Trauma Systems in the United States: An Examination of Structural Development." *Social Science and Medicine* 46 (9): 1137–49.

Black, R. S., and P. Brocklehurst. 2003. "A Systematic Review of Training in Acute Obstetric Emergencies." *BJOG: An International Journal of Obstetrics and Gynaecology* 110 (9): 837–41.

Bollig, G., A. G. Myklebust, and K. Ostringen. 2011. "Effects of First Aid Training in the Kindergarten: A Pilot Study." *Scandinavian Journal of Trauma, Resuscitation and Emergency Medicine* 19 (1): 13.

Bollig, G., H. A. Wahl, and M. V. Svendsen. 2009. "Primary School Children Are Able to Perform Basic Life-Saving First Aid Measures." *Resuscitation* 80 (6): 689–92.

Bose, S. K., K. D. Bream, F. K. Barg, and R. A. Band. 2012. "Willingness to Pay for Emergency Referral Transport in a Developing Setting: A Geographically Randomized Study." *Academic Emergency Medicine* 19 (7): 793–800. doi:10.1111/j.1553-2712.2012.01382.x.

Bossyns, P., R. Abache, M. S. Abdoulaye, and W. V. Lerberghe. 2005. "Unaffordable or Cost-Effective?: Introducing an Emergency Referral System in Rural Niger." *Tropical Medicine and International Health* 10 (9): 879–87.

Chandy, H., M. Steinholt, and H. Husum. 2007. "Delivery Life Support: A Preliminary Report on the Chain of Survival for Complicated Deliveries in Rural Cambodia." *Nursing and Health Sciences* 9 (4): 263–69.

Desmet, M., A. Q. Chowdhury, and M. K. Islam. 1999. "The Potential for Social Mobilisation in Bangladesh: The Organisation and Functioning of Two Health Insurance Schemes." *Social Science and Medicine* 48 (7): 925–38.

Essien, E., D. Ifenne, K. Sabitu, A. Musa, M. Alti-Mu'azu, and others. 1997. "Community Loan Funds and Transport Services for Obstetric Emergencies in Northern Nigeria." *International Journal of Gynaecology and Obstetrics* 59 (Suppl 2): S237–44.

Fiander, S. 2001. *Anyone Can Save a Life: Road Accidents and First Aid.* London: British Red Cross.

Geduld, H., and L. Wallis. 2011. "Taxi Driver Training in Madagascar: The First Step in Developing a Functioning Prehospital Emergency Care System." *Emergency Medicine Journal* 28 (9): 794–96.

GFHR (Global Forum for Health Research) and WHO (World Health Organization). 2002. *The 10/90 Report on Health Research 2001–2002.* Geneva: Global Forum for Health Research.

Gomes, E., R. Araujo, A. Carneiro, C. Dias, A. Costa-Pereira, and others. 2010. "The Importance of Pre-trauma Centre Treatment of Life-Threatening Events on the Mortality of Patients Transferred with Severe Trauma." *Resuscitation* 81 (4): 440–45.

Hauswald, M., and E. Yeoh. 1997. "Designing a Prehospital System for a Developing Country: Estimated Cost and Benefits." *American Journal of Emergency Medicine* 15 (6): 600–03.

Henry, J. A., and A. L. Reingold. 2012. "Prehospital Trauma Systems Reduce Mortality in Developing Countries: A Systematic Review and Meta-Analysis." *Journal of Trauma and Acute Care Surgery* 73 (1): 261–68.

Hsia, R. Y., N. A. Mbembati, S. MacFarlane, and M. E. Kruk. 2012. "Access to Emergency and Surgical Care in Sub-Saharan Africa: The Infrastructure Gap." *Health Policy and Planning* 27 (3): 234–44.

Husum, H., M. Gilbert, and T. Wisborg. 2003. "Training Pre-Hospital Trauma Care in Low-Income Countries: The 'Village University' Experience." *Medical Teacher* 25 (2): 142–48.

Husum, H., M. Gilbert, T. Wisborg, Y. Van Heng, and M. Murad. 2003. "Rural Prehospital Trauma Systems Improve Trauma Outcome in Low-Income Countries: A Prospective Study from North Iraq and Cambodia." *Journal of Trauma* 54 (6): 1188–96.

Ismail, M. S., A. B. Hasinah, M. N. Syaiful, H. B. Murshidah, T. J. Thong, and others. 2012. "Study on Advanced Life Support Devices in the Ambulances for Emergency Cases in Klang Valley, Malaysia." *La Clinica Terapeutica* 163 (2): 115–22.

Jamison, D. T., J. G. Bremen, A. R. Measham, G. Alleyne, M. Claeson, D. B. Evans, P. Jha, A. Mills, and P. Musgrove, eds. 2006. *Disease Control Priorities in Developing Countries.* 2nd ed. Washington, DC: World Bank and Oxford University Press.

Jayaraman, S., J. R. Mabweijano, M. S. Lipnick, N. Caldwell, J. Miyamoto, and others. 2009a. "Current Patterns of Prehospital Trauma Care in Kampala, Uganda and the Feasibility of a Lay-First-Responder Training Program." *World Journal of Surgery* 33 (12): 2512–21.

———. 2009b. "First Things First: Effectiveness and Scalability of a Basic Prehospital Trauma Care Program for Lay First-Responders in Kampala, Uganda." *PLoS One* 4 (9): e6955.

Jayaraman, S., and D. Sethi. 2010. "Advanced Trauma Life Support Training for Ambulance Crews." *Cochrane Database of Systematic Reviews* 1: CD003109. doi:10.1002/14651858 .CD003109.pub2.

Joshipura, M. K., H. S. Shah, P. R. Patel, P. A. Divatia, and P. M. Desai. 2003. "Trauma Care Systems in India." *Injury* 34 (9): 686–92.

Kane, G., N. C. Wheeler, S. Cook, R. Englehardt, B. Pavey, and others. 1992. "Impact of the Los Angeles County Trauma System on the Survival of Seriously Injured Patients." *Journal of Trauma* 32 (5): 576–83.

Khorasani-Zavareh, D., B. J. Haglund, R. Mohammadi, M. Naghavi, and L. Laflamme. 2009. "Traffic Injury Deaths in West Azarbaijan Province of Iran: A Cross-Sectional Interview-Based Study on Victims' Characteristics and Prehospital Care." *International Journal of Injury Control and Safety Promotion* 16 (3): 119–26.

Kirsch, T. D. 1998. "Emergency Medicine around the World." *Annals of Emergency Medicine* 32 (2): 237–38.

Kobusingye, O. C., D. Guwatudde, G. Owor, and R. R. Lett. 2002. "Citywide Trauma Experience in Kampala, Uganda: A Call for Intervention." *Injury Prevention* 8 (2): 133–36.

Kobusingye, O. C., A. A. Hyder, D. Bishai, E. R. Hicks, C. Mock, and others. 2005. "Emergency Medical Systems in Low- and Middle-Income Countries: Recommendations for Action." *Bulletin of the World Health Organization* 83 (8): 626–31. http://www.ncbi.nlm.nih.gov/pmc/articles /PMC2626309/.

Kobusingye, O. C., A. A. Hyder, D. Bishai, M. Joshipura, E. R. Hicks, and others. 2006. "Emergency Medical Services." In *Disease Control Priorities in Developing Countries*, edited by D. T. Jamison, J. G. Bremen, A. R. Measham, G. Alleyne, M. Claeson, D. B. Evans, P. Jha, A. Mills, and P. Musgrove, 2nd ed. 1261–80. Washington, DC: World Bank and Oxford University Press.

Leigh, B., H. B. Kandeh, M. S. Kanu, M. Kuteh, I. S. Palmer, and others. 1997. "Improving Emergency Obstetric Care at a District Hospital, Makeni, Sierra Leone: The Freetown/ Makeni PMM Team." *International Journal of Gynaecology and Obstetrics* 59 (Suppl 2): S55–65.

Liberman, M., D. Mulder, A. Lavoie, R. Denis, and J. S. Sampalis. 2003. "Multicenter Canadian Study of Prehospital Trauma Care." *Annals of Surgery* 237 (2): 153–60.

Lungu, K., V. Kamfose, J. Hussein, and H. Ashwood-Smith. 2001. "Are Bicycle Ambulances and Community Transport Plans Effective in Strengthening Obstetric Referral Systems in Southern Malawi?" *Malawi Medical Journal* 12: 16–18.

Macintyre, K., and D. R. Hotchkiss. 1999. "Referral Revisited: Community Financing Schemes and Emergency Transport in Rural Africa." *Social Science and Medicine* 49 (11): 1473–87.

Mahadevan, S., M. Strehlow, A. Chiao, G. Ramana Rao, D. Shelke, and others. 2009. *Development of a Self-Sustaining Paramedic Educational Program in India.* Guwahati, India: EMCON.

Mantha, A., A. Gupta, M. Strehlow, and S. Mahadevan. 2009. *Development of a Focused Leadership Curriculum for Paramedic Students in India.* Guwahati, India: EMCON.

McClure, E. M., W. A. Carlo, L. L. Wright, E. Chomba, F. Uxa, and others. 2007. "Evaluation of the Educational Impact of the WHO Essential Newborn Care Course in Zambia." *Acta Paediatrica* 96 (8): 1135–38.

McSwain, N. 1991. "Prehospital Emergency Medical Systems and Cardiopulmonary Resuscitation." In *Trauma*, edited by E. Moore, K. Mattox, and D. Feliciano. Norwalk, CT: Appleton and Lange.

Mock, C. N., G. J. Jurkovich, D. nii-Amon-Kotei, C. Arreola-Risa, and R. V. Maier. 1998. "Trauma Mortality Patterns in Three Nations at Different Economic Levels: Implications for Global Trauma System Development." *Journal of Trauma* 44 (5): 804–12; discussion 812–14.

Mock, C. N., M. Tiska, M. Adu-Ampofo, and G. Boakye. 2002. "Improvements in Prehospital Trauma Care in an African Country with No Formal Emergency Medical Services." *Journal of Trauma* 53 (1): 90–97.

Mullins, R. J., J. Veum-Stone, M. Helfand, M. Zimmer-Gembeck, J. R. Hedges, and others. 1994. "Outcome of Hospitalized Injured Patients after Institution of a Trauma System in an Urban Area." *Journal of the American Medical Association* 271 (24): 1919–24.

Murad, M. K., and H. Husum. 2010. "Trained Lay First Responders Reduce Trauma Mortality: A Controlled Study of Rural Trauma in Iraq." *Prehospital and Disaster Medicine* 25 (6): 533–39.

Murad, M. K., D. B. Issa, F. M. Mustafa, H. O. Hassan, and H. Husum. 2012. "Prehospital Trauma System Reduces Mortality in Severe Trauma: A Controlled Study of Road Traffic Casualties in Iraq." *Prehospital and Disaster Medicine* 27 (1): 36–41.

Murad, M. K., S. Larsen, and H. Husum. 2012. "Prehospital Trauma Care Reduces Mortality. Ten-Year Results from a Time-Cohort and Trauma Audit Study in Iraq." *Scandinavian Journal of Trauma, Resuscitation and Emergency Medicine* 20: 13.

Nguyen, T. L., T. H. Nguyen, S. Morita, and J. Sakamoto. 2008. "Injury and Pre-hospital Trauma Care in Hanoi, Vietnam." *Injury* 39 (9): 1026–33.

Nurok, M. 2001. "The Death of a Princess and the Formulation of Medical Competence." *Social Science and Medicine* 53 (11): 1427–38.

Oyesola, R., D. Shehu, A. T. Ikeh, and I. Maru. 1997. "Improving Emergency Obstetric Care at a State Referral Hospital, Kebbi State, Nigeria: The Sokoto PMM Team." *International Journal of Gynaecology and Obstetrics* 59 (Suppl 2): S75–81.

Ramanujam, P., and M. Aschkenasy. 2007. "Identifying the Need for Pre-hospital and Emergency Care in the Developing World: A Case Study in Chennai, India." *Journal of the Association of Physicians of India* 55: 491–95.

Reines, H. D., R. L. Bartlett, N. E. Chudy, K. R. Kiragu, and M. A. McKnew. 1988. "Is Advanced Life Support Appropriate for Victims of Motor Vehicle Accidents: The South Carolina Highway Trauma Project." *Journal of Trauma* 28 (5): 563–70.

Rutledge, R., J. Messick, C. C. Baker, S. Rhyne, J. Butts, A. Meyer, and others. 1992. "Multivariate Population-Based Analysis of the Association of County Trauma Centers with per Capita County Trauma Death Rates." *Journal of Trauma* 33 (1): 29–37; discussion 37–28.

Sampalis, J. S., S. Boukas, A. Lavoie, A. Nikolis, P. Frechette, and others. 1995. "Preventable Death Evaluation of the Appropriateness of the On-Site Trauma Care Provided by Urgences-Sante Physicians." *Journal of Trauma* 39 (6): 1029–35.

Sampalis, J. S., A. Lavoie, M. Salas, A. Nikolis, and J. I. Williams. 1994. "Determinants of On-Scene Time in Injured Patients Treated by Physicians at the Site." *Prehospital and Disaster Medicine* 9 (3): 178–88; discussion 189.

Sampalis, J. S., H. Tamim, R. Denis, S. Boukas, S. A. Ruest, and others. 1997. "Ineffectiveness of On-Site Intravenous Lines: Is Prehospital Time the Culprit?" *Journal of Trauma* 43 (4): 608–15; discussion 615–07.

Sangowawa, A. O., and E. T. Owoaje. 2012. "Building Capacity of Drivers in Nigeria to Provide First Aid for Road Crash Victims." *Injury Prevention* 18 (1): 62–65.

Sasser, S., M. Varghese, A. Kellerman, and J.-D. Lormand, eds. 2005. *Prehospital Trauma Care Systems.* Geneva: World Health Organization.

Shehu, D., A. T. Ikeh, and M. J. Kuna. 1997. "Mobilizing Transport for Obstetric Emergencies in Northwestern Nigeria. The Sokoto PMM Team." *International Journal of Gynaecology and Obstetrics* 59 (Suppl 2): S173–80.

Solagberu, B. A., C. K. Ofoegbu, L. O. Abdur-Rahman, A. O. Adekanye, U. S. Udoffa, and others. 2009. "Pre-hospital Care in Nigeria: A Country without Emergency Medical Services." *Nigerian Journal of Clinical Practice* 12 (1): 29–33.

Stiell, I. G., L. P. Nesbitt, W. Pickett, D. Munkley, D. W. Spaite, and others. 2008. "The OPALS Major Trauma Study: Impact of Advanced Life-Support on Survival and Morbidity." *Canadian Medical Association Journal* 178 (9): 1141–52. doi:10.1503/cmaj.071154.

Sun, J. H., R. Shing, M. Twomey, and L. A. Wallis. 2012. "A Strategy to Implement and Support Pre-hospital Emergency Medical Systems in Developing, Resource-Constrained Areas of South Africa." *Injury* 45 (1): 31–38.

Sun, J. H., M. Twomey, J. Tran, and L. A. Wallis. 2012. "The Need for a Usable Assessment Tool to Analyse the Efficacy of Emergency Care Systems in Developing Countries: Proposal to Use the TEWS Methodology." *Emergency Medicine* 29 (11): 882–86.

Sun, J. H., and L. Wallis. 2011. "The Psychological Effects of Widespread Emergencies and a First Responder Training Course on a Violent, Developing Community." *African Journal of Emergency Medicine* 1 (4): 166–73.

Tannebaum, R. D., J. L. Arnold, A. De Negri Filho, and V. S. Spadoni. 2001. "Emergency Medicine in Southern Brazil." *Annals of Emergency Medicine* 37 (2): 223–28.

Tiska, M. A., M. Adu-Ampofo, G. Boakye, L. Tuuli, and C. N. Mock. 2004. "A Model of Prehospital Trauma Training for Lay Persons Devised in Africa." *Emergency Medicine* 21 (2): 237–39.

Varghese, M., and P. Mohan. 1998. *When Someone Is Hurt: A First Aid Guide for Laypersons and Community Workers.* New Delhi: The Other Media Communications.

WHO (World Health Organization). 2010. *Strengthening Care for the Injured: Success Stories and Lessons Learned from around the World.* Geneva: WHO.

———. 2013. "Global Health Estimates for Deaths by Cause, Age, and Sex for Years 2000–2011." WHO, Geneva. http://www.who.int/healthinfo/global_burden_disease/en/.

WHO and UNICEF (United Nations International Children's Emergency Fund). 2000. *Management of the Child with a Serious Infection or Severe Malnutrition: Guidelines for Care at the First-Referral Level in Developing Countries.* Geneva: WHO.

Wilkinson, D., and M. Skinner. 2000. *Primary Trauma Care Manual: A Manual for Trauma Management in District and Remote Locations.* Oxford: Primary Trauma Care Foundation. http://www.primarytraumacare.org/wp-content/uploads/2011/09/PTC_ENG.pdf.

Wisborg, T., M. K. Murad, O. Edvardsen, and B. S. Brinchmann. 2008. "Life or Death: The Social Impact of Paramedics and First Responders in Landmine-Infested Villages in Northern Iraq." *Rural and Remote Health* 8 (1): 816.

Wisborg, T., M. K. Murad, O. Edvardsen, and H. Husum. 2008. "Prehospital Trauma System in a Low-Income Country: System Maturation and Adaptation During 8 Years." *Journal of Trauma* 64 (5): 1342–48.

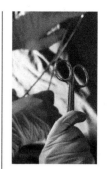

Chapter **15**

Anesthesia and Perioperative Care

Kelly McQueen, Thomas Coonan, Andrew Ottaway,
Richard P. Dutton, Florian R. Nuevo,
Zipporah Gathuya, and Iain H. Wilson

INTRODUCTION

In the not-so-distant past, the impact of safe anesthesia on surgical outcomes often went unrecognized. Beginning in the 1950s, as surgical techniques advanced, strategies to improve patient safety and surgical outcomes were emphasized; physician anesthesia providers were recognized as essential members of surgical teams in high-income countries (HICs). Most low- and middle-income countries (LMICs), which have the greatest unmet surgical need, have not been able to apply the anesthesia advances in patient care and monitoring that have proven so successful in HICs. The availability of anesthesia providers is limited in LMICs, and many lack requisite training and supervision.

Although many of the advances that improved outcomes in anesthesia and surgery are technology based and expensive, several early interventions are feasible in all settings. As surgical intervention expands in LMICs to fill the growing and largely unmet treatment needs, an anesthesia crisis looms.

This chapter reviews the historical, remote, and recent global data that reveal the contributions of anesthesia to surgical and perioperative outcomes, as well as the anesthesia-associated morbidity and mortality rates, where available. It emphasizes the role of outcomes analysis and quality improvement, and it discusses the global cost and cost-effectiveness data, as well as the limited data from LMICs on human

resources, education, and outcomes. Finally, this chapter proposes effective and responsible policy and funding solutions for the anesthesia crisis in most of these countries.

ANESTHESIA AND THE GLOBAL BURDEN OF DISEASE

Global Burden of Disease Averted by Safe Anesthesia for Surgical Interventions

The anesthesia crisis significantly affects the global gap between the surgical burden of disease and access to surgical services. The World Health Organization's (WHO's) Global Health Estimates documented substantial premature death and disability from trauma, cancer, and pregnancy and childbirth worldwide (WHO 2013a) and the inadequate surgical resources to meet these burgeoning surgical needs (Notrica and others 2011; Penoyar and others 2012). The unmet anesthesia and patient safety needs are generally correlated with the level of a country's development, with the greatest needs in South Asia and Sub-Saharan Africa (map 15.1).

Noncommunicable diseases are eclipsing infectious diseases as the leading global health issue and are projected to be the most important cause of mortality by 2020. Many of these conditions are potentially amenable to surgical treatment. Although providing adequate

Corresponding author: Kelly McQueen, MD, MPH, Vanderbilt University Medical Center, kelly.mcqueen@vanderbilt.edu

Map 15.1 Global Development and Surgical Need

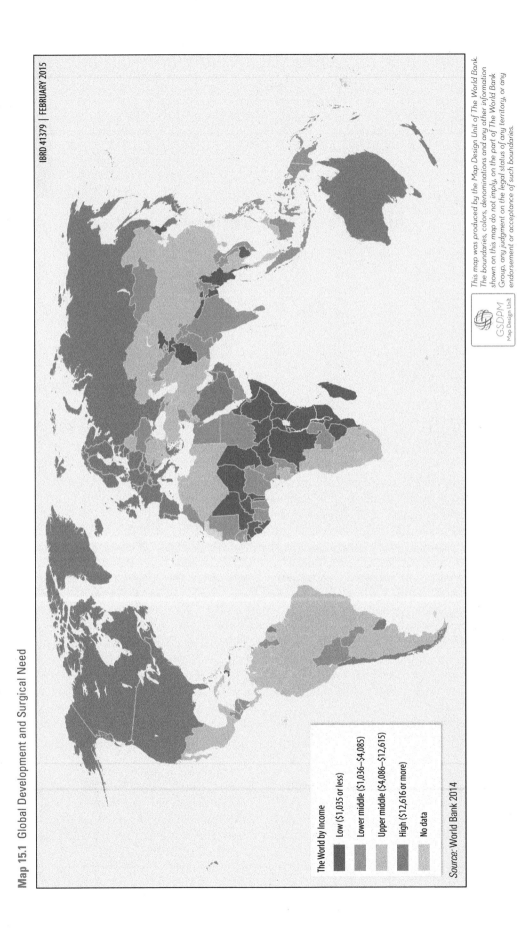

The World by Income

■ Low ($1,035 or less)
■ Lower middle ($1,036–$4,085)
■ Upper middle ($4,086–$12,615)
■ High ($12,616 or more)
■ No data

Source: World Bank 2014

IBRD 41379 | FEBRUARY 2015

This map was produced by the Map Design Unit of The World Bank.
The boundaries, colors, denominations and any other information
shown on this map do not imply, on the part of The World Bank
Group, any judgment on the legal status of any territory, or any
endorsement or acceptance of such boundaries.

GSDPM
Map Design Unit

resources is a daunting task, it is no more impossible than addressing the HIV/AIDS crisis in the past 25 years. Cost-effective and attainable surgical solutions exist (WHO 2008) but will only be valuable if safe anesthesia is simultaneously supported. The contribution of anesthesia to the burden of surgical disease is difficult to measure, but it is integral to surgery and an equal contributor to disability and death. Without safe anesthesia, current anesthesia practice will contribute to additional disability and death, even when surgery is provided.

Definitions essential to understanding the contributions that anesthesia makes to patient safety and outcomes include the following:

- **Anesthesia machine:** A machine specifically designed for the delivery of anesthesia that includes the ability to provide oxygen and ventilation.
- **Patient safety:** A phrase that describes processes in place in hospitals and operating rooms to ensure the best possible outcomes for patients; these processes include policies and monitors that focus on preventing adverse outcomes and on alerting personnel to situations requiring urgent attention.
- **Precordial stethoscope:** A modified stethoscope for the purpose of listening to heart and breath sounds; it may be modified to become an esophageal stethoscope that amplifies sounds.
- **Perioperative period:** The days and weeks immediately preceding and following a surgical intervention. In this period, optimization of the patient's health may occur preoperatively, and complications are observed. In HICs, the postoperative period at 24 hours and at 30 days is specifically noted for critical events, including death.
- **Perioperative Mortality Rates (POMRs):** The mortality rates in the operating room or within 24 hours of a surgical intervention and anesthesia. In HICs, these rates are reported and followed as indicators of safety.
- **Vigilance:** The continuous presence of and monitoring by providers, without distraction or time lapses.

Global Anesthesia Crisis

In LMICs, poor perioperative care has several causes: few trained providers; unreliable access to essential medications, including oxygen; limited safety monitoring; and limited options for postoperative care, including pain management.

In these truly austere situations, most anesthetics are administered with intravenous or intramuscular ketamine, with no safety monitoring and no oxygen, by attendants with limited training. Airway protection with a tracheal tube is often not an option, even during general anesthesia, because of a lack of provider skills and the absence of a laryngoscope required for intubation. Equipment is antiquated, broken, or absent. Frequently there are no pressurized gasses, no anesthesia circuitry or other requisite disposables, and no medications for hemodynamic rescue.

Causes of the Crisis. Many factors contribute to the crisis (McQueen 2010). Inadequate numbers of trained anesthesiologists and the brain drain to other specialties or higher resource countries are important contributors.[1] Understandably, available resources—human, capital, and pharmaceutical—were diverted away from surgically treatable diseases and toward HIV/AIDS.

A correlation exists between surgical access, anesthesia capacity, and patient safety on the one hand and mortality on the other hand. Few studies speak directly to this correlation. Several studies strikingly reveal specific risks of anesthesia in LMICs. Anesthesia-related mortality is unacceptably high in these countries and is amplified in the maternal and pediatric populations (Bosenberg 2007; Fenton, Whitty, and Reynolds 2003; Hodges and Hodges 2000; Hodges and others 2007; Jochberger and others 2008; Kushner and others 2010; Walker and Wilson 2008; Walker and others 2010). Globally, 2 billion people lack access to surgical treatment (Funk and others 2010), and 85 percent of children in LMICs are likely to require treatment for a surgical condition by age 15 years (Bickler, Telfer, and Sanno-Duanda 2003). In Uganda in 2010, 17 percent of anesthesia providers had no formal training (Walker and others 2010). The absence of trained providers for children is a matter of particular concern.

Barriers to Safe Anesthesia Services. The greatest barriers to access to safe anesthesia are the lack of adequate training and supervision for providers, safety monitoring capacity, sustainable organizational structure, and a modern system of quality review. The state of the crisis has been largely underestimated as a result of the lack of outcomes measurement, including perioperative mortality, and the overall absence of patient follow-up. Assessments of anesthesia-related mortality rates, when available, are indicative of poor patient care and safety (Bosenberg 2007; Fenton, Whitty, and Reynolds 2003; Hodges and Hodges 2000; Hodges and others 2007; Jochberger and others 2008; Kushner and others 2010; Walker and Wilson 2008; Walker and others 2010).

The shortage in the number of anesthesiologists is exacerbated by the fact that the available anesthesia providers spend only 60 percent of their time in clinical care. The remainder is spent dealing with broken equipment and the bureaucracy necessary to improve conditions for providers and patients (Dubowitz, Detlefs, and McQueen 2010).

SAFE ANESTHESIA FOR SURGICAL INTERVENTIONS

Patient Safety

Successful initiatives directed at patient safety and improved outcomes include airway management, cardiac outcomes, and perioperative care.

Airway Management. Safe anesthesia requires the skills to maintain an open airway and to provide breathing and oxygenation. The lack of such skills is at the core of patient safety issues in LMICs.

Pulse oximetry and continuous capnography have undoubtedly improved results in HICs, although ethical practice has forestalled a true scientific study comparing anesthesia safety with and without these monitors. Pulse oximetry, a noninvasive monitoring of oxygen saturation, has been in use since 1981. Capnography is the monitoring of carbon dioxide in the respiratory gases. Anesthesia-related mortality rates declined in HICs with the mandatory use of both of these monitors. Both pulse oximetry and capnography require the continuous vigilance of an anesthesia provider with appropriate skills to respond to deviations. Such providers are more important than the monitors (Beecher and Todd 1954; Merry and others 2010; Pedersen and others 2014).

The contributory role of neuromuscular blocking agents administered to facilitate intubation or surgery in poor outcomes related to airway management is well known. In a seminal examination of perioperative mortality in a cohort of American hospitals, Beecher and Todd (1954) document a twofold increase in death when these agents were used. Neuromuscular blocking agents are included in the *WHO Model List of Essential Medicines* (WHO 2013b) but are often unavailable in LMICs, which is perhaps fortunate for patient safety. However, as surgical interventions become increasingly available and surgical techniques advance, these medications have the potential to contribute to poor outcomes.

Cardiac Perturbations. Myocardial depression is a common side effect of anesthesia medications and can prove lethal in patients with underlying disease or those with hemorrhage or hemodynamic instability. The older anesthetics still commonly in use in most LMICs, including halothane, cause more myocardial depression than more modern agents. Unfortunately, in these same settings, standard rescue medications, including epinephrine, are not routinely available to treat these predictable side effects.

One major study found that in HICs approximately 5 percent of patients have perioperative myocardial infarctions following major noncardiac surgery (Devereaux and others 2011). This event was associated with a fivefold increase in 30-day mortality. Evidence suggests that changes in the perioperative management initiated by anesthetists at the time of surgery can significantly reduce mortality related to these anticipated cardiac events (Canty and others 2012).

Perioperative Care. The perioperative period—extending from the initial preoperative evaluation of the patient's general health and comorbidities to 30 days postoperatively—is an important window for patient evaluation and significantly affects patient outcomes. Perioperative evaluation provides valuable information to providers planning optimal anesthesia management. An inexpensive screening test, such as hemoglobin measurement, contributes to improved outcomes.

Comorbidities. Ideally, the perioperative period should be used to alter or improve comorbidities and to improve perioperative health status. The current situation in most LMICs does not often allow for this advance preparation; as surgical systems evolve, planning for perioperative evaluation will become necessary.

Pain Management. Pain management is not only basic to the right to health (MacIntyre and Scott 2010; Morriss and Goucke 2011; Size, Soyannwo, and Justins 2007), but inadequately treated pain contributes to morbidity and, in some rare cases, to mortality. Uncontrolled acute pain also increases the incidence of chronic pain (MacIntyre and Scott 2010), potentially imposing a degree of suffering and disability that may last for years. The tragic reality in LMICs is that pain medicines, opioids, or nonsteroidal anti-inflammatory medications are often unavailable, even though they are included on the *WHO Model List of Essential Medicines* (WHO 2013b) and are inexpensive and effective.

In HICs, the initial postoperative care of patients is provided by anesthesia providers and thereafter by surgeons and other physicians; this approach has improved outcomes. In LMICs, postoperative care is often administered by family members, even in the immediate postoperative period. Although the impact of the absence of professional care in the postoperative period is unknown, it is likely to be associated with increased POMRs.

Perioperative- and Anesthesia-Related Mortality

Systematic review of perioperative and anesthesia-related mortality demonstrates global improvements in outcomes during the past five decades, primarily in HICs (Bainbridge and others 2012). Overall mortality from anesthesia fell from 357 per million before the 1970s to 34 per million during 1990–2010, despite the growing number of patients with increased anesthetic risks. Analysis demonstrated not only an increased risk of anesthesia in higher-risk patients but also a correlation between anesthesia risk, mortality, and the human development index (HDI), an index related to life expectancy, education, and income (Bainbridge and others 2012). In countries with high HDIs, anesthesia mortality has fallen from 357 per million to 25 per million. In low-HDI countries, no figure from before the 1970s is available; in recent decades, the estimate of 141 per million has been reported (Bainbridge and others 2012).

Studies of perioperative mortality are difficult to conduct and infrequent in LMICs. However, a series of small anesthesia outcome studies in Sub-Saharan Africa from the 1980s to the 2000s has reported consistent and shocking rates of mortality in otherwise healthy patients in countries with similar HDIs. In 1988, a study from a hospital in Zambia reported an anesthesia mortality rate of 1 in 1,925; in Malawi in 2000, a rate of 1 in 504; in Zimbabwe in 2005, a rate of 1 in 482; in Togo in 2005, a rate of 1 in 133; in Nigeria in 2006, a rate of 1 in 387 in mothers undergoing cesarean section; and in Benin in 2010, a rate of 1 in 97 in pediatric anesthesia patients (Enohuman and Imarengiaye 2006; Glenshaw and Madzimbamuto 2005; Hansen, Gausi, and Merikebu 2000; Heywood, Wilson, and Sinclair 1989; Ouro-Bang'na Maman and others 2005; Zoumenou and others 2010). In comparison, the perioperative mortality in the United States in the 1950s was 1 in 1,500 (Beecher and Todd 1954). In each study, deaths from anesthesia were most commonly due to undetected hypoxia or hypovolemia. Inadequate equipment, training and supervision, and safety monitoring—particularly pulse oximetry—were cited as contributors to these poor outcomes. Several of these studies shared a similar methodology; despite being relatively small, they are important because of the consistently high rates of mortality reported.

During the past 30 years, anesthesia mortality and morbidity have decreased significantly, primarily in HICs, as a result of aggressive implementation of clinical adjuvants, monitoring capacity, and the imprint of a culture of safety (Eichorn 1989; Merry and others 2010). For example, 50 years of intense commitment in Australia has reduced avoidable anesthesia-related mortality from 1 in 5,000 to 1 in 100,000—and 1 in 180,000 in cases in which anesthesia is the sole cause of mortality and morbidity (Mackay and Cousins 2006). Unfortunately, LMICs lag far behind; mortality rates solely related to anesthesia are 100 to 1,000 times higher than in HICs, especially in obstetric and pediatric populations (Hansen, Gausi, and Merikebu 2000; Heywood, Wilson, and Sinclair 1989; Kushner and others 2010; McKenzie 1996; Ouro-Bang'na Maman and others 2005; Vasdev and others 2008). Information related to perioperative morbidity is more difficult to obtain because of the lack of postoperative care units and postsurgical patient follow-up. Solutions to this information gap are possible based on HIC models, but the feasibility of these solutions may be decades away.

As the anesthesia and surgical resources of a country improve, gains in absolute perioperative mortality are likely to be reinvested in operating on patients with more serious conditions and comorbidities. Figure 15.1 provides a graphic representation of this hypothesis. Low-HDI countries with high POMRs today might be expected to make rapid progress in the short term, perhaps based on a few highly cost-effective interventions. In time, however, the improvements in mortality will plateau. Further gains will require exponentially greater investments, and progress might be more apparent in the increased acuity of patients taken to the operating room rather than in improved overall survival.

Figure 15.1 Perioperative Mortality versus National Resources

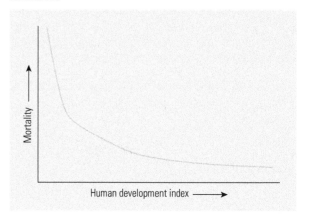

Reporting POMRs and benchmarking outcomes will be essential to improving patient safety and to better anesthesia and surgical outcomes in LMICs. Preventable, anesthesia-specific mortality rates will only be affected when common inciting events are documented and stratified using the American Society of Anesthesiologists (ASA) physical status, age, and the social determinants of health related to living in LMICs (Doorley and others 2013).

COST, EFFECTIVENESS, AND COST-EFFECTIVENESS OF SAFE ANESTHESIA

Improvements in monitoring, and the increased availability of medications and screened blood products, have elevated the effectiveness and safety of anesthesia. These improvements have occurred in the context of a platform of professional education and training, clinical excellence, and professionalism. Safety innovation has not always occurred under circumstances of rigorous validation of efficacy and cost-effectiveness. The pulse oximeter, for instance, was rapidly embraced as mandatory safety technology and included as a required monitor for sedation and anesthesia by organizations and societies throughout the world; to date, however, it has not been evaluated for cost-effectiveness (Pedersen and others 2014). The most compelling argument for the effectiveness of anesthesia safety initiatives is evident in a comparison of the mortality rates over time in HICs (table 15.1), and between countries that commonly use standard safety measures and those that do not (Bainbridge and others 2012; Fenton, Whitty, and Reynolds 2003; Hodges and Hodges 2000; Hodges and others 2007).

Costs of Adequate Resources and Patient Safety

Safety measures since 1970 include the required vigilance of anesthesia providers, improved pharmacology to support hemodynamic stability, and safety monitoring to provide early warning of the common risks of anesthesia—hypoxemia, inadvertent esophageal intubation, and cardiac depression. The mortality rates

Table 15.1 Global Perioperative Mortality, per 1 Million Population

	Before 1970	Since 1990
Anesthesia-related mortality	357	34
Perioperative mortality	10,600	1,170

Source: Bainbridge and others 2012.

in table 15.1 suggest that these improvements and interventions have been effective. The determination of cost-effectiveness is more arduous. Even in HICs, cost-effectiveness analyses have not been applied to the standard monitoring of patients undergoing anesthesia.

Absolute Costs. The absolute cost of providing safe anesthesia is a complex equation that varies by country and is affected by market variables such as the required use of medical-grade equipment, nongeneric medications, and changing technology. Every variable, from the cost of training a physician anesthesiologist to providing oxygen, is affected by local access, government, and regional availability of resources. Table 15.2 illustrates the spectrum of costs in HICs for necessary infrastructure and the required safety equipment to provide continuous information on patients' vital functions.

The comprehensive list of medications, solutions, and blood products for anesthesia are included in the *WHO Model List of Essential Medicines* (WHO 2013b); the World Federation of Societies of Anaesthesiologists (WFSA) considers these to be the minimum for the safe administration of anesthesia (Merry and others 2010). The WHO's selection process for essential medicines ensures cost-effectiveness and promotes quality (Manikandan and Gitanjali 2012), but it requires appropriate resourcing and procurement by governments. The medicines for anesthesia and pain management included on the *WHO Model List of Essential Medicines* identifies inexpensive and cost-effective choices, agreed upon by international experts for local, regional, and general anesthesia as well as for acute and chronic pain management (table 15.3).[2]

Efficacy and Cost-Effectiveness

An evolving library of literature is evaluating anesthesia efficacy and cost-effectiveness, applicable mostly to upper-middle-income countries and HICs (Nakada and others 2010; Rando and others 2011). Some of these studies will have applicability for LMICs when trained providers and advanced pharmacology are available and adequate monitoring is in place. Until then, the most compelling analyses are those comparing general, regional, and local anesthesia for specific procedures (Borendal Wodlin and others 2011; Doberneck 1980; Duh and others 1999; Gonano and others 2009; Schuster and others 2005; Shillcutt, Clarke, and Kingsnorth 2010; Shillcutt and others 2013; Song and others 2000; Wilhelm and others 2006). Much of this research was undertaken in HICs, and more research specific to LMICs is needed. Local and regional techniques provide nearly equivalent

Table 15.2 Required Patient Safety Monitors and Medications in High-Resource Settings

Improvement or intervention	Year introduced	Cost (US$)
Professionalism in anesthesiology	1950s	$1,000–$148,000[a]
Sphygmomanometer	1881	Less than $20
Electrocardiogram (three-lead machine)	1901	More than $1,000
Smartphone monitor (AliveCor)		$199 + phone
Precordial stethoscope	1950s	Less than $20
Capnography	1990	$1,600–$2,500
Pulse oximetry	1980	
Durable, portable unit (Lifebox)		$250
Smartphone monitor (Masimo)		$100 + phone
Anesthetic agent monitoring	1980s	$350 to $2,500
Oxygen:	1903	$40/6,000 liters + $100 flowmeter + more than $10,000 per 20 beds
Cylinders		$500–$1,500
Hospital piping system[b]		
Concentrator[c]		
Rescue medicines	1902	Less than $1

a. Estimated training costs per anesthesiologist based on country of training.
b. Initial capital costs for systems and equipment.
c. Electricity must be available and energy costs must be considered for operating a concentrator.

Table 15.3 World Health Organization's List of Essential Medicines for Anesthesia and Pain Management, 2013

Medication class	Specific medication listed
Inhaled gas	Oxygen, halothane, isoflurane, nitrous oxide
Muscle relaxant	Suxamethonium, atracurium
Sedative/hypnotic	Ketamine, propofol or thiopental, midazolam, diazepam
Narcotic	Morphine, codeine
Local anesthetic	Lidocaine, bupivacaine
Anti-inflammatory	Ibuprofen, paracetamol
Antiemetic	Ondansetron
Chronic pain relief	Amitriptyline
Reversal agent	Neostigmine, naloxone
Rescue medicines	Epinephrine, atropine, ephedrine

Source: WHO 2013b.

surgical conditions, hemodynamics, and patient comfort, compared with general anesthesia (Faisy and others 1996). Where providers have limited training and rescue medicines are often unavailable, the safety profile for these approaches is greater (Edomwonyi and others 2000; Fenton, Whitty, and Reynolds 2003; Glenshaw and Madzimbamuto 2005; Hansen, Gausi, and Merikebu 2000; Heywood, Wilson, and Sinclair 1989; McKenzie 1996; Ouro-Bang'na Maman and others 2005; Vasdev and others 2008; Walker and others 2010; Zoumenou and others 2010).

Both local and regional anesthetic techniques are low cost and low technology; they offer achievable proficiency and have a good safety record when basic sterile techniques are employed and key safety steps are observed. Few direct comparisons of local anesthesia versus neuroaxial anesthesia, such as spinal anesthesia, have been performed in LMICs; however, Vaz and others (2010) report no increase in operative time, and significant reductions in recovery room time and immediate postoperative pain, in a group receiving local anesthesia and intravenous sedation for loop colostomy. This technique was cost saving when compared with spinal anesthesia for the same procedure.

Comparisons between local anesthetic classes (amide vs. ester) reveal no difference in efficacy in endodontic treatment and a statistically significant cost savings when the amide lidocaine is used (Li and others 2000; Maniglia-Ferreira and others 2009). The risk profiles of local anesthetics vary significantly, as do the costs of treating toxicity for an accidental intravascular injection of an amide or an ester (Harmatz 2009).

Intralipid, the treatment for intravascular injection of bupivacaine (Mirtallo and others 2010) is approximately US$100–US$300 per dose and not routinely available in LMICs; for this reason alone, lidocaine is cost saving in LMICs.

Literature from HICs compares regional, local, and general anesthesia safety and outcomes; on balance, there is no consensus that regional and local anesthesia are superior to general anesthesia (Lin and others 2013). However, there is no evidence that regional and local anesthesia are inferior. Studies conducted in HICs have consistently shown lower costs and at least equal efficacy with regional anesthesia compared with general anesthesia (Neuman and others 2012).

The situation is quite different in LMICs. Reliable equipment for general anesthesia, including airway equipment and the medications necessary to manage circulatory challenges, is limited and frequently not available. Regional and especially local anesthesia are therefore preferable, when feasible (Schnittger 2007; Wilhelm and others 2006).

The systematic literature review of anesthesia cost-effectiveness revealed no cost-effectiveness analysis of general anesthesia, and no comparisons between general anesthesia and regional anesthesia in LMICs. Logical conclusions can be drawn from the comparative costs of general anesthesia and regional anesthesia, especially when the costs are inclusive of an anesthesia machine specific for this purpose (Beringer and Eltringham 2008; Read and Taylor 2012). Anesthesia machines for general anesthesia deliver anesthetic gases and frequently have a ventilator component, essential to providing oxygenation and ventilation when pharmaceutical paralytics are used for some types of surgical intervention. However, if based only on known mortality rates related to anesthesia in adults, children, and parturients, the cost-effectiveness of local and regional anesthesia exceeds that of general anesthesia (Bosenberg, Jöhr, and Wolf 2011; Fecho and others 2008; Luger and others 2010; Wilhelm and others 2006). General anesthesia is uniquely related to malignant hyperthermia, a genetic condition for which anesthesia gases are the trigger, requiring prompt treatment with dantrolene for survival. Dantrolene is expensive and not available in most LMICs, and this rare but reported event is uniformly fatal in these countries.

Although the general anesthesia medications on the *WHO Model List of Essential Medicines* (WHO 2013b) are cost-effective, the overall costs are substantially affected by the additional supplies, delivery systems, and related complications. When general anesthesia is indicated, it is possible to deliver a cost-responsible option with available medications and other resources.

However, in LMICs, the skill of providers and the lack of safety monitors contribute to the overall greater risk for complications. The quality and type of anesthesia provided for the surgical intervention, particularly regional versus general, and the adequacy of postoperative analgesia have a major impact on the incidence of complications, and thereby the overall cost-effectiveness of the technique (Duggan and Kavanagh 2010; MacIntyre and Scott 2010). The relationship between general anesthesia and complication incidence is one reason that ketamine is ubiquitously and uniquely used in LMICs. Ketamine, which can be used alone or as an adjuvant therapy for postoperative or chronic pain management, can be safely used for general anesthesia for many surgical interventions without the additional infrastructure required for general anesthesia secondary to inhaled gases (Green, Clem, and Rothrock 1996).

Developing markets in LMICs are driving the availability of cost-appropriate equipment, anesthesia machines, and safety monitors. The nearly ubiquitous availability of smartphones has encouraged manufacturers to produce pulse oximetry and electrocardiogram (ECG) attachments and apps for use wherever smartphones are functional (Dawson and others 2013).[3] These solutions have yet to be tested and compared with standard monitors, but the trend is encouraging for patient safety in LMICs (McCormick and Eltringham 2007). It is timely that an initiative is underway for the creation of an International Organization for Standardization (ISO) standard for equipment being marketed to LMICs (Walker and others 2010).

The best evidence of the cost-effectiveness of successful interventions is likely to be the prevention of ASA category 1 or 2 perioperative deaths or permanent disability secondary to hypoxemia or sustained hypotension. Modeling has shown that overall risk is reduced by a checklist (WHO 2006) that includes the use of a pulse oximeter and the ability to identify risks related to surgery, anesthesia, and the presence of patient allergies.

Cost of Training Anesthesia Providers

Until trained and credentialed providers are present and vigilant for every surgical intervention, it is unlikely that the addition of technology, machines, or advanced medications will significantly affect outcomes in the short term; even the addition of cost-appropriate monitors and equipment must be carefully balanced with the simultaneous addition of education and training. Investments in training and evaluating existing providers will have the greatest impact on patient safety and outcomes in LMICs. The costs of training vary, and the effectiveness of training in anesthesia is likely to be revealed by the anesthesia-related mortality rates.

The shortage of physician anesthesiologists has led to task-shifting to nurses and technicians as the most feasible workforce alternative in many LMICs (Hoyler and others 2014; Rosseel and others 2010). This practical measure can mitigate the crisis but does not replace the long-term need for physician anesthesia providers for leadership, oversight, and education. The critical need and dangerous situation require accepting a functional model for the provision of anesthesia that specifically addresses barriers to patient safety and unacceptable outcomes. Building on existing in-country models will facilitate the transition to safe patient care if education and credentialing are provided at all levels.

Comprehensive information on types of and costs of training for anesthesia providers in LMICs is still widely unavailable. Increasingly, however, reports are available from surveys (Hoyler and others 2014) and from several training programs in East Asia and the Pacific and in Sub-Saharan Africa (table 15.4). The training required, costs incurred, and external support received vary considerably across countries and regions; the absence of a related metric or indicator limits comparison of effectiveness and resulting patient safety.

Many countries train their own anesthesia providers, even if only in the form of on-the-job training at the hospital level. Countries that provide training outside of physician training programs usually offer two tiers of training (Cherian, Merry, and Wilson 2007; Collins 2011; Dubowitz, Detlefs, and McQueen 2010; Dubowitz and Evans 2012; Hodges and others 2007; Notrica and others 2011; Rosseel and others 2010). At a basic level, anesthesia officers often originate from a nursing or medical background and train for 6 to 24 months. Graduates of these programs commonly provide basic anesthesia in second- and third-level hospitals, under varying degrees of supervision, and frequently without supervision. Several LMICs offer a higher level of training to medical practitioners for two to four years; these providers function in third-level referral hospitals providing complex anesthesia and supervision of anesthesia officers at all levels (Dubowitz, Detlefs, and McQueen 2010; Dubowitz and Evans 2012; Newton and Bird 2010; Notrica and others 2011).

Anesthesia training in HICs is evidence based and includes theoretical knowledge and clinical, practical experience. At its most basic level, four practical skills are required of anesthesia providers:

- Intravenous cannulation
- Bag-mask ventilation
- Tracheal intubation
- Initiation of neuroaxial (spinal or epidural) or peripheral nerve block anesthesia.

Table 15.4 Training and Education Levels, Time Commitment, and Costs in Selected Countries, 2013

| Country | Physician anesthetists | | Anesthesia officers | | | External support | |
	Duration of training	Cost of tuition (US$ per year)	Duration of training	Cost of tuition (US$ per year)	Resident salary (per year)	Financial (per year)	Teaching (months per year)
Rwanda	4 years	$0	2 years	—	$8,400	$500,000	18
Zambia	—	—	2 years	—	$9,700	$24,000	—
Uganda	—	$2,000	18–24 months	$400	Variable, may be $0	$2,000+	—
Kenya	4 years	$2,500	18–24 months	$2,500	$0	—	—
Lao PDR	3 years	$0	6–12 months	$0	$0	$2,500	3
Mongolia	2 years	$1,000	—	—	$0	$0	4
Fiji	4 years for a master's	$0	1 year for a diploma	$0	—	—	18
Canada	5 years	$0	—	—	$60,000–$80,000	—	—

Sources: Personal communications with local professionals providing and administering education: Dr. Paulin Ruhato, Rwanda; Dr. Sarah Hodges, Zambia; Dr. Gerald Dubowitz, Uganda; Dr. Mark Newton, Kenya; Dr. Simon Hendle, Fiji, the Lao People's Democratic Republic, and Mongolia; and Dr. Tom Coonan, Canada.
Note: — = not available.

All providers must also understand basic physiology and a few interventions to improve life-threatening alterations in physiology, including hypoxemia and hypotension. An intricate knowledge of patient physiology, pharmacology, and therapeutics is essential, of course, for physicians and nurses with advanced training. Access to leaders with this knowledge is important to the implementation of a system of safe anesthesia care and patient safety.

The costs of theoretical and clinical teaching vary. Ideally, anesthesia education is provided by physicians with years of clinical experience. In some LMICs, such as Kenya and Rwanda, senior nurses and technicians have become effective clinical teachers. However, the importance of physicians in ensuring the quality and accuracy of the information imparted cannot be discounted. Costs are a consideration for the teaching model chosen; any system must be benchmarked and monitored for acceptable patient outcomes, including perioperative mortality.

Administrative costs are incurred when providing educational materials, as well as when examinations or assessment processes are conducted. In LMICs, living expenses are often required to enable trainees to participate in the program; these expenses may include food, accommodation, and travel. The estimated costs of providing safe anesthesia in LMICs must include the investment in training. These specific costs are program and country specific, and are attainable through several models (table 15.4). Similarly the costs of accreditation will vary by country, and this important component of a system of trained providers is unlikely to add significant costs to the required education and training described.

FUTURE DIRECTIONS FOR MITIGATING THE GLOBAL ANESTHESIA CRISIS

Patient Safety

Improving patient safety and access to surgery requires an investment across health care systems, especially outside of the second- and third-level hospitals in urban areas. Strategies for patient safety will need to be tailored and sufficiently flexible to meet diverse training needs. However, the goal of vigilance must be uniform, even where safety monitors vary. This systemic approach has the potential to improve the entire health system through access to appropriate technology and diagnostics required for surgery and safe anesthesia with dual purposes for other disease states.

Education and Training

Investments in education, training, and credentialing for anesthesia providers are essential to improving patient safety and surgical outcomes. Anesthesia-specific education in LMICs will involve the training of future anesthesia providers as well as the ongoing education and support of those already providing services. *Task-shifting or task-sharing* is often applied to the global surgical and anesthesia crises as a means to expand the workforce responsibly and more rapidly than traditional educational tracks allow. This practice is already widespread in LMICs out of necessity (table 15.5). Ensuring that providers at all levels have education, training, and credentials will be important to ensuring patient safety and creating a culture of vigilance and best practice.

Table 15.5 Surgical and Anesthesia Tasks for Task-Sharing

Health workers	Level of care	Procedures performed
Surgeon-anesthesiologist	Third-level hospital	Complex airway procedures, neurosurgery, thoracic and vascular surgery, pediatric surgery, complex orthopedic surgery, reconstruction surgery, endocrine surgery, critical care
General doctor; nonphysician clinician with surgical or anesthesia skills (nurse or technician anesthesia provider)	Second-level hospital	Cesarean section (elective and emergency), emergency airway management, abscess drainage, wound debridement, circumcision, hernia repair, dilation and curettage, exploratory laparotomy—bowel resection, ectopic pregnancy, ovarian torsion, hysterectomy, appendectomy, limb amputation, skin grafts, skeletal traction, acute burn care
Community health worker	First-level hospital	Prehospital transport of trauma patients, basic wound care, resuscitation, emergency cesarean section

Source: Adapted from Chu and others 2009.

The WFSA regards anesthesia as a medical specialty to be provided by medically trained and accredited physicians. Where this is not possible—and it often is not—the WFSA recommends that medically qualified anesthetists supervise nonmedical anesthesia providers (Merry and others 2010). Although the pros and cons of this position have been debated (Dubowitz, Detlefs, and McQueen 2010; Jacob 2009; Walker 2009), the reality remains that medical anesthetists are often rare in LMICs. What is needed is the development of a coordinated anesthesia workforce led by fully trained physician anesthesiologists who train, supervise, and monitor nonphysician anesthesia providers.

There is no central, international classification of anesthesia providers. Many countries, even at the level of the Ministry of Health, have incomplete knowledge of the anesthesia providers functioning in remote settings. Planning for a spectrum of training and credentialing is recommended, and providing practical guidelines for anesthesia safety will empower even the providers functioning with the fewest resources without compromising progress.

A focus on the ongoing education and training of anesthesia providers will generate benefits, including increased surgical capacity within LMICs, improved patient outcomes, respect for the specialty of anesthesia among other health care providers, and the potential for better staff retention. Creating high levels of patient safety and access to quality anesthesia in the context of the current crisis will require a comprehensive approach:

- Developing and implementing national training programs for anesthesia providers at all levels supported by the national health care system and the Ministries of Health
- Credentialing of trained anesthesia providers that allows for the tracking of providers and ensures a minimum qualification level
- Creating national and global professionalism within the anesthesia community through continuing medical education and the support of national societies for representation and growth.

Quality Improvement

Efforts to improve anesthesia and perioperative care will be influenced by measurement of the outcomes in LMICs similar to the influence of quality improvement programs in Europe and the United States. The observation that surgical outcomes are substantially better in the high HDI world, despite a generally older population of patients with greater comorbidity, confirms the pivotal role of the quality process.

One approach is to pursue quality management metrics for perioperative care that are attainable for LMICs as a tiered process. The most fundamental outcomes to pursue would be simple recording of the surgical procedure performed and the short-term survival of the patient in every setting in which surgical procedures are provided. When possible, additional collection of data, including patient demographics such as age, gender, illness, and the acuity of the planned procedure, will augment the value of the quality metric. Additional stratification of the fundamental outcomes, through capture of the ASA Physical Status, is internationally defined and of value in every setting when outcomes are analyzed (box 15.1). The ASA's five-point scale is intended to capture multiple objective and subjective assessments of patients' states of health before surgery and correlates strongly with perioperative mortality.

Perioperative Mortality Rate. A nonspecific indicator of patient safety during anesthesia and surgery amenable to the tiered process and of value to LMICs is the POMR at 24 hours. This rate, defined as unexpected death within 24 hours of surgery, is often captured even in the most austere circumstances for two reasons: the existence of an operative log book, and the fact that most surgical patients in LMICs remain in the hospital for 24 hours. Consistent with the tiered quality-management process described above, the fundamental outcomes are

---

Box 15.1

American Society of Anesthesiologists' Physical Status

1 = A normal, healthy patient

2 = A patient with a stable chronic disease, for example, diabetes or asthma

3 = A patient with an active disease process, for example, new onset angina or shortness of breath

4 = A patient with a severe medical condition that is life threatening, for example, liver failure

5 = A patient not expected to survive the surgical procedure

Source: American Society of Anesthesiologists (https://www.asahq.org/For-Members/Clinical-Information/ASA-Physical-Status-Classification-System.aspx).

uniformly available for capture. Although the data captured in the first step of the process are minimal, similar to the maternal mortality rate the POMR is a benchmark of surgical and anesthesia safety, and an initial indicator that is easy to track and report (McQueen 2013; Watters and others 2014).

Stratification and Data Capture. As the data collection capabilities of the hospital or nation advance, more information should be collected and reported related to the outcomes of surgery and anesthesia and the population of patients treated. Anesthesia-related disability or morbidity includes the occurrence of any permanent injury, such as renal failure, myocardial infarction, stroke, or peripheral neurologic injury. Also included at this level of data capture should be the occurrence of perioperative events that carry a high risk of death or major morbidity: malignant hyperthermia, anaphylaxis, intraoperative cardiac arrest, major transfusion reaction, and wrong-site or wrong-side surgery. On the preoperative side, more detailed coding of patient comorbidities (for example, the International Classification of Diseases [ICD] codes) and patient physical examination (for example, body mass index and airway) will allow for improved risk adjustment of quality-management results.

Research

Capturing surgical and anesthesia complications and related mortality rates is not yet a global health priority. As noncommunicable diseases increasingly contribute to the global burden of disease, the need for access to surgical services and safe anesthesia will increase. Related mortality rates are important to benchmark progress and document improved patient safety in LMICs. The only perioperative complication currently recorded on a routine basis is intraoperative death; after the event is recorded in the operating theater log book, it is rarely reviewed.

Perioperative mortality in the operating theater and within 24 hours is reemphasized here because of the ease of data collection and existence of an example of similar reporting—the maternal mortality rate, which is required by the WHO and performed by every member nation on an annual basis.

Finding solutions for collecting meaningful data in LMICs is an important prerequisite to addressing the global anesthesia crisis. Acknowledging that finding solutions may be a stepwise process, and agreeing on an initial indicator that is logistically possible and ultimately meaningful, are the first steps. Several

independent groups have suggested the POMR as a low-technology option (McQueen 2013; Watters 2014). Initially nonspecific, the POMR at 24 hours could be stratified and expanded to 30 days as the surgical system grows.

CONCLUSIONS

Safe anesthesia is effective, beneficial, and inexpensive when essential medicines are routinely available, appropriate technology is used, and sustained investments are made in training and credentialing.

The scope of global mortality that would be modified by enhanced surgical capacity is staggering. Safe anesthesia is critical to improving access to surgery, achieving acceptable outcomes for the spectrum of surgical interventions, and mitigating the global burden of disease.

The scale of the global burden of surgical disease in LMICs and the critical role of safe anesthesia in averting disability and death through surgical intervention has led to the following recommendations:

- Prioritize patient safety and safe anesthesia to secure a foundation of quality anesthesia and monitor the impact of surgical intervention on the rates of premature death from surgically treatable diseases
- Maintain functional workforces through patient safety education, training, and credentialing for existing and future anesthesia providers, including technicians, nurses, and physicians
- Create a culture committed to vigilance, and provide appropriate safety monitoring
- Ensure that oxygen and rescue medicines are reliably available
- Collect and report POMRs for benchmarking patient safety and quality improvement
- Recommend universal reporting of POMRs by the WHO as part of the initiative for global patient safety.

NOTES

The World Bank classifies countries according to four income groupings. Income is measured using gross national income (GNI) per capita, in U.S. dollars, converted from local currency using the *World Bank Atlas* method. Classifications as of July 2014 are as follows:

- Low-income countries (LICs) = US$1,045 or less in 2013
- Middle-income countries (MICs) are subdivided:
  - Lower-middle-income = US$1,046 to US$4,125
  - Upper-middle-income (UMICs) = US$4,126 to US$12,745
- High-income countries (HICs) = US$12,746 or more.

1. World Federation of Societies of Anaesthesiologists, http://www.wfsahq.org/.
2. The process by which medicines are added to or deleted from the model list, and the related applications, is available at http://www.who.int/features/2013/essential_medicines_list/en/.
3. "Masimo Launches iPhone-Compatible Pulse Oximeter," Damian Garde, December 13, 2012. http://www.fiercemedicaldevices.com/story/masimo-launches-iphone-compatible-pulse-oximeter/2012-12-13.

REFERENCES

Bainbridge, D., J. Martin, M. Arango, D. Cheng, and Evidence-based Peri-operative Clinical Outcomes Research. 2012. "Perioperative and Anaesthetic-Related Mortality in Developed and Developing Countries: A Systematic Review and Meta-Analysis." *Lancet* 380 (9847): 1075–81.

Beecher, H. K., and D. P. Todd. 1954. "A Study of the Deaths Associated with Anesthesia and Surgery: Based on a Study of 599,548 Anesthesias in Ten Institutions 1948–1952, Inclusive." *Annals of Surgery* 140 (1): 2–35.

Beringer, R. M., and R. J. Eltringham. 2008. "The Glostavent: Evolution of an Anaesthetic Machine for Developing Countries." *Anaesthesia and Intensive Care* 36 (3): 442–48.

Bickler, S. W., M. L. Telfer, and B. Sanno-Duanda. 2003. "Need for Paediatric Surgery Care in an Urban Area of The Gambia." *Tropical Doctor* 33 (2): 91–94.

Borendal Wodlin, N., L. Nilsson, P. Carlsson, and P. Kjolhede. 2011. "Cost-Effectiveness of General Anesthesia vs Spinal Anesthesia in Fast-Track Abdominal Benign Hysterectomy." *American Journal of Obstetrics and Gynecology* 205 (4): e321–27.

Bosenberg, A. T. 2007. "Pediatric Anesthesia in Developing Countries." *Current Opinion in Anaesthesiology* 20 (3): 204–10.

Bosenberg, A. T., M. Jöhr, and A. R. Wolf. 2011. "Pro Con Debate: The Use of Regional vs Systemic Analgesia for Neonatal Surgery." *Paediatric Anaesthesia* 21 (12): 1247–58.

Canty, D. J., C. F. Royse, D. Kilpatrick, A. Bowyer, and A. G. Royse. 2012. "The Impact on Cardiac Diagnosis and Mortality of Focused Transthoracic Echocardiography in Hip Fracture Surgery Patients with Increased Risk of Cardiac Disease: A Retrospective Cohort Study." *Anaesthesia* 67 (11): 1202–09.

Cherian, M. N., A. F. Merry, and I. H. Wilson. 2007. "The World Health Organization and Anaesthesia." *Anaesthesia* 62 (Suppl 1): 65–66.

Chu, K., P. Rosseel, P. Gielis, and N. Ford. 2009. "Surgical Task Shifting in Sub-Saharan Africa." *PLoS Medicine* 6 (5): e1000078. doi:10.1371/journal.pmed.1000078. http://www.plosmedicine.org/article/info:doi/10.1371/journal.pmed.1000078.

Collins, S. B. 2011. "Model for a Reproducible Curriculum Infrastructure to Provide International Nurse Anesthesia Continuing Education." *AANA Journal* 79 (6): 491–96.

Dawson, J. A., A. Saraswat, L. Simionato, M. Thio, C. O. Kamlin, and others. 2013. "Comparison of Heart Rate and Oxygen Saturation Measurements from Masimo and Nellcor Pulse Oximeters in Newly Born Term Infants." *Acta Paediatrica* 102 (10): 955–60.

Devereaux, P. J., D. Xavier, J. Pogue, G. Guyatt, A. Sigamani, and others. 2011. "Characteristics and Short-Term Prognosis of Perioperative Myocardial Infarction in Patients Undergoing Noncardiac Surgery: A Cohort Study." *Annals of Internal Medicine* 154 (8): 523–28.

Doberneck, R. C. 1980. "Breast Biopsy: A Study of Cost-Effectiveness." *Annals of Surgery* 192 (2): 152–56.

Doorley, S. L., N. C. Doohan, S. Kodali, and K. McQueen. 2013. "Social Determinants of the Impact of Surgical Disease on Health." *Tropical Medicine and Surgery* 1: 113–18.

Dubowitz, G., S. Detlefs, and K. A. McQueen. 2010. "Global Anesthesia Workforce Crisis: A Preliminary Survey Revealing Shortages Contributing to Undesirable Outcomes and Unsafe Practices." *World Journal of Surgery* 34 (3): 438–44.

Dubowitz, G., and F. M. Evans. 2012. "Developing a Curriculum for Anaesthesia Training in Low- and Middle-Income Countries." *Best Practice and Research Clinical Anaesthesiology* 26 (1): 17–21.

Duggan, M., and B. P. Kavanagh. 2010. "Perioperative Modifications of Respiratory Function." *Best Practice and Research Clinical Anaesthesiology* 24 (2): 145–55.

Duh, Q. Y., A. L. Senokozlieff-Englehart, Y. S. Choe, A. E. Siperstein, K. Rowland, and others. 1999. "Laparoscopic Gastrostomy and Jejunostomy: Safety and Cost with Local vs General Anesthesia." *Archives of Surgery* 134 (2): 151–56.

Edomwonyi, N. P., M. O. Obiaya, S. O. Imasuen, and A. S. Weerasinghe. 2000. "A Study of Co-induction of Anaesthesia U.B.T.H. Experience." *West African Journal of Medicine* 19 (2): 132–36.

Eichorn, J. H. 1989. "Prevention of Intraoperative Anesthesia Accidents and Related Severe Injury through Safety Monitoring." *Anesthesiology* 70 (4): 572–77.

Enohumah, K. O., and C. O. Imarengiaye. 2006. "Factors Associated with Anaesthesia-Related Maternal Mortality in a Tertiary Hospital in Nigeria." *Acta Anaesthesiologica Scandinavica* 50 (2): 206–10.

Faisy, C., G. Gueguen, M. Lanteri-Minet, A. Blatt, and J. Iloumbou. 1996. "Cost Effectiveness of Local Regional Anesthesia in a Remote Area." *Médecine Tropicale (Mars)* 56 (4): 367–72.

Fecho, K., A. T. Lunney, P. G. Boysen, P. Rock, and E. A. Norfleet. 2008. "Postoperative Mortality after Inpatient Surgery: Incidence and Risk Factors." *Therapeutics and Clinical Risk Management* 4 (4): 681–88.

Fenton, P. M., C. J. Whitty, and F. Reynolds. 2003. "Caesarean Section in Malawi: Prospective Study of Early Maternal and Perinatal Mortality." *BMJ* 327 (7415): 587.

Funk, L. M., T. G. Weiser, W. R. Berry, S. R. Lipsitz, A. F. Merry, and others. 2010. "Global Operating Theatre Distribution and Pulse Oximetry Supply: An Estimation from Reported Data." *Lancet* 376 (9746): 1055–61.

Glenshaw, M., and F. D. Madzimbamuto. 2005. "Anaesthesia Associated Mortality in a District Hospital in Zimbabwe: 1994 to 2001." *Central African Journal of Medicine* 51 (3–4): 39–44.

Gonano, C., S. C. Kettner, M. Ernstbrunner, K. Schebesta, A. Chiari, and others. 2009. "Comparison of Economical Aspects of Interscalene Brachial Plexus Blockade and General Anaesthesia for Arthroscopic Shoulder Surgery." *British Journal of Anaesthesia* 103 (3): 428–33.

Green, S. M., K. J. Clem, and S. G. Rothrock. 1996. "Ketamine Safety Profile in the Developing World: Survey of Practitioners." *Academic Emergency Medicine* 3 (6): 598–604.

Hansen, D., S. C. Gausi, and M. Merikebu. 2000. "Anaesthesia in Malawi: Complications and Deaths." *Tropical Doctor* 30 (3): 146–49.

Harmatz, A. 2009. "Local Anesthetics: Uses and Toxicities." *Surgical Clinics of North America* 89 (3): 587–98.

Heywood, A. J., I. H. Wilson, and J. R. Sinclair. 1989. "Perioperative Mortality in Zambia." *Annals of the Royal College of Surgeons of England* 71 (6): 354–58.

Hodges, S. C., and A. M. Hodges. 2000. "A Protocol for Safe Anasthesia for Cleft Lip and Palate Surgery in Developing Countries." *Anaesthesia* 55 (5): 436–41.

Hodges, S. C., C. Mijumbi, M. Okello, B. A. McCormick, I. A. Walker, and others. 2007. "Anaesthesia Services in Developing Countries: Defining the Problems." *Anaesthesia* 62 (1): 4–11.

Hoyler, M., S. R. Finlayson, C. D. McClain, J. G. Meara, and L. Hagander. 2014. "Shortage of Doctors, Shortage of Data: A Review of the Global Surgery, Obstetrics, and Anesthesia Workforce Literature." *World Journal of Surgery* 38 (2): 269–80.

Jacob, R. 2009. "Pro: Anesthesia for Children in the Developing World Should Be Delivered by Medical Anesthetists." *Paediatric Anaesthesia* 19 (1): 35–38.

Jochberger, S., F. Ismailova, W. Lederer, V. D. Mayr, G. Luckner, and others. 2008. "Anesthesia and Its Allied Disciplines in the Developing World: A Nationwide Survey of the Republic of Zambia." *Anesthesia and Analgesia* 106 (3): 942–48.

Kushner, A. L., M. N. Cherian, L. Noel, D. A. Spiegel, S. Groth, and C. Etienne. 2010. "Addressing the Millennium Development Goals from a Surgical Perspective: Essential Surgery and Anesthesia in 8 Low- and Middle-Income Countries." *Archives of Surgery* 145 (2): 154–59.

Li, S., M. Coloma, P. F. White, M. F. Watcha, J. W. Chiu, and others. 2000. "Comparison of the Costs and Recovery Profiles of Three Anesthetic Techniques for Ambulatory Anorectal Surgery." *Anesthesiology* 93 (5): 1225–30.

Lin, R., A. Hingorani, N. Marks, E. Ascher, R. Jimenez, and others. 2013. "Effects of Anesthesia versus Regional Nerve Block on Major Leg Amputation Mortality Rate." *Vascular* 21 (2): 83–86.

Luger, T. J., C. Kammerlander, M. Gosch, M. F. Luger, U. Kammerlander-Knauer, and others. 2010. "Neuroaxial versus General Anaesthesia in Geriatric Patients for Hip Fracture Surgery: Does It Matter?" *Osteoporosis International* 21 (Suppl 4): S555–72.

MacIntyre, P. E., and D. A. Scott, eds. 2010. *Acute Pain Management: Scientific Evidence.* 3rd ed. Sydney: Australian and New Zealand College of Anaesthetists and Faculty of Pain Medicine. http://www.anzca.edu.au.

Mackay, P., and M. Cousins. 2006. "Safety in Anaesthesia." *Anaesthesia and Intensive Care* 34 (3): 303–04.

Maniglia-Ferreira, C., F. Almeida-Gomes, B. Carvalho-Sousa, A. V. Barbosa, C. C. Lins, and others. 2009. "Clinical Evaluation of the Use of Three Anesthetics in Endodontics." *Acta Odontológica Latinoamericana* 22 (1): 21–26.

Manikandan, S., and B. Gitanjali. 2012. "National List of Essential Medicines of India: The Way Forward." *Journal of Postgraduate Medicine* 58 (1): 68–72.

McCormick, B. A., and R. J. Eltringham. 2007. "Anaesthesia Equipment for Resource-Poor Environments." *Anaesthesia* 62 (Suppl 1): 54–60.

McKenzie, A. G. 1996. "Mortality Associated with Anaesthesia at Zimbabwean Teaching Hospitals." *South African Medical Journal* 86 (4): 338–42.

McQueen, K. A. 2010. "Anesthesia and the Global Burden of Surgical Disease." *International Anesthesiology Clinics* 48 (2): 91–107.

———. 2013. "Global Surgery: Measuring the Impact." *World Journal of Surgery* 37 (11): 2505–6. doi:10.1007/s00268-013-2198-z.

Merry, A. F., J. B. Cooper, O. Soyannwo, I. H. Wilson, and J. H. Eichhorn. 2010. "International Standards for a Safe Practice of Anesthesia 2010." *Canadian Journal of Anesthesia* 57 (11): 1027–34.

Mirtallo, J. M., J. F. Dasta, K. C. Kleinschmidt, and J. Varon. 2010. "State of the Art Review: Intravenous Fat Emulsions: Current Applications, Safety Profile, and Clinical Implications." *Annals of Pharmacotherapy* 44 (4): 688–700.

Morriss, W., and R. Goucke. 2011. "Essential Pain Management: A Workshop for Health Workers." Sydney: Australian and New Zealand College of Anaesthetists and Faculty of Pain Medicine. http://www.fpm.anzca.edu.au/fellows/essential-pain-management/pdfs/EPM-Manual-2012-04-19.pdf.

Nakada, T., D. Ikeda, M. Yokota, and K. Kawahara. 2010. "Analysis of the Cost-Effectiveness of Remifentanil-Based General Anesthesia: A Survey of Clinical Economics under the Japanese Health Care System." *Journal of Anesthesia* 24 (6): 832–37.

Neuman, M. D., J. H. Silber, N. M. Elkassabany, J. M. Ludwig, and L. A. Fleisher. 2012. "Comparative Effectiveness of Regional versus General Anesthesia for Hip Fracture Surgery in Adults." *Anesthesiology* 117 (1): 72–92.

Newton, M., and P. Bird. 2010. "Impact of Parallel Anesthesia and Surgical Provider Training in Sub-Saharan Africa: A Model for a Resource-Poor Setting." *World Journal of Surgery* 34 (3): 445–52.

Notrica, M. R., F. M. Evans, L. M. Knowlton, and K. A. Kelly McQueen. 2011. "Rwandan Surgical and Anesthesia Infrastructure: A Survey of District Hospitals." *World Journal of Surgery* 35 (8): 1770–80.

Ouro-Bang'na Maman, A. F., K. Tomta, S. Ahouangbevi, and M. Chobli. 2005. "Deaths Associated with Anaesthesia in Togo, West Africa." *Tropical Doctor* 35 (4): 220–22.

Pedersen, T., A. Nicholson, K. Hovhannisyan, A. M. Moller, A. F. Smith, and others. 2014. "Pulse Oximetry for Perioperative Monitoring." *Cochrane Database of Systematic Reviews* 3: CD002013.

Penoyar, T., H. Cohen, P. Kibatala, A. Magoda, G. Saguti, and others. 2012. "Emergency and Surgery Services of Primary Hospitals in the United Republic of Tanzania." *BMJ Open* 2 (1): e000369.

Rando, K., C. U. Niemann, P. Taura, and J. Klinck. 2011. "Optimizing Cost-Effectiveness in Perioperative Care for Liver Transplantation: A Model for Low- to Medium-Income Countries." *Liver Transplantation* 17 (11): 1247–78.

Read, E., and E. Taylor. 2012. "Portable Diamedica Glostavent: An Anaesthetic Machine for the Itinerant Anaesthetist." *British Journal of Anaesthesia* 109 (4): 648–49.

Rosseel, P., M. Trelles, S. Guilavogui, N. Ford, and K. Chu. 2010. "Ten Years of Experience Training Non-physician Anesthesia Providers in Haiti." *World Journal of Surgery* 34 (3): 453–58.

Schnittger, T. 2007. "Regional Anaesthesia in Developing Countries." *Anaesthesia* 62 (Suppl 1): 44–47.

Schuster, M., A. Gottschalk, J. Berger, and T. Standl. 2005. "A Retrospective Comparison of Costs for Regional and General Anesthesia Techniques." *Anesthesia and Analgesia* 100 (3): 786–94.

Shillcutt, S. D., M. G. Clarke, and A. N. Kingsnorth. 2010. "Cost-Effectiveness of Groin Hernia Surgery in the Western Region of Ghana." *Archives of Surgery* 145 (10): 954–61.

Shillcutt, S. D., D. L. Sanders, M. Teresa Butron-Vila, and A. N. Kingsnorth. 2013. "Cost-Effectiveness of Inguinal Hernia Surgery in Northwestern Ecuador." *World Journal of Surgery* 37 (1): 32–41.

Size, M., O. A. Soyannwo, and D. M. Justins. 2007. "Pain Management in Developing Countries." *Anaesthesia* 62 (Suppl 1): 38–43.

Song, D., N. B. Greilich, P. F. White, M. F. Watcha, and W. K. Tongier. 2000. "Recovery Profiles and Costs of Anesthesia for Outpatient Unilateral Inguinal Herniorrhaphy." *Anesthesia and Analgesia* 91 (4): 876–81.

Vasdev, G. M., B. A. Harrison, M. T. Keegan, and C. M. Burkle. 2008. "Management of the Difficult and Failed Airway in Obstetric Anesthesia." *Journal of Anesthesia* 22 (1): 38–48.

Vaz, F. A., R. A. Abreu, P. C. Soarez, M. B. Speranzini, L. C. Fernandes, and others. 2010. "Cost-Effectiveness Analysis on Spinal Anesthesia versus Local Anesthesia Plus Sedation for Loop Colostomy Closure." *Arquivos de Gastroenterologia* 47 (2): 159–64.

Walker, I. A. 2009. "Con: Pediatric Anesthesia Training in Developing Countries Is Best Achieved by Out of Country Scholarships." *Paediatric Anaesthesia* 19 (1): 45–49.

———, A. D. Obua, F. Mouton, S. Ttendo, and I. H. Wilson. 2010. "Paediatric Surgery and Anaesthesia in South-Western Uganda: A Cross-Sectional Survey." *Bulletin of the World Health Organization* 88 (12): 897–906.

Walker, I. A., and I. H. Wilson. 2008. "Anaesthesia in Developing Countries: A Risk for Patients." *Lancet* 371 (9617): 968–69.

Watters D. A., M. J. Hollands, R. L. Gruen, K. Maoate, H. Perndt, and others. 2014. "Perioperative Mortality Rate: A Global Indicator of Access to Safe Surgery and Anesthesia." *World Journal of Surgery*. Electronic publication ahead of print. doi:10.1007/s00268-014-2638-4.

WHO (World Health Organization). 2006. "Surgical Safety Checklist." WHO, Geneva. http://www.who.int /patientsafety/safesurgery/ss_checklist/en.

———. 2008. *World Health Report 2008*. Geneva: WHO. http://www.who.int/whr/2008/en.

———. 2013a. "Global Health Estimates for Deaths by Cause, Age, and Sex for Years 2000–2011." WHO, Geneva. http:// www.who.int/healthinfo/global_health_estimates/en/.

———. 2013b. *WHO Model List of Essential Medicines*. 18th List (April 2013) Final Amendments—October 2013. http://www.int/medicines/publications/essentialmedicines /en/index.html.

Wilhelm, T. J., S. Anemana, P. Kyamanywa, J. Rennie, S. Post, and others. 2006. "Anaesthesia for Elective Inguinal Hernia Repair in Rural Ghana: Appeal for Local Anaesthesia in Resource-Poor Countries." *Tropical Doctor* 36 (3): 147–49.

World Bank. 2014. *World Development Indicators*. Washington, DC: World Bank.

Zoumenou, E., S. Gbenou, P. Assouto, A. F. Ouro-Bang'na Maman, T. Lokossou, and others. 2010. "Pediatric Anesthesia in Developing Countries: Experience in the Two Main University Hospitals of Benin in West Africa." *Paediatric Anaesthesia* 20 (8): 741–47.

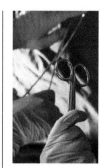

Chapter 16

Excess Surgical Mortality: Strategies for Improving Quality of Care

Thomas G. Weiser and Atul Gawande

GLOBAL VOLUME AND SAFETY OF SURGICAL CARE

The World Health Organization (WHO) has estimated that 234 million operations are performed worldwide each year (Weiser and others 2008). The WHO's analysis establishes three significant findings:

- Surgical interventions take place on a massive and previously unrecognized scale in all countries and resource settings.
- The inequity in service provision among countries and settings is dramatic.
- Little is known about the indications for, and the quality, safety, and outcomes of, surgical care.

Much has since been done to investigate these issues. The WHO has provided guidance for measuring surgical services and capacity through a set of standardized metrics for surgical surveillance (Weiser and others 2009). In addition, a situational analysis tool has been constructed and deployed in a number of countries to help assess surgical capacity (WHO 2010). Yet the logistics of performing surgery are complex and demand standardization. Surgical services must also continuously measure patient outcomes to identify shortcomings, inform improvements, and maintain high levels of quality care.

Mortality Following Surgery

The annual volume of surgery is almost twice that of obstetrical deliveries, and surgical death rates far surpass maternal mortality rates. Global estimates suggest that at least 7 million people suffer complications following surgery each year, including at least 1 million deaths, a magnitude that exceeds both maternal and AIDS-related mortality. As many as 50 percent of these deaths and complications are preventable (Weiser and others 2008). Surgical care is fraught with hazards in every setting; patients face immediate danger from both the technical risks of the procedures themselves and the anesthesia needed to induce insensibility and sedation.

Studies from high-income countries (HICs) confirm high rates of postoperative mortality and high variability in those rates. In the Netherlands, a review of 3.7 million inpatient surgical procedures at 102 hospitals over 15 years reveals a perioperative mortality rate of 1.85 percent (Noordzij and others 2010). A similar inpatient surgical death rate has been noted in the United States, with all-cause postoperative mortality in 2006 estimated to be 1.14 percent to 1.32 percent (Semel and others 2012; Weiser and others 2011). Pearse and others (2012) studied the outcomes of one week of inpatient surgery (excluding cardiac, neurosurgical, radiological, and obstetric procedures) in 498 hospitals in 28 European countries. The in-hospital crude

Corresponding author: Thomas G. Weiser, MD, Stanford University Medical Center, tweiser@stanford.edu postoperative mortality ranged from 1.2 percent in Iceland to 21.5 percent in Latvia. After adjusting for patient age, the American Society of Anesthesiologists's score of patient fitness for surgery, the urgency of surgery, the extent of surgery (minor, intermediate, or major), the specialty, and the presence of metastatic disease or cirrhosis, the odds ratios for death following surgery—using the United Kingdom as reference—ranged from a low of 0.44 in Finland to a high of 6.92 in Poland (figure 16.1). Overall, the researchers noted a 4 percent in-hospital crude mortality rate in this sample of more than 46,000 surgical cases, a previously unreported and unexpectedly high number.

Disparity of Service Provision

Nearly 60 percent of all operations take place in HICs, where 15 percent of the world's population lives (table 16.1). Low-income countries (LICs) account for nearly 35 percent of the global population, yet only 3.5 percent of all surgical interventions (Weiser and others 2008). This lack of equity in access to surgical interventions demands further investigation.

Figure 16.1 Adjusted Odds Ratio for In-Hospital Mortality Following Surgery in 28 European Countries, 2011

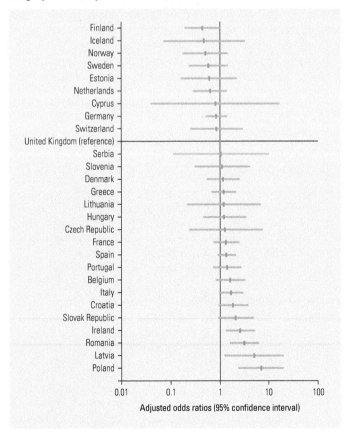

Source: Pearse and others 2012.

The extent of unmet need in resource-poor settings remains unclear, but basic surgical services are increasingly recognized as essential for relieving suffering and sustaining health. Surgery is critical for obstetrical emergencies; common congenital conditions, such as clubfoot; traumatic injuries, including orthopedic injuries; and treatment of abscesses, cancers, hernias, and cataracts. Maternal health advocates estimate that an optimum rate of cesarean section is at least 5 percent of all births to avert high rates of death of mothers and children (Dumont and others 2001), but similar minimum criteria have not been proposed for basic surgical services to address the disease burden in a population.

It has, however, become clear that surgical care is an essential component of effective health delivery systems and vital for enabling long and healthy life. In a population-based survey in Sierra Leone, one of the poorest countries in the world, one in every four respondents reported needs that might benefit from surgical consultation (Groen and others 2012). In addition, almost one in three households had experienced a death within the past year; of these households, one in four had a condition within the week preceding death that likely could have been treated surgically: abdominal distention, bleeding or complications following childbirth, an acute or chronic wound, a mass, or an acquired or congenital deformity. This survey indicates a tremendous unaddressed disease burden that might be mitigated with improved access to surgical care.

Limitations in the Scope of Practice in LMICs

Surgical interventions are performed at much lower frequency in the resource-poor settings of low- and middle-income countries (LMICs) and under more limited circumstances. Typically, rural first-level hospitals and even third-level public hospitals have a high-percentage of urgent cases; these facilities focus on a limited set of interventions, given their resource constraints. For example, studies from LMICs have shown very high ratios of cesarean section compared with other types of surgical procedures. Cesarean section has been found to represent a substantially higher proportion of all surgical interventions in Sierra Leone (42 percent), Zambia (40 percent), Uganda (34 percent), Niger (26 percent), Malawi (23 percent), and Haiti (12 percent) than in Organisation for Economic Co-operation and Development countries (3 percent) (Bowman 2013; Hughes and others 2012; Kushner, Groen, and Kingham 2010). At least one study suggests that the higher the surgical capacity, the lower the observed proportion of cesarean section, indicating that improved skills, materials, and capacity allow the

Table 16.1 Average National Rate of Surgery for Countries by Category of Health Expenditure, and Total Surgical Volume by Category, 2004

	Mean estimated surgical rate per 100,000 population (standard errors in parentheses)	Estimated volume of surgery in millions (%; 95% confidence interval)	Share of global population (%)
Expenditure			
Poor-expenditure countries (N = 47)	295 (53)	8.1 (3.5; 3.4–12.8)	34.8
Low-expenditure countries (N = 60)	2,255 (342)	53.8 (23.0; 9.8–97.4)	35.0
Middle-expenditure countries (N = 47)	4,248 (524)	34.3 (14.6; 23.6–43.3)	14.6
High-expenditure countries (N = 38)	11,110 (1,300)	138.0 (58.9; 132.5–143.9)	15.6
Overall			
Total global volume of surgery	n.a.	234.2 (187.2–281.2)	n.a.
Average surgical rate	4,016 (431)	n.a.	n.a.

Source: Weiser and others 2008.

Note: Expenditures are adjusted to 2004 U.S. dollars. Poor-expenditure countries = per capita total expenditure on health US$100 or less; low-expenditure countries = US$101 to US$400; middle-expenditure countries = US$401 to US$1,000; high-expenditure countries > US$1,000. n.a. = not applicable.

$p < 0.0001$ for difference between expenditure groups.

provision of a more comprehensive range of surgical services (Petroze, Mehtsun, and others 2012).

The WHO has identified a set of emergency and essential surgical interventions that all first-level hospitals with surgical capacity should be able to perform. Besides cesarean section, these procedures encompass uterine evacuation, circumcision, wound care, chest drainage, basic laparotomy, amputation, hernia repair, tubal ligation, closed or temporary reduction of fractures, cataract surgery, removal of foreign bodies, and emergency airway management and ventilation. This guideline for essential surgical services is based on the typical capacity of health facilities in remote, resource-constrained settings. These conditions involve relatively straightforward interventions, requiring less complex skills, resources, and postoperative management. Surgical providers at first-level hospitals appear to refer patients to higher-level facilities due to lack of training and experience rather than lack of resources (Bowman and others 2013; Petroze, Nzayisenga, and others 2012). The WHO recommends that referral facilities ensure capacity to provide facial and intracranial surgery, complex bowel surgery, pediatric and neonatal surgery, thoracic surgery, major ophthalmic surgery, and complex gynecologic surgery (WHO 2009c).

MORTALITY FOLLOWING SURGERY IN LMICs

As explained in chapter 2, increasing basic surgical capacity at first-level hospitals could potentially avert loss of 77.2 million disability-adjusted life years every year.

However, improvements in appropriateness, safety, and quality must accompany any increase in surgical volume in LMICs to minimize harm and secure patient trust in care. Currently, resource-poor settings place little emphasis on safety or quality, effectively constraining the value of improving access to surgical care. Earlier chapters of this volume focus on the lack of services and the unmet need for surgical care; this chapter assesses the magnitude of harm from surgical interventions under these circumstances and evaluates strategies to mitigate it.

The analysis was performed in three phases. We first evaluated the unmet surgical volume using data previously gathered for a study assessing the global volume of surgery (Weiser and others 2008). We then sought to estimate potential excess harm by ascertaining postsurgical mortality rates for three procedures common in LMICs: cesarean section, appendectomy, and inguinal hernia repair. Finally, we combined these two analyses to estimate the theoretical risks if surgical capacity were increased to meet minimum estimates of delivery without concurrent improvements in mortality rates. By quantifying excess mortality across countries and settings, we demonstrate large gaps in safety and the impact these have on outcomes and postoperative mortality.

Methodology

Estimates of Minimum Surgical Rates. Using previously estimated national surgical rates for 192 countries (Weiser and others 2008), we performed an incremental surgical effectiveness analysis comparing surgical rates with average life expectancy (Goldie 2003). We eliminated "strongly dominated" nations—those that either provided more operations for equal or lesser life expectancy or provided the same amount as a nation with greater life expectancy—and then arrayed the remaining nations in ascending order by surgical rate. Incremental surgical rates and life expectancy, and the incremental surgical system effectiveness ratio were then calculated by comparing the surgical rates and life expectancy of each country with the one above it. Countries whose surgical system effectiveness ratio was greater than an adjacent, higher-rate country (that is, one in which the incremental gain in life expectancy per increase in surgery was less than its comparator) was considered "weakly dominated" and was discarded, leaving only countries with maximally "efficient" systems, that is, those with the lowest surgical rate for the highest life expectancy (table 16.2). We estimated the minimum per capita surgical rates from an "efficiency frontier" line plotted from these countries (figure 16.2).

We then created a regression model for these maximally efficient countries and extrapolated a provisional minimum surgical rate based on life expectancies of 70, 75, and 80 years. We estimated the surgical gap by determining the deficit of surgery for countries whose rates were below these minimum surgical rates at each life expectancy. Confidence intervals for the surgical deficit were calculated taking into account the error of the imputed country-specific rates.

Estimates of Surgical Mortality in LMICs. We reviewed the published literature from LMICs that reported death and complication rates following three operations commonly performed in first-level hospitals: cesarean section, appendectomy, and hernia repair. Our inclusion criteria were articles published since 2000 from countries classified by the World Bank as LICs or middle-income countries in either 2005 or 2012 that reported either morbidity or mortality following one of these interventions, regardless of preoperative status, indication for intervention, or cause of death. We reviewed SCOPUS, MedLine, and PubMed, as well as other studies identified by their references or bibliographies (see annex 16A for search terms and identified references). We discarded studies that appeared to be duplicate analyses of the same data. We aggregated studies by country to create larger data samples for analysis.

Estimates of Theoretical Death Following Increased Surgical Service Delivery. We applied our estimates of surgical mortality to the volume of surgery needed to close the gap in surgical care and bring all countries falling below our minimum surgical rate up to the calculated minimum. We assumed a conservative midrange mortality rate estimate, even though we presumed that this low surgical volume continues to reflect a similar proportion of urgent cases with a correspondingly high mortality rate.

Table 16.2 Countries with the Lowest Surgical Rates and Highest Life Expectancies Based on an Incremental Cost-Effectiveness Selection Strategy

	Life expectancy (years)	Surgical rate (per 100,000 people)
Tajikistan	63	181
Korea, Dem. People's Rep.	66	303
Panama	76	1,637
New Zealand	80	4,547
Italy	81	7,768
Japan	82	11,741

Figure 16.2 Surgical Efficiency Curve Based on Countries Whose Health Systems Provide the Lowest Surgical Rates and the Highest Life Expectancies

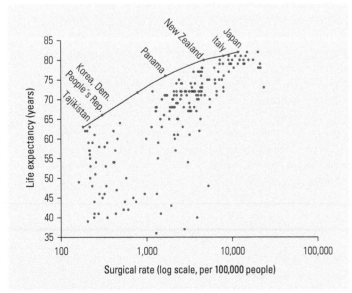

Note: Any particular life expectancy can be associated with a minimum estimated surgical rate based on this efficiency frontier. In this example, a life expectancy of 75 years is associated with a surgical rate of at least 1,504 per 100,000 people.

Results

Minimal Annual Surgical Rates. Six countries defined the efficiency frontier with a combination of the lowest rates of surgery and the highest life expectancies (table 16.2 and figure 16.2). Using this surgical efficiency calculation, minimum annual surgical rates observed at life expectancies of 70, 75, and 80 years were 836, 1,504, and 4,547 operations per 100,000 people, respectively. In 2004, 49 countries had rates of less than 836 per 100,000, and 65 had rates of less than 1,504 per 100,000; the vast majority of countries with rates of less than 836 were LICs. Most countries with rates higher than 4,547 per 100,000 were upper-middle-income (UMICs) or high-income countries (HICs). For LMICs to deliver at least 836 operations per 100,000 people, an additional 10.9 million operations per year (95 percent confidence interval of 3.9 million to 30.7 million) would need to be performed in these settings. To achieve a rate of 1,504 operations per 100,000 people would require an additional 28.4 million (95 percent confidence interval of 11.3 million to 71.2 million) operations annually in these countries.

Variable Mortality Rates. Based on the results of our estimates of surgical mortality, however, increased surgical capacity will exact a substantial toll in postsurgical harm and risk for adverse events. The literature search

identified 131 articles that met the inclusion criteria and evaluated either mortality or morbidity from cesarean section, appendectomy, and inguinal hernia repair in LMICs. We summarize these results in tables 16.3, 16.4, and 16.5. Crude mortality rates following cesarean section ranged from 0.5 per 1,000 operations to 51.3 per 1,000. For appendectomy, the rates of death were 0 to 88.6 per 1,000 operations; and for inguinal hernia repair, rates of death ranged from 0 to 411.8 per 1,000 operations. For comparison, historical death rates following cesarean section in Sweden and the Netherlands are 0.4 and 0.53 per 1,000, respectively (Hogberg 1989; Schuitemaker and others 1997); for appendectomy they are 2.4 and 3.0 per 1,000 (Blomqvist and others 2001; Noordzij and others 2010). The mortality rate for elective inguinal hernia repair in Sweden is 1.1 per 1,000, but the rate rises to 29.5 for emergency operations; overall mortality following inguinal hernia repair is 2.4 per 1,000 in Sweden (Nilsson and others 2007). The death rate following elective inguinal hernia repair in Denmark is calculated to be 2.2 per 1,000; however, for urgent cases it is substantially higher at 70.1, with an overall mortality rate of 5.2 per 1,000 operations (Bay-Nielsen and others 2001).

Table 16.3 Published Mortality and Morbidity Rates in Selected Countries Following Cesarean Section

Country	Cesarean section rate (percent)	Total number of cesarean sections	Total number of deaths	Total number of complications	Crude mortality per 1,000 cesarean sections	Crude morbidity per 1,000 cesarean sections
Afghanistan	1.0	565	29	—	51.3	—
Brazil	45.9	371,981	202	—	0.5	—
Burkina Faso	0.7	15,279	58	206	3.8	56.0
Chad	0.4	275	11	—	40.0	—
Ethiopia	1.0	267	2	20	7.5	88.9
India	8.5	8,893	25	35	2.8	18.7
Malawi	3.1	10,201	108	151	10.6	70.9
Morocco	5.4	3231	9	165	2.8	51.1
Nigeria	1.8	4215	41	11	9.7	67.1
Pakistan[a]	7.3	14,257	39	—	2.7	—
Rwanda	2.9	896	9	—	10.0	—
Senegal	3.3	370	7	—	18.9	—
South Africa	20.6	904	1	—	1.1	—
Tanzania	3.2	6,765	7	—	1.0	—
Thailand	17.4	187	0	7	0	37.4
Uganda	3.1	500	7	77	14.0	154.0
Zimbabwe	4.8	3,147	25	—	7.9	—

table continues next page

Table 16.3 Published Mortality and Morbidity Rates in Selected Countries Following Cesarean Section **(continued)**

Country	Cesarean section rate (percent)	Total number of cesarean sections	Total number of deaths	Total number of complications	Crude mortality per 1,000 cesarean sections	Crude morbidity per 1,000 cesarean sections
Bangladesh, China, Indonesia, Mongolia, Myanmar, Nepal, Thailand, Sri Lanka, and Vietnam	0.4	7,390	14	1,137	1.9	153.9
Cambodia, China, India, Japan, Nepal, Philippines, Sri Lanka, Thailand, and Vietnam	0.3	29,428	35	2,895	1.2	98.4
Congo, Dem. Rep.; Burundi; and Sierra Leone	—	1,276	7	93	5.5	72.9
Côte d'Ivoire, Mali, Niger, Mauritania, Burkina Faso, and Senegal	—	335	13	—	38.8	—
Senegal and Mali	0.1	11,255	157	536	13.9	47.6
Argentina, Brazil, Cuba, Ecuador, Nicaragua, Mexico, Paraguay, and Peru	0.3	31,803	16	984	0.5	30.9

Source: Authors' calculations based on Abbassi and others 2000; Bano and others 2011; Basak and others 2011; Bouvier-Colle and others 2001; Briand and others 2012; Chilopora and others 2007; Chongsuvivatwong and others 2010; Chu and others 2012; Fauveau 2007; Fenton and others 2003; Fesseha and others 2011; Glenshaw and Madzimbamuto 2005; Imbert and others 2003; Kaboro and others 2012; Kambo and others 2002; Kandasamy and others 2009; Kelly and others 2010; Kilsztajn and others 2007; Kim and others 2012; Kor-Anantakul and others 2008; Lumbiganon and others 2010; Ministère de la Santé Burkina Faso 2013; Okafor and Okezie 2005; Okafor and others 2009; Okezie and others 2007; Oladapo and others 2007; Ozumba and Anya 2002; Rahlenbeck and Hakizimana 2002; Rutgers and van Eygen 2008; Seal and others 2010; Sekirime and Lule 2008; Sorbye and others 2011; Tshibangu and others 2002; and Villar and others 2007. Cesarean section rates for Afghanistan and The Gambia are from Kim and others 2012 and Fauveau 2007, respectively. All other cesarean section rates are from Gibbons and others 2010.
Note: Denominators of mortality and morbidity may differ due to different studies from the same country using separate patient populations. — = not available.
a. Total number of cesarean sections in Pakistan obtained from Naheed Bano, Rawalpindi Medical College, and Holy Family Hospital, Rawalpindi, Pakistan.

Table 16.4 Published Mortality and Morbidity Rates in Selected Countries Following Appendectomy

Country	Total number of appendectomies	Total number of deaths	Total number of complications	Crude mortality per 1,000 appendectomies	Crude morbidity per 1,000 appendectomies
Bangladesh	30	0	7	0	233.3
Bolivia	55	1	4	18.2	72.7
Burkina Faso	789	0	—	0	—
Cameroon	323	2	33	6.2	102.2
Central African Republic	158	14	19	88.6	188.1
China	1,269	3	143	2.4	112.7
Congo, Rep.	56	1	4	17.9	71.4
Ethiopia	200	8	64	40.0	320.0
Ghana	789	13	114	16.5	178.7
India	749	0	39	0	52.1
Iran, Islamic Rep.	450	0	17	0	37.8
Kenya	301	0	43	0	142.9
Nepal	536	3	38	5.6	102.2
Nigeria	2,220	14	492	6.3	222.8
Pakistan	516	1	58	1.9	112.4
Peru	104	0	23	0	221.2

table continues next page

Table 16.4 Published Mortality and Morbidity Rates in Selected Countries Following Appendectomy (continued)

Country	Total number of appendectomies	Total number of deaths	Total number of complications	Crude mortality per 1,000 appendectomies	Crude morbidity per 1,000 appendectomies
Senegal	100	0	—	0	—
South Africa	960	12	96	12.5	183.2
Thailand	2,139	0	26	0	12.2
Turkey	183	10	36	54.6	235.0

Source: Authors' calculations, based on Abantanga and others 2009; Adisa and others 2012; Ali and Aliyu 2012; Asefa 2002; Ayoade and others 2006; Batajoo and Hazra 2012; Chamisa 2009; Chavda and others 2005; Chung and others 2000; Cunnigaiper and others 2010; Ekenze and others 2010; Fahim and Shirjeel 2005; Farthouat and others 2005; Fashina and others 2009; Gavilan-Yodu 2010; Gurleyik and Gurleyik 2003; Ibis and others 2010; Kargar and others 2011; Kasatpibal and others 2006; Khalil and others 2011; Khan and others 2012; Khiria and others 2011; Kong and others 2012; Kumar and Jain 2004; Liu and others 2007; Mabiala-Babela and others 2006; Malik and others 2009; Mehrabi Bahar and others 2010; Ming and others 2009; Ministère de la Santé Burkina Faso 2013; Ngowe Ngowe and others 2008; Ohene-Yeboah and Togbe 2006; Okafor and others 2003; Osifo and Ogiemwonyi 2009; Paudel and others 2003; Peralta Vargas and others 2004; Pokharel and others 2011; Rogers and others 2008; Saha and others 2010; Salahuddin and others 2012; Séréngbé and others 2002; Shaikh and others 2009; Terzi and others 2010; Utpal 2005; Willmore and Hill 2001; H. S. Wu and others 2011; S. C. Wu and others 2011; and Zoguereh and others 2001. See annex 16A for a list of citations by country.

Note: Denominators of mortality and morbidity may differ due to multiple different studies from the same country using separate patient populations.

— = not available.

LICs and lower-middle-income countries have rates of death that are orders of magnitude greater than those of HICs and UMICs. Compared with Sweden, a country with historically low death rates following these three operations, cesarean section mortality is at least 2 to 4 times higher in Latin America and the Caribbean, 6 to 10 times higher in South Asia, and 100 times higher in Sub-Saharan Africa. The ranges of mortality rates following both appendectomy and inguinal hernia repair are much narrower, but there is frequently a 40-fold mortality increase in Sub-Saharan Africa, and in some cases more than a 100-fold increased risk of death for the same intervention. If LICs and lower-middle-income countries closed the gap in surgical rates to attain a minimum rate of 836 operations per 100,000 people, but surgical mortality remained at 4 percent—a number well within the range of that in Europe—436,000 people would die annually following surgery in these settings. With rates of surgery reaching 1,504 per 100,000 people in LICs and lower-middle-income countries, a postoperative mortality rate of 4 percent would increase this number to 1.14 million deaths per year. Reducing variability in mortality and bringing postoperative mortality to 1.5 percent would prevent more than 200,000 and 700,000 deaths, respectively, for these two surgical rates.

Although these estimates do not control for comorbidities or other demographic, patient, or facility factors, they suggest tremendous excess mortality following surgical interventions. The excessively high death rates following essential surgical interventions such as cesarean section, appendectomy, and hernia repair indicate that safety concerns are justified and demand attention. The variability in mortality in HICs in Europe and North America has been well established, both among and

within countries; it is not surprising that this variability is more pronounced in LICs and lower-middle-income countries. However, the extreme rates of death and disability are so dramatic that health systems in these settings need to adopt strategies to improve survival and reduce complications if surgical interventions are to be acceptable and have a meaningful health impact.

CHALLENGES TO SURGICAL SERVICES IN LICs AND LMICs

The causes of the disparities in mortality described in the previous section are multifactorial and include access to care, transportation options, behaviors, and attitudes. Financial barriers in particular are substantial, especially for the poor and near poor. Catastrophic health expenditure is a major cause of impoverishment, and surgical care can quickly deplete a family's financial resources (Kruk, Goldmann, and Galea 2009; Nguyen and others 2013; Van Minh and others 2013; Xu and others 2007). Geographic and transportation barriers present a challenge for populations who live at distances from health centers and first-level hospitals. Delays in care-seeking behaviors are exacerbated when populations lack knowledge of health risks or when poor care has led to severe mistrust in health systems (Gauthier and Wane 2011; Kahabuka and others 2011; Kruk and others 2009; Yaffee and others 2012).

These factors pose difficult challenges when evaluating outcomes of surgical care. Delays in presentation for care translate into higher morbidity and mortality, particularly for surgically treatable conditions. Patients may arrive septic, malnourished, physiologically stressed, dehydrated, and anemic; many may arrive moribund. Yet those with life- or limb-threatening conditions tend

Table 16.5 Published Mortality and Morbidity Rates in LMICs Following Inguinal Hernia Repair

Country	Total number of patients undergoing hernia repair	Total number of deaths	Total number of complications	Crude mortality per 1,000 hernia repairs	Crude morbidity per 1,000 hernia repairs
Burkina Faso	7,421	36	0	4.9	0
Cameroon and Mali	524	0	5	0	9.5
China	4,072	0	13	0	3.2
Colombia	13	0	0	0	0
Côte d'Ivoire	128	1	1	7.8	7.8
Dominican Republic	239	0	0	0	0
Ecuador	102	0	0	0	0
Ghana	973	9	29	9.2	33.1
Haiti	17	0	1	0	58.8
India	358	0	31	0	86.6
Jamaica	314	0	—	0	—
Nepal	61	0	5	0	82.0
Nicaragua	10	0	0	0	0
Niger	34	14	16	411.8	470.6
Nigeria	5,451	26	275	4.8	50.5
Pakistan	605	8	25	13.2	41.3
Sierra Leone	45	5	—	111.1	—
Sudan	64	4	7	62.5	109.4
Tanzania	452	44	24	97.3	53.1
Thailand	24	0	1	0	41.7
Tunisia	595	4	—	6.7	—
Turkey	970	11	31	11.3	37.7

Source: Authors' calculations; based on Abantanga 2003; Aderounmu and others 2008; Adesunkanmi and others 2000; Akcakaya and others 2000; Akinci and others 2010; Ameh 2002; Awojobi and Ayantunde 2004; Chauhan and others 2007; Cingi and others 2005; Clarke and others 2009; Diarra and others 2001; ElRashied and others 2007; Freudenberg and others 2006; Gao and others 2009; Gil and others 2012; Harouna and others 2001; Huang and others 2005; Jani 2005; Kingsnorth and others 2006; Lagoo and others 2012; Lau and others 2002; Lohsiriwat and others 2007; Mabula and Chalya 2012; Malik and others 2010; Mbah 2007; McConkey 2002; Memon and others 2013; Ministère de la Santé Burkina Faso 2013; Mungadi 2005; Obalum and others 2008; Ohene-Yeboah 2003; Osifo and Irowa 2008; Pradhan and others 2011; Ramyil and others 2000; Samaali and others 2012; Sanders and Kingsnorth 2007; Scarlett and others 2007; Shaikh and others 2012; Shi and others 2010; Shillcutt and others 2010; Shillcutt and others 2013; Taqvi and others 2006; Turaga and others 2006; Usang and others 2008; Walk and others 2012; Wu and others 2008; Yeung and others 2002; and Zhou 2013. See annex 16A for a list of citations by country.
Note: Denominators of mortality and morbidity may differ due to multiple different studies from the same country using separate patient populations.
— = not available.

to derive the greatest benefit from interventions, but at a cost of poorer overall outcomes. The physiologic insults of surgery and anesthesia are substantial, and patients that arrive with only minimal physiological reserves fare poorly. Thus, even situations that might be considered low risk from a population perspective—such as cesarean section in otherwise young, healthy women or appendectomy in healthy young children—demonstrate high levels of complications and mortality compared with similar conditions in HICs. When addressing issues of harm from surgery, providing constructive improvement strategies to health systems and providers who

work under less-than-ideal circumstances and operate on patients with more severe, life-threatening comorbid conditions are important.

As demonstrated throughout this volume, LMICs do not meet the basic surgical needs of their populations. Estimating minimum surgical rates using a surgical rate efficiency methodology indicates that most LMICs fall far short of minimum need. In addition, death rates following common operations are substantial and exceed what would be considered acceptable in HICs. If health systems in LMICs improve their surgical numbers without concurrently improving the safety, quality, and transparency of their services, they jeopardize the health of patients seeking care and risk exacerbating mistrust.

Barriers to Surgical Care

Multiple factors contribute to the risks that surgical patients face in resource-constrained environments. Patients, particularly those whose conditions require urgent surgical interventions, encounter significant barriers to effective and timely care. These conditions can rapidly become fatal, and delays in care are associated with significantly worse outcomes. Emergency surgery carries an added risk of mortality due to the extenuating circumstances of the condition, the inability to adequately plan or prepare for the procedure, the inability to control or modify patient-specific risk factors, the logistical difficulties rallying appropriate human or infrastructure resources, and the challenge of intervening with incomplete information. Accordingly, outcomes are worse for emergency interventions compared with elective or semielective procedures. Emergency operations constitute a higher proportion of operations in resource-limited settings, and any barrier that delays presentation imposes a tremendous burden on patients and the health system.

Delays in care have been categorized into three phases: delays in deciding to seek care; delays in reaching adequate health facilities; and delays in receiving adequate, appropriate, and timely care (Thaddeus and Maine 1994). Because access to and delivery of surgical care presents particular challenges in LICs and LMICs, it is especially important to understand the barriers that contribute to delays in definitive interventional care. These barriers can generally be divided into three dimensions: availability, affordability, and acceptability (Grimes and others 2011; McIntyre, Thiede, and Birch 2009). Each of these dimensions causes delays experienced by patients in need of surgical care (figure 16.3).

Availability of Care. *Availability* refers to the following:

- The relationship between the location of health care facilities with the capacity to provide appropriate services, the location of the population needing them, and the transport opportunities available
- The ability and willingness of care providers to serve the population in accordance with the type and severity of the presenting condition
- The timing and hours of available services and the times patients seek care

Figure 16.3 Relationship of Barriers to Care and Delays in Obtaining Care

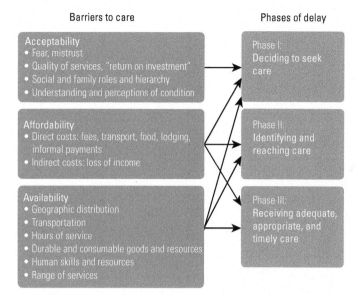

Source: Adapted from Thaddeus and Maine 1994.

- The range, quantity, and quality of services provided and the nature and extent of the health needs of people seeking care

A tremendous obstacle to early presentation is the geographic distribution of health facilities with the capacity to recognize and deal with surgical issues (Dye and others 2010; Hang and Byass 2009; Macharia and others 2009; Mock, nii-Amon-Kotei, and Maier 1997; Parkhurst, Rahman, and Ssengooba 2006). Health centers with the sophistication to provide surgical care tend to be located in more populous areas, and LMICs with the lowest surgical volumes frequently have large rural populations. Timely transport to surgical care is critical, yet road and transportation infrastructure can be lacking or intermittent (Macharia and others 2009; Mock, nii-Amon-Kotei, and Maier 1997; Seljeskog, Sundby, and Chimango 2006). Finally, social norms can prevent early presentation; consultation with traditional healers, village elders, or heads of family may delay access to the formal health care system (Briesen and others 2010; Hang and Byass 2009; Mock, nii-Amon-Kotei, and Maier 1997; Parkhurst, Rahman, and Ssengooba 2006; Seljeskog, Sundby, and Chimango 2006).

Once patients do arrive at facilities, the requisite durable and consumable supplies and equipment are often inadequate (Lebrun, Chackungal, and others 2013; Lebrun, Dhar, and others 2014; Macharia and others 2009). The availability of personnel and services is often intermittent, particularly at night. Above all, the human resources for health are frequently lacking. Surgical skill requires education, training, and experience; trained clinicians are not always available or capable of performing specific surgical tasks; the status of anesthesia services, as discussed in chapter 15, is even more dire. Providers' confidence in their skills is particularly important for the provision of surgical care; recent research has indicated that lack of confidence—due to lack of training, experience, or surgical assistance—may be a primary cause of triage and transfer, as well as a major barrier preventing immediate intervention (Bowman and others 2013; Petroze, Nzayisenga, and others 2012).

Affordability of Care. *Affordability*, the match between costs of services and the ability of individuals to pay, presents a major challenge because of the following factors:

- Price of services at the point of delivery
- Direct costs associated with transportation, food, and lodging
- Indirect costs, such as lost income or productivity

The ability of individuals to pay also relates to their personal wealth and assets, eligibility for financial support from financing mechanisms, and amount of indirect costs incurred. Transportation costs can be unaffordable, and, when combined with prohibitive out-of-pocket expenses, frequently delays early consultation (Afsana 2004; Mock, nii-Amon-Kotei, and Maier 1997; Nwameme, Phillips, and Adongo 2013). In addition, affordability refers not just to the ability of an individual or family to pay for care but also the potential impact of that payment on the household, and the manner and timing of payment. For example, up-front charges may prevent early assessment and definitive management as families seek to secure necessary funds for payment for services (Kruk, Goldmann, and Galea 2009).

Acceptability of Care. *Acceptability* refers to the expectations, behaviors, perceptions, and attitudes inherent in medical encounters. Providers' attitudes are affected by stereotypes, chief complaints, and the manner of presentation. Patients' attitudes are similarly affected by stereotypes, as well as by perceptions of respect, efficiency of care, and trust in the integrity of the system. Of particular concern with surgical intervention is the personal security of clinicians; deaths following surgery may be blamed directly on surgical providers, and family and community members may seek retribution, regardless of premorbid conditions or cause of demise (Burch and others 2011; Malik and others 2010).

Many of these domains interact in ways that magnify delays. Concerns about financial commitments, compounded by mistrust of the health care system, a lack of transparency, and poor quality, lead to long delays in treatment-seeking behavior. People in many LMICs may justifiably perceive surgical care to be a poor investment of resources.

Anesthesia Safety

The safe provision of anesthesia is a critical consideration in establishing and expanding the capacity for surgical care. Improvements in anesthetic monitoring and techniques have led to dramatic improvements in its safety profile in HICs and UMICs. In many settings with low levels of human resources, however, anesthesia is provided by nonphysician clinicians or technicians, or even by the operating surgeons. Poor training, supervision, and monitoring standards all contribute to high mortality from the administration of anesthesia.

Although the rate of overall deaths due to anesthesia is estimated to be 34 per 1 million anesthetics administered, profound differences exist among countries and settings. Bainbridge and others (2012) report that in low human development index countries, deaths solely attributable to anesthesia are estimated to be 141 per million, compared with 25 per million in high human development index countries. Critically, anesthesia mortality in LMICs continues to be a major problem, with death rates as high as one per 500 (Walker and Wilson 2008). Anesthesia in HICs and UMICs has improved only relatively recently, with changes in monitoring and increased standardization responsible for a 100-fold reduction in mortality over the past 40 years—34 deaths per million instances of anesthetics administered in the 1990s and 2000s, down from 357 deaths per million before 1970 (figure 16.4). Low professional standing, inadequate basic monitoring equipment, and a lack of professional standards all contribute to the current disparity between HICs and other countries.

Perioperative Safety

Surgical intervention, by its nature, involves risks. High-quality and high-resource systems still fail to provide proven interventions every time for every patient.

In the United States, the failure to adhere to basic WHO standards occurs in 6 percent to 20 percent of operations, indicating substantial room for improvement (Stulberg and others 2010). Individual care standards are being used in pay-for-performance initiatives to help improve quality by linking it to reimbursement. When individual standards are evaluated in isolation, however, they frequently fail to demonstrate improvements in outcomes with improving levels of compliance (table 16.6) (Stulberg and others 2010). Multiple care standards need to be evaluated as a composite whole; partial completion of tasks does not always deliver a partial benefit, and improvements often require total compliance to result in improved outcomes (Nolan and Berwick 2006).

This all-or-none compliance likely indicates that systems able to achieve high compliance rates with multiple standards-of-care processes are highly organized and functioning efficiently; accordingly, they are able to deliver on difficult-to-measure but essential components of care, such as communication and information transfer (Weiser 2010). In LMICs, lack of compliance may be especially germane—poorly used or misallocated

Figure 16.4 Meta-Regression for Risk of Death due Solely to Anesthesia, 1939–2009

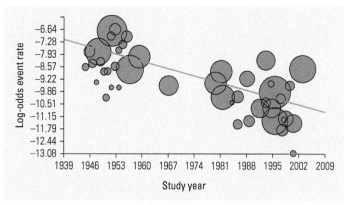

Source: Bainbridge and others 2012.
Note: Every circle represents a study; the circle size is representative of the weight of that study in the analysis. The relationship between mortality and year of study was significant, with a significant decline over the decades (slope –0.053; 95 percent confidence interval of –0.058 to –0.049; $p = 0.000001$).

Table 16.6 Surgical Care Improvement Project: Infection-Prevention Process Measures

	Nonadherent discharges		Adherent discharges			
	Postoperative infections	Discharges	Postoperative infections	Discharges	Adjusted odds ratio (95% CI)	
Individual SCIP measures						
Prophylactic antibiotic received within 1 hour prior to surgical incision	251	18,147	1,394	190,925	0.89 (0.75–1.06)	
Prophylactic antibiotic selection for surgical patients	266	12,670	1,486	198,002	0.83 (0.69–1.00)	
Prophylactic antibiotics discontinued within 24 hours after surgery end time	310	26,499	1,024	173,228	0.94 (0.78–1.13)	
Cardiac surgery patients with controlled postoperative morning blood glucose	65	4,168	362	31,512	0.93 (0.68–1.27)	
Surgery patients with appropriate hair removal	194	21,308	3,539	360,111	1.00 (0.85–1.19)	
Colorectal surgery patients with immediate postoperative normothermia	181	4,564	676	18,101	1.00 (0.81–1.23)	
Composite measures						
SCIP Antibiotic Measures (1st three above) performed	511	44,417	816	154,963	0.86 (0.74–1.01)	
At least 2 of the above SCIP measures recorded in a single visit	843	59,356	1,070	158,304	0.85 (0.76–0.95)	

Source: Stulberg and others 2010.
Note: Each estimate accounts for the surgical procedure performed, patient characteristics, and hospital characteristics. CI = confidence interval; SCIP = Surgical Care Improvement Project.

resources constitute a drain on an already stressed health system.

Compliance with care standards in LMICs is frequently poor. In a study in India, Das and others (2012) selected a random sample of health care providers in rural Madhya Pradesh and urban Delhi to receive a visit from a "standardized patient" trained to present one of three scenarios: unstable angina, asthma, or a parent describing dysentery in a child at home. These standardized patients were then debriefed following their clinic visit to assess the quality of care and compliance with care checklists and best practices. Providers in both locations did poorly in asking appropriate questions and performing appropriate examinations (33.7 percent and 31.8 percent in Madhya Pradesh and Delhi, respectively); making the correct diagnosis (12.2 percent and 21.8 percent in Madhya Pradesh and Delhi, respectively); and identifying pertinent clinical issues and making appropriate recommendations for treatment (30.4 percent and 45.6 percent in Madhya Pradesh and Delhi, respectively) (figure 16.5). The rate of unnecessary or harmful treatments exceeded 40 percent in Madhya Pradesh. Despite the range of provider education, from no formal medical education to fully licensed physician, only a small difference was observed in adherence to care standards; no difference was observed in arriving at the correct diagnosis or providing the correct treatment.

Such studies point to troubling discrepancies between what is known and taught about care standards, on the one hand, and actual practice patterns, on the other hand. Adherence to known practice standards is a hallmark of high-quality health organizations; yet, similar to what is found in primary care and general practice settings, surgical delivery in HICs and LMICs alike frequently fails to follow standards of care, despite well-described strategies and techniques for improvement.

Postoperative Care and Safety

In addition to the risks during surgery, patients are at high risk during postoperative recovery. The two most common causes of complications within the first week of surgery are bleeding and infections. Additional causes of delayed morbidities include blood clots, heart attacks, pneumonia, and stroke. Anticipating potential complications, and either preventing them (for example, by prophylaxis for venous thromboembolism) or identifying the signs and symptoms and intervening early and aggressively, are essential to reduce these risks.

An important study established the prominent role of a mature system of postoperative care in managing complications and preventing them from resulting in death (also known as *failure to rescue*). Ghaferi, Birkmeyer, and Dimick (2009a, 2009b) found that although baseline complications rates were strikingly similar in institutions across the United States, mortality rates following these complications varied dramatically (figure 16.6 and table 16.7). These findings confirm earlier research suggesting that the primary difference in outcomes among hospitals is not due to differences in complication rates but to differences in the rates of failure to rescue (Silber and others 1992).

Further research has demonstrated that higher-volume hospitals appear to have a better ability to recognize, intervene, and save patients undergoing high-risk procedures from death and complications following surgery (Ghaferi, Birkmeyer, and Dimick 2011). Complications must be anticipated following high-risk procedures; the ability to recognize, diagnose, and treat complications separates the high performers from the poor performers. The quality of communication and the systems of care, and the skills and capacity of ancillary services—such as availability of intensive care and the presence and experience of specialized services—appear to be important factors for improving outcomes following complications.

Figure 16.5 Adherence to Checklist of Questions and Examinations for Unstable Angina, Madhya Pradesh, 2010

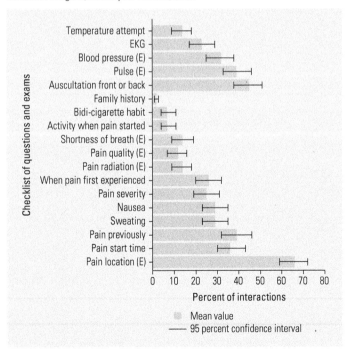

Source: Das and others 2012.
Note: All items listed are recommended; those marked (E) are essential. "Temperature attempt" refers to checking temperature either by touch or with a thermometer. EKG = electrocardiogram and refers to either an electrocardiogram performed by practitioners or referrals for electrocardiograms.
"Bidi-cigarette habit" indicates whether the doctor asked about tobacco use; a bidi is an Indian cigarette consisting of tobacco wrapped in a leaf. "Pain start time" is asked to ascertain a specific time of day.

STRATEGIES FOR IMPROVING SURGICAL CARE

Several effective strategies have been identified for improving surgical outcomes in LMICs. These strategies include the adoption and use of basic technologies, the development of monitoring standards, and the use of surgical safety checklists. Organizational and management strategies also appear to be important. Essential to all of these interventions is a mandate to measure the delivery of care and its impact on health. These low-cost interventions, which can dramatically lower postsurgical mortality rates, demand prioritization by health systems seeking to improve access and surgical service provision.

Anesthetic Monitoring and Safety

One of the most important contributions to improved surgical safety has been the development of basic standards of anesthetic monitoring. The Harvard monitoring

Figure 16.6 Rates of All Postsurgical Complications, Major Complications, and Deaths after Major Complications, According to Hospital Quintile of Mortality

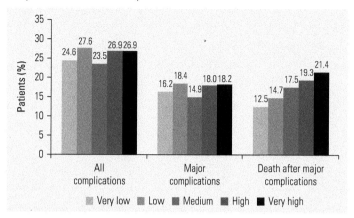

Source: Ghaferi and others 2009b.
Note: Although rates of all complications and major complications did not vary significantly across hospital mortality quintiles, the rate of death in patients with major complications was almost twice as high in hospitals with very high overall mortality as in those with very low overall mortality (21.4 percent versus 12.5 percent, $p < 0.001$).

Table 16.7 Rates of Deaths, Complications, and Death after Major Complications for Five Operations with the Highest Number of Deaths, According to Hospital Quintile of Mortality, 2005–07

Type of surgery	Very low mortality (percent of patients)	Very high mortality (percent of patients)	Odds ratio for very high versus very low mortality (95% confidence interval)
Colectomy			
Overall mortality	2.5	5.6	2.29 (1.76–2.98)
All complications	24.7	28.1	1.19 (0.95–1.50)
Major complications	15.4	17.6	1.17 (0.94–1.46)
Mortality after major complications	11.4	20.5	2.08 (1.54–2.82)
Abdominal-aortic-aneurysm repair			
Overall mortality	3.1	7.3	2.49 (1.63–3.81)
All complications	17.4	19.3	1.13 (0.87–1.46)
Major complications	13.6	15.5	1.26 (0.86–1.56)
Mortality after major complications	15.6	26.3	1.94 (1.04–3.62)
Above-knee amputation			
Overall mortality	10.0	15.0	1.59 (1.00–2.53)
All complications	25.7	26.6	1.05 (0.75–1.47)
Major complications	18.9	18.6	0.98 (0.67–1.43)
Mortality after major complications	20.8	35.2	2.08 (0.94–4.60)
Lower-extremity bypass			
Overall mortality	1.9	2.9	1.55 (0.92–2.60)
All complications	24.0	23.6	0.97 (0.81–1.17)
Major complications	11.5	11.1	0.95 (0.75–1.22)
Mortality after major complications	8.2	12.7	1.63 (0.76–3.53)

table continues next page

Table 16.7 Rates of Deaths, Complications, and Death after Major Complications for Five Operations with the Highest Number of Deaths, According to Hospital Quintile of Mortality, 2005–07 **(continued)**

Type of surgery	Very low mortality (percent of patients)	Very high mortality (percent of patients)	Odds ratio for very high versus very low mortality (95% confidence interval)
Below-knee amputation			
Overall mortality	4.2	8.4	2.07 (1.18–3.63)
All complications	23.7	25.4	1.09 (0.82–1.46)
Major complications	15.5	17.3	1.14 (0.81–1.60)
Mortality after major complications	14.5	29.7	2.49 (1.10–5.63)

Source: Ghaferi, Birkmeyer, and Dimick 2009b.

standards for intraoperative anesthesia care formalized a set of medical standards of practice that have become de facto international standards endorsed by the World Federation of Societies of Anaesthesiologists (Eichhorn and others 1986; WFSA 2008). The standards include the continuous presence of trained anesthesia providers and the uninterrupted monitoring of oxygenation, ventilation, and perfusion. Today, adherence to these standards in HICs is essentially universal; however, this was not the case a mere three decades ago, and it is far from standard practice in many LMICs.

In addition to continuous monitoring techniques, anesthesia delivery systems have been standardized, with safety engineered into the instruments themselves. Inhalational anesthetic machines are now engineered to be redundant; safety features, such as auto-lock mechanisms, prevent lethal hypoxic gas mixtures. Despite the 100-fold plunge in anesthetic-related mortality rates in HICs and UMICs during the past 40 years, anesthetic mortality in LMICs is a major problem due to lack of professional stature, training, and credentialing of anesthesia providers; deficiencies in basic monitoring equipment; and failure to adhere to strict standards of care.

One critical mechanism for anesthesia monitoring is the use of pulse oximetry. Although the continuous monitoring of blood oxygen levels using a pulse oximeter is considered an essential standard, more than 77,000 operating rooms worldwide do not have this basic monitoring device (Funk and others 2010). Pulse oximetry can alert anesthesia personnel to drops in oxygenation before clinical signs become apparent, allowing for corrective actions before hemodynamic instability or lethal arrhythmias occur. In Moldova, an implementation program supplying pulse oximetry equipment in conjunction with provider training on the use of a surgical safety checklist reduced postoperative deaths and complications (Kwok and others 2013). Use of pulse oximetry is highly cost-effective as well,

with the cost per DALY averted from anesthetic mishaps due to improved monitoring at US$374 for a standard commercial oximeter and US$115 for a smaller hand held device (Burn and others 2014). A concerted effort is underway through the Lifebox Foundation to provide pulse oximetry monitoring capabilities to every operating theater in the world (http://www.lifebox.org).

Surgical Checklists

Standardization of care is essential because of the tremendous magnitude of interactions and care processes that occur during even simple surgical procedures. Complex patient characteristics, therapeutic options, technical demands, and team dynamics require specific strategies for organizing care protocols and service delivery. The effective use of checklists by teams during surgery has cut mortality rates by up to 50 percent.

In 2008, the WHO codified a set of basic surgical standards into guidelines for safe surgery. Researchers transformed these guidelines into a simple, 19-item checklist to be used during the perioperative period and conducted a multicenter trial assessing the efficacy of this safety tool on postoperative morbidity and mortality (figure 16.7). In a pre- and postanalysis of nearly 8,000 surgical patients, use of this checklist nearly doubled adherence to basic perioperative safety standards, including confirmation of the procedure and operative site, administration of antibiotics, use of pulse oximetry for monitoring, objective airway assessment, and completion of instrument and sponge counts at the conclusion of the operation. Use of the checklist reduced deaths by more than 47 percent and cut complication rates by 35 percent (Haynes and others 2009). This beneficial effect was maintained in a subanalysis of urgent and emergency cases (Weiser, Haynes, Dziekan, and others 2010).

Several other large, well-designed studies have confirmed the substantial enhancements to surgical safety

Figure 16.7 World Health Organization Surgical Safety Checklist

Before induction of anesthesia	Before skin incision	Before patient leaves operating room
(with at least nurse and anesthetist)	(with nurse, anesthetist, and surgeon)	(with nurse, anesthetist, and surgeon)

Before induction of anesthesia

Has the patient confirmed his/her identity, site, procedure, and consent?
☐ Yes

Is the site marked?
☐ Yes
☐ Not applicable

Is the anesthesia machine and medication check complete?
☐ Yes

Is the pulse oximeter on the patient and functioning?
☐ Yes

Does patient have a:

Known allergy?
☐ No
☐ Yes

Difficult airway or aspiration risk?
☐ No
☐ Yes, and equipment/assistance available

Risk of >500ml blood loss (7ml/kg in children)?
☐ No
☐ Yes, and two IVs/central access and fluids planned

Before skin incision

☐ Confirm all team members have introduced themselves by name and role.

☐ Confirm the patient's name, procedure, and where the incision will be made.

Has antibiotic prophylaxis been given within the last 60 minutes?
☐ Yes
☐ Not applicable

Anticipated critical events

To surgeon:
☐ What are the critical or nonroutine steps?
☐ How long will the case take?
☐ What is the anticipated blood loss?

To anesthetist:
☐ Are there any patient-specific concerns?

To nursing team:
☐ Has sterility (including indicator results) been confirmed?
☐ Are there equipment issues or any concerns?

Is essential imaging displayed?
☐ Yes
☐ Not applicable

Before patient leaves operating room

Nurse verbally confirms:

☐ The name of the procedure

☐ Completion of instrument, sponge, and needle counts

☐ Specimen labeling (read specimen labels aloud, including patient name)

☐ Whether there are any equipment problems to be addressed

To surgeon, anesthetist, and nurse:

☐ What are the key concerns for recovery and management of this patient?

Source: WHO 2009b.

Note: This checklist is not intended to be comprehensive. Additions and modifications to fit local practice are encouraged. IV = intravenous therapy; kg = kilogram; ml = milliliter.

that checklists provide. Following the introduction of a comprehensive perioperative checklist in six hospitals in the Netherlands, postoperative complications and deaths dropped by 30 percent and 47 percent, respectively; in five control hospitals, no improvements were noted during the same period (de Vries and others 2010). A second study in the Netherlands virtually repeated the original multinational WHO investigation, demonstrating improvements in postoperative mortality that strongly correlated with checklist compliance (van Klei and others 2012).

Just as a pilot's checklist does not instruct a pilot how to fly a plane, surgical checklists do not dictate how clinicians should deliver care; instead, checklists help confirm critical steps, prompt consideration of extenuating or unusual factors, and stimulate or facilitate team communication. These processes are particularly important in the complex and multidisciplinary environment of surgery. Checklists are often a critical part of crew resource management, a method of team training that promotes shared mental models for care and conduct that has been implemented in many

organizations and sectors in which high reliability and fidelity are paramount, such as aviation and nuclear power. This method has been extended to surgical teams; it has been observed, for example, that cardiac surgery teams that consistently work together are more efficient and have better outcomes than those with rotating members (Carthey, de Leval, and Reason 2001; de Leval and others 2000). Because this method is often not possible in urgent circumstances or when human resources are limited, checklists can play an essential role in promoting consistent processes of care. A study conducted at 74 Veterans Administration hospitals in the United States demonstrated significant improvements in mortality compared to controls following a full-day team training program that included implementation and training in the use of checklist-guided briefings and debriefings (Neily and others 2010).

Checklists have become an established standard of surgical care globally (Birkmeyer 2010). Their effectiveness has demonstrated the accuracy of previous estimates suggesting that at least 50 percent of existing surgical mortality is preventable. Checklists are most effective when they are implemented, not as a tickbox exercise, but as a means to reinforce communication, prompt genuine dialogue and discussion of critical information, and facilitate prospective feedback and quality improvement (Weiser, Haynes, Lashoher, and others 2010). Large-scale regulatory mandates alone appear not to be effective in fostering effective adoption (Urbach and others 2014). Implementation has been found to require local champions from all disciplines, support from leadership, monitoring of progress, and involvement of frontline clinicians (such as through team training) and not just administrators. Such an approach has been followed in Scotland, leading to a statistically significant drop in inpatient surgical death rates from 2011 after three years of flat mortality rates. The Scottish government has documented more than 9,000 lives saved (Leitch 2012).

The challenge of conducting multidisciplinary implementation programs in LMICs raises legitimate concerns about ability to scale up such programs globally. However, a follow-up WHO study in Honduras, Moldova, and Zambia confirms the ability to implement and replicate large improvements in safety and outcomes (Kim and others 2012).

Management Practices

Effective and efficient management strategies are an essential component in the smooth functioning of health facilities. Numerous econometric studies have looked at management practices in industry and business and identified characteristics that affect productivity. Two economists from Stanford University and the London School of Economics conducted a series of interviews with midlevel managers from a range of medium-sized manufacturing firms in France, Germany, the United Kingdom, and the United States, using a survey to assess four domains of management: operations, monitoring, targets, and incentives (Bloom and van Reenen 2007). High scores in these domains were strongly related to higher productivity and profitability, as well as to the longevity of the company.

In LMICs, however, multiple factors affect the performance of industry, particularly for the worse. Management practices are suboptimal for various reasons, including lack of knowledge of optimal management practices, reduced competition, high proportion of family ownership, lack of delegation of decision making because of fear or mistrust, reduced incentives, and poorly allocated financing. Bloom and van Reenen (2010) and Bloom and others (2010) note that similarly sized local firms in LMICs were severely lacking in management practices, with correspondingly lower overall productivity. Although economic environments and organizational factors played a role (Bloom, Sadun, and van Reenen 2012), introducing management practices through an intensive consulting process resulted in massive improvements in efficiency and productivity (Bloom and others 2010; Bloom and others 2013).

In health care, the management practices evaluated by Bloom and van Reenen (2010) roughly translate to operations management, quality evaluation, goal-setting, and talent management. Their scoring mechanism has been used to evaluate hospital management practices and its subsequent correlation with patient outcomes across Brazil, Europe, India, and the United States. They find tremendous variability in management practices within countries, as well as a particularly large proportion of poorly managed hospitals in LMICs. A McKinsey study looking at hospitals in the United Kingdom and the United States determined that an increase of 1 point on Bloom's management practice survey scale is associated with a decrease of 6 percent to 7 percent in 30-day mortality following acute myocardial infarction, an increase in hospital earnings of 14 percent to 33 percent, and an overall improvement in patient satisfaction (Bury and others 2007).

Although there is a paucity of research in the area of hospital management in LMICs, it is reasonable to infer that management practices affect the organizational structure, efficiency, and even safety of the health system. In one of the first studies of this kind, Funk and others (2013) suggest that more robust management practices are associated with enhanced surgical productivity. Unfortunately, many first-level rural and urban referral hospitals in LMICS are likely to be plagued by poor management practices similar to their business and manufacturing counterparts. Such problems lead to waste and poor resource allocation, and potentially even to fraud and abuse. It remains to be seen whether improvements in management translate into improved surgical productivity in these settings and, if so, the mechanisms by which such improvements occur.

One essential mechanism that management uses to enhance the quality of care is the implementation of surveillance and evaluation practices, allowing quality improvement (QI) programs to be targeted to identified weaknesses. These practices range from very simple outcome assessments, such as Morbidity and Mortality Conferences (M&M), to more complex monitoring, such as ongoing surveillance of complications, adverse events, and errors, and use of risk-adjusted mortality. Many hospitals in LMICs have some type of QI activity, even if limited to periodic M&M conferences. Often, the effectiveness of these efforts could be increased by simple measures, such as better recording of problems discussed, more purposeful enactment of corrective action, and monitoring of the outcome of the corrective action. A WHO review of the effectiveness of QI programs for trauma care identifies 36 studies, 34 of which report improvements in patient outcomes (including mortality) or process of care after a new QI program or method is introduced (Juillard and others 2009). Two articles report no change, and no articles report a worsening of any outcome; five articles also report cost savings. Most of the articles were from HICs; two were from Thailand. A summary of the model QI program in Thailand is provided in chapter 3 on trauma care in this volume. The WHO has outlined a multimodal approach to QI processes for trauma systems through the use of morbidity and mortality, preventable death panel reviews, audit filters, and the establishment of trauma data bases and surveillance systems (WHO 2009a).

Measurement Strategies

The measurement of outcomes of intervention, regardless of the service provided, is essential to ensure that the effects of care are aligned with intent and that resources are used efficiently, effectively, and with the least harm to patients. Practitioners, facilities, and health systems require information on surgical capacity, throughput, and results to determine how such service lines perform. Other notable public health successes, such as improvements in maternal and neonatal health, HIV care, and control of poliomyelitis and malaria, have been dependent on surveillance (Ceesay and others 2008; Ronsmans and Graham 2006; WHO 2000, 2005, 2007). Surveillance is equally essential in optimizing access to and the safety of surgical care; the absence of data on surgical delivery and outcomes perpetuates the neglect such therapy receives in resource-constrained settings (Weiser and others 2008, 2009).

The WHO has proposed a set of standardized metrics for surgical surveillance at the national level that have been tested and validated (WHO 2009d), and is included in annex 16B. These metrics include the number of operating rooms in each country, the numbers of trained surgeons and trained anesthetists in each country, the number of procedures performed in operating rooms in each country, the number of deaths on the day of surgery, and the number of in-hospital deaths after surgery (Weiser and others 2009) (table 16.8). Although each

Table 16.8 Standardized Statistics for Surgery: Definitions, Rationale, and Data Sources

	Definition	Rationale for use	Data sources	Comments
Number of operating rooms	Operating rooms are rooms used specifically for surgical procedures and equipped to deliver anesthesia	The number of operating rooms available to a population is a structural indicator of the ability to provide surgical interventions.	Administrative records based on reported data by inpatient and outpatient facilities; censuses of health facilities	Minor procedure rooms that are not suitable for invasive operations and are not equipped to deliver anesthesia should not be included in the total number of operating rooms.
Number of accredited surgeons and number of accredited anesthesia professionals	Accredited surgeons are physicians who have achieved certification in a surgical specialty as recognized by the accepted national standards of the state or national professional organizations. Accredited anesthesia professionals are physicians, nurses, and other practitioners who have achieved certification in the provision of anesthesia as recognized by the accepted national standards of the state or national professional organizations	The availability and composition of human resources for health is an important indicator of the strength of the health system.	Facility surveys, labor force surveys, and records from professional and administrative sources	Each country can define the acceptable national standards for accreditation of surgeons and anesthesia professionals. The word *professional* in anesthesia professional recognizes the important contribution nonphysician anesthesia practitioners provide in all countries. Individuals who perform surgery or administer anesthesia but are not accredited, including those still in training, should not be included in this measure.

table continues next page

	Definition	Rationale for use	Data sources	Comments
Number of surgical procedures done in an operating room per year	The absolute number of all surgical procedures, defined as the incision, excision, or manipulation of tissue that requires regional or general anesthesia, or profound sedation to control pain, undertaken in an operating room	Surgical volume is an indication of the access to and use of health care, particularly surgical services.	Hospital records and routine health service statistics	Invasive procedures that meet the definition but that are done in a procedure room not suitable for more extensive operations should not be considered in the total number of surgical procedures. If, however, they are done in the operating room, they should be counted.
Day-of-surgery death ratio	Number of deaths on the day of surgery, irrespective of cause, divided by the number of surgical procedures in a given year or period, reported as a percentage	Day-of-surgery death ratios allow the health system to assess its performance and the state of health of the population.	Administrative and hospital records based on health service statistics	Death on the day of surgery often reflects the comorbidities and physiological disorders of the patient, the quality and complexity of surgical care, or the risks of anesthesia. This measure cannot be used to compare one site, facility, or country with another without appropriate, validated, and time-consuming risk adjustment.
Postoperative in-hospital death ratio	Number of deaths in the hospital following surgery, irrespective of cause and limited to 30 days, divided by the number of surgical procedures done in a given year or period, reported as a percentage	The in-hospital death ratio after surgery provides insight into the risks associated with surgical intervention.	Administrative and hospital records based on health service statistics	Patients who undergo surgery and die outside a health facility or after readmission to the same or a different facility are important to record in postoperative mortality assessments. Facilities should be encouraged to gather such information. Neither circumstance is included in this statistic, however.

Source: Weiser and others 2009.

of these metrics has important weaknesses that must be acknowledged, all can be obtained and reported in a straightforward manner.

National-level metrics nonetheless require the interest, investment, and commitment of the central government or agency responsible for collecting, analyzing, and disseminating such information. Local efforts at QI should not be limited to crude, population-level data collected to measure health system performance. Several basic metrics must be adopted by facilities and health systems to improve the quality and delivery of care (table 16.9). These could include the following:

- *Structural metrics,* such as the availability of essential monitors like pulse oximetry; equipment, such as anesthetic machines and autoclaves; and consumable and reusable materials, such as surgical equipment, devices, and antibiotics

- *Process metrics,* such as hours of operation, duration of operations, number of operations per operating room, appropriate administration of antibiotics, and use of and compliance with checklists
- *Outcome metrics beyond mortality,* such as surgical infections and reoperation, and other perioperative complications such as pneumonia, renal failure, heart attack, or stroke

One of the issues of greatest concern is the misuse of such metrics to deny care to the most frail and vulnerable populations. Health systems that manipulate their outcomes by increasing inappropriate services, failing to intervene, and underreporting mortality succumb to perverse, negative incentives that divert essential resources and inhibit care for the sickest patients. Under ideal circumstances, surgical statistics should help health systems improve the delivery

Table 16.9 Proposed Facility-Level Metrics for Quality Improvement, in Addition to the Standardized Statistics Described in Table 16.8

Structural metrics	Process metrics	Outcome metrics
Number of pulse oximeters per operating room	Number of cases performed with pulse oximetry in place for entirety of operation	Surgical-site infection rates
Number of functional anesthetic machines	Number of cases delayed because of lack of equipment or supplies	Percentage of cases requiring reoperation
	Number of cases delayed because of lack of personnel	Other complication rates, for example, transfusion or renal insufficiency
Number of functioning autoclaves	Percentage of cases in full checklist compliance	
	Percentage of cases with appropriate antibiotic administration	
	Percentage of essential surgical procedures transferred to another facility	

and safety of surgical care by creating benchmarks for improvement rather than being used for punishment or comparison across fundamentally different organizations, environments, and populations (WHO 2009b). Attempts at comparisons across systems, countries, and health settings ignore variations in patient condition and complexity of procedure. Hospitals and health systems that wish to evaluate differences between facilities and practitioners must account for the characteristics of the patients, case mix, and urgency—all of which require robust and sophisticated data collection that is frequently beyond the capacity of overworked or underfinanced health systems. However, countries and health systems in LMICs that are able to collect such metrics will have a foundation of information upon which they can improve and sustain surgical care to the betterment of their nation's health.

Any complete discussion of quality clearly encompasses more than simple measures of mortality and complications. Important outcomes also include, among others, the nuanced measures of functional recovery, control of pain, and satisfaction with care. While meaningful, these issues are beyond the scope of this chapter, as are the potentially important strategies for improving surgical capacity through the use of physician extenders and task sharing, and the aggregation and centralization of cases to take advantage of volume-outcome relationships.

Much work is needed to strengthen surgical systems of care, and the investments are likely to be considerable. Given the barriers to access and delivery of needed surgical services, investments are necessary at the facility and institutional level, as well as for the progressive financing of health protection and communication and transportation infrastructure. Improving anesthetic monitoring and safety, implementing surgical checklists, refining

management practices, and instituting measurement and surveillance techniques could dramatically improve care within existing health systems. However, designing, implementing, and scaling these interventions in LMICs will take considerable resources because each strategy for improvement requires training, infrastructure, an information management system, and political will. Even though little is currently known about the actual investment and recurrent costs of introducing and scaling up these strategies, they are likely to be highly cost-effective.

CONCLUSIONS

To avoid premature death, disability, and suffering from the time of birth through adulthood, most human beings require surgical care at some point in their lives. Strategies to increase access to surgical care, however, must also increase the safety and quality of care. Profound consequences, including massively high rates of disability and death, ensue when health systems neglect to use strategies known to improve surgical safety. Profound indirect consequences also follow that are harder to measure but that are also extremely important, including loss of confidence in the health system, late patient presentation, and cost inefficiencies that add to an overburdened and underfunded health system. Well-established interventions have proven effective in reducing surgical risk and provide promising strategies to further reduce harm from surgical care.

ACKNOWLEDGMENTS

The authors would like to thank Charles N. Mock, University of Washington, for his help and guidance with this chapter; Pablo Uribe Leitz, Lydia Maurer, and Joshua Jaramillo, Stanford University, for help with data extraction and analysis; and Marissa Wagner, University of Texas, Houston, and Kimberly Brayton, Stanford University, for their assistance with the initial creation and structuring of the database. They also would like to extend appreciation to Rebecca Kim and Lyen Huang, Stanford University Medical Center; Luke Funk, University of Wisconsin Medical Center; and Kendra Bowman, Brigham and Women's Hospital, for their willingness to share preliminary data. Kristan Staudenmayer, Stanford University, helped review and proof drafts. Riti Shimkhada and John Peabody, Qure Healthcare, provided insightful feedback on metrics for measurement; and Nick Bloom, Stanford University, offered invaluable insights regarding his work on management practices.

ANNEXES

The annexes to this chapter are as follows. They are available at http://www.dcp-3.org/surgery.

- Annex 16A. Search Terms and Bibliographic References per Country
- Annex 16B. WHP Guidelines for Safe Surgery 2009, Objective 10: Hospitals and Public Health Systems Will Establish Routine Surveillance of Surgical Capacity, Volume, and Results

NOTE

The World Bank classifies countries according to four income groupings. Income is measured using gross national income (GNI) per capita, in U.S. dollars, converted from local currency using the *World Bank Atlas* method. Classifications as of July 2014 are as follows:

- Low-income countries (LICs) = US$1,045 or less in 2013
- Middle-income countries (MICs) are subdivided:
  - Lower-middle-income = US$1,046 to US$4,125
  - Upper-middle-income (UMICs) = US$4,126 to US$12,745
- High-income countries (HICs)= US$12,746 or more

REFERENCES

Abantanga, F. A. 2003. "Groin and Scrotal Swellings in Children Aged 5 Years and Below: A Review of 535 Cases." *Pediatric Surgery International* 19 (6): 446–50.

Abantanga, F. A., B. Nimako, and M Amoah. 2009. "The Range of Abdominal Surgical Emergencies in Children Older Than 1 Year at the Komfo Anokye Teaching Hospital, Kumasi, Ghana." *Annals of African Medicine* 8 (4): 236–42.

Abbassi, H., A. Aboulfalah, F. Morsad, N. Matar, A. Himmi, and A. E. Mansouri. 2000. "Maternal Complications of Cesarean Section: Retrospective Analysis of 3,231 Interventions at the Casablanca University Hospital, Morocco." [In French.] *Santé* 10 (6): 419–23.

Aderounmu, A. O., S. A. Afolayan, T. A. Nasiru, J. A. Olaore, M. L. Adeoti, and M. Adelasoye. 2008. "Rotational Rural Surgery for the Poor in Developing Countries." *Tropical Doctor* 38 (3): 141–44.

Adesunkanmi, A. R., T. A. Badmos, and A. A. Salako. 2000. "Groin Hernias in Patients 50 Years of Age and Above Pattern and Outcome of Management in 250 Consecutive Patients." *West African Journal of Medicine* 19 (2): 142–47.

Adisa, A. O., O. I. Alatise, O. A. Arowolo, and O. O Lawal. 2012. "Laparoscopic Appendectomy in a Nigerian Teaching Hospital." *Journal of the Society of Laparoendoscopic Surgeons* 16 (4): 576–80.

Afsana, K. 2004. "The Tremendous Cost of Seeking Hospital Obstetric Care in Bangladesh." *Reproductive Health Matters* 12 (24): 171–80.

Akcakaya, A., et al. 2000. "Mechanical Intestinal Obstruction Caused by Abdominal Wall Hernias." [In Turkish.] *Ulusal Travma Dergisi* [Turkish journal of trauma and emergency surgery] 6 (4): 260–265.

Akinci, M., Z. Ergül, B. Kulah, K. B. Yilmaz, and H. Kulacoğlu. 2010. "Risk Factors Related with Unfavorable Outcomes in Groin Hernia Repairs." *Hernia* 14 (5): 489–93.

Ali, N., and S. Aliyu 2012. "Appendicitis and Its Surgical Management Experience at the University of Maiduguri Teaching Hospital Nigeria." *Nigerian Journal of Medicine* 21 (2): 223–26.

Ameh, E. A. 2002. "Morbidity and Mortality of Inguinal Hernia in the Newborn." *Nigerian Postgraduate Medical Journal* 9 (4): 233–34.

Asefa, Z. 2002. "Acute Appendicitis in Yirgalem Hospital, Southern Ethiopia." *Ethiopian Medical Journal* 40 (2): 155–62.

Awojobi, O. A., and A. A. Ayantunde 2004. "Inguinal Hernia in Nigeria." *Tropical Doctor* 34(3): 180–81.

Ayoade, B. A., O. A. Olawoye, B. A. Salami, and A. A. Banjo. 2006. "Acute Appendicitis in Olabisi Onabanjo University Teaching Hospital Sagamu: A Three-Year Review." *Nigerian Journal of Clinical Practice* 9 (1): 52–56.

Bainbridge, D., J. Martin, M. Arango, and D. Cheng. 2012. "Perioperative and Anaesthetic-Related Mortality in Developed and Developing Countries: A Systematic Review and Meta-Analysis." *The Lancet* 380 (9847): 1075–81.

Bano, N., R. Chaudhri, L. Yasmeen, F. Shafi, and L. Ejaz. 2011. "A Study of Maternal Mortality in 8 Principal Hospitals in Pakistan in 2009." *International Journal of Gynecology and Obstetrics* 114 (3): 255–59.

Basak, S., S. Kanungo, and C. Majhi. 2011. "Symphysiotomy: Is It Obsolete?" *Journal of Obstetrics and Gynaecology Research* 37 (7): 770–74.

Batajoo, H., and N. K. Hazra 2012. "Laparoscopic versus Open Appendectomy in Acute Appendicitis." *Journal of Nepal Health Research Council* 10 (22): 239–42.

Bay-Nielsen, M., H. Kehlet, L. Strand, J. Malmstrom, F. H. Andersen, and others. 2001. "Quality Assessment of 26,304 Herniorrhaphies in Denmark: A Prospective Nationwide Study." *The Lancet* 358 (9288): 1124–28.

Birkmeyer, J. D. 2010. "Strategies for Improving Surgical Quality: Checklists and Beyond." *New England Journal of Medicine* 363 (20): 1963–65.

Blomqvist, P. G., R. E. Andersson, F. Granath, M. P. Lambe, and A. R. Ekbom. 2001. "Mortality after Appendectomy in Sweden, 1987–1996." *Annals of Surgery* 233 (4): 455–60.

Bloom, N., B. Eifert, A. Mahajan, D. McKenzie, and J. Roberts. 2013. "Does Management Matter? Evidence from India." *Quarterly Journal of Economics* 128 (1): 1–51.

Bloom, N., A. Mahajan, D. McKenzie, and J. Roberts. 2010. "Why Do Firms in Developing Countries Have Low Productivity?" *American Economic Review: Papers and Proceedings* 100 (2): 619–23.

Bloom, N., R. Sadun, and J. van Reenen. 2012. "The Organization of Firms across Countries." *Quarterly Journal of Economics* 127 (4): 1663–705.

Bloom, N., and J. van Reenen. 2007. "Measuring and Explaining Management Practices across Firms and Countries." *Quarterly Journal of Economics* 122 (4): 1351–408.

———. 2010. "Why Do Management Practices Differ across Firms and Countries?" *Journal of Economic Perspectives* 24 (1): 203–24.

Bouvier-Colle, M. H., C. Ouedraogo, A. Dumont, C. Vangeenderhuysen, B. Salanave, and C. Decam. 2001. "Maternal Mortality in West Africa: Rates, Causes, and Substandard Care from a Prospective Survey." *Acta Obstetricia et Gynecologica Scandinavica* 80 (2): 113–19.

Bowman, K. G., G. Jovic, S. Rangel, W. R. Berry, and A. A. Gawande. 2013. "Pediatric Emergency and Essential Surgical Care in Zambian Hospitals: A Nationwide Study." *Journal of Pediatric Surgery* 48 (6): 1363–70.

Briand, V., A. Dumont, M. Abrahamowicz, A. Sow, M. Traore, P. Rozenberg, L. Watier, and P. Fournier. 2012. "Maternal and Perinatal Outcomes by Mode of Delivery in Senegal and Mali: A Cross-Sectional Epidemiological Survey." *PLoS One* 7 (10): e47352.

Briesen, S., R. Geneau, H. Roberts, J. Opiyo, and P. Courtright. 2010. "Understanding Why Patients with Cataract Refuse Free Surgery: The Influence of Rumours in Kenya." *Tropical Medicine and International Health* 15 (5): 534–39.

Burch, V. C., D. McKinley, J. van Wyk, S. Kiguli-Walube, D. Cameron, and others. 2011. "Career Intentions of Medical Students Trained in Six Sub-Saharan African Countries." *Education for Health (Abingdon)* 24 (3): 614.

Burn S., P. Chilton, A. Gawande, and R. Lilford. 2014. "Perioperative Pulse Oximetry in Low-Income Countries: A Cost-Effectiveness Analysis." *Bulletin of the World Health Organization* 92: 858–67.

Bury, E., K. Carter, M. Feigelman, and J. Grant. 2007. "How Service-Line Management Can Improve Hospital Performance." *Health International* 7: 54–65. http://www.mckinsey.it/storage/first/uploadfile/attach/140188/file/hi08_5slm_final.pdf.

Carthey, J., M. R. de Leval, and J. T. Reason. 2001. "The Human Factor in Cardiac Surgery: Errors and Near Misses in a High Technology Medical Domain." *Annals of Thoracic Surgery* 72 (1): 300–05.

Ceesay, S. J., C. Casals-Pascual, J. Erskine, S. E. Anya, N. O. Duah, and others. 2008. "Changes in Malaria Indices between 1999 and 2007 in The Gambia: A Retrospective Analysis." *The Lancet* 372 (9649): 1545–54.

Chauhan, A., S. Tiwari, and A. Gupta. 2007. "Study of Efficacy of Bilayer Mesh Device versus Conventional Polypropelene Hernia System in Inguinal Hernia Repair: Early Results." *World Journal of Surgery* 31 (6): 1356–59; discussion 1360–61.

Chamisa, I. 2009. "A Clinicopathological Review of 324 Appendices Removed for Acute Appendicitis in Durban, South Africa: A Retrospective Analysis." *Annals of the Royal College of Surgeons of England* 91 (8): 688–92.

Chavda, S. K., S. Hassan, and G. A. Magoha. 2000. "Appendicitis at Kenyatta National Hospital, Nairobi." *East African Medical Journal* 82 (10): 526–30.

Chilopora, G., C. Pereira, F. Kamwendo, A. Chimbiri, E. Malunga, and S. Bergström. 2007. "Postoperative Outcome of Caesarean Sections and Other Major Emergency Obstetric Surgery by Clinical Officers and Medical Officers in Malawi." *Human Resources for Health* 5: 17.

Chongsuvivatwong, V., H. Bachtiar, M. E. Chowdhury, S. Fernando, C. Suwanrath, O. Kor-Anantakul, A. Tuan le, A. Lim, P. Lumbiganon, B. Manandhar, M. Muchtar, L. Nahar, N. T. Hieu, P. X. Fang, W. Prasertcharoensuk, E. Radnaabarzar, D. Sibuea, K. K. Than, P. Tharnpaisan, T. S. Thach, and P. Rowe. 2010. "Maternal and Fetal Mortality and Complications Associated with Cesarean Section Deliveries in Teaching Hospitals in Asia." *Journal of Obstetrics and Gynaecology Research* 36 (1): 45–51.

Chu, K., H. Cortier, F. Maldonado, T. Mashant, N. Ford, and M. Trelles. 2012. "Cesarean Section Rates and Indications in Sub-Saharan Africa: A Multi-Country Study from Medecins sans Frontieres." *PLoS One* 7 (9): e44484.

Chung, C. H., et al. 2000. "Delays by Patients, Emergency Physicians, and Surgeons in the Management of Acute Appendicitis: Retrospective Study." *Hong Kong Medical Journal* 6 (3): 254–59.

Cingi, A., et al. 2005. "Use of Resterilized Polypropylene Mesh in Inguinal Hernia Repair: A Prospective, Randomized Study." *Journal of the American College of Surgeons* 201 (6): 834–40.

Clarke, M. G., et al. 2009. "The Use of Sterilised Polyester Mosquito Net Mesh for Inguinal Hernia Repair in Ghana." *Hernia* 13 (2): 155–59.

Cunnigaiper, N. D., et al. 2010. "Does Ochsner-Sherren Regimen Still Hold True in the Management of Appendicular Mass?" *Ulusal Travma Ve Acil Cerrahi Dergisi-Turkish Journal of Trauma & Emergency Surgery* 16 (1): 43–46.

Das, J., A. Holla, V. Das, M. Mohanan, D. Tabak, and others. 2012. "In Urban and Rural India, a Standardized Patient Study Showed Low Levels of Provider Training and Huge Quality Gaps." *Health Affairs (Millwood)* 31 (12): 2774–84.

de Leval, M. R., J. Carthey, D. J. Wright, V. T. Farewell, and R. T. Reason. 2000. "Human Factors and Cardiac Surgery: A Multicenter Study." *Journal of Thoracic and Cardiovascular Surgery* 119 (4 Pt 1): 661–72.

de Vries, E. N., H. A. Prins, R. M. Crolla, A. J. den Outer, G. van Andel, and others. 2010. "Effect of a Comprehensive

Surgical Safety System on Patient Outcomes." *New England Journal of Medicine* 363 (20): 1928–37.

Diarra, B., et al. 2001. "Experience with Preperitoneal Hernioplasty Using Stoppa's Procedures in the Ivory Coast." [In French.] *Annales de Chirurgie* 126 (4): 325–29.

Dumont, A., L. de Bernis, M. H. Bouvier-Colle, and G. Breart. 2001. "Caesarean Section Rate for Maternal Indication in Sub-Saharan Africa: A Systematic Review." *The Lancet* 358 (9290): 1328–33.

Dye, T. D., S. Bogale, C. Hobden, Y. Tilahun, V. Hechter, and others. 2010. "Complex Care Systems in Developing Countries: Breast Cancer Patient Navigation in Ethiopia." *Cancer* 116 (3): 577–85.

Eichhorn, J. H., J. B. Cooper, D. J. Cullen, W. R. Maier, J. H. Philip, and others. 1986. "Standards for Patient Monitoring during Anesthesia at Harvard Medical School." *Journal of the American Medical Association* 256 (8): 1017–20.

Ekenze, S. O., P. A. Anyanwu, U. O. Ezomike, and T. Oguonu. 2010. "Profile of Pediatric Abdominal Surgical Emergencies in a Developing Country." *International Surgery* 95 (4): 319–24.

ElRashied, M., A. H. Widatalla, and M. E. Ahmed. 2007. "External Strangulated Hernia in Khartoum, Sudan." *East African Medical Journal* 84 (8): 379–82.

Fahim, F., and S. Shirjeel. 2005. "A Comparison between Presenatation Time and Delay in Surgery in Simple and Advanced Appendicitis." *Journal of Ayub Medical College Abbottabad* 17 (2): 37–39.

Farthouat, P., O. Fall, M. Ogougbemy, A. Sow, A. Millon, and others. 2005. "Appendicectomy in the tropics: Prospective study at Hopital Principal in Dakar." [In French.] *Médecine tropicale (Mars)* 65 (6): 549–53.

Fashina, I. B., A. A. Adesanya, O. A. Atoyebi, O. O. Osinowo, and C. J. Atimomo. 2009. "Acute Appendicitis in Lagos: A Review of 250 Cases." *Nigerian Postgraduate Medical Journal* 16 (4): 268–73.

Fauveau, V. 2007. "Using UN Process Indicators to Assess Needs in Emergency Obstetric Services: Gabon, Guinea-Bissau, and The Gambia." *International Journal of Gynaecology and Obstetrics* 96 (3): 233–40.

Fenton, P. M., C. J. Whitty, and F. Reynolds. 2003. "Caesarean Section in Malawi: Prospective Study of Early Maternal and Perinatal Mortality." *BMJ* 327 (7415): 587.

Fesseha, N., A. Getachew, M. Hiluf, Y. Gebrehiwot, and P. Bailey. 2011. "A National Review of Cesarean Delivery in Ethiopia." *International Journal of Gynecology and Obstetrics* 115 (1): 106–11.

Freudenberg, S., D. Sano, E. Ouangré, C. Weiss, and T. J. Wilhelm. 2006. "Commercial Mesh versus Nylon Mosquito Net for Hernia Repair. A Randomized Double-Blind Study in Burkina Faso." *World Journal of Surgery* 30 (10): 1784–89; discussion 1790.

Funk, L. M., D. M. Conley, W. R. Berry, and A. A. Gawande. 2013. "Hospital Management Practices and Availability of Surgery in Sub-Saharan Africa: A Pilot Study of Three Hospitals." *World Journal of Surgery* 37 (11): 2520–28.

Funk, L. M., T. G. Weiser, W. R. Berry, S. R. Lipsitz, A. F. Merry, and others. 2010. "Global Operating Theatre Distribution and Pulse Oximetry Supply: An Estimation from Reported Data." *The Lancet* 376 (9746): 1055–61.

Gao, J. S., Z. J. Wang, B. Zhao, S. Z. Ma, G. Y. Pang, and others. 2009. "Inguinal Hernia Repair with Tension-Free Hernioplasty under Local Anesthesia." *Saudi Medical Journal* 30 (4): 534–36.

Gauthier, B., and W. Wane. 2011. "Bypassing Health Providers: The Quest for Better Price and Quality of Health Care in Chad." *Social Science and Medicine* 73 (4): 540–49.

Gavilan-Yodu, R. L. 2010. "Morbilidad y mortalidad por apendicitis aguda en el hospital integral comunitario del municipio Monteagudo (2006–2008)." *MEDISAN* 14: 2010–2016.

Ghaferi, A. A., J. D. Birkmeyer, and J. B. Dimick. 2009a. "Complications, Failure to Rescue, and Mortality with Major Inpatient Surgery in Medicare Patients." *Annals of Surgery* 250 (6): 1029–34.

———. 2009b. "Variation in Hospital Mortality Associated with Inpatient Surgery." *New England Journal of Medicine* 361 (14): 1368–75.

———. 2011. "Hospital Volume and Failure to Rescue with High-Risk Surgery." *Medical Care* 49 (12): 1076–81.

Gibbons, L., J. M. Belizán, J. A. Lauer, A. P. Betrán, M. Merialdi, and others. 2010. "The Global Numbers and Costs of Additionally Needed and Unnecessary Caesarean Sections Performed per Year: Overuse as a Barrier to Universal Coverage." World Health Report Background Paper 30, World Health Organization, Geneva.

Gil, J., J. M. Rodríguez, Q. Hernández, E. Gil, M. D. Balsalobre, and others. 2012. "Do Hernia Operations in African International Cooperation Programmes Provide Good Quality?" *World Journal of Surgery* 36 (12): 2795–801.

Glenshaw, M., and F. D. Madzimbamuto. 2005. "Anaesthesia-Associated Mortality in a District Hospital in Zimbabwe: 1994 to 2001." *Central African Journal of Medicine* 51 (3–4): 39–44.

Goldie, S. J. 2003. "Chapter 15: Public Health Policy and Cost-Effectiveness Analysis." *Journal of the National Cancer Institute Monograph* 31: 102–10.

Grimes, C. E., K. G. Bowman, C. M. Dodgion, and C. B. Lavy. 2011. "Systematic Review of Barriers to Surgical Care in Low-Income and Middle-Income Countries." *World Journal of Surgery* 35 (5): 941–50.

Groen, R. S., M. Samai, K. A. Stewart, L. D. Cassidy, T. B. Kamara, and others. 2012. "Untreated Surgical Conditions in Sierra Leone: A Cluster Randomised, Cross-Sectional, Countrywide Survey." *The Lancet* 380 (9847): 1082–87.

Gurleyik, G., and E. Gurleyik. 2003. "Age-Related Clinical Features in Older Patients with Acute Appendicitis." *European Journal of Emergency Medicine* 10 (3): 200–03.

Hang, H. M., and P. Byass. 2009. "Difficulties in Getting Treatment for Injuries in Rural Vietnam." *Public Health* 123 (1): 58–65.

Harouna, Y., H. Yaya, I. Abdou, and L. Bazira. 2001. "Prognosis of Strangulated Hernia in Adult With Necrosis of Small Bowel: A 34 Cases Report." *Bulletin de la Societe de Pathologie Exotique* 93 (5): 317–20.

Haynes, A. B., T. G. Weiser, W. R. Berry, S. R. Lipsitz, A. H. Breizat, and others. 2009. "A Surgical Safety Checklist to Reduce Morbidity and Mortality in a Global Population." *New England Journal of Medicine* 360 (5): 491–99.

Hogberg, U. 1989. "Maternal Deaths Related to Cesarean Section in Sweden, 1951–1980." *Acta Obstetricia et Gynecologica Scandinavica* 68 (4): 351–57.

Huang, C. S., C. C. Huang, and H. H. Lien. 2005. "Prolene Hernia System Compared with Mesh Plug Technique: A Prospective Study of Short- to Mid-term Outcomes in Primary Groin Hernia Repair." *Hernia* 9 (2): 167–71.

Hughes, C. D., C. D. McClain, L. Hagander, J. H. Pierre, R. S. Groen, and others. 2012. "Ratio of Cesarean Deliveries to Total Operations and Surgeon Nationality Are Potential Proxies for Surgical Capacity in Central Haiti." *World Journal of Surgery* 37 (7): 1526–29. doi:10.1007/s00268-012-1794-7.

Ibis, C., D. Albayrak, A. R. Hatipoglu, and N. Turan. 2010. "The Amount of Comorbidities as a Single Parameter Has No Effect in Predicting the Outcome in Appendicitis Patients Older Than 60 Years." *Southern Medical Journal* 103 (3): 202–06.

Imbert, P., F. Berger, N. S. Diallo, C. Cellier, M. Goumbala, A. S. Ka, and R. Petrognani. 2003. "Maternal and Infant Prognosis of Emergency Cesarean Section: Prospective Study of the Principal Hospital in Dakar, Senegal." [In French.] *Médecine tropicale: Revue du Corps de santé colonial* 63 (4–5): 351–57.

Jani, K. 2005. "Prospective Randomized Study of Internal Oblique Aponeurotic Flap Repair for Tension-Free Reinforcement of the Posterior Inguinal Wall: A New Technique." *International Surgery* 90 (3): 155–59.

Juillard, C. J., C. Mock, J. Goosen, M. Joshipura, and I. Civil. 2009. "Establishing the Evidence Base for Trauma Quality Improvement: A Collaborative WHO-IAtypesetterIC Review." *World Journal of Surgery* 33 (5): 1075–86.

Kaboro, M., M. A. Djibril, E. Zoumendou, P. Assouto, T. Lokossou, and M. Chobli. 2012. "L'anesthésie en urgence à la maternité de l'hôpital général de réfence national de N'Djaména (Tchad)." *Médecine-afrique-noire* 4 (59): 211–20.

Kahabuka, C., G. Kvale, K. M. Moland, and S. G. Hinderaker. 2011. "Why Caretakers Bypass Primary Health Care Facilities for Child Care: A Case from Rural Tanzania." *BMC Health Services Research* 11: 315.

Kambo, I., N. Bedi, B. S. Dhillon, and N. C. Saxena. 2002. "A Critical Appraisal of Cesarean Section Rates at Teaching Hospitals in India." *International Journal of Gynecology and Obstetrics* 79 (2): 151–58.

Kandasamy, T., M. Merialdi, R. J. Guidotti, A. P. Betran, J. Harris-Requejo, F. Hakimi, P. F. van Look, and F. Kakar. 2009. "Cesarean Delivery Surveillance System at a Maternity Hospital in Kabul, Afghanistan." *International Journal of Gynecology and Obstetrics* 104 (1): 14–17.

Kargar, S., M. H. Mirshamsi, M. Zare, S. Arefanian, E. Shadman Yazdi, and A. Aref. 2011. "Laparoscopic versus Open Appendectomy; Which Method to Choose? A Prospective Randomized Comparison." *Acta Medica Iranica* 49 (6): 352–56.

Kasatpibal, N., M. Nørgaard, H. T. Sørensen, H. C. Schønheyder, S. Jamulitrat, and V. Chongsuvivatwong. 2006. "Risk of Surgical Site Infection and Efficacy of Antibiotic Prophylaxis: A Cohort Study of Appendectomy Patients in Thailand." *BMC Infectious Diseases* 6: 111.

Kelly, J., E. Kohls, P. Poovan, R. Schiffer, A. Redito, H. Winter, and C. MacArthur. 2010. "The Role of a Maternity Waiting Area (MWA) in Reducing Maternal Mortality and Stillbirths in High-Risk Women in Rural Ethiopia." *BJOG: An International Journal of Obstetrics and Gynaecology* 117 (11): 1377–83.

Khalil, J., R. Muqim, M. Rafique, and M. Khan. 2011. "Laparoscopic versus Open Appendectomy: A Comparison of Primary Outcome Measures." *Saudi Journal of Gastroenterology* 17 (4): 236–40.

Khan, K. I., S. Mahmood, M. Akmal, and A. Waqas. 2012. "Comparison of Rate of Surgical Wound Infection, Length of Hospital Stay and Patient Convenience in Complicated Appendicitis between Primary Closure and Delayed Primary Closure." *Journal of the Pakistan Medical Association* 62 (6): 596–98.

Khiria, L. S., R. Ardhnari, N. Mohan, P. Kumar, and R. Nambiar. 2011. "Laparoscopic Appendicectomy for Complicated Appendicitis: Is It Safe and Justified? A Retrospective Analysis." *Surgical Laparoscopy, Endoscopy, and Percutaneous Techniques* 21 (3): 142–45.

Kilsztajn, S., M. S. Carmo, L. C. Machado Jr., E. S. Lopes, and L. Z. Lima. 2007. "Caesarean Sections and Maternal Mortality in São Paulo." *European Journal of Obstetrics and Gynecology and Reproductive Biology* 132 (1): 64–69.

Kim, Y. M., H. Tappis, P. Zainullah, N. Ansara, C. Evans, and others. 2012. "Quality of Caesarean Delivery Services and Documentation in First-Line Referral Facilities in Afghanistan: A Chart Review." *BMC Pregnancy and Childbirth* 12: 14. doi:10.1186/1471-2393-12-14.

Kingsnorth, A. N., C. Oppong, J. Akoh, B. Stephenson, and R. Simmermacher. 2006. "Operation Hernia to Ghana." *Hernia* 10 (5): 376–79.

Kong, V. Y., B. Bulajic, N. L. Allorto, J. Handley, and D. L. Clarke. 2012. "Acute Appendicitis in a Developing Country." *World Journal of Surgery* 36 (9): 2068–73.

Kor-Anantakul, O., C. Suwanrath, A. Lim, and V. Chongsuviwatwon. 2008. "Comparing Complications in Intended Vaginal and Caesarean Deliveries." *Journal of Obstetrics and Gynaecology Research* 28 (1): 64–68.

Kruk, M. E., E. Goldmann, and S. Galea. 2009. "Borrowing and Selling to Pay for Health Care in Low- and Middle-Income Countries." *Health Affairs (Millwood)* 28 (4): 1056–66.

Kruk, M. E., G. Mbaruku, C. W. McCord, M. Moran, P. C. Rockers, and others. 2009. "Bypassing Primary Care Facilities for Childbirth: A Population-Based Study in Rural Tanzania." *Health Policy and Planning* 24 (4): 279–88.

Kumar, S. and S. Jain. 2004. "Treatment of Appendiceal Mass: Prospective, Randomized Clinical Trial." *Indian Journal of Gastroenterology* 23 (5): 165–67.

Kushner, A. L., R. S. Groen, and T. P. Kingham. 2010. "Percentage of Cesarean Sections among Total Surgical Procedures in Sub-Saharan Africa: Possible Indicator of the Overall Adequacy of Surgical Care." *World Journal of Surgery* 34 (9): 2007–08.

Kwok, A. C., L. M. Funk, R. Baltaga, S. R. Lipsitz, A. F. Merry, and others. 2013. "Implementation of the World Health Organization Surgical Safety Checklist, Including Introduction of Pulse Oximetry, in a Resource-Limited Setting." *Annals of Surgery* 257 (4): 633–39.

Lagoo, J., J. Wilkinson, J. Thacker, M. Deshmukh, S. Khorgade, and R. Bang. 2012. "Impact of Anemia on Surgical Outcomes: Innovative Interventions in Resource-Poor Settings." *World Journal of Surgery* 36 (9): 2080–89.

Lau, H., C. Wong, L. C. Goh, N. G. Patil, and F. Lee. 2002. "Prospective Randomized Trial of Pre-emptive Analgesics Following Ambulatory Inguinal Hernia Repair: Intravenous Ketorolac versus Diclofenac Suppository." *ANZ Journal of Surgery* 72 (10): 704–07.

Lebrun, D. G., S. Chackungal, T. E. Chao, L. M. Knowlton, A. F. Linden, and others. 2014. "Prioritizing Essential Surgery and Safe Anesthesia for the Post-2015 Development Agenda: Operative Capacities of 78 District Hospitals in 7 Low- and Middle-Income Countries." *Surgery* 155 (3): 365–73.

Lebrun, D. G., D. Dhar, M. I. Sarkar, T. M. Imran, S. N. Kazi, and others. 2013. "Measuring Global Surgical Disparities: A Survey of Surgical and Anesthesia Infrastructure in Bangladesh." *World Journal of Surgery* 37 (1): 24–31.

Leitch, J. 2012. "Measuring Outcomes across a Nation: The Scottish Experience." Presentation to the International Society for Quality in Healthcare International Conference, Geneva, October 21–24, 2012. http://www.isqua.org/docs /geneva-presentations/b16-jason-leitch.pdf.

Levy, S. M., C. E. Senter, R. B. Hawkins, J. Y. Zhao, K. Doody, and others. 2012. "Implementing a Surgical Checklist: More Than Checking a Box." *Surgery* 152 (3): 331–36.

Liu, Z. F., J. C. Yu, H. F. Hsieh, and C. H. Lin. 2007. "Perforated Appendicitis: Urgency or Interval Surgery?" *Zentralblatt für Chirurgie* 132 (6): 539–41

Lohsiriwat, V., W. Sridermma, T. Akaraviputh, W. Boonnuch, V. Chinsawangwatthanakol, and others. 2007. "Surgical Outcomes of Lichtenstein Tension-Free Hernioplasty for Acutely Incarcerated Inguinal Hernia." *Surgery Today* 37 (3): 212–14.

Lumbiganon, P., M. Laopaiboon, A. M. Gulmezoglu, J. P. Souza, S. Taneepanichskul, P. Ruyan, D. E. Attygalle, N. Shrestha, R. Mori, D. H. Nguyen, T. B. Hoang, T. Rathavy, K. Chuyun, K. Cheang, M. Festin, V. Udomprasertgul, M. J. Germar, G. Yanqiu, M. Roy, G. Carroli, K. Ba-Thike, E. Filatova, and J. Villar. 2010. "Method of Delivery and Pregnancy Outcomes in Asia: the WHO Global Survey on Maternal and Perinatal Health 2007–08." *The Lancet* 375 (9713): 490–99.

Mabiala-Babela, J. R., N. Pandzou, E. Koutaba, S. Ganga-Zandzou, and P. Senga. 2006. "Retrospective Study of Visceral Surgical Emergencies in Children at the University Hospital Center of Brazzaville (Congo)." [In French.] *Médecine tropicale (Mars)* 66 (2): 172–76.

Mabula, J. B. and P. L. Chalya. 2012. "Surgical Management of Inguinal Hernias at Bugando Medical Centre in Northwestern Tanzania: Our Experiences in a Resource-Limited Setting." *BMC Research Notes* 5: 585.

Macharia, W. M., E. K. Njeru, F. Muli-Musiime, and V. Nantulya. 2009. "Severe Road Traffic Injuries in Kenya, Quality of Care and Access." *African Health Sciences* 9 (2): 118–24.

Malik, A. A., S. S. Yamamoto, A. Souares, Z. Malik, and R. Sauerborn. 2010. "Motivational Determinants among Physicians in Lahore, Pakistan." *BMC Health Services Research* 10: 201.

Malik, A.M., A.H. Talpur, and A.A. Laghari. 2009. "Video-Assisted Laparoscopic Extracorporeal Appendectomy versus Open Appendectomy." *Journal of Laparoendoscopic and Advanced Surgical Techniques* 19 (3): 355–59.

Malik, A. M., A. Khan, K. A. Talpur, and A. A. Laghari. 2010. "Factors Influencing Morbidity and Mortality in Elderly Population Undergoing Inguinal Hernia Surgery." *Journal of the Pakistan Medical Association* 60 (1): 45–47.

Mbah, N. 2007. "Morbidity and Mortality Associated with Inguinal Hernia in Northwestern Nigeria." *West African Journal of Medicine* 26 (4): 288–92.

McConkey, S. J. 2002. "Case Series of Acute Abdominal Surgery in Rural Sierra Leone." *World Journal of Surgery* 26 (4): 509–13.

McIntyre, D., M. Thiede, and S. Birch. 2009. "Access as a Policy-Relevant Concept in Low- and Middle-Income Countries." *Health Economics, Policy and Law* 4 (Pt 2): 179–93.

Mehrabi Bahar, M., A. Jangjoo, A. Amouzeshi, and K. Kavianifar. 2010. "Wound Infection Incidence in Patients with Simple and Gangrenous or Perforated Appendicitis." *Archives of Iranian Medicine* 13 (1): 13–16.

Memon, A. A., F. G. Siddiqui, A. H. Abro, A. H. Agha, S. Lubna, and A. S.Memon. 2013. "Management of Recurrent Inguinal Hernia at a Tertiary Care Hospital of Southern Sindh, Pakistan." *World Journal of Surgery* 37 (3): 510–15.

Ming, P. C., T. Y. Yan, and L. H. Tat. 2009. "Risk Factors of Postoperative Infections in Adults with Complicated Appendicitis." *Surgical Laparoscopy, Endoscopy, and Percutaneous Techniques* 19 (3): 244–48.

Ministère de la Santé Burkina Faso. 2013. "Annuaire statistique 2012." http://www.sante.gov.bf/index.php/publications -statistiques/file/338-annuaire-statistique-2012. (Accessed March 5, 2014.)

Mock, C. N., D. nii-Amon-Kotei, and R. V. Maier. 1997. "Low Utilization of Formal Medical Services by Injured Persons in a Developing Nation: Health Service Data Underestimate the Importance of Trauma." *Journal of Trauma* 42 (3): 504–11.

Mungadi, I. A. 2005. "Quality Surgical Care for Rural Dwellers: The Visiting Option." *Tropical Doctor* 35 (3): 151–53.

Neily, J., P. D. Mills, Y. Young-Xu, B. T. Carney, P. West, and others. 2010. "Association between Implementation of a Medical Team Training Program and Surgical Mortality." *Journal of the American Medical Association* 304 (15): 1693–700.

Ngowe Ngowe, M., J. Bissou Mahop, R. Atangana, V. C. Eyenga, C. Pisoh-Tangnym, and A. M. Sosso. 2008. "Current Clinical Features of Acute Appendicitis in Adults in Yaounde, Cameroon." [In French.] *Bulletin de la Société de pathologie exotique* 101 (5): 398–99.

Nguyen, H., R. Ivers, S. Jan, A. Martiniuk, and C. Pham. 2013. "Catastrophic Household Costs Due to Injury in Vietnam." *Injury* 44 (5): 684–90.

Nilsson, H., G. Stylianidis, M. Haapamaki, E. Nilsson, and P. Nordin. 2007. "Mortality after Groin Hernia Surgery." *Annals of Surgery* 245 (4): 656–60.

Nolan, T., and D. M. Berwick. 2006. "All-or-None Measurement Raises the Bar on Performance." *Journal of the American Medical Association* 295 (10): 1168–70.

Noordzij, P. G., D. Poldermans, O. Schouten, J. J. Bax, F. A. Schreiner, and others. 2010. "Postoperative Mortality in the Netherlands: A Population-Based Analysis of Surgery-Specific Risk in Adults." *Anesthesiology* 112 (5): 1105–15.

Nwameme, A. U., J. F. Phillips, and P. B. Adongo. 2013. "Compliance with Emergency Obstetric Care Referrals among Pregnant Women in an Urban Informal Settlement of Accra, Ghana." *Maternal and Child Health Journal*. Advance online publication. doi:10.1007/s10995-013-1380-0.

Obalum, D. C., S. U. Eyesan, C. N. Ogo, and O. A. Atoyebi. 2008. "Day-Case Surgery for Inguinal Hernia: A Multi-Specialist Private Hospital Experience in Nigeria." *Nigerian Quarterly Journal of Hospital Medicine* 18 (1): 42–44.

Ohene-Yeboah, M. 2003. "Strangulated External Hernias in Kumasi." *West African Journal of Medicine* 22 (4): 310–13.

Ohene-Yeboah, M., and B. Togbe. 2006. "An Audit of Appendicitis and Appendicectomy in Kumasi, Ghana." *West African Journal of Medicine* 25 (2): 138–43.

Okafor, P. I., J. C. Orakwe, and G. U. Chianakwana. 2003. "Management of Appendiceal Masses in a Peripheral Hospital in Nigeria: Review of Thirty Cases." *World Journal of Surgery* 27 (7): 800–803.

Okafor, U. V., H. U. Ezegwui, and K. Ekwazi. 2009. "Trends of Different Forms of Anaesthesia for Caesarean Section in South-Eastern Nigeria." *Journal of Obstetrics and Gynaecology Research* 29 (5): 392–95.

Okafor, U. V. and O. Okezie 2005. "Maternal and Fetal Outcome of Anaesthesia for Caesarean Delivery in Preeclampsia/Eclampsia in Enugu, Nigeria: A Retrospective Observational Study." *International Journal of Obstetric Anesthesia* 14 (2): 108–13.

Okezie, A. O., B. Oyefara, and C. O. Chigbu. 2007. "A 4-year Analysis of Caesarean Delivery in a Nigerian Teaching Hospital: One-Quarter of Babies Born Surgically." *Journal of Obstetrics and Gynaecology* 27 (5): 470–74.

Oladapo, O. T., M. A. Lamina, and A. O. Sule-Odu. 2007. "Maternal Morbidity and Mortality Associated with Elective Caesarean Delivery at a University Hospital in Nigeria." *Australian and New Zealand Journal of Obstetrics and Gynaecology* 47 (2): 110–14.

Osifo, O. D., and O. O. Irowa. 2008. "Indirect Inguinal Hernia in Nigerian Older Children and Young Adults: Is Herniorrhaphy Necessary?" *Hernia* 12 (6): 635–39.

Osifo, O. D., and S. O. Ogiemwonyi. 2009. "Appendicitis in Children: An Increasing Health Scourge in a Developing Country." *Pakistan Journal of Medical Sciences* 25 (3): 490–95.

Ozumba, B. C., and S. E. Anya. 2002. "Maternal Deaths Associated with Cesarean Section in Enugu, Nigeria." *International Journal of Gynecology and Obstetrics* 76 (3): 307–9.

Parkhurst, J. O., S. A. Rahman, and F. Ssengooba. 2006. "Overcoming Access Barriers for Facility-Based Delivery in Low-Income Settings: Insights from Bangladesh and Uganda." *Journal of Health, Population and Nutrition* 24 (4): 438–45.

Paudel, R. K., B. K. Jain, S. Rani, S. K. Gupta, and S. R. Niraula. 2003. "Acute Appendicitis: A Quality Assurance Study." *Tropical Gastroenterology* 24 (2): 83–86.

Pearse, R. M., R. P. Moreno, P. Bauer, P. Pelosi, P. Metnitz, and others. 2012. "Mortality after Surgery in Europe: A 7 Day Cohort Study." *The Lancet* 380 (9847): 1059–65.

Peralta Vargas, C. E., A. López, J. R. Díaz Gil, R. M. Rodríguez Montoya, and W. R. Angulo Guzmán. 2004. "Surgical Wound Infection in Appendectomized Patients in the Surgical Service of Hospital III Essalud-Chimbote." [In Spanish.] *Revista de gastroenterología del Perú* 24 (1): 43–49.

Petroze, R. T., W. Mehtsun, A. Nzayisenga, G. Ntakiyiruta, R. G. Sawyer, and others. 2012. "Ratio of Cesarean Sections to Total Procedures as a Marker of District Hospital Trauma Capacity." *World Journal of Surgery* 36 (9): 2074–79.

Petroze, R. T., A. Nzayisenga, V. Rusanganwa, G. Ntakiyiruta, and J. F. Calland. 2012. "Comprehensive National Analysis of Emergency and Essential Surgical Capacity in Rwanda." *British Journal of Surgery* 99 (3): 436–43.

Pokharel, N., P. Sapkota, B. Kc, S. Rimal, S. Thapa, and R. Shakya. 2011. "Acute appendicitis in Elderly Patients: A Challenge for Surgeons." *Nepal Medical College Journal* 13 (4): 285–88.

Pradhan, G. B., D. Shrestha, S. Shrestha, and C. L. Bhattachan. 2011. "Inguinal Herniotomy in Children: A One Year Survey at Nepal Medical College Teaching Hospital." *Nepal Medical College Journal* 13 (4): 301–2.

Ramyil, V. M., D. Iya, B. C. Ogbonna, and N. K. Dakum. 2000. "Safety of Daycare Hernia Repair in Jos, Nigeria." *East African Medical Journal* 77 (6): 326–28.

Rahlenbeck, S., and C. Hakizimana. 2002. "Deliveries at a District Hospital in Rwanda, 1997–2000." *International Journal of Gynecology and Obstetrics* 76(3): 325–28.

Rogers, A. D., M. I. Hampton, M. Bunting, and A. K. Atherstone. 2008. "Audit of Appendicectomies at Frere Hospital, Eastern Cape." *South African Journal of Surgery* 46 (3): 74–77.

Ronsmans, C., and W. J. Graham. 2006. "Maternal Mortality: Who, When, Where, and Why." *The Lancet* 368 (9542): 1189–200.

Rutgers, R. A., and L. van Eygen. 2008. "Mortality Related to Caesarean Section in Rural Matebeleland North Province, Zimbabwe." *Central African Journal of Medicine* 54 (5–8): 24–27.

Saha, N., D. K. Saha, M. A. Rahman, M. K. Islam, and M. A. Aziz. 2010. "Comparison of Post Operative Morbidity between Laparoscopic and Open Appendectomy in Children." *Mymensingh Medical Journal: MMJ* 19 (3): 348–52.

Salahuddin, O., M. A. Malik, M. A. Sajid, M. Azhar, O. Dilawar, and A. Salahuddin. 2012. "Acute Appendicitis in the Elderly; Pakistan Ordnance Factories Hospital, Wah Cantt. Experience." *Journal of the Pakistan Medical Association* 62 (9): 946–49.

Samaali, I., S. Ben Osman, R. Bedoui, I. Bouasker, Y. Chaker, and others. 2012. "Spinal Anesthesia versus General Anesthesia for Inguinal Hernia Repair: Propensity Score Analysis." [In French.] *Tunisie Médicale* 90 (10): 686–91.

Sanders, D. L., and A. N. Kingsnorth. 2007. "Operation Hernia: Humanitarian Hernia Repairs in Ghana." *Hernia* 11 (5): 389–91.

Scarlett, M., A. Crawford-Sykes, M. Thomas, and N. D. Duncan. 2007. "Paediatric Day Surgery: Revisiting the University Hospital of the West Indies Experience." *West Indian Medical Journal* 56 (4): 320–25.

Schuitemaker, N., J. van Roosmalen, G. Dekker, P. van Dongen, H. van Geijn, and J. B. Gravenhorst. 1997. "Maternal Mortality after Cesarean Section in the Netherlands." *Acta Obstetricia et Gynecologica Scandinavica* 76 (4): 332–34.

Seal, S. L., G. Kamilya, J. Mukherji, S. K. Bhattacharyya, A. De, and A. Hazra. 2010. "Outcome in Second- versus First-Stage Cesarean Delivery in a Teaching Institution in Eastern India." *American Journal of Perinatology* 27 (6): 507–12.

Sekirime, W. K., and J. C. Lule. 2008. "Maternal Morbidity Following Emergency Caesarean Section in Asymptomatic HIV-1 Infected Patients in Mulago Hospital Kampala, Uganda." *Journal of Obstetrics and Gynaecology Research* 28 (7): 703–9.

Seljeskog, L., J. Sundby, and J. Chimango. 2006. "Factors Influencing Women's Choice of Place of Delivery in Rural Malawi: An Explorative Study." *African Journal of Reproductive Health* 10 (3): 66–75.

Semel, M. E., S. R. Lipsitz, L. M. Funk, A. M. Bader, T. G. Weiser, and others. 2012. "Rates and Patterns of Death after Surgery in the United States, 1996 and 2006." *Surgery* 151 (2): 171–82.

Séréngbé, B. G., A. Gaudeuille, A. Soumouk, J. C. Gody, S. Yassibanda, and J. L. Mandaba. 2002. "Acute Abdominal Pain in Children at the Pediatric Hospital in Bangui (Central African Republic). Epidemiological, Clinical, Paraclinical, Therapeutic and Evolutive Aspects." [In French.] *Archives des pédiatrie* 9 (2): 136–41.

Shaikh, A. R., A. M. Rao, and A. Muneer. 2012. "Inguinal Mesh Hernioplasty under Local Anaesthesia." *Journal of the Pakistan Medical Association* 62 (6): 566–69.

Shaikh, A. R., A. K. Sangrasi, and G. A. Shaikh. 2009. "Clinical Outcomes of Laparoscopic versus Open Appendectomy." *Journal of the Society of Laparoendoscopic Surgeons* 13 (4): 574–80.

Shi, Y., Z. Su, L. Li, H. Liu, and C. Jing. 2010. "Comparing the Effects of Bassini versus Tension-Free Hernioplasty: Three Years' Follow-Up." *Frontiers of Medicine in China* 4 (4): 463–68.

Shillcutt, S. D., M. G. Clarke, and A. N. Kingsnorth. 2010. "Cost-Effectiveness of Groin Hernia Surgery in the Western Region of Ghana." *Archives of Surgery* 145 (10): 954–61.

Shillcutt, S. D., D. L. Sanders, M. Teresa Butrón-Vila, and A. N. Kingsnorth. 2013. "Cost-Effectiveness of Inguinal Hernia Surgery in Northwestern Ecuador." *World Journal of Surgery* 37 (1): 32–41.

Silber, J. H., S. V. Williams, H. Krakauer, and J. S. Schwartz. 1992. "Hospital and Patient Characteristics Associated with Death after Surgery: A Study of Adverse Occurrence and Failure to Rescue." *Medical Care* 30 (7): 615–29.

Sorbye, I. K., S. Vangen, O. Oneko, J. Sundby, and P. Bergsjo. 2011. "Caesarean Section among Referred and Self-Referred Birthing Women: A Cohort Study from a Tertiary Hospital, Northeastern Tanzania." *BMC Pregnancy and Childbirth* 11 (55).

Stulberg, J. J., C. P. Delaney, D. V. Neuhauser, D. C. Aron, P. Fu, and S. M. Koroukian. 2010. "Adherence to Surgical Care Improvement Project Measures and the Association with Postoperative Infections." *Journal of the American Medical Association* 303 (24): 2479–85.

Taqvi, S. R., J. Akhtar, T. Batool, R. Tabassum, and F. Mirza. 2006. "Complications of Inguinal Hernia Surgery in Children." *Journal of the College of Physicians and Surgeons, Pakistan* 16 (8): 532–35.

Terzi, A., F. Yildiz, M. Vural, S. Coban, H. Cece, and M. Kaya. 2010. "A Case Series of 46 Appendectomies during Pregnancy." *Wien Klin Wochenschr* 122 (23–24): 686–690.

Thaddeus, S., and D. Maine. 1994. "Too Far to Walk: Maternal Mortality in Context." *Social Science and Medicine* 38 (8): 1091–110.

Tshibangu, K. C., M. A. de Jongh, D. J. de Villiers, J. J. du Toit, and S. M. Shah. 2002. "Incidence and Outcome of Caesarean Section in the Private Sector--3-Year Experience at Pretoria Gynaecological Hospital." *South African Medical Journal* 92 (12): 956–59.

Turaga, K. K., N. Garg, M. Coeling, K. Smith, B. Amirlak, and others. 2006. "Inguinal Hernia Repair in a Developing Country." *Hernia* 10 (4): 294–98.

Urbach, D. R., A. Govindarajan, R. Saskin, A. S. Wilton, and N. N. Baxter. 2014. "Introduction of Surgical Safety Checklists in Ontario, Canada." *New England Journal of Medicine* 370 (11): 1029–38.

Usang, U. E., O. A. Sowande, O. Adejuyigbe, T. I. Bakare, and O. A. Ademuyiwa. 2008. "The Role of Preoperative Antibiotics in the Prevention of Wound Infection after Day Case Surgery for Inguinal Hernia in Children in Ile Ife, Nigeria." *Pediatric Surgery International* 24 (10): 1181–85.

Utpal, D. 2005. "Laparoscopic versus Open Appendectomy in West Bengal, India." *Chinese Journal of Digestive Diseases* 6 (4): 165–69.

van Klei, W. A., R. G. Hoff, E. E. van Aarnhem, R. K. Simmermacher, L. P. Regli, and others. 2012. "Effects of the Introduction of the WHO Surgical Safety Checklist on In-Hospital Mortality: A Cohort Study." *Annals of Surgery* 255 (1): 44–9.

Van Minh, H., N. T. Kim Phuong, P. Saksena, C. D. James, and K. Xu. 2013. "Financial Burden of Household Out-of Pocket Health Expenditure in Viet Nam: Findings from the National Living Standard Survey 2002–2010." *Social Science and Medicine* 96: 258–63.

Villar, J., G. Carroli, N. Zavaleta, A. Donner, D. Wojdyla, A. Faundes, A. Velazco, V. Bataglia, A. Langer, A. Narvaez, E. Valladares, A. Shah, L. Campodonico, M. Romero, S. Reynoso, K. S. de Padua, D. Giordano, M. Kublickas, and A. Acosta. 2007. "Maternal and Neonatal Individual Risks and Benefits Associated with Caesarean Delivery: Multicentre Prospective Study." *BMJ* 335 (7628): 1025.

Walk, R. M., J. Glaser, L. M. Marmon, T. F. Donahue, J. Bastien, and S. D. Safford. 2012. "Continuing Promise 2009-Assessment of a Recent Pediatric Surgical Humanitarian Mission." *Journal of Pediatric Surgery* 47 (4): 652–57.

Walker, I. A., and I. H. Wilson. 2008. "Anaesthesia in Developing Countries: A Risk for Patients." *The Lancet* 371 (9617): 968–69.

Weiser, T. G. 2010. "Health Policy: All-or-None Compliance is the Best Determinant of Quality of Care." *Nature Reviews Urology* 7 (10): 541–42.

Weiser, T. G., A. B. Haynes, G. Dziekan, W. R. Berry, S. R. Lipsitz, and others. 2010. "Effect of a 19-Item Surgical Safety Checklist during Urgent Operations in a Global Patient Population." *Annals of Surgery* 251 (5): 976–80.

Weiser, T. G., A. B. Haynes, A. Lashoher, G. Dziekan, D. J. Boorman, and others. 2010. "Perspectives in Quality: Designing the WHO Surgical Safety Checklist." *International Journal for Quality in Health Care* 22 (5): 365–70.

Weiser, T. G., M. A. Makary, A. B. Haynes, G. Dziekan, W. R. Berry, and others. 2009. "Standardised Metrics for Global Surgical Surveillance." *The Lancet* 374 (9695): 1113–17.

Weiser, T. G., S. E. Regenbogen, K. D. Thompson, A. B. Haynes, S. R. Lipsitz, and others. 2008. "An Estimation of the Global Volume of Surgery: A Modelling Strategy Based on Available Data." *The Lancet* 372 (9633): 139–44.

Weiser, T. G., M. E. Semel, A. E. Simon, S. R. Lipsitz, A. B. Haynes, and others. 2011. "In-Hospital Death Following Inpatient Surgical Procedures in the United States, 1996–2006." *World Journal of Surgery* 35 (9): 1950–56.

WFSA (World Federation of Societies of Anesthesiologists). 2008. "2008 International Standards for Safe Practice of Anaesthesia." WFSA, London. http://www.anaesthesiologists .org.

WHO (World Health Organization). 2000. "Millennium Development Goals." WHO, Geneva.

———. 2005. *Make Every Mother and Child Count: The World Health Report 2005.* Geneva: WHO.

———. 2007. *World Health Statistics 2007.* Geneva: WHO.

———. 2009a. "Guidelines for Trauma Quality Improvement Programmes." WHO, Geneva.

———. 2009b. *Implementation Manual: Surgical Safety Checklist,* edited by A. A. Gawande and T. G. Weiser, first edition. Geneva: WHO.

———. 2009c. "Integrated Management of Essential and Emergency Surgical Care (IMEESC) Tool Kit." Geneva: WHO. http://www.who.int/surgery/publications/imeesc/en/.

———. 2009d. *WHO Guidelines for Safe Surgery: Safe Surgery Saves Lives,* edited by A. A. Gawande and T. G. Weiser. Geneva: WHO. http://whqlibdoc.who.int/publications /2009/9789241598552_eng.pdf.

———. 2010. "Tool for Situational Analysis to Assess Emergency and Essential Surgical Care." Geneva: WHO. http://www.who.int/surgery/publications /QuickSitAnalysisEESCsurvey.pdf.

Willmore, W. S., and A. G. Hill. 2001. "Acute Appendicitis in a Kenyan Rural Hospital." *East African Medical Journal* 78 (7): 355–57.

Wu, H. S., H. W. Lai, S. J. Kuo, Y. T. Lee, D. R. Chen, and others. 2011. "Competitive Edge of Laparoscopic Appendectomy versus Open Appendectomy: A Subgroup Comparison Analysis." *Journal of Laparoendoscopic and Advanced Surgical Techniques, Part A* 21 (3): 197–202.

Wu, S. C., C. C. Wang, and C. C. Yong. 2008. "Quadrapod Mesh for Posterior Wall Reconstruction in Adult Inguinal Hernias." *ANZ Journal of Surgery* 78 (3): 182–84.

Wu, S. C., Y. C. Wang, C. Y. Fu, R. J. Chen, H. C. Huang, and others. 2011. "Laparoscopic Appendectomy Provides Better Outcomes Than Open Appendectomy in Elderly Patients." *American Surgeon* 77 (4): 466–70.

Xu, K., D. B. Evans, G. Carrin, A. M. Aguilar-Rivera, P. Musgrove, and others. 2007. "Protecting Households from Catastrophic Health Spending." *Health Affairs (Millwood)* 26 (4): 972–83.

Yaffee, A. Q., L. K. Whiteside, R. A. Oteng, P. M. Carter, P. Donkor, and others. 2012. "Bypassing Proximal Health Care Facilities for Acute Care: A Survey of Patients in a Ghanaian Accident and Emergency Centre." *Tropical Medicine and International Health* 17 (6): 775–81.

Yeung, Y. P., M. S. Cheng, K. L. Ho, and A. W. Yip. 2002. "Day-Case Inguinal Herniotomy in Chinese Children: Retrospective Study." *Hong Kong Medical Journal* 8 (4): 245–48.

Zhou, X. L. 2013. "Comparison of the Posterior Approach and Anterior Approach for a Kugel Repair of Treatment of Inguinal Hernias." *Surgery Today* 43 (4): 403–7.

Zoguereh, D. D., X. Lemaître, J. F. Ikoli, J. Delmont, A. Chamlian, and others. 2001. "Acute Appendicitis at the National University Hospital in Bangui, Central African Republic: Epidemiologic, Clinical, Paraclinical and Therapeutic Aspects." [In French.] *Santé* 11 (2): 117–25.

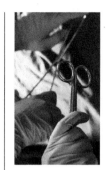

Chapter 17

Workforce Innovations to Expand the Capacity for Surgical Services

Staffan Bergström, Barbara McPake, Caetano Pereira, and Delanyo Dovlo

INTRODUCTION

Surgical interventions are often considered complex procedures to be undertaken by highly trained surgeons, but such specialists are rare in many low-income countries (LICs). However, many common surgical problems in resource-limited settings do not require the intervention of specialized staff. Significant documentation demonstrates that cost-effective surgical interventions can be undertaken in LICs with the innovative use and deployment of trained staff, including emergency care for trauma and obstetrical needs. Despite this documentation, surgical workforce innovations that use nonspecialized cadres often meet with resistance from established surgeons and their professional associations.

The most important barrier to the safe provision of preoperative, intraoperative, and postoperative surgical and anesthesia services in LICs is the shortage of trained staff. The well-documented reasons for this scarcity include the following (Chu and others 2009; FAIMER Institute 2008):

- Low number of medical school graduates
- Inadequate initial and ongoing training
- Poor salaries and working conditions
- Inability to motivate and retain staff in remote and rural areas

- Staff attrition due to retirement, death, or resignation, and the consequences of brain drain

The reluctance of governments to invest in human resources compounds the effects of these factors. Current financial constraints, such as those in Tanzania, for example, have forced governments to announce freezes in employing new human resources for health.

Sub-Saharan Africa is most affected by the global shortage of human resources for health (Chankova, Muchiri, and Kombe 2009; Mills and others 2008; WHO 2006). Two countries profiled in this chapter, Mozambique and Tanzania, experienced this crisis some years ago (Liese and Dussault 2004; Mills and others 2008; Smith and Henderson-Andrade 2006). In other countries, despite years of interventions to overcome the scarcity of doctors, the shortage has worsened as the result of population growth, presenting a major challenge to the ability of these countries to achieve the health-related Millennium Development Goals (MDGs) (Anand and Barnighausen 2004; Liese and Dussault 2004) (box 17.1). Available doctors tend to concentrate and work in urban areas and in regional or even national hospitals, limiting access for rural populations, who often constitute up to 75 percent of national populations.

A major reason for Sub-Saharan Africa's high maternal mortality is that few infants are born in the presence

Corresponding author: Staffan Bergström, MD, PhD, Karolinska Institutet, staffan.bergstrom@ki.se

Millennium Development Goals (MDGs) for Health

Goal 4: Reduce the under-five mortality rate by two-thirds between 1990 and 2015.

Goal 5: Reduce the maternal mortality ratio by three-quarters; achieve universal access to reproductive health.

Goal 6: Have halted and begun to reverse the spread of HIV/AIDS by 2015; achieve universal access to treatment for HIV/AIDS by 2010 for all those who need it; have halted and begun to reverse by 2015 the incidence of malaria and other major diseases.

A review of progress on the MDGs is available at http://www.hrh-observatory.afro.who.int/en/data-and-statistics/hrh-statistics.html.

Source: United Nations, http://www.un.org/millenniumgoals.

of skilled attendants. The lack of skilled birth attendants contributes to the 5 million to 6 million maternal deaths, stillbirths, and newborn deaths each year worldwide. In 19 of the 52 Sub-Saharan African countries that reported data, fewer than 50 percent of births were attended by skilled health personnel. The World Health Organization (WHO) estimates that 80 percent of births need to be attended by an adequately equipped and skilled birth attendant to reach the fifth MDG target of reducing maternal mortality by three-quarters (UNECA, African Commission, African Development Bank, and UNDP n.d.).

One colleague in Tanzania expressed his frustrations in the following way:

> ... [We] are fed up with the government's commitments and the politicians' alleged devotion to the problem of maternal deaths in Tanzania. Our work burden is increasing tremendously, but there are no signs of real support. Imagine: If I am up during the night to make one to two cesarean sections, I have to work the full day the morning after. We are entitled to a symbolic call allowance of US$6 (six!) per night, but we do not receive even that! The government says "there is no money." This is not true.

The AIDS epidemic in Sub-Saharan Africa may have aggravated this crisis by depriving health systems of a significant proportion of their trained staff (Chen and others 2004). Sub-Saharan Africa has 11 percent of the world's population and 24 percent of the total estimated

global burden of disease; yet it has 3 percent of the global health workforce (Chen and others 2004), only a small percentage of whom are qualified surgeons. Sub-Saharan Africa has less than 1 percent of the number of surgeons that the United States has, despite having a population that is three times as large (Ozgediz, Riviello, and Rogers 2008). Expanding the human workforce is clearly essential to improving the performance of health systems (de Bertodano 2003; Chankova, Muchiri, and Kombe 2009; Liese and Dussault 2004; WHO 2000; World Bank 2004) and improving outcomes, even under difficult circumstances (Chu and others 2009; EQUINET 2007; FAIMER Institute 2008; Mills and others 2008).

In Mozambique, the scarcity of human resources for health 30 years ago was alarming; the country had fewer than 5 physicians per 100,000 population. Our research estimated that there are 33 registered nurses and midwives per 100,000 population (Pereira 2010). In Tanzania, the health workforce shortage was disastrous, according to the report of the Joint Learning Initiative (Chen and others 2004). A study by the London School of Hygiene and Tropical Medicine suggests that the number of health care providers would need to increase by more than 58,000 to provide necessary interventions to meet the health-related MDGs for Tanzania (Anyangwe and Mtonga 2007).

In most countries in Sub-Saharan Africa, the scarcity of human resources for health existed before independence, as a result of colonial training policies and, in some cases, the massive exodus of colonial professionals after independence (Ministry of Health, Mozambique 2008; Ozgediz and others 2008). In Mozambique, a civil war provoked by neighboring South Africa in the early 1980s worsened the situation. Both Mozambique and Tanzania suffered from the consequences of the brain drain, either externally as health professionals moved to high-income countries (HICs) or internally as they migrated from rural to urban areas (Dodani and LaPorte 2005; McKinsey and Company 2006; Mullan and Frehywot 2007).

NONPHYSICIAN CLINICIANS

The literature uses a number of terms to describe categories of health professionals who may serve as substitutes for physicians in providing health care. The most common are *nonphysician clinicians* (NPCs)—nowadays referred to as *associate clinicians*—and *midlevel providers* (MLPs), although others such as *substitute health workers* have been used (Dovlo 2005).

The terms appear to be used interchangeably, although there is inconsistency across the literature in the ways in which the terms are used. In the Sub-Saharan African literature, the characteristics of the nontraditional cadres of health professionals are generally as follows:

- They have been created as a response to physician scarcity.
- They have a lower initial level of education.
- They receive a shorter period of preservice training than physicians, with the training often limited to a specific set of clinical skills.

These cadres include the Tanzanian *assistant medical officers* (AMOs) and the Mozambican *técnicos de cirurgia* (TCs), whose experiences particularly inform this chapter. Other countries use the terms *medical assistants* (Ghana) or *clinical officers* (Kenya and Uganda) to denote similar cadres.

Studies and commentators differ in their inclusion or exclusion of traditional health professional cadres, including nurses, midwives, pharmacists, and other allied health professionals, who have distinct and complementary clinical roles to play. For example, Warriner and others (2006, 1) define *MLPs* as "health care providers who are not doctors, such as nurses, midwives, and doctor-assistants" in their review of the options for providing induced abortion services in South Africa and Vietnam. Similarly, the American Osteopathic Association, Division of State Government Affairs (2003), based in the United States, counts both new and traditional health professional cadres in the definition of the term NPC. In contrast, Bradley and McAuliffe (2009, n.p.) define MLPs as "cadres of health workers who undertake roles and tasks that are more usually the province of internationally recognized cadres, such as doctors and nurses," implying that nurses are not included among MLPs. This definition is similar to that of NPCs according to Mullan and Frehywot (2007), who list *health officers, clinical officers, physician assistants, nurse practitioners,* and *nurse clinicians* as the labels by which NPCs are known.

This chapter focuses on the role of NPCs or MLPs— AMOs and TCs in particular—in surgical services in Sub-Saharan Africa in situations characterized by physician shortages. These cadres have been central to the debate about ensuring adequate staffing for essential surgery and other physician-delivered services in such environments, although growing interest has been expressed in the greater use of midwives and nurse-midwives in obstetric surgery, and countries have been building on their experiences in such expanded uses (Berer 2009; Warriner and others 2006).

In recent years, a welcome terminological shift has occurred, from the NPC concept (which actually is a negation) to the concept of *associate clinician*. A growing network—the African Network of Associate Clinicians (ANAC)—has developed and is based at the Chainama College of Health Sciences in Lusaka, Zambia, a lower-middle-income country. The ANAC is significant; for the first time, differently titled MLPs from a large number of Sub-Saharan African countries have formed a major international association. This development will facilitate the recognition of this category of key health staff for advanced care, including surgery, in rural settings that lack access to physicians.

TASK-SHIFTING AND TASK-SHARING

The literature indicates that informal or formal delegation of tasks from one cadre to another is not a new concept. *Task-shifting* implies the delegation of certain medical responsibilities to less specialized health workers (McCord and others 2009). This is the direct substitution of new and different cadres for an existing traditional profession (Pereira and others 2007; Pereira and others 2011). In surgery, such health workers may provide many of the diagnostic and clinical functions usually performed by physicians. However, opinions have diverged; some experts suggest that *task-sharing* may be a more appropriate concept. These two expressions, however, seem to signify two different realities. Where no physicians are available, the tasks of physicians must be shifted to nonphysicians. Where a few physicians are available, their range of tasks may be shared with nonphysicians.

Training for Safe and Effective Care

In most Sub-Saharan countries, the use of substitute health workers started as a temporary measure until more doctors could be trained. However, in the face of the persisting human resources crisis, this strategy has become permanent. More of these countries have embarked on the expanded training of midlevel health professionals and nonphysician cadres to promote access to care and to contain costs (Dovlo 2004; Ministry of Health, Mozambique 2008; Pereira and others 2011).

This trend to delegate procedures to lower cadres has often met with resistance for various reasons. Surgery is considered a highly specialized field that requires several years of training; hence, it is important to define the boundaries of surgical task-shifting considered essential to ensure quality of care. The WHO has established a list of surgical procedures performed at first-level hospitals that facilitates the classification of various interventions and can help training schools establish which essential interventions could be safely shifted to NPCs (Lehmann, Dieleman, and

Martineau 2008; McCord and others 2009). A district or first-level hospital is usually the most remote, rurally situated hospital with inpatient care and a theater for limited major surgery interventions, such as cesarean sections, open fractures, and bowel resections for strangulated hernias (Chilopora and others 2007).

In Mozambique, the training of NPCs in surgery is well structured and is followed by a formal internship. The recruitment focus is on candidates with previous job experience in peripheral health units or first-level hospitals (Pereira 2010). Studies have shown that NPCs in Mozambique are well appreciated by other professionals, doctors, nurses, and midwives (Cumbi and others 2007). Approximately 90 percent of physicians and other health staff gave positive ratings to the strong practical skills and the critical roles played by NPCs in saving the lives of mothers and newborns at first-level hospitals. With accumulated surgical experience among these NPCs, young doctors deployed in rural areas are increasingly trained in surgery by TCs (Hounton and others 2009). An assessment of the outcomes of cesarean sections between TCs and physicians at the Maputo Central Hospital showed no clinically significant differences between the two cadres (Cherian and others 2004).

In Tanzania, AMOs are selected from among the *clinical officers* who have a minimum of three years of working experience in peripheral health units or first-level hospitals. Their subsequent training is for two years and includes three months each of surgery and obstetrics. Studies show no significant differences in the clinical outcomes, risk indicators, or quality of care indicators for major obstetric operations performed by AMOs and nonspecialized physicians (McKinsey and Company 2006). For example, despite logistic and material resource problems in all the hospitals, the aggregate maternal case fatality rate was acceptable at 1 percent to 2 percent.

Ghana, a lower-middle-income country, initiated its program for training medical assistants, consisting of one year of postnursing qualification training, in 1969. In 2007, this program was converted into a physician assistants program, consisting of four years of direct training after high school. The students were trained to perform only limited surgical procedures and tasks. A nurse anesthetist (now called *anesthetist physician assistant*) program has become the backbone of surgical procedures, even in regional third-level hospitals. The surgical tasks of these cadres remain limited to performing incisions, draining abscesses, suturing wounds, and immobilizing fractures. Most obstetric tasks beyond normal delivery are not part of their responsibilities. According to the director of the College of Health and Well-Being in Kintampo, a move is underway to change the procedures and allow these cadres to perform life-saving surgery and obstetric procedures.

In both Mozambique and Tanzania, the real challenge in providing quality care is not primarily in the practical skills in the operating room. The difficult aspect of emergency obstetrics and surgery is rather in the decision-making process, specifically, whether and how to intervene. It is easy to solve most emergency problems in obstetrics by resorting to cesarean section, a simple technique that is easy to learn. Any health worker, NPC (assistant medical officer, clinical officer, or other category of midlevel health worker), or physician who has not been trained in properly assisting vaginal delivery in general and in vacuum extraction in particular would tend to solve many obstetric problems by performing a cesarean section—whether justified or not.

Most often—in practice—no one would blame a health care provider for having performed a cesarean section; however, health care providers would be blamed for not having performed a cesarean section if the mother or the baby died or suffered a serious complication. This reality increases the number of medically unnecessary cesarean sections. This problem has one solution: the careful auditing of cesarean section decision making. This auditing practice is already routine in efforts in Tanzania to reduce maternal mortality rates. Cesarean section auditing has proven to be a necessary corollary to the task-shifting of major obstetric surgery. The audit scrutinizes the circumstances leading to the cesarean section; it then questions each step by examining the details of the partogram to determine whether oxytocin augmentation of labor should have been undertaken, or if assisted vaginal delivery should have been considered to be the preferred option.

Treatment Areas for Task-Sharing or Task-Shifting

Our studies and other literature show that midlevel health professionals carry out the majority of surgical procedures outside urban areas in a number of Sub-Saharan African countries and can be indispensable when physicians are scarce (Chankova and others 2009; Cumbi and others 2007; Dovlo 2004; McCord and others 2009). The studies indicate that TCs in Mozambique perform 92 percent of cesarean sections in first-level hospitals (Pereira 2010; Pereira and others 2007); in Tanzania, AMOs perform 85 percent of cesarean sections, 94 percent of repairs of ruptured uterus, 86 percent of removals of ectopic pregnancy, and 70 percent of hysterectomies in the Mwanza and Kigoma regions in Tanzania (McCord and others 2009; Pereira 2010).

ACCEPTANCE OF MIDLEVEL PROVIDERS FOR MAJOR SURGERY

The literature highlights the problem of reluctance and even resistance among doctors and other professionals to consider task-shifting in surgery (Lehman, Dieleman, and Martineau 2008; McCord and others 2009). Since the inception in 1984 of training of TCs in Mozambique, this reluctance has gradually disappeared; members of this cadre are now well accepted and recognized among physicians. They are also acknowledged to be important for the training and support of recently graduated and inexperienced physicians assigned to first-level hospitals (Cumbi and others 2007). One physician in our research in Mozambique expressed his opinion as follows:

> … [O]ur TC is good, because without him I don't know what would be in terms of the rural hospital [where] he is the surgeon; here in the provincial hospital he works in shifts in equal terms with the other specialists [surgeon, obstetrician, and orthopedist]; when one specialist goes on vacation, she or he is replaced by the TC. At rural hospital level, they [TCs] provide all [types of] care and they decrease the provincial hospital workload, [can you] imagine without their presence [in the districts], what would be the workload at the provincial hospital?

The TCs have been trained and deployed for a quarter of a century, and the young physicians are taught in school to respect these cadres, given that new physicians themselves have limited exposure to surgical interventions.

In Tanzania, this issue has not yet been studied scientifically. Forthcoming research into attitudinal problems related to perceived threats to conventional areas of professional competence in surgical practice by task-shifting will be useful. In Ghana, physician assistants were, until recently, not under any regulatory authority, which may have contributed to their lack of acceptance by physicians and the reluctance to shift certain tasks to them. Associate physicians in Ghana are now registered and regulated by the Medical and Dental Council and may soon be permitted to perform life-saving surgical procedures.

IMPROVING WORKING CONDITIONS AND PROMOTING RETENTION OF MIDLEVEL PROVIDERS

The need to develop policies and programs to improve health worker motivation and retention in rural locations is a crucial area in addressing the health resource crisis,

especially in LICs and lower-middle-income countries (Mills and others 2008; Pereira and others 1996). Both motivation and retention are directly influenced by poor remuneration and working conditions, suboptimal management of human resources, and limited opportunities for career progression (Pereira 2010). These challenges are issues for both physicians and NPCs.

In Mozambique, the same factors resulting in poor motivation also prevail (Cumbi and others 2007). A key issue behind the dissatisfaction that TCs express is the heavy workload; they can rarely leave the workplace to attend training in referral hospitals or attend specific seminars to enhance their knowledge. In addition, the scarcity of surgical specialists at the provincial level limits the capacity to provide and receive adequate supervision (Hounton and others 2009).

The NPCs in Ghana and Tanzania face a similar situation, with motivation reportedly weak (Hongoro and McPake 2004). AMOs are overworked, face poor working conditions, and experience a lack of supervision. Unlike nurses and midwives, they are rarely invited to attend professional meetings and workshops, despite their crucial roles. They are seldom moved to referral hospitals for job training to improve their skills and performance. Limited career prospects and opportunities for upward mobility increase their levels of dissatisfaction (Pereira 2010).

Financial Incentives

In Mozambique, the lower salary level for TCs than for other midlevel professionals has been a significant cause of dissatisfaction. The training of TCs was initially controversial, largely due to physician resistance, resulting in the unclear definition of career paths by the Ministry of Health, since TCs were considered midlevel professionals without specialization. This designation affects their position on the salary scale, which has a significant impact on their motivation (Pereira 2010). During the past decade, the salaries of TCs have improved.

Nonfinancial Incentives

Improving Supervision. Initiatives to improve the capacity to provide adequate supervision and management can improve work satisfaction, performance, and quality of work in remote settings (Maestad 2006; Pang, Lansang, and Haines 2002; Pereira and others 2007). Our studies did not specifically address supervision, but the literature reviewed indicates that supervision is irregular or nonexistent in most districts in the two countries (Anyangwe and Mtonga 2007; Dovlo 2005). In Ghana, annual meetings have become popular and important sources for updating skills and providing forums for professional networking.[1]

Improving Working and Living Conditions. Working and living conditions are important determinants of motivation and retention in HICs, lower-middle-income countries, and LICs (Douglas 1991; Lavy and others 2007; Pereira and others 2007; Stringhini and others 2009). Our studies did not address these issues further, because in the majority of districts, the housing for TCs had been assessed beforehand, a prerequisite to deployment of these cadres at first-level hospitals. In Mozambique, the government is implementing a decentralization program to partner with local authorities and communities to better respond to the health resource problems in remote areas. This consultative process is expected to generate better accommodations for staff, more electricity, better roads, and improvements to health and educational facilities (Loevinsohn and others 1995). The impact of this program has not yet been evaluated.

In Tanzania, the health sector reform strategy, which aims to influence changes in the health system to improve the health status of all citizens, has focused on district decentralization, improvement of the health system, health management, and financing and human resource development (Cavanagh and Coffin 1992; Kunaviktikul and others 2001). An evaluation reveals that the impact on the general health status of the population was unsatisfactory (Lambert and Lambert 2001).

Improving Staff Satisfaction. Staff satisfaction has a large influence on motivation, which affects the performance and retention of health workers (Ministério da Administração Estatal 2001). Training, study leave, the opportunity to work in a team, support from supervisors, and provision of housing and transport increase staff satisfaction and consequently motivation (Dominick and Kurowski 2005; Munishi 2003). In both Mozambique and Tanzania, a widespread opinion among health workers is that the situation is difficult because their salaries do not adequately cover the cost of living. Health workers consider administrative management to be weak (Anyangwe and Mtonga 2007; Dovlo 2005; Ministry of Health, Tanzania 2007).

Improving Retention. According to the literature, the retention of human resources for health, particularly in rural areas, is a major and complex problem in most LICs (Pereira and others 2007; Stilwell and others 2001; WHO 2004; Wilbulpolprasert 1999), and no single solution applies in all settings. Comparatively low salaries are the primary source of dissatisfaction. However, socioeconomic status—implying a set of appreciating and depreciating circumstances—such as access or lack of access to housing, positive or negative working conditions, an enabling or disabling work environment, and the availability or lack of availability of further training are the decisive factors in whether to stay in or leave remote areas.

Our results in Mozambique show that 88 percent of TCs remained in rural areas seven years after graduation, while none of the physicians remained after graduation (the first assignment always being in a rural area) (Pereira 2010; Pereira and others 2007). Another study indicates that retention may be related to the recruitment system. If candidates are selected from each region of the country, are mainly from rural areas, and are integrated into scholarship schemes at the provincial level with the commitment to return after completion of training, then the distribution of cadres and their retention may be improved.[2]

Retention is also a major issue in Tanzania (Anyangwa and Mtonga 2007; Ministry of Health, Tanzania 2007), with migratory flows from rural to urban areas and from the public to the private sectors. Most of the skilled health workforce, particularly physicians and specialists, are concentrated in urban areas, where only 20 percent of the population lives. As early as 1982, Tanzania started a decentralization reform that was designed to empower local authorities to recruit health workers. Decentralized recruitment was supposed to be effective in improving retention because the responsibility for hiring was transferred to the local governments. The assessment of the potential impact of this decentralization program is underway, but the initial findings reveal that decentralization enhanced the retention of the lower-cadre health workers in the districts.[3] In Ghana, approximately 75 percent of medical assistants and physician assistants work in rural areas.[4]

COST-EFFECTIVENESS OF SURGICAL TRAINING OF MIDLEVEL PROVIDERS

Few studies have addressed the issue of the cost-effectiveness of training NPCs, associate clinicians, general practitioners, and specialists (Dovlo 2004). In Burkina Faso, NPCs are trained for two years in surgery (*attachés de santé*), and general practitioners receive six months of training to perform emergency surgery in rural areas. These personnel are cost-effective compared with specialists (Hounton and others 2009). In Mozambique, the cost-effectiveness of general practitioners was not addressed in our studies, given that this cadre does not receive additional training in surgery. Such a scheme would increase the training of general practitioners to a total of nine years after secondary school, which the Ministry of Health did not deem advisable. A comparison of the cost-effectiveness of TCs in relation to physicians demonstrates that the former are significantly more cost-effective if the costs of training and deployment are considered (Kruk and others 2007). In Mozambique, most physicians, after initial rural assignments of a few years, move to urban areas to meet administrative commitments or to start their specialization at teaching hospitals (Pereira 2010). In Tanzania, the literature review shows that training AMOs is less expensive than training physicians (Anyangwe and Mtonga 2007).

ESTABLISHING ENABLING ENVIRONMENTS

The governments of Mozambique and Tanzania have made strong commitments in recent decades to address the crisis in human resources for health. Solving the problem of inadequate numbers of health professionals, however, is not the solution to improving access to health care. Other problems have to be addressed simultaneously. An environment conducive to quality surgical care, as perceived by the health workers, requires that trained NPCs be able to execute their skills in settings that foster and value their professional services. This environment, which is required for well-trained health workers in sufficient numbers to perform optimally, is needed both at the central level of the Ministry of Health and at the provincial and district levels.

Mozambique

In Mozambique, the Instituto Superior de Ciências de Saúde (Higher Institute of Health Sciences) was created to clarify the career path for TCs (ISCISA 2003). The initiation of the national human resources program is a positive step in counteracting the human resources crisis (Pereira 2010). In Ghana, a similar school is under the medical faculty of a university and the program has been upgraded, measures that have improved the environment for task enhancement.[5]

To begin to reduce TCs' heavy workload in Mozambique, a program to train midwives to perform major obstetric surgery has been initiated (Enfermeiras de Saùde Materna) to strengthen teamwork at first-level hospitals.[6] This new training, which results in a licentiate degree, comprises three-and-a-half years of theoretical and practical training, in addition to six months of internship in first- or second-level hospitals. The training is grounded in nursing but emphasizes diagnostic and treatment skills, the practice of

major emergency obstetric surgery, and the concept of teamwork. The Ministry of Health expects that more effective teamwork and, consequently, improvement of the quality of work can be achieved because TCs will be relieved of much of the workload of obstetrical and gynecological emergency surgery.

Emergency obstetrics and gynecology constitutes the predominant work burden for TCs. The task-shifting scenario, however, is changing; NPCs, in all likelihood, will handle more elective surgery in general surgery, as well as in obstetrics and gynecology. Two examples are bilateral tubal ligation and a growing number of planned cesarean sections, whether clinically indicated or not. In middle-class Sub-Saharan Africa, the trend to request cesarean sections is, unfortunately, clearly on the rise.

In Mozambique, the government plan for 2005–09 focused on capacity building, including the rehabilitation of infrastructure and theaters in the whole health system; the timely supply and deployment of human resources in general, and in peripheral areas in particular; the development of norms and guidelines for obstetric emergency care and essential care to newborns; the implementation of a formative system of supervision; and the strengthening of the ability to communicate with radios and to transport patients (ISCISA 2003). The plan from 2010 onward aims to strengthen the system and the previously existing plan (Ministry of Health, Mozambique 2008).

The human resources plan approved by the Ministry of Health for implementation incorporates four main strategic areas:

- Organization of services and a functioning system of rules
- Expanded capacity of management at different levels
- Improved distribution and retention of human resources for health
- Expansion of the institutional capacity to provide training and continuous education

Tanzania

In Tanzania, facilitating the establishment of an enabling environment has received increasing attention (Munga and others 2009; Nyamtema and others 2011). The government recognizes the importance of improving health care and expanding the supply of human resources. It has made a commitment to address the shortage of human resources for health, particularly the skilled workforce. Tanzania has established relationships with other governments, donors, and agencies that are potential partners in these approaches (Anyangwe and Mtonga 2007).

CONCLUSIONS

The shortage of skilled human resources in surgical health care is a major health system problem in Mozambique and Tanzania, as well as in other LICs. Innovative and multi-faceted workforce solutions offer viable options for alleviating the consequences of the shortage and building the capacity of countries to provide skilled surgical care. Task-shifting and task-sharing are feasible strategies and should be seriously considered to address the human resources crisis in Mozambique and Tanzania, as well as in other countries facing the same human resources problems.

NPCs perform approximately 90 percent of major emergency obstetric surgeries in rural areas where most of the population live in both Mozambique and Tanzania. A comparison of the quality of care provided by medical doctors and that provided by TCs and AMOs demonstrates no clinically significant differences in outcomes in major obstetric surgery. In Mozambique, physicians (general practitioners and specialists), nurses, and midwives rate TCs and AMOs positively.

In Mozambique, NPCs have a high retention rate in rural areas. NPCs are cost-effective, and the training and deployment of TCs is three times more cost-effective than the training and deployment of medical doctors. Motivation is a problem among NPCs in general and among TCs in particular, for multiple reasons, and programs are being developed to address some of the causes.

Challenges continue for many countries in physician acceptance of midlevel clinicians; the development and implementation of training and regulatory mechanisms; the expansion of the capacity for skills development and improvement, as well as supervision; and better financial and nonfinancial compensation. Initiatives to improve accuracy in decision making in obstetric cases by different professional categories deserve a more specific approach.

NOTES

One of the authors of this chapter is a WHO staff member. The authors alone are responsible for the views expressed in this publication and they do not necessarily represent the decisions or policies of the World Health Organization.

The World Bank classifies countries according to four income groupings. Income is measured using gross national income (GNI) per capita, in U.S. dollars, converted from local currency using the *World Bank Atlas* method. Classifications as of July 2014 are as follows:

- Low-income countries (LICs) = US$1,045 or less in 2013
- Middle-income countries (MICs) are subdivided:
  - Lower-middle-income = US$1,046 to US$4,125
  - Upper-middle-income (UMICs) = US$4,126 to US$12,745

- High-income countries (HICs) = US$12,746 or more
1. Delanyo Dovlo, personal communication.
2. Caetano Pereira, personal communication.
3. Caetano Pereira, personal communication.
4. Delanyo Dovlo, personal communication.
5. Delanyo Dovlo, personal communication.
6. Caetano Pereira and Staffan Bergström, personal communication.

REFERENCES

American Osteopathic Association. 2003. "Support Needed for Clinical Faculty in Osteopathic Emergency Residencies." 103 (12): 575–76. http://www.jaoa.org/content/103/12/575 .full.pdf.

Anand, S., and T. Barnighausen. 2004. "Human Resources and Health Outcomes: Cross-Country Econometric Study." *The Lancet* 364 (9445): 1603–09.

Anyangwe, S. C., and C. Mtonga. 2007. "Inequities in the Global Health Workforce: The Greatest Impediment to Health in Sub-Saharan Africa." *International Journal of Environmental Research and Public Health* 4 (2): 93–100.

Berer, M. 2009. "Provision of Abortion by Mid-level Providers: International Policy, Practice and Perspectives." *Bulletin of the World Health Organization* 97: 1.

Bradley, S., and E. McAuliffe. 2009. "Mid-Level Providers in Emergency Obstetric and Newborn Health Care: Factors Affecting Their Performance and Retention within the Malawian Health System." *Human Resources for Health* 7: 14.

Cavanagh, S. J., and D. A. Coffin. 1992. "Staff Turnover among Hospital Nurses." *Journal of Advanced Nursing* 17 (11): 1369–76.

Chankova, S., S. Muchiri, and G. Kombe. 2009. "Health Workforce Attrition in the Public Sector in Kenya: A Look at the Reasons." *Human Resources for Health* 7: 58.

Chen, L., T. Evans, S. Anand, J. B. Ivey, H. Brown, and others. 2004. "Human Resources for Health: Overcoming the Crisis." *The Lancet* 364 (9449): 1984–90.

Cherian, M. N., L. Noel, Y. B. Jargan, and G. Salil. 2004. "Essential Emergency Surgical Procedures in Resource-Limited Facilities: A WHO Workshop in Mongolia." *World Hospital Health Services* 40 (4): 24–29.

Chilopora, G., F. Kamwendo, E. Malunga, C. Pereira, S. Bergström, and others. 2007. "Postoperative Outcome of Caesarean Sections and Other Major Emergency Obstetric Surgery by Clinical Officers and Medical Officers in Malawi." *Human Resources for Health* 5: 17.

Chu, K., P. Rosseel, P. Gielis, and N. Ford. 2009. "Surgical Task Shifting in Sub-Saharan Africa." *PLoS Med* 6 (5): e1000078.

Cumbi, A., C. Pereira, R. Malalane, F. Vaz, C. McCord, and others. 2007. "Major Surgery Delegation to Mid-level Health Practitioners in Mozambique: Health Professionals' Perceptions." *Human Resources for Health* 5: 27.

de Bertodano, I. 2003. "The Costa Rican Health System: Low Cost, High Value." *Bulletin of the World Health Organization* 81 (8): 626–27.

Dodani, S., and R. E. LaPorte. 2005. "Brain Drain from Developing Countries: How Can Brain Drain Be Converted into Wisdom Gain?" *Journal of the Royal Society of Medicine* 98 (11): 487–91.

Dominick, A., and C. Kurowski. 2005. "Human Resources for Health: An Appraisal of the Status Quo in Tanzania Mainland." Working Paper, Ifakara Health Research and Development Centre and World Bank, Washington, DC.

Douglas, M. 1991. "Supervision of Rural Health Centres in Papua New Guinea: Consolidation of the Delivery of Health Services." *Papua New Guinea Medical Journal* 34 (2): 144–48.

Dovlo, D. 2004. "Using Mid-level Cadres as Substitutes for Internationally Mobile Health Professionals in Africa: A Desk Review." *Human Resources for Health* 2 (1): 7.

———. 2005. "Wastage in the Health Workforce: Some Perspectives from African Countries." *Human Resources for Health* 3: 6.

EQUINET. 2007. "Health Worker Retention and Migration in East and Southern Africa." Regional meeting report from the Regional Network for Equity in Health in East and Southern Africa (EQUINET/ECSA-CH), Training and Research Support Center, Arusha, March 17–19. http://www.equinetafrica.org/bibl/docs/REPMTG0307HRH.pdf.

FAIMER (Foundation for Advancement of International Medical Education and Research) Institute. 2008. "International Medical Directory." FAIMER Institute, New York.

Hongoro, C., and B. McPake. 2004. "How to Bridge the Gap in Human Resources for Health." *The Lancet* 364 (9443): 451–56.

Hounton, S. H., D. Newlands, N. Meda, and V. D. Brouwere. 2009. "A Cost-Effectiveness Study of Caesarean-Section Deliveries by Clinical Officers, General Practitioners and Obstetricians in Burkina Faso." *Human Resources for Health* 7: 34.

ISCISA. 2003. *Estatuto Orgânico do Instituto Superior de Ciências de Saúde*. Instituto Superior de Ciências de Saúde, Maputo, Mozambique.

Kruk, M., C. Pereira, F. Vaz, S. Bergström, and S. Galeae. 2007. "Economic Evaluation of Surgically Trained Assistant Medical Officers in Performing Major Obstetric Surgery in Mozambique." *BJOG: An International Journal of Obstetrics and Gynaecology* 1 (14): 1253–60.

Kunaviktikul, W., R. Anders, W. Srisuphan, R. Chontawan, R. Nuntasupawat, and others. 2001. "Development of Quality of Nursing Care in Thailand." *Journal of Advanced Nursing* 36 (6): 776–84.

Lambert, V. A., and C. E. Lambert. 2001. "Literature Review of Role Stress/Strain on Nurses: An International Perspective." *Nursing and Health Sciences* 3 (3): 161–72.

Lavy, C., A. Tindall, C. Steinlechner, N. Mkandawire, and S. Chimageni. 2007. "Surgery in Malawi: A National Survey of Activity in Rural and Urban Hospitals." *Annals of the Royal College of Surgeons* 89 (7): 722–24.

Lehmann, U., M. Dieleman, and T. Martineau. 2008. "Staffing Remote Rural Areas in Middle- and Low-Income Countries: A Literature Review of Attraction and Retention." *Biomed Central Health Services Research* 8: 19.

Liese, B., and G. Dussault. 2004. "The State of the Health Workforce in Sub-Saharan Africa: Evidence of Crisis and Analysis of Contributing Factors." Africa Region Human Development Working Paper 32804, World Bank, Washington, DC.

Loevinsohn, B., P. Erlinda, T. Guerrero, and S. P. Gregorio. 1995. "Improving Primary Health Care through Systematic Supervision: A Controlled Field Trial." *Health Policy and Planning* 10 (2): 144–53.

Maestad, O. 2006. "Human Resources for Health in Tanzania: Challenges, Policy Options and Knowledge Gaps." CMI Report, CHR Michelsen Institute, Bergen, Norway.

McCord, C., G. Mbaruku, C. Pereira, C. Nzabuhakwam, and S. Bergström. 2009. "The Quality of Emergency Obstetrical Surgery by Assistant Medical Officers in Tanzanian District Hospitals." *Health Affairs (Millwood)* 28 (5): w876–85.

McKinsey and Company. 2006. "Investing in Tanzanian Human Resources for Health." Human Resources for Health Report, TOUCH Foundation, New York.

Mills, E. J., W. A. Schabas, J. Volmink, R. Walker, N. Ford, and others. 2008. "Should Active Recruitment of Health Workers from Sub-Saharan Africa Be Viewed as a Crime?" *The Lancet* 371 (9613): 685–88.

Ministério da Administração Estatal. 2001. "Documento: Estrategia Global da Reforma Sector Publico 2001–2011." http://www.Portaldogoverno.gov.mz.

Ministry of Health, Tanzania. 2007. "Joint External Evaluation of the Health Sector in Tanzania." Inception Report 13–18. Dar es Salaam, Tanzania: Ministry of Health.

Ministry of Health, Mozambique. 2008. "Plano Nacional de Desenvolvimento dos Recursos Humanos da Saúde." PNRHS 2008–2015. National Directorate of Human Resources, Maputo, Mozambique.

Mullan, F., and S. Frehywot. 2007. "Non-physician Clinicians in 47 Sub-Saharan African Countries." *The Lancet* 370 (9605): 2158–63.

Munga, M. A., N. G. Songstad, A. Blystad, and O. Mæstad. 2009. "The Decentralisation-Centralisation Dilemma: Recruitment and Distribution of Health Workers in Remote Districts of Tanzania." *BioMed Central International Health and Human Rights* 9 (1): 9.

Munishi, G. K. 2003. "Intervening to Address Constraints through Health Sector Reforms in Tanzania: Some Gains and the Unfinished Business." *Journal of International Development* 15 (1): 115–31.

Nyamtema, A. S., S. K. Pemba, G. Mbaruku, F. D. Rutasha, and J. van Roosmalen. 2011. "Tanzanian Lessons in Using Non-physician Clinicians to Scale Up Comprehensive Emergency Obstetric Care in Remote and Rural Areas." *Human Resources for Health* 9: 28.

Ozgediz, D., R. Riviello, and S. O. Rogers. 2008. "The Surgical Workforce Crisis in Africa: A Call to Action." *Bulletin of the American College of Surgeons* 93 (8): 10–16.

Pang, T., M. A. Lansang, and A. Haines. 2002. "Brain Drain and Health Professionals." *British Medical Journal* 324 (7336): 499–500.

Pereira, C. 2010. "Task-Shifting of Major Surgery to Midlevel Providers of Health Care in Mozambique and Tanzania: A Solution to the Crisis in Human Resources to Enhance

Maternal and Neonatal Survival." PhD thesis, Karolinska Institutet, Stockholm.

Pereira, C., A. Bugalho, F. Vaz, M. Cotiro, and S. Bergström. 1996. "A Comparative Study of Caesarean Deliveries by Assistant Medical Officers and Obstetricians in Mozambique." *BJOG: An International Journal of Obstetrics and Gynaecology* 103 (6): 508–12.

Pereira, C., A. Cumbi, R. Malalane, F. Vaz, C. McCord, and others. 2007. "Meeting the Need for Emergency Obstetric Care in Mozambique: Work Performance and Histories of Medical Doctors and Assistant Medical Officers Trained for Surgery." *BJOG: An International Journal of Obstetrics and Gynaecology* 114 (12): 1530–33.

Pereira, C., G. Mbaruku, C. Nzabuhakwa, S. Bergström, and C. McCord. 2011. "Emergency Obstetric Surgery by Non-physician Clinicians in Tanzania." *International Journal of Gynecology and Obstetrics* 114 (2): 180–83.

Smith, M. K., and N. Henderson-Andrade. 2006. "Facing the Health Worker Crisis in Developing Countries: A Call for Global Solidarity." *Bulletin of the World Health Organization* 84 (6): 426–27.

Stilwell, B., K. Diallo, P. Zurn, M. Vujicic, O. Adams, and others. 2001. "Health Worker Motivation in Zimbabwe." Internal Report for the Department of Organization of Health Care Delivery, World Health Organization, Geneva.

Stringhini, S., S. Thomas, P. Bidwell, T. Mtui, and A. Mwisongo. 2009. "Understanding Informal Payments in Health Care: Motivation of Health Workers in Tanzania." *Human Resources for Health* 7: 53.

UN (United Nations). "Millennium Development Goals." http://www.un.org/millenniumgoals.

UNECA (United Nations Economic Commission for Africa), African Union, African Development Bank Group, and UNDP (United Nations Development Programme). n.d. *Executive Summary, MDG Report 2013, Assessing Progress in Africa toward the Millennium Development Goals— Food Security in Africa: Issues, Challenges and Lessons.* Addis Ababa, Ethiopia: United Nations Economic Commission for Africa. http://www.undp.org/content /dam/undp/library/MDG/english/MDG%20Regional%20 Reports/Africa/MDG%20report%202013%20summary _EN.pdf.

Warriner, I. K., O. Meirik, M. Hoffman, C. Morroni, J. Harries, and others. 2006. "Rates of Complication in First-Trimester Manual Vacuum Aspiration Abortion Done by Doctors and Mid-level Providers in South Africa and Vietnam: A Randomized Controlled Equivalence Trial." *The Lancet* 368 (9551): 1965–72.

WHO (World Health Organization). 2000. *World Health Report 2000: Health Systems—Improving Performance.* Geneva: WHO.

———. 2004. "Migration of Health-Care Workers from Developing Countries: Strategic Approaches to Its Management." *Bulletin of the World Health Organization* 82 (8): 595–600.

———. 2006. *The World Health Report 2006: Working Together for Health.* Geneva: WHO.

Wilbulpolprasert, S. 1999. "Inequitable Distribution of Doctors: Can It Be Solved?" *Human Resources for Health* 3: 2–22.

World Bank. 2004. *World Development Report 2004: Making Services Work for Poor People.* Washington, DC: Oxford University Press and World Bank.

Costs, Effectiveness, and Cost-Effectiveness of Selected Surgical Procedures and Platforms

Shankar Prinja, Arindam Nandi, Susan Horton, Carol Levin,
and Ramanan Laxminarayan

INTRODUCTION

This volume has shown that universal provision of a package of essential surgical services would avert an estimated 1.5 million deaths per year, or 6–7 percent of all avertable deaths in LMICs (Debas and others 2006; Mock and others 2015). Although approximately 234 million surgeries are performed worldwide each year, the distribution is very inequitable (Funk and others 2010). Nearly two billion people live in areas with a density of less than one operating room per 100,000 population (Funk and others 2010); in high-income countries (HICs), the density is 14 per 100,000. With this scarcity of surgical services in low- and middle-income countries (LMICs), the need for scaling up is imperative.

Challenges to the implementation of surgical services in resource-limited environments are substantial and include limited human resources, transportation systems, and access to electricity and water (Hsia and others 2012; Kruk and others 2010). Moreover, evidence on the different attributes of scaling up is insufficient. Scaling up requires increasing the share of current income devoted to spending on health, as well as major investments in facilities and human resources.

Priority interventions in LMICs are those that are cost-effective and reasonable in cost; *reasonable* is defined relative to the prevalence of the condition and size of the government health budget. Feasibility is important, particularly in low-income countries (LICs), which lack many health systems resources. Some deficiencies can be remedied if cost and cost-effectiveness considerations identify additional investments that provide good value. For example, purchasing more radiotherapy equipment or training additional personnel may make a substantial difference. Other deficiencies are harder to remedy. LMICs typically have limited ability to manage resources, which restricts how referral or organized screening systems work.

In this chapter, we discuss evidence showing that some types of surgery can be both highly cost-effective—saving lives or improving the quality of life—and affordable. We focus on a set of surgical interventions that can be undertaken at first-level hospitals, or in some cases, in clinics or mobile facilities. These interventions include selected emergency surgeries, surgeries associated with reproductive functions, and nonemergency surgeries. We do not cover other types of surgery that also may be cost-effective and even modest in cost but that are more suited to referral hospitals in LMICs, namely, surgery for cardiovascular disease, cancer, organ transplantation, and neurosurgery.

Surgical interventions for cardiovascular disease, such as left main coronary artery bypass graft surgery and percutaneous transluminal coronary angioplasty, have

Corresponding author: Shankar Prinja, MD, Post Graduate Institute of Medical Education and Research, shankarprinja@gmail.com been very cost-effective in certain population groups in HICs, compared with medical management (Tengs and others 1995); this outcome is likely to apply to some population groups in LMICs. Basic surgical interventions for cancer treatment are likely to be cost-effective and, in some cases, feasible at the first-level hospital, for example, oophorectomy, simple hysterectomy, radical mastectomy, and colectomy. Very few cost-effectiveness results are available on these interventions, surveyed in Horton and Gauvreau (2015) and not discussed further here. Kidney transplants, although relatively costly, may be cost-effective (Tengs and others 1995). We do not cover neurosurgery, such as surgery to treat epilepsy or to treat infant hydrocephalus, although Warf and others (2011) show that such surgeries can be cost-effective in Sub-Saharan Africa. Cost-effectiveness of reproductive surgery is considered in volume 2, *Reproductive, Maternal, Newborn, and Child Health* (Black and others forthcoming). Dental surgery is not covered because of a lack of studies using quality-adjusted life year (QALY), disability-adjusted life year (DALY), life year saved (LYS), and death-averted outcome measures.

The set of conditions covered in the chapter is listed in annex 18A and includes interventions discussed in other chapters in this volume; chapter 1 provides a more comprehensive list of the detailed procedures considered. These are surgery types that can feasibly be undertaken at first-level hospitals, although they may also be undertaken at second-level hospitals, often when urgent cases arrive at these emergency units. Some can be undertaken in specialized facilities, for example, a cataract hospital, a specialized mobile facility, a short-term surgical mission focused on specific surgical conditions, or a trauma center.

We briefly summarize the literature on the cost-effectiveness of different ways of organizing facilities for surgery. Equity and affordability are important considerations when prioritizing care. We review both of these issues before discussing data limitations and presenting conclusions. This chapter uses World Health Organization (WHO) geographical regions: Africa, the Americas, South-East Asia, Europe, Eastern Mediterranean, and Western Pacific.

WHY ARE COST-EFFECTIVENESS DATA USEFUL FOR SURGERY?

Conditions potentially treatable by surgery constitute a significant proportion of the global burden of disease. Bickler and others (chapter 2) estimate that scaling up the recommended list of procedures at first-level hospitals could prevent 1.4 million deaths annually—3.2 percent of the global number—taking into account the proportion for which treatment can be expected to be successful. An additional 0.9 percent of deaths could be averted by advanced surgical care delivered at specialized clinics to treat nonemergency conditions, such as cataracts, cleft lip and palate, congenital heart anomalies, neural tube defects, and obstetric fistula. In addition, surgery could reduce the substantial burden of disabilities.

Cost-effectiveness data can provide important support for additional investments in surgical facilities at first-level hospitals. The data can help identify high-priority procedures from a cost-effectiveness perspective, leading to an analysis of the resources required to expand their availability.

The cost-effectiveness data have limitations. In the United States, a major expansion of access to surgical facilities occurred after the 1930s (chapter 4), while cost-effectiveness analysis in health became widespread only during the 1970s. By the 1970s, it was not easy to conduct cost-effectiveness studies of many basic and nonelective surgical techniques because they had become "usual care." Much of the more recent cost-effectiveness literature for HICs focuses on refinements, such as minimally invasive techniques, for example, laparoscopic surgery; new types of surgery that become more relevant in aging populations, for example, joint arthroplasty; or new, and often disposable, technologies, such as mesh or stents, and compares these newer interventions with more basic forms of surgery. This literature is of less immediate interest to policy makers in LMICs.

Cost-effectiveness data are more feasibly obtained in LMICs as services expand, given that "usual care" can mean "no intervention" in areas with little or no access to surgery. In LMICs, however, there are fewer studies of emergency procedures and a greater number of studies of elective procedures and nonurgent procedures. Much of the evidence is from surgical missions or nongovernment surgical facilities, and this evidence has limitations. Mission data tend to underestimate costs, because the costs of facilities and follow-up care tend not to be included; nongovernment facilities often have foreign support or foreign personnel, and their costs are not representative.

The organization of surgical services affects cost-effectiveness; in particular, the cost effectiveness of first-level hospitals differs from that of second-level hospitals, specialty hospitals, and surgical missions. Cost-effectiveness of government hospitals may differ from that in hospitals operated by charitable organizations. We briefly summarize some comparative cost-effectiveness data for surgical missions compared with first-level hospitals, specialized hospitals compared with first-level hospitals, and one example of a government-run hospital compared with a nongovernment-run hospital. Shrime and others (chapter 13) discuss in more detail the cost-effectiveness of surgical missions compared with first-level hospitals.

COST-EFFECTIVENESS OF SURGICAL INTERVENTIONS

Methods

Several different metrics can be used to measure the cost-effectiveness of surgical interventions. For LMICs, the cost per DALY averted is often used, as are older variants, such as cost per life year saved (LYS) or cost per death averted. For HICs, the cost per QALY gained is often used. The DALY and QALY measures allow comparisons to be made between interventions that do not necessarily save lives but may substantially improve the quality of life or reduce disabilities; deaths averted or LYS only allow comparisons to be made between life-saving interventions. Some studies do not assess disability and measure only LYS. We have to be cautious because studies do not use the same outcome measures; the underlying methodologies and assumptions also vary. Accordingly, we use such data to illustrate broad tendencies.

The studies cited mainly use DALYs averted or QALYs gained. Although DALYs and QALYs are not identical (the weights attached to different conditions are not the same), we treat them as roughly equivalent. We have

converted all published cost data if expressed in another currency into U.S. dollars, using the market exchange rate of the year the data were collected. We have also converted costs to 2012 U.S. dollars to allow comparisons, first inflating local currency units to 2012 using the consumer price index of the relevant country, and then converting using the average exchange rate for 2012. Throughout the discussion, we refer to the costs and cost-effectiveness in 2012 U.S. dollars.

There is a large literature on methodology (see, for example, Drummond and others 2005), and the debates continue. For example, many of the studies surveyed use discounting to weight costs and benefits occurring further in the future, commonly using the 3 percent social discount rate. More recently, some have argued that discounting is not appropriate (Murray and others, 2012). Past efforts applied different preference weights at different ages, weighting deaths of prime-age working adults more heavily than those of children or the elderly, but this is no longer common practice. Differences in methodology can change the cost-effectiveness ranking of different procedures; for example, the decision as to whether, and by how much, to discount the future has major impacts on interventions affecting children.

The data in tables 18.1 through 18.4 come from various sources. A systematic search of the literature on all surgical costs was undertaken from March through July 2013, with a supplemental search in 2014 in PubMed since 2000 in English. The search combined

Table 18.1 Cost-Effectiveness of Trauma and Emergency Surgery, Excluding Obstetric Emergencies

Source	Condition	Country	Cost per outcome US$	Unit of outcome	Currency, US$	Cost per outcome, 2012 US$
Gosselin and Heitto 2008[a]	Trauma	Cambodia	$77	DALY averted	2006	87
Gosselin, Maldonado, and Elder 2010[b]	Trauma	Haiti	$223	DALY averted	2008	302
	Trauma including burns	Nigeria	$172	DALY averted	2008	218
Gosselin, Gialamas, and Atkin 2011[c]	Acute orthopedic conditions	Haiti	$343	DALY averted	2010	362
Kong and others 2013[d]	Acute appendicitis	South Africa	$1,714	LYS	2011	1,611

Note: DALY = disability-adjusted life year; LYS = life year saved; n.a. = not applicable.

a. Modeled based on costs and estimated DALYs saved for all admissions during a three-month period for a trauma hospital, excluding outpatients.

b. Modeled based on costs and estimated DALYs saved associated with all admissions for a trauma hospital during a three-month period. A higher proportion in Nigeria was life-saving surgery; Haiti includes burns.

c. Included 93 patients during 5 one-week relief missions following earthquake, all acute conditions (debridements, amputation, stump revision, few fixations).

d. Microcosting of appendicitis surgery, combined with estimate from Jha, Bangoura, and Ranson (1998) that appendectomy saves 1.86 life years, based on mortality risks for complicated appendicitis. In South Africa, 36 percent were uncomplicated, 57 percent had perforation, 8 percent had other pathologies and were excluded.

terms for specific surgical interventions listed in annex 18A with economic terms as well as with names of all LMICs and regions containing groups of LMICs. Items determined to be relevant included outcomes such as cost per LYS, per QALY gained, or per DALY averted. From the 124 articles found on all surgeries, we included 29 cost studies that were for essential surgeries covered in this chapter. The search for LMICs identified 36 cost-effectiveness studies, of which 17 were also captured in a systematic survey by Grimes and others (2014) that used slightly different search criteria. We augmented our search with another systematic survey by Chao and others (2014), which added three articles not obtained from either of the searches. Of these, we omitted 16 studies that were not related to essential surgeries, or that focused on circumcision, which is treated in volume 2 of this series. The result was a total of 25 cost-effectiveness studies included in this review. Databases other than PubMed were not included and would have potentially yielded additional studies. Additional articles published between the time of the original search and the publication date of this chapter were not included.

This systematic search was augmented by selective searches of the literature for HICs using more limited search terms for potentially important interventions for which little or no literature turned up for LMICs, such as trauma centers. Results for HICs are discussed in the text but not included in the tables. Other useful published systematic searches, including studies of HICs, include Brauer and others (2005) and Dougherty and Howard (2013), both for orthopedic surgery in HICs, and Lansingh, Carter, and Martens (2007) for cataracts in LMICs and HICs. Annex 18B provides the search statistics.

Articles included were also graded using the Drummond and others (2005) checklist, as used by Chao and others (2014), to provide a quality score for each article (annex 18c). The quality score data are included in the tables. Most of the studies were graded as 7 or above out of 10, with the one exception of nonemergency surgery, where three of the seven articles were graded lower than 7 out of 10. The checklist is similar but not identical to the Consolidated Health Economic Evaluation Reporting Standards checklist (Husereau and others 2013). Some variations occurred across the studies with regard to methodology. For example, although many adopt a societal perspective for the analysis, others use the health system perspective.

Articles chosen for inclusion typically compare a surgical intervention with usual care, that is, no surgical intervention. Comparisons of two different surgical interventions were generally not included.

The focus was on identifying a base set of candidate interventions that are cost-effective at first-level hospitals and another set that are not cost-effective. In HICs, where surgical capacity is much more broadly available and the interventions described have become usual care, the focus of recent literature has shifted to comparisons between different surgical interventions for the same condition or sometimes surgical interventions in comparison with other treatment, for example, a surgical versus a medical approach to cardiovascular disease, or surgery for a musculoskeletal condition versus a corrective device. We reference some of these studies in the text but do not include them in the tables.

We use the term *cost-effectiveness*. Unless otherwise specified, we use incremental cost-effectiveness ratios (ICERs); when comparing surgical treatment to "no intervention," this can readily be described as cost-effectiveness. When we start comparing two different interventions, we need to be more precise. The cost-effectiveness ratios presented are point estimates, but individual studies often conduct sensitivity analysis and provide ranges for their estimates.

How can we compare cost-effectiveness results across a range of countries? How transferable are these results across different environments? Care must be taken in extrapolating results. Costs of interventions vary considerably across countries. The same intervention may have different effectiveness when implemented in different environments. Disease prevalence differs, comorbidities differ, and usual care may be vastly different.

The approach suggested by the Commission on Macroeconomics and Health (WHO 2001) is that interventions costing less than the per capita gross domestic product (GDP) in LMICs are "very cost-effective," and those costing less than triple the per capita GDP are "cost-effective." Although this approach has not typically been applied to HICs, a major study of Australia (Vos and others 2010) categorized a cost per QALY gained of less than $A 50,000 as cost-effective, and less than $A 10,000 as very cost-effective. Studies of the United States have used a similar yardstick for cost-effectiveness; a threshold of £20,000–£30,000 has sometimes been used for the United Kingdom (NICE 2008).

Trauma and Emergency Surgery

Trauma Care

Trauma care saves lives; 77 percent of the deaths preventable by surgery are from injuries, representing 1.04 million deaths annually (chapter 2). Every year, 20–50 million injury survivors are left permanently disabled, most often because of musculoskeletal injuries (Debas and others 2006).

Trauma care can be very cost-effective (table 18.1). Gosselin and Heitto (2008) show that at US$87 per DALY averted, pure trauma hospitals in Cambodia could be very cost-effective. Gosselin, Maldonado, and Elder (2010) evaluate two trauma hospitals in Haiti and Nigeria to find cost-effectiveness ratios of US$302 and US$218 per DALY averted, respectively. The differences in cost-effectiveness were mainly due to different labor cost structures, as well as differences in case mix: the hospital in Haiti includes a burn unit, whereas the one in Nigeria does not. A study of five short relief missions to Haiti following the 2010 earthquake suggested that the cost per DALY averted was US$362 for acute orthopedic conditions (Gosselin, Gialamas, and Atkin 2011).

Emergency Surgery

Although emergency surgery is life saving, it is more difficult to find cost-effectiveness estimates for interventions such as obstructed airway, bowel obstruction, perforation, and cholecystectomy. Appendectomy may be emergency surgery, depending on whether there are complications and sepsis. Kong and others (2013; see table 18.1) estimate that appendectomy costs were US$1,611 per LYS for South Africa. A study for Guinea by Jha, Bangoura, and Ranson (1998) finds appendectomy to be very cost-effective for emergency cases.

Reproductive Surgery

Selected maternal and neonatal conditions avertable by surgery account for 234,000 deaths annually (Bickler and

others, chapter 2 of this volume). The major conditions included are maternal hemorrhage, obstructed labor, abortion, and neonatal encephalopathy. Table 18.2 summarizes some of the cost-effectiveness results for reproductive surgery.

Abortion and Early Pregnancy Loss

Early pregnancy failure is a common occurrence that affects one-third of early pregnancies (Wilcox and others 1988) and one-fourth of all women (Warburton and Fraser 1964). Although the traditional treatment option for such pregnancies has been surgical evacuation of the uterus, medical treatment with misoprostol has been gaining popularity as a noninvasive alternative. Both surgical and nonsurgical treatments are acceptable in practice (Chen and Creinin 2008), but determining the best regimen to use in a given clinical scenario is not always clear. With regard to the cost-effectiveness of different methods, four strategies have been evaluated:

- Hospital-based dilatation and curettage (D&C)
- Hospital-based manual vacuum aspiration (MVA)
- Clinic-based MVA
- Medical abortion using misoprostol.

The World Health Organization (WHO) recommends vacuum aspiration (manual or electric) and medical abortion as the preferred methods for first-trimester abortion (Grimes and others 2006; WHO 2003a). Findings from economic evaluations generally support these recommendations and suggest clinic-based MVA is the most cost-effective option for safe, first-trimester induced abortion. In Mexico and Nigeria, clinic-based MVA was found to be least costly and most effective, compared with D&C; in Ghana,

Table 18.2 Cost-Effectiveness of Reproductive Surgery

Source	Condition	Country	Cost per outcome	Unit of outcome	Currency (unless noted otherwise)	Cost per outcome 2012 US$
First trimester pregnancy termination						
Hu and others 2009[a]	First trimester pregnancy termination	Mexico	n.a.		Clinic-based MVA dominated	n.a.
Hu and others 2010[b]	First trimester pregnancy termination	Nigeria	n.a.		Clinic-based MVA is most cost-effective and cost saving	n.a.
		Ghana	n.a.		Medical abortion is most cost-effective and cost saving	n.a.

table continues next page

Table 18.2 Cost-Effectiveness of Reproductive Surgery (continued)

Source	Condition	Country	Cost per outcome	Unit of outcome	Currency (unless noted otherwise)	Cost per outcome 2012 US$
Intrapartum care						
Hu and others 2007[c]	Intrapartum care	Mexico	$300	DALY averted	2001 US$	$308
Goldie and others 2010[d]	Intrapartum care	India	$150–$350	LYS	2010 US$	$211–$492
Erim, Resch, and Goldie 2012[d]	Intrapartum care	Nigeria	< $550	LYS	2008 US$	< $696
Carvalho, Salehi, and Goldie 2013[d]	Intrapartum care	Afghanistan	$143–$178 (national model)	LYS	2006 US$	$215–$268 (national model)
			$100–$400 (subnational model)			$151–$602 (subnational model)
Obstructed labor or cesarean section						
Adam and others 2005[e]	Management of obstructed labor	Southeast Asia	$38	DALY averted	2000 US$	$72
		Sub-Saharan Africa	$28			$82
Hounton and others 2009	Surgically trained medical officers for cesarean section	Burkina Faso	Obstetrician: $11,757 Clinical officer: $3,235 General practitioner: $200	Newborn life saved	2006 I$	Obstetrician: $5,080 Clinical officer: $1,398 General practitioner: $86
Alkire and others 2012[f]	Cesarean section for obstructed labor	49 LMICs	$304 (median) $251–$3,462 (range)	DALY averted	2008 US$	$384
McCord and Chowdhury 2013[g]	Emergency obstetric care	Bangladesh	$11	DALY averted	1995 US$	$15

Note: DALY = disability-adjusted life year; D&C = dilation and curettage; I$ = international dollar; LMIC = low- to middle-income country; LYS = life year saved; MVA = manual vacuum aspiration; n.a. = not applicable.

a. Model-based comparative analysis of three methods for first-trimester pregnancy termination: D&C, MVA, and medical abortion using a regimen of vaginal misoprostol.

b. Computer-based decision analytic model of induced abortion and its complications comparing unsafe abortion and three methods for safe, first trimester pregnancy: D&C, MVA, and medical abortion using misoprostol.

c. Maternal health policy model used to evaluate a package of care that includes safe abortion and surgical treatment of emergency obstetric care.

d. Maternal health policy model.

e. WHO-CHOICE cost-effectiveness analysis of a package of interventions that includes treatment of emergency obstetric care. Skilled attendance to allow appropriate early recognition and treatment of complications and timely referral to hospitals for more complex care require considerably more resources than community-based and antenatal care packages, but are effective in reducing maternal and neonatal morbidity and mortality and are highly cost-effective.

f. Modeling study.

g. Includes all emergency care at a hospital in Bangladesh for three months: obstetric emergencies are a large proportion and have higher cost-effectiveness than other emergency surgeries.

medical abortion using misoprostol was most cost-effective. In addition to being cost-effective, similar to studies in the United States, shifting to MVA outpatient services has been found to be cost saving (Levin and others 2009; Rausch and others 2012; Rocconi and others 2005). The promotion of medical abortion may have additional benefits by increasing access to safe abortion services, given the challenges of providing surgical services in many low-resource settings, and reducing overall costs of care. It also frees up surgical resources for other essential services for which there may be no nonsurgical options.

The overall implications of these findings from economic evaluations of the management of early pregnancy loss can be summarized as follows:

- The provision of safe abortion is the single most influential factor on health and economic outcomes.
- All else equal, shifting services from D&C to clinic-based MVA will provide equivalent or greater benefits and will result in fewer complications and lower costs.

Institutional Delivery: Emergency Obstetric Care

Overall, achievement of the Millennium Development Goals for the reduction of maternal mortality hinges on the extent of the provision of institutional care during the intrapartum period. Evidence shows that the best intrapartum care strategy is likely to be one in which women routinely choose to deliver in health centers, with midwives as the main providers but with other attendants working with them. Such care is variously referred to as *basic, primary, routine, basic essential obstetric care*, and most recently, *skilled care at the first level* (WHO 2005). Two cost-effectiveness analyses of maternal and neonatal care packages and means of distribution emphasize the potential of close-to-client care for normal and complicated cases—essentially encompassing basic essential obstetric care and basic emergency obstetric care, finding them among the most cost-effective options (Adam and others 2005; Bale and others 2003). More widespread availability of proximate services would increase the likelihood that women would have access if the need for emergency care were to arise in the antenatal or postpartum period (Campbell and Wendy 2006).

Moreover, because health centers are part of the health system, the affordability and sustainability of a health center intrapartum-care strategy are likely to surpass those of strategies distributed outside of the health system, such as traditional birth attendants or volunteer community workers. Accordingly, it is likely that a health center intrapartum-care strategy would be adequate to deal with most births and that this level fits well with the district approach to health systems. Minor variations on the strategy might be needed in some contexts. These variations relate to the cadre of skilled attendants—midwives or doctors—and the case for a hospital intrapartum-care strategy (Campbell and Wendy 2006).

Safe motherhood strategies, such as intrapartum care consisting of normal or assisted delivery, or comprehensive emergency obstetric care, are usually delivered as a package of services. The literature evaluates the cost-effectiveness of such strategies using packages of care. Family planning interventions and safe abortion services are central to reducing the maternal mortality rate in Afghanistan, India, and Nigeria (Carvalho, Salehi, and Goldie 2013; Erim, Resch, and Goldie 2012; Goldie and others 2010). However, these studies consistently find that further reductions would not occur without increasing access to high-quality intrapartum and emergency obstetrical care.

For example, in India, attainment of the fifth Millennium Development Goal of a 75 percent reduction in maternal mortality by 2015 would require investments targeting the intrapartum period, in addition to family planning and safer abortion. Including surgery in a package of maternal care also includes family planning, safe abortion facilities, facility-based basic emergency obstetric care, and quality comprehensive emergency obstetric care. The ICERs for increased coverage were in the range of US$211–US$492 per LYS, that is, 14 percent to 33 percent of GDP per capita in India and hence very cost-effective (Goldie and others 2010; table 18.2). The same package of care costs less than US$696 per LYS in Nigeria (Erim, Resch, and Goldie 2012) and less than US$268 in Afghanistan (Carvalho, Salehi, and Goldie 2013).

Adam and others (2005) find skilled care at birth consisting of basic emergency obstetric care and comprehensive emergency obstetric care to be cost-effective in LMICs, such as those in South and Southeast Asia and Sub-Saharan Africa. In 2000, a package of care consisting of basic antenatal care and skilled attendance at birth had an incremental cost of US$21.72 in Sub-Saharan Africa and US$36.64 in South and Southeast Asia, compared with the option of antenatal care without skilled attendance at birth. This package amounted to an additional US$67.3 million and US$96.2 million, respectively, in the entire Sub-Saharan African and Southeast Asian regions, including South Asia, for universal access (Adam and others 2005).

Two studies explore increasing access through task-shifting and the training of lower-level general practitioners to overcome staff shortages of physicians for performing emergency care and surgical services. Kruk and others (2007) show that lower-level cadres can provide surgical services at a reasonable cost in rural Mozambique. Hounton and others (2009) look at the cost-effectiveness of training different cadres of health workers to perform cesarean sections, finding that training of general practitioners appeared effective and cost-effective.

Nonemergency Surgery

Nonemergency surgery, although less often life saving, can still alleviate a considerable proportion of the global burden of disease. Cost-effectiveness data are summarized in table 18.3, panels a (congenital defects, hernia, and nonemergency orthopedic conditions) and b (selected types of eye surgery).

Congenital Defects

Cleft lip/palate is one of the more common birth defects, occurring in 1 out of 500–700 births (Magee, Vander Burg, and Hatcher 2010). If untreated, it can lead to problems with eating, language development, and hearing; in severe cases, it is associated with higher mortality in early childhood. Data from surgical missions for cleft lip/palate surgery in four countries (Magee, Vander Burg, and Hatcher 2010; Moon, Perry, and Baek 2012) suggest that this surgery is very cost-effective. Moon, Perry, and Baek (2012) estimate the average cost for a mission in Vietnam was US$86/DALY averted; Magee, Vander Burg, and Hatcher (2010) estimate that the cost over eight missions to four countries ranged from US$9 to US$108 per DALY averted. Surgical mission data do not typically account for the costs of the surgeon's time or the facilities.

Table 18.3 Cost-Effectiveness of Nonemergency Surgeries

a. Selected surgeries

Source	Condition	Country	Cost per outcome	Unit of outcome	Currency	Cost per outcome, 2012 US$
Congenital defects						
Corlew 2010[a]	Cleft lip, cleft palate	Nepal	$29	DALY averted	2005 US$	$40
Magee, Vander Burg, and Hatcher 2010[b]	Cleft lip, cleft palate	8 missions (5 Vietnam, 1 each Nicaragua, Kenya, Russian Federation)	$7–$96	DALY averted	2008 US$	$9–$108
Moon, Perry, and Baek 2012[c]	Cleft lip, cleft palate	Vietnam	$68 ($87 imputing volunteer time)	DALY averted	2003 US$	$67 ($86 imputing volunteer time)
Hernia						
Shillcutt, Clarke, and Kingsnorth 2010[d]	Inguinal hernia	Ghana	$13	DALY averted	2008 US$	$11
Shillcutt and others 2013[e]	Inguinal hernia	Ecuador	$96	DALY averted	2011 US$	$101
Nonemergency orthopedic surgery						
Gosselin, Gialamas, and Atkin 2011[f]	Various	Dominican Republic, Nicaragua	$362	DALY averted	2009/10 US$	$359
Chen and others 2012[g]	Various	Nicaragua	$476	DALY averted	2011 US$	$540

Source:

Note: DALY = disability-adjusted life year.

a. Calculated from one center in Kathmandu specializing in cleft lip (402 cases) and palate (166 cases) in one year.

b. Only includes mission costs, not local hospital costs.

c. Based on costs of 16 missions from Korea to Vietnam during 1996–2010. Excludes cost of hospital space and depreciation of hospital facilities.

d. Based on five-day mission to four first-level hospitals in Ghana. Used Liechtenstein repair, day surgery.

e. Based on 2 two-week missions. Used Liechtenstein repair, day surgery.

f . Volunteer surgical mission of one week, 30 patients (knee osteoarthritis, fractures, dislocations, amputations, injured nerves); excludes building costs, maintenance, utilities. Cost-effectiveness from Nicaraguan provider perspective.

g. Some 117 patients over three missions 2009–10; less than 10 percent were acute conditions; congenital malformations (club foot, developmental dysplasia of hip) were 32 percent. No salary cost for surgical volunteers, but travel and lodging cost is included.

b. Cataract Surgery and Similar Eye Surgeries

Source	Condition	Country	Cost per outcome	Unit of outcome	Currency	Cost per outcome, 2012 US$
Baltussen and others 2005[a]	Trachoma	Seven WHO subregions AFR-E (lowest cost per DALY averted) to EMRO-D	$13–$78	DALY averted	2000 I$	$7–$28
Lansingh, Carter, and Martens 2007[b]	Cataracts	Nine LMICs	$4–$253	QALY gained	2004 US$	$6–$423
Wittenborn and Rein 2011[c]	Laser surgery for glaucoma	Barbados	$1,528	DALY averted	2005 US$	$2,314
		Ghana	$1,771			$1,989
Baltussen and Smith 2012[d]	Trachoma (trichiasis surgery)	Sub-Saharan Africa (AFR-E); South Asia (SEA-D)	$71–$90 AFR-E $285–$374 SEA-D (80–95% coverage)	DALY averted	2005 I$	$31–$40 AFR-E $106–$140 SEA-D
	Cataracts		$116 AFR-E $97 SEA-D	DALY averted	2005 I$	$36 AFR-E $51 SEA-D

Note: AFR-E = the WHO subregion in Africa with the highest mortality rates; DALY = disability-adjusted life year; EMRO-B = the WHO subregion in the Eastern Mediterranean with the highest mortality rates; I$ = international dollar; n.a. = not applicable; QALY = quality-adjusted life year; SEA-D = the WHO subregion in Southeast Asia (including South Asia) with the highest mortality rates.

a. WHO-CHOICE model; extracapsular cataract extraction for cataracts.

b. Literature survey 1996–2006. The authors find 5 studies with calculated cost-effectiveness for first eye (4 countries), and use cost data from another 11 countries to calculate cost-effectiveness.

c. Laser surgery only for syndromic referral; treatment with full American Academy of Ophthalmology guidelines is more costly, as is treatment on incidence, and screen and treat.

d. Newer version of model in Baltussen and others (2005).

An estimate by Corlew (2010) for a nongovernment-supported program at Katmandu Model Hospital, using local physicians, was US$40 per DALY averted for Nepal; these DALYs were age weighted. The program also provides orthodontic services and speech therapy, which are not included in the short-term missions. Cost data from a permanent facility are likely to be a better guide for ongoing programs than cost data from missions. All of these estimates are in the very cost-effective range.

Clubfoot is a less common condition, and can be treated nonsurgically as well as surgically. One estimate of surgical cost for New Zealand (Halanski and others 2009) yielded an estimated cost per DALY averted that would fall in the very cost-effective range for New Zealand; however, no cost-effectiveness results were found for LMICs.

Hernia

Repair of inguinal hernia is one of the most commonly performed operations in the Americas (Shillcutt and others 2013). In Sub-Saharan Africa, 175 people per 100,000 need this operation each year (Shillcutt, Clarke, and Kingsnorth 2010). The lack of access to timely care leads to complications and ultimately more expensive emergency surgery, and it increases mortality and morbidity. Estimates from surgical missions suggest that the repair was very cost-effective in Ecuador at US$101 per DALY averted (Shillcutt and others 2013) and Ghana at US$11 per DALY averted (Shillcutt, Clarke, and Kingsnorth 2010).

Estimates from HICs confirm the findings that surgery for abdominal, inguinal, umbilical, and femoral hernia is very cost-effective (Coronini-Cronberg, Appleby, and Thompson 2013). A comparative study of three different options for inguinal hernia repair for the United States (Stylopoulos, Gazelle, and Rattner 2003) suggests that laparoscopic repair was more cost-effective than open methods, each compared with no intervention, largely because the greater effectiveness possibly offset the higher cost. However, laparoscopic methods are not widely available in LMICs at first-level hospitals. One study for the United States (Stroupe and others 2006) points out that cost-effectiveness depends on the population considered; repair is much less cost-effective for men with asymptomatic or minimally symptomatic hernia.

Recent literature in HICs examines the cost-effectiveness of devices and technologies that may require expensive purchased inputs. Most LMICs cannot afford these inputs. In India, Gundre, Iyer, and Subramaniyan (2012) have shown that using polyethylene mesh for inguinal hernia meshplasty is equally safe and effective but 2,808 times cheaper compared with the use of commercially available polypropylene mesh.

Nonemergency Orthopedic Procedures

In 1990, an estimated 1.7 million people worldwide had hip fractures, a number that is expected to increase to 6 million annually by 2050 (chapter 3). Estimates for 2002 were that osteoarthritis was the fourth most important source of disability, mainly due to osteoarthritis of the hip and knee (chapter 3). As populations in large LMICs age, the demand for nonemergency orthopedic procedures is expected to grow dramatically.

Estimates of the cost per DALY averted for nonemergency surgical missions are similar to those for trauma surgery. One study of 30 patients (Chen and others 2012, table 18.3A) estimates the cost of a mission to Nicaragua to be US$540 per DALY averted; another study of 117 patients and three missions estimates the costs for the Dominican Republic and Nicaragua to be US$359 per DALY averted (Gosselin, Gialamas, and Atkin 2011). Both studies likely underestimate the costs of such treatment on an ongoing basis. The former study does not include costs for space, maintenance, and utilities; the latter does not include salary costs, although it includes travel costs for the volunteers. These costs per DALY averted are similar to those of the emergency surgery missions and likely suffer from similar methodological issues in costing. However, the costs per DALY averted are so modest that even if all costs are included these interventions are likely to remain very cost-effective. Mission data in general are likely to be somewhat artificial. To take maximum advantage of the availability of surgeons, it is likely that a significant amount of organization has to occur before the mission to line up a suitable number of surgical appointments. Similarly, following the mission, follow-up is likely to be required by the local hospitals and health facilities. Neither of these inputs is generally included in the mission cost. The caseload and case mix for missions is not representative of that seen in a regular hospital. Missions may aim not to have downtime, while ongoing surgical facilities in LMICs may have more downtime. Missions have the advantage of economies of scale, that is, a number of similar surgeries are grouped together. Nonspecialized hospitals could conceivably try to do similar grouping, for example, perform orthopedic surgery on one specific day of the week, but doing so requires managerial capacity that is scarce in many of these settings.

Data from HICs confirm that there are cost-effective, nonemergency orthopedic procedures. Hip arthroplasty is very cost-effective in the United States (Chang, Pellissier, and Hazen 1996), although some of the assumptions, such as the cost savings anticipated in the United States from custodial care in the absence of surgery, are unlikely to apply in LMICs. Dougherty and Howard (2013) show similar findings for the United Kingdom, but the costs per QALY gained are higher than for the United States; James, St Leger, and Rowsell (1996) find that hip arthroplasty is very cost-effective in the United Kingdom. This operation is likely to become increasingly common in LMICs as populations age.

Knee arthroplasty costs at least twice as much as hip arthroplasty per DALY averted in both the United Kingdom and the United States, but it may also be cost-effective (Chang, Pellissier, and Hazen 1996; James, St Leger, and Rowsell 1996; Lavernia, Guzman, and Gachupin-Garcia 1997). However, Dougherty and Howard (2013) find that hip arthroplasty in the United Kingdom is twice as costly as knee arthroplasty, although their work is a literature survey and the underlying studies may not all use the same methodology. James, St Leger, and Rowsell (1996) suggest that other interventions in the United Kingdom, including those for spinal discectomy, carpal tunnel syndrome, and Dupuytren's contracture, were also very cost-effective, but that flexor tenosynovectomy costs more per DALY averted, and some operations had negative cost-effectiveness. The sample numbers in this study for interventions other than knee and hip arthroscopy were fairly small. Dougherty and Howard (2013) also provide cost-effectiveness results for other orthopedic procedures for the United States.

Cataracts

The number of blind persons globally increased from 38 million in 1990 to 124 million in 2002 (Resnikoff and others 2004; Thylefors and others 1995). Cataract disease is the cause of approximately 48 percent of the cases of total blindness worldwide (Resnikoff and others 2004); a rapidly aging population in many countries will continue to exacerbate the prevalence of visual impairment as a result of cataract disease. The WHO and the International Agency for the Prevention of Blindness joined forces in 1999 to respond to the problem, resulting in the launch of VISION 2020: The Right to Sight global initiative (Pizzarello and others 2004). The chief goal of this program is to eliminate avoidable blindness by 2020; if the planned interventions succeed, an estimated 52 million persons will have their sight saved, with the concurrent avoidance of 429 million blind person-years and an economic gain of US$102 billion (Frick and Foster 2003). To achieve this lofty target, one of VISION 2020's specific objectives is to increase the availability of cataract surgery globally by raising output and training ophthalmic surgeons, especially in LMICs.

Cataract surgery is a routine intervention, and demand is expected to increase substantially as populations age. Knowledge of the cost-effectiveness of cataract surgery is essential if decisions on health care spending are to be as objective as possible.

Baltussen and Smith (2012, table 18.3B) estimate the cost-effectiveness of cataract surgery via extracapsular cataract extraction (ECCE) with posterior chamber intraocular lens implantation compared with no intervention, and find it to be very cost-effective in various WHO subregions, as is trichiasis surgery for trachoma. Another review (Lansingh, Carter, and Martens 2007) finds that cataract surgery, irrespective of country, is very cost-effective in all 15 countries considered (including 9 LMICs). The study also shows that cataract surgery is cheaper in an outpatient setting than with an overnight stay, and the phacoemulsification technique is costlier than either ECCE or manual small-incision cataract surgery. This review assesses the affordability of cataract surgery, defined as cost compared with per capita income, and finds that it is more affordable in Western Europe than in the United States; India is one country where it is most affordable among the LMICs of Asia (Lansingh, Carter, and Martens 2007).

A study in Nepal (Marseille 1996) confirms that cataract surgery is very cost-effective, although this particular study may not have fully incorporated all costs.

Several issues affect the cost-effectiveness of cataract surgery. Cost-effectiveness tends to be higher in the first eye treated than in the second, and the worse eye is usually prioritized. Most of the studies include a short follow-up period. Lundström and Wendel (2005) find that in Sweden, 80 percent of patients still enjoyed improved visual function seven years after surgery. This finding implies that a lifetime study horizon would be most appropriate for evaluating economic impact. With the rising life expectancy of populations, patients who receive the surgery are likely to live longer and enjoy a better quality of life with better vision for a longer period. This finding implies that the ICERs for cataract surgery are likely to be lower in the future, and cataract surgery will become even more cost-effective.

Wittenborn and Rein (2011) find that one-time surgery for self-referring patients was very cost-effective for

both Barbados and Ghana; screening and using the full United States guideline treatment was not cost-effective in Ghana.

Organization of Surgical Services

The volume of surgeries undertaken is important. Effectiveness is higher and mortality rates are lower for surgeons who undertake the same operation many times in a year or in their careers; the same holds true for facilities and hospitals. In most cases, costs will likely be lower per operation at higher volumes because standardization typically reduces costs and allows the cost of any specialized equipment to be spread over a larger volume of patients.

For nonemergency surgery, specialized units that focus on specific types of surgery can be considered. These include specialized units performing cataract surgery, such as the Lumbini Zone eye hospital in Nepal (Marseille 1996); cleft lip and palate surgery, such as the one in Nepal (Corlew 2010); and fistula repair, such as centers in Ethiopia, Ghana, Nigeria, and Rwanda. To increase access, specialized units can be brought to local areas periodically, for example, through camps.

Cataract camps occur in South Asia with some regularity. Singh and others (2000) review the cost-effectiveness of three different types of facility offering cataract surgery in Karnataka state, India. They compare government camps, which were the least expensive for patients; nongovernment facilities, in which costs to patients were double that of the camps; and a government medical college hospital, in which costs to patients were three times that of the camps. The total costs of the camps and the nongovernment facility were similar; the cost of the medical college hospital was more than twice that of the others. The most cost-effective facility was the nongovernment one because of higher quality; the camps were intermediate, and the medical college the least cost-effective.

Specialized facilities bring tradeoffs. The facilities may offer greater effectiveness due to the specialized team and facilities, possibly even a lower cost due to economies of scale, but they may be more distant and hence be more costly to patients. To address the accessibility issue, it may be possible to bring specialized teams closer to more decentralized populations by offering a mobile camp, or by bringing specialized teams to first-level hospitals one day a week or one week every few months; however, doing so requires additional organizational capacity.

Finally, international surgical missions are a particular version of increasing access by bringing in specialized resources. Surgical missions occur in all areas: trauma

(Gosselin and Heitto 2008, table 18.1; Gosselin, Heitto, and Zirkle 2009); congenital defects (Magee, Vander Burg, and Hatcher 2010; Moon, Perry, and Baek 2012; hernia (Shillcutt, Clarke, and Kingsnorth 2010; Shillcutt and others 2013); cataract surgery (Marseille 1996); and nonemergency orthopedic surgery (Chen and others 2012; Gosselin, Gialamas, and Atkin 2011). Missions can increase capacity, and many surgical missions assist in building local capacity by helping train local surgical teams.

Shrime and others (chapter 13) examine the cost-effectiveness of surgical missions, as well as that of specialty hospitals supported by charitable organizations. Their conclusion is that short-term missions should be used only if no other option is available because evidence suggests that effectiveness is not as high as in more fixed facilities. This result is not surprising given that preoperative care and follow-up after surgery are not to the usual standard because of the logistics. They also examine the limited cost-effectiveness data on specialty hospitals, identifying the same study of cataract surgery (Singh, Garner, and Floyd 2000) discussed in this chapter, which shows that the charitable hospital had the most cost-effective outcomes of the three modalities considered. Cost-effectiveness data are available for other such facilities (Corlew 2010) for cleft palate, but no comparison is made to other facilities in the same country.

Trauma care is different from other surgical interventions. The emergency nature of this care, which also applies to obstetric emergencies, makes specialized trauma care facilities more difficult to establish. Urban areas in HICs can support trauma centers, provided that adequate rapid transportation is available. Trauma centers do exist in LMICS, for example, the ones analyzed by Gosselin, Maldonado, and Elder (2010) in Nigeria and Haiti.

Several studies for the United States have documented the effectiveness of a regionalized approach to trauma care, where critically injured patients are treated in a limited number of designated trauma centers (Durham and others 2006; MacKenzie and others 2010; Nathens and others 2000). Risk of death is 25 percent lower when care is provided in a regional, third-level trauma center than when it is provided in a nontrauma center hospital (MacKenzie and others 2010).

MacKenzie and others (2010) find that the cost-effectiveness ratio for treatment in a trauma center versus a nontrauma center in the United States fell in the cost-effective range. It is more cost-effective to treat more severely injured patients and those patients younger than age 55 years in a trauma center. This study uses comprehensive data available on both the effectiveness and the costs incurred in the year after injury for 5,043

patients treated at 69 trauma centers and nontrauma centers in 14 states of the United States (MacKenzie and others 2010).

WHO BENEFITS FROM SURGICAL SERVICES?

Major health shocks often lead to large out-of-pocket medical expenditures, induced borrowing, or the forced selling of assets and resulting in impoverishment in LMICs. Using data from 89 countries, Xu and others (2007) estimate that annually 150 million households across the world experience *catastrophic* health spending, defined as 40 percent or more of their nonfood expenditure on health care. Leive and Xu (2008) analyze household health care financing in 15 Sub-Saharan African countries; they find that in Burkina Faso, as many as 68 percent of households that had out-of-pocket health spending had borrowed money or sold assets to finance medical expenditures in the past year. In a larger study, Kruk, Goldmann, and Galea (2009) use data from 40 LMICs and find that more than 25 percent of households were forced to borrow money or sell assets to pay for health care costs. Other multicountry studies report similar large household financial costs associated with major health shocks (van Doorslaer and others 2007; Xu and others 2007).

Additional factors—such as access to care, willingness to pay, and the ability to pay—are important. As Weiser and others (2008) estimate, LMICs account for about 70 percent of the world's population but only perform about 26 percent of the 234 million annual surgeries. The large and often prohibitive costs of surgery are likely to be the greatest deterrent to obtaining care (Malhotra and others 2005). Accordingly, the majority of the literature on surgery in LMICs focuses on the barriers to access.

A few studies have examined the economic benefits of providing access to surgical care, particularly for poor people. For example, poverty and blindness are often found to be highly correlated (Gilbert and others 2008; Zimmer 2008). Accordingly, cataract surgery that prevents blindness may also prevent impoverishment. Kuper and others (2010) conducted a case-control study of cataract surgery in Bangladesh, Kenya, and the Philippines. The authors find that cataract surgery successfully increased the standard of living, as measured by monthly per capita expenditure, in the intervention group. The average increase in monthly per capita expenditure among patients who received the surgery was 36 percent in Kenya, 44 percent in Bangladesh, and 88 percent in the Philippines, compared with the control group, whose income did not change in Kenya and the Philippines and fell slightly in Bangladesh. Although the economic benefits reached patients in all socioeconomic groups, the positive effect of blindness prevention was the greatest among the poorest participants.

Finger and others (2012), in a similar study in south India, find that cataract surgery was associated with higher standards of living and gainful economic activities. At least 45 percent of the participants receiving cataract surgery reported higher income levels after surgery, and the share of participants engaged in economic activities increased from 44 percent to 77 percent. The authors also found that the surgery improved the social status of widowed participants by increasing the rates of remarriage.

Two studies have modeled the economic benefits from cleft lip and palate surgery but without using household data on actual effects. Corlew (2010) for Nepal and Alkire and others (2011) for Sub-Saharan Africa estimate that considerable potential economic benefits were realized.

SURGICAL INTERVENTION COSTS[1]

The unit cost data in LMICs are not robust, but they have grown since the publication of Disease Control Priorities in Developing Countries, second edition, in 2006. Noting the paucity of literature on surgical costs and cost-effectiveness, Debas and others (2006) estimate costs of surgical services offered by first-level hospitals and community clinics that were not specific to interventions. The number of studies presenting economic information on surgical services and intervention-specific surgeries has increased since 2000; the majority of articles were published after 2006, and more than two-thirds were published after 2009. Most studies were conducted in South Asia and Sub-Saharan Africa, with the greatest body of literature emerging from India, followed by Bangladesh and Pakistan. Box 18.1 summarizes results for one such study, for Nepal. Much of the recent literature captures costs from third-level hospitals and focuses on specific diseases, surgical procedures, or platforms, with fewer studies providing estimates of surgical facility or ward costs from first-level hospitals.

Surgical Costs, by Type of Hospital

Total program costs for surgical care are driven by several factors, including the type and size of the hospital; whether it is public or privately owned and operated; and the surgical platform for delivering services, bed occupancy, and differences in salary structures. A study of five hospitals in India finds a range of annual program costs for different types of hospitals,

including US$295,556 in a 60-bed charitable hospital; US$321,887 in a 400-bed first-level public hospital; US$1,314,935 in a private teaching hospital with 655 beds; and US$2,019,260 in a public third-level care hospital with 778 beds (Chatterjee and Laxminarayan 2013). In Ghana, a first-level hospital with 117 beds had annual surgical costs of US$66,492, which was two-and-a-half times less than a 200-bed mission hospital and four times less than a 110-bed third-level hospital (Aboagye, Degboe, and Obuobi 2010). These surgical program costs in India and Ghana vary considerably from previous regional estimates attributable to surgical patients, based on a standardized first-level hospital of 100 beds, which was US$1,124,728 for South Asia and US$1,471,575 for Sub-Saharan Africa (Debas and others 2006).

In LMICs, nongovernment surgical hospitals are a popular strategy for providing specialty care for trauma and orthopedics, especially among the urban poor who have limited access to surgical services. Nongovernmental hospitals are often characterized by higher costs because expatriate surgeons are working closely with national counterparts in a well-staffed and supplied facility, and the throughput of patients and surgical procedures performed throughout the year is higher. Two nongovernment surgical hospitals with 70 beds in Sierra Leone and 106 beds in Cambodia had annual operating budgets of US$214,113 and US$118,228, respectively (Gosselin, Thind, and Bellardinelli 2006; Gosselin and Heitto 2008). Labor costs constituted the major share of total surgical costs, with expatriate staff alone accounting for 30 percent of total costs in Cambodia. Medical surgical trauma centers operated by Médecins Sans Frontières cost US$1,112,665 per year in Nigeria's 70-bed urban hospital and US$1,864,822 per year in two surgical sites in Haiti, with one urban hospital with 60 beds and a second facility with 48 beds (Gosselin, Maldonado, and Elder 2010). Surgical unit costs are also available for platforms that deliver specialized services for cataract, cleft palate, or orthopedics through short-term outreach or medical missions; costs for these services are typically provided on a per trip or per person basis, and the services reach between 30 and 2,000 patients per year through time-limited medical missions (Chen and others 2012; Kandel and others 2010; Moon, Perry, and Baek 2012).

Surgical Unit Costs, by Condition

Recently published studies provide costs for disease-specific surgeries rather than surgical programs, adding an additional layer of variability depending on the

Financial Sustainability of Scaling Up Surgical Services in a First-Level Facility: Case Study of Bayalpata Hospital in Nepal

Bayalpata Hospital in Nepal offers a unique case study for understanding the financial issues of scaling up (Maru and others 2011). This hospital serves as the referral hospital for the Achham district's primary health care centers, as well as for populations from two adjacent districts. It has three sources of funding:

- The government of Nepal (25 percent)
- Individual donors via the U.S.-based parent organization, Nyaya Health (approximately 50 percent)
- Foundation grants (25 percent).

The hospital includes outpatient and inpatient services and 24-hour emergency and delivery services, as well as laboratory and radiological (x-ray and ultrasound) diagnostic services. It has an onsite pharmacy and ambulance, and it implements community health programs. Its staff performs minor surgeries, such as repair of lacerations, abscess drainage, closed reductions, casting, and manual vacuum aspiration. It has two physicians and a nursing and midwifery staff but no surgeon. Without an operating room, there is no capacity for major surgeries.

The WHO developed an Integrated Management of Emergency and Essential Surgical Care (IMEESC) program in LMICs (WHO 2006). Bayalpata Hospital in Nepal upgraded its services under the IMEESC-Plus program (Maru and others 2011). This upgrade included the list of essential services proposed under IMEESC and two other components: community follow-up of surgical cases and quality improvement of hospital care. A general physician was trained

to perform surgery, and visiting senior surgeons, both national and international, provided ongoing training.

The list of essential surgical services to be provided under IMEESC-Plus includes the following:

- Amputation of distal or proximal limbs
- Appendectomy
- Cesarean section
- Cholecystectomy
- Exploratory laparotomy
- Hernia repair
- Hydrocele reduction
- Surgical correction of head, chest, and abdominal trauma
- Surgical management of acute closed and open fractures
- Surgical management of wounds and burns.

A financial costing of this basic package of surgical services was undertaken. Based on Bayalpata Hospital's costing model, it was proposed that the overall construction and two-year operating costs of implementing the IMEESC-Plus model would be US$0.50 per capita in the district, which has a population of 266,000 (Maru and others 2011). The reported per capita health expenditure in Nepal in 2008–09 was US$24.8. Nearly 24 percent of this expenditure, or US$6, was borne by the government. If this incremental cost of US$0.50 were entirely publicly financed and scaled up across the country, it would amount to an 8.4 percent increase in the government's health budget.

Source: Maru and others 2011.

disease condition treated, the number and frequency of surgeries performed for a particular condition during a given period, and the surgical technique used. Table 18.4 provides a summary for four reproductive surgeries, two types of nonemergency surgeries, and cardiothoracic surgery.

Information is available on the costs of specific conditions for obstetric and gynecological services

because of research and advocacy interest in increasing access to reproductive and maternal health services, including access to safe surgical abortion. In addition, obstetric and gynecological services typically constitute a large share of total inpatient activity at hospitals. Although variations across studies are typical, several studies have shown variations in the cost of procedures, such as cesarean section, within the same study (Levin

Table 18.4 Variations in Cost of Selected Surgical Procedures

Type of surgery	Location	Range of costs (2012 US$)	Source
Reproductive surgery			
Cesarean section	Africa	$41–$202	Honda, Randaoharison, and Matsui 2011; Hounton and others 2009; Kruk and others 2007; Levin and others 2003
	East Asia and Pacific	$548	Quayyum and others 2010
	South Asia	$121–$195	Khan and Zaman 2010; Sarowar and others 2010
Emergency obstetric surgery	Africa	$158–$202	Kruk and others 2007; Richard and others 2007
Surgical abortion	Various countries, types of hospital (public, private), and procedures	$8–$158 (D&C) $8–$103 (MVA)	Banerjee, Andersen, and Warvadekar 2012; Benson and others 2012; Henshaw and others 2008; Hu and others 2010; Koontz and others 2003; Levin and others 2009; PATH and M. O. H. Reproductive Health Department 2006; Sarowar and others 2010; Xia, She, and Lam 2011
Postabortion complications	Various countries; various procedures (cervical or vaginal lacerations less costly than vaginal perforations)	$58 (median) $18–$2,368	Asante, Avotri, and d'Almeida 2004; Erim, Resch, and Goldie 2012; Hu and others 2010; Levin and others 2003; Levin and others 2009; Rehan 2011; Vlassoff and others 2012; Vlassoff and others 2014
Nonemergency surgery			
Cataract surgery	India, various techniques	$30–$47	Muralikrishnan and others 2004
	Nepal, different camps	$63–$94	Kandel and others 2010
Hernia repair	Lichtenstein tension-free repair, various countries	$114 (Ghana), US$1,212 (China)	Gong and others 2011; Shillcutt, Clarke, and Kingsnorth 2010
	India, different hospitals and techniques	$270 (first-level)–$1,047 (third-level hospital, laparoscopic method)	Bansal and others 2012; Chatterjee and Laxminarayan 2013; Krishna and others 2012
Cardiothoracic surgery	India, public hospital	$3,315	Chatterjee and Laxminarayan 2013

and others 2003; Quayyum and others 2010). Some differences could be explained by differences in cost components.

In general, labor was the single largest component of total direct costs for all public hospital types, and indirect costs were the largest driver of costs for charitable and private hospitals. For some procedures, such as hernia repair and external fixations, drugs and materials constituted the largest share of direct costs. In general, costs tend to be lower at first-level hospitals than at second-level hospitals, probably because the more costly and specialized facilities are not available at the first-level hospital; private hospitals may be more costly than public; more specialized procedures and procedures using additional medical technologies are more costly;

and costs are generally lower in countries with lower per capita incomes.

LIMITATIONS IN THE EVIDENCE BASE

As this review suggests, cost-effectiveness data for LMICs are scarce and may be affected by reporting bias. The data that do exist are heavily dominated by studies of surgical missions and nongovernment facilities. The data for missions likely understate the costs of ongoing services, and the effectiveness of government hospitals may be lower than that of hospitals run by charitable foundations. We have used data from HICs to supplement that from LMICs and to fill gaps. Cost-effectiveness findings depend on the context, methodology, and assumptions made. However, there is reason to believe that a range of surgical interventions are cost-effective for LMICs.

The data limitations include the following:

- First, despite the increase in the number of economic evaluations, cost estimations, especially of unit cost data from first-level hospitals covering some or all of the recommended essential surgeries, are deficient. Specifically, most cost estimations have been disease specific and typically do not provide the costs of surgical wards. In addition, whatever cost estimates are available pertain to localized geographic areas and are typically derived from one or several hospitals, but they are not representative of the national health care system. In addition to heterogeneity in costs due to geography or conditions treated, inconsistency in data-collection methods and reporting formats limit the comparability of the data.
- Second, limited availability of empirical disability weights for various conditions in international health is an issue, mentioned, for example, in Shillcutt, Clarke, and Kingsnorth (2010) and Shillcutt and others (2013).
- Third, reliable information is critical if any attempt is to be made to base medical decisions on health and monetary considerations. The value of economic analysis is compromised if the quality of the data is poor. Methodologies for economic analyses appeared in the medical literature as early as the 1970s, with refinements over time (Blackmore and Smith 1998; Detsky and Naglie 1990; Jefferson, Demicheli, and Vale 2002). Although these methods are intended to reduce bias and improve the validity of economic analyses, these methodological principles are used infrequently (Blackmore and Smith 1998; Doubilet, Weinstein, and McNeil 1986). Calls have been made to standardize economic analysis methodology and for adherence to these principles in the medical literature (Doubilet, Weinstein and McNeil 1986; Drummond and Jefferson 1996; Jefferson, Demicheli, and Vale 2002).

Research that assesses the quality of cost-effectiveness data in specialties is available, including for gynecologic oncology (Manuel and others 2004), pharmacoeconomics (Iskedjian and others 1997), pediatrics (Ungar and Santos 2005), and nuclear medicine (Gambhir and Schwimmer 2000). These assessments, along with more generalized ones, systematically review studies to verify compliance with methodological criteria. Studies use various scoring methods; however, many check compliance with methodological principles thought to represent the minimum standards for medical economic analysis. Kruper, Kurichi, and Sonnad (2007) searched MEDLINE for 1995 to 2004 to identify articles that included economic analyses of surgical procedures. Their review indicates that published economic evaluations of surgical procedures in general do not follow accepted methodological standards, with fewer than half of the basic principles met by any given analysis. A comparison of nonsurgical versus surgical journals demonstrates a significant difference in compliance with methodological criteria, with much lower compliance in surgical journals. The average proportion of criteria met in the nonsurgical journals was slightly more than half, whereas in the surgery journals it was less than one-third. The surgical journals were also consistently lower in compliance with each individual criterion as compared with the nonsurgical journals, with less than 20 percent compliance for five criteria.

To defend the use of surgical interventions and treatment strategies in an environment that is becoming progressively more cost conscious, quality data become increasingly important. Those performing analyses in surgical areas need to increase their awareness of methodological standards so that the quality of surgical economic evaluations can improve, especially those evaluations in surgical journals. Wider promulgation of the methodological criteria in surgical journals or at surgical meetings may significantly improve the quality of economic analysis published in surgical journals or concerning surgical interventions.

Evidence gaps exist in the literature. No studies for LMICs were found for several conditions relevant for cancer, including mastectomy, hysterectomy, and blockages of the colon, or for obstetric fistula, despite the existence of some specialized units providing surgery for this condition in LMICs.

CONCLUSIONS

Disease Control Priorities in Developing Countries, second edition (DCP2), drew attention to the importance of surgical interventions in LMICs (Debas and others 2006). The authors showed that particular examples of surgical packages and platforms, such as providing cataract surgery, training lower-level medical staff for emergency obstetric surgery, and delivering surgery at first-level hospitals, were very cost-effective in many countries in South Asia and Sub-Saharan Africa.

Inclusion in Primary Health Care

Many countries are considering including surgical care in comprehensive primary health care. This primary care initiative, described in *World Health Report* (WHO 2008), focuses on strengthening health systems through a series of reforms under the umbrella of primary health care. It is increasingly recognized that the provision and maintenance of a quality surgical service can strengthen the capacity to deliver other health services. Surgery is an essential component of efforts to reduce maternal mortality in childbirth, and it is of growing importance as the burden of noncommunicable diseases increases.

Global Initiatives

In response to the deficiencies in the capacity to deliver basic surgical services in LMICs, the WHO launched the Emergency and Essential Surgical Care (EESC) Project in 2004 (Bickler and Spiegel 2010). The IMEESC toolkit, supplemented by the text *Surgical Care at the District Hospital* (WHO 2003b), was developed to provide a basic training package. These teaching materials are based on the WHO's minimum standards and technologies for emergency and essential surgical care, and they are designed to strengthen the delivery of surgical and anesthetic services at primary health facilities.

The Global Initiative for Emergency and Essential Surgery Care (GIEESC) was established in 2005 to promote the EESC program and to address deficiencies in capacity for surgical care at the primary referral level in LMICs. The overall objective of the GIEESC is to stimulate collaboration among organizations, agencies, and institutions involved in reducing death and disability from surgically treatable conditions.

Future Priorities

Future priorities include development of appropriate surgical care models for all levels of care, based on local and regional characteristics and surgical needs. Cost-effectiveness and cost-benefit analyses of health systems implementation need to be undertaken. Further research on different modalities for provision of surgery, for example, the use of mobile clinics to reach underserviced areas, as well as the possibilities of task-shifting to reduce costs and increase affordability, would be useful. The evaluation of surgery as a prevention strategy in public health should include cost-effectiveness analysis of adequate, prompt, initial surgical treatment of injuries to prevent chronic disability from poorly diagnosed and treated survivable injuries, as well as elective treatment of hernia, hydrocele, otitis media, cataract, clubfoot, and nonemergency orthopedic conditions to prevent complications and disabilities.

This chapter has shown the potential for these interventions to be cost-effective and reasonable in cost. More work needs to be done to determine how best to organize these services to use economies of scale to reduce costs and increase effectiveness when specialized surgical interventions are consolidated. More work also needs to be done to estimate the investment costs of setting up these facilities, including training surgeons, providing specialty training, and equipping facilities appropriately.

ANNEXES

The annexes to this chapter are as follows. They are available at http://www.dcp-3.org/surgery:

- Annex 18A. Search Terms Used to Identify Relevant Literature.
- Annex 18B. Flow Chart of Identification, Screening, and Eligibility of Included Cost Studies: Surgery.
- Annex 18C. List of Studies, Results, and Quality Scores

NOTES

The World Bank classifies countries according to four income groupings. Income is measured using gross national income (GNI) per capita, in U.S. dollars, converted from local currency using the *World Bank Atlas* method. Classifications as of July 2014 are as follows:

- Low-income countries (LICs) = US$1,045 or less in 2013
- Middle-income countries (MICs) are subdivided:
  - Lower-middle-income = US$1,046 to US$4,125
  - Upper-middle-income (UMICs) = US$4,126 to US$12,745
- High-income countries (HICs)= US$12,746 or more

1. All intervention costs in this section have been converted into 2012 U.S. dollars using the World Bank consumer price index or regional inflation rates, unless otherwise noted.

REFERENCES

Aboagye, A. Q. Q., A. N. K. Degboe, and A. A. D. Obuobi. 2010. "Estimating the Cost of Healthcare Delivery in Three Hospitals in Southern Ghana." *Ghana Medical Journal* 44 (3): 82.

Adam, T., S. S. Lim, S. Mehta, Z. A. Bhutta, H. Fogstad, and others. 2005. "Cost Effectiveness Analysis of Strategies for Maternal and Neonatal Health in Developing Countries." *British Medical Journal* 331 (7525): 1107.

Alkire, B., C. D. Hughes, K. Nash, J. R. Vincent, and J. G. Meara. 2011. "Potential Economic Benefit of Cleft Lip and Palate Repair in Sub-Saharan Africa." *World Journal of Surgery* 35 (6): 1194–201.

Alkire, B., J. R. Vincent, C. T. Burns, I. S. Metzler, P. E. Farmer, and others. 2012. "Obstructed Labor and Caesarean

Delivery: The Cost and Benefit of Surgical Intervention." *PLoS One* 7 (4): e34595. doi:10.1371/journal.pone.0034595.

Asante, F. A., T. S. Avotri, and S. A. d'Almeida. 2004. "Costing of Safe Motherhood (Making Pregnancy Safer) Initiative in Ghana: A Case Study of Wassa West District." WHO Regional Office for Africa, Harare, Zimbabwe.

Bale, J., B. Stoll, A. Mack, and A. Lucas. 2003. *Improving Birth Outcomes: Meeting the Challenges in the Developing World.* Washington, DC: National Academy of Sciences and Institute of Medicine.

Baltussen, R., and A. Smith. 2012. "Cost Effectiveness of Strategies to Combat Vision and Hearing Loss in Sub-Saharan Africa and South East Asia: Mathematical Modelling Study." *British Medical Journal* 344: E615.

Baltussen, R., M. Sylla, K. D. Frick, and S. P. Mariotti. 2005. "Cost-Effectiveness of Trachoma Control in Seven World Regions." *Ophthalmic Epidemiology* 12 (2): 91–101.

Banerjee, S. K., K. L. Andersen, and J. Warvadekar. 2012. "Pathways and Consequences of Unsafe Abortion: A Comparison among Women with Complications after Induced and Spontaneous Abortions in Madhya Pradesh, India." *International Journal of Gynecology and Obstetrics* 118: S113–20.

Bansal, V. K., M. C. Misra, D. Babu, P. Singhal, K. Rao, and others. 2012. "Comparison of Long-Term Outcome and Quality of Life after Laparoscopic Repair of Incisional and Ventral Hernias with Suture Fixation with and without Tacks: A Prospective, Randomized, Controlled Study." *Surgical Endoscopy* 26 (12): 3476–85.

Benson, J., M. Okoh, K. Krennhrubec, M. A. Lazzarino, and H. B. Johnston. 2012 "Public Hospital Costs of Treatment of Abortion Complications in Nigeria." *International Journal of Gynecology and Obstetrics* 118: S134–40.

Bickler, S. W., and D. Spiegel. 2010. "Improving Surgical Care in Low- and Middle-Income Countries: A Pivotal Role for the World Health Organization." *World Journal of Surgery* 34 (3): 386–90.

Black, R., R. Laxminarayan, M. Temmerman, and N. Walker, eds. Forthcoming. *Reproductive, Maternal, Newborn, and Child Health.* Vol. 2 in *Disease Control Priorities in Developing Countries,* third edition, edited by D. T. Jamison, H. Gelband, S. Horton, P. Jha, R. Laxminarayan, and R. Nugent. Washington, DC: World Bank.

Blackmore, C. C., and W. J. Smith. 1998. "Economic Analyses of Radiological Procedures: A Methodological Evaluation of the Medical Literature." *European Journal of Radiology* 27 (2): 123–30.

Brauer, C. A., A. B. Rosen, N. V. Olchanski, and P. J. Neumann. 2005. "Cost-Utility Analyses in Orthopaedic Surgery." *Journal of Bone and Joint Surgery* 87-A (6): 1253–59.

Campbell, O., and J. Wendy. 2006. "Strategies for Reducing Maternal Mortality: Getting on with What Works." *The Lancet* 368 (9543): 1284–99.

Carvalho, N., A. S. Salehi, and S. J. Goldie. 2013. "National and Sub-National Analysis of the Health Benefits and Cost-Effectiveness of Strategies to Reduce Maternal Mortality in Afghanistan." *Health Policy and Planning* 28: 62–74.

Chang, R. W., J. M. Pellissier, and G. B. Hazen. 1996. "A Cost-Effectiveness Analysis of Total Hip Arthroplasty for Osteoarthritis of the Hip." *Journal of the American Medical Association* 275 (11): 858–65.

Chao, T. E., K. Sharma, M. Mandigo, L. Hagander, S. C. Resch, and others. 2014. "Cost-Effectiveness of Surgery and Its Policy Implications for Global Health: A Systematic Review and Analysis." *The Lancet Global Health* 2: e334–45.

Chatterjee, S., and R. Laxminarayan. 2013. "Costs of Surgical Procedures in Indian Hospitals." *BMJ Open* 3 (6).

Chen, A. T., A. Pedtke, J. K. Kobs, G. S. Edwards, R. R. Coughlin, and R. A. Gosselin. 2012. "Volunteer Orthopedic Surgical Trips in Nicaragua: A Cost-Effectiveness Evaluation." *World Journal of Surgery* 35 (12): 951–55.

Chen, B., and M. Creinin. 2008. "Medical Management of Early Pregnancy Failure: Efficacy." *Seminars in Reproductive Medicine* 26 (5): 411–22.

Corlew, D. 2010. "Estimation of Impact of Surgical Disease through Economic Modeling of Cleft Lip and Palate Care." *World Journal of Surgery* 34 (3): 391–96.

Coronini-Cronberg, S., J. Appleby, and J. Thompson. 2013. "Application of Patient-Reported Outcome Measures (PROMs) Data to Estimate Cost-Effectiveness of Hernia Surgery in England." *Journal of the Royal Society of Medicine* 106 (7): 278–87.

Debas, H., R. Gosselin, C. McCord, and A. Thind. 2006. "Surgery." In *Disease Control Priorities in Developing Countries,* 2nd edition, edited by D. T. Jamison, J. G. Breman, A. R. Measham, G. Alleyne, M. Claeson, and others, 1245–59. Washington, DC: World Bank and Oxford University Press.

Detsky, A. S., and I. G. Naglie. 1990. "A Clinician's Guide to Cost-Effectiveness Analysis." *Annals of Internal Medicine* 113 (2): 147–54.

Doubilet, P., M. C. Weinstein, and B. J. McNeil. 1986. "Use and Misuse of the Term 'Cost Effective' in Medicine." *New England Journal of Medicine* 314 (4): 253–56.

Dougherty, C., and T. Howard. 2013. "Cost-Effectiveness in Orthopedics: Providing Essential Information to Both Physicians and Health Care Policy Makers for Appropriate Allocation of Medical Resources." *Sports Medicine and Arthroscopy Review* 21 (3): 166–68.

Drummond, M. F., and T. O. Jefferson. 1996. "Guidelines for Authors and Peer Reviewers of Economic Submissions to the BMJ: The BMJ Economic Evaluation Working Party." *British Medical Journal* 313 (7052): 275–83.

Drummond, M. F., M. J. Schulpher, G. W. Torrance, D. J. O'Brien, and G. L. Stoddart. 2005. *Methods for the Economic Evaluation of Health Care Programmes,* 3rd edition. New York: Oxford University Press.

Durham, R., E. Pracht, B. Orban, L. Lottenburg, J. Tepas, and others. 2006. "Evaluation of a Mature Trauma System." *Annals of Surgery* 243 (6): 775–83; discussion 83–5.

Erim, D. O., S. C. Resch, and S. G. Goldie. 2012. "Assessing Health and Economic Outcomes of Interventions to Reduce Pregnancy-Related Mortality in Nigeria." *BMC Public Health,* September 14. doi: 10.1186/1471-2458-12-786.

Finger, R. P., D. G. Kupitz, E. Fenwick, B. Balasubramaniam, R. V. Ramani, and others. 2012. "The Impact of Successful Cataract Surgery on Quality of Life, Household Income and Social Status in South India." *PloS One* 7 (8): E44268.

Frick, K. D., and A. Foster. 2003. "The Magnitude and Cost of Global Blindness: An Increasing Problem That Can Be Alleviated." *American Journal of Ophthalmology* 135 (4): 471–76.

Funk, L. M., T. G. Weiser, W. R. Berry, S. R. Lipsitz, A. F. Merry, and others. 2010. "Global Operating Theatre Distribution and Pulse Oximetry Supply: An Estimation from Reported Data." *The Lancet* 376 (9746): 1055–61.

Gambhir, S. S., and J. Schwimmer. 2000. "Economic Evaluation Studies in Nuclear Medicine: A Methodological Review of the Literature." *Quarterly Journal of Nuclear Medicine* 44 (2): 121–37.

Gilbert, C. E., S. P. Shah, M. Z. Jadoon, R. Bourne, B. Dineen, and others. 2008. "Poverty and Blindness in Pakistan: Results from the Pakistan National Blindness and Visual Impairment Survey." *British Medical Journal* 336 (7634): 29–32.

Goldie, S. J., S. Sweet, N. Carvalho, U. C. Natchu, and D. Hu. 2010. "Alternative Strategies to Reduce Maternal Mortality in India: A Cost-Effectiveness Analysis." *PloS Medicine* 7 (4): e1000264.

Gong, K., N. Zhang, Y. Lu, B. Zhu, Z. Zhang, and others. 2011. "Comparison of the Open Tension-Free Mesh-Plug, Transabdominal Preperitoneal (TAPP), and Totally Extraperitoneal (TEP) Laparoscopic Techniques for Primary Unilateral Inguinal Hernia Repair: A Prospective Randomized Controlled Trial." *Surgical Endoscopy* 25 (1): 234–39. doi:10.1007/s00464-010-1165-0.

Gosselin, R. A., G. Gialamas, and D. M. Atkin. 2011. "Comparing the Cost-Effectiveness of Short Orthopedic Missions in Elective and Relief Situations in Developing Countries." *World Journal of Surgery* 35 (5): 951–55.

Gosselin, R. A., and M. Heitto. 2008. "Cost-Effectiveness of a District Trauma Hospital in Battambang, Cambodia." *World Journal of Surgery* 32 (11): 2450–53.

———, and L. Zirkle. 2009. "Cost-Effectiveness of Replacing Skeletal Traction by Interlocked Intramedullary Nailing for Femoral Shaft Fractures in a Provincial Trauma Hospital in Cambodia." *International Orthopaedics* 33 (5): 1445–58.

Gosselin, R. A., A. Maldonado, and G. Elder. 2010. "Comparative Cost-Effectiveness Analysis of Two MSF Surgical Trauma Centers." *World Journal of Surgery* 34 (3): 415–19.

Gosselin, R. A., A. Thind, and A. Bellardinelli. 2006. "Cost/DALY Averted in a Small Hospital in Sierra Leone: What Is the Relative Contribution of Different Services?" *World Journal of Surgery* 30 (4): 505–11.

Grimes, C. E., J. A. Henry, J. Maraka, N. C. Mkandawire, and others. 2014. "Cost-Effectiveness of Surgery in Low- and Middle-Income Countries: A Systematic Review." *World Journal of Surgery* 38 (1): 252–63.

Grimes, D., J. Benson, S. Singh, M. Romero, B. Ganatra, and others. 2006. "Unsafe Abortion: The Preventable Pandemic." *The Lancet* 368 (9550): 1908–19.

Gundre, N. P., S. P. Iyer, and P. Subramaniyan. 2012. "Prospective Randomized Controlled Study Using Polyethylene Mesh for Inguinal Hernia Meshplasty as a Safe and Cost-Effective Alternative to Polypropylene Mesh." *Updates in Surgery* 64 (1): 37–42.

Halanski, M. A., J.-C. Huang, S. J. Walsh, and H. A. Crawford. 2009. "Resource Utilization in Clubfoot Management." *Clinical Orthopaedics and Related Research* 467 (5): 1171–79.

Henshaw, S. K., I. Adewole, S. Singh, A. Bankole, B. Oye-Adeniran, and others. 2008. "Severity and Cost of Unsafe Abortion Complications Treated in Nigerian Hospitals." *International Family Planning Perspectives* 34 (1): 40–50.

Honda, A., P. G. Randaoharison, and M. Matsui. 2011. "Affordability of Emergency Obstetric and Neonatal Care at Public Hospitals in Madagascar." *Reproductive Health Matters* 19 (37): 10–20.

Horton, S., and C. Gauvreau. 2015. "Economic Overview: Cancer in Low and Middle-Income Countries." In *Disease Control Priorities in Developing Countries (third edition): Volume 3, Cancer,* edited by H. Gelband, P. Jha, R. Sankaranarayanan, and S. Horton. Washington, DC: World Bank.

Hounton, S. H., D. Newlands, N. Meda, and V. De Brouwere. 2009. "A Cost-Effectiveness Study of Caesarean-Section Deliveries by Clinical Officers, General Practitioners and Obstetricians in Burkina Faso." *Human Resources for Health* 7: 34–45.

Hsia, R., N. Mbembate, S. Macfarlane, and M. Kruk. 2012. "Access to Emergency and Surgical Care in Sub-Saharan Africa: The Infrastructure Gap." *Health Policy and Planning* 27 (3): 234–44.

Hu, D., S. M. Bertozzi, E. Gakidou, S. Sweet, and S. Goldie. 2007. "The Costs, Benefits, and Cost-Effectiveness of Interventions to Reduce Maternal Morbidity and Mortality in Mexico." *PLoS One:* e750. doi:10.1371/Journal. Pone.0000750.

Hu, D., D. Grossman, C. Levin, K. Blanchard, and S. J. Goldie. 2009. "Cost-Effectiveness Analysis of Alternative First-Trimester Pregnancy Termination Strategies in Mexico City." *British Journal of Obstetrics and Gynaecology* 116 (6): 768–79.

Hu, D., D. Grossman, C. Levin, K. Blanchard, R. Adanu, and others. 2010. "Cost-Effectiveness Analysis of Unsafe Abortion and Alternative First-Trimester Pregnancy Termination Strategies in Nigeria and Ghana." *African Journal of Reproductive Health* 14 (2): 85–103.

Husereau, D., M. Drummond, S. Petrou, C. Carswell, D. Moher, and others. 2013. "Consolidated Health Economic Evaluation Reporting Standards (CHEERS)–Explanation and Elaboration: An ISPOR Task Force Report." ISPOR Health Economic Evaluation Publication Guidelines: CHEERS Good Reporting Practices Task Force. *Value in Health* 16 (2): 231–50.

IHME (Institute for Health Metrics and Evaluation). 2013. *The Global Burden of Disease: Generating Evidence, Guiding Policy.* Seattle, WA: IHME.

Iskedjian, M., K. Trakas, C. A. Bradley, A. Addis, K. Lanctot, and others. 1997. "Quality Assessment of Economic Evaluations

Published in Pharmacoeconomics. The First Four Years (1992 to 1995)." *Pharmacoeconomics* 12 (6): 685–94.

James, M., S. St Leger, and K. V. Rowsell. 1996. "Prioritising Elective Care: A Cost Utility Analysis of Orthopaedics in the North West of England." *Journal of Epidemiology and Community Health* 50 (2): 182–89.

Jefferson, T., V. Demicheli, and L. Vale. 2002. "Quality of Systematic Reviews of Economic Evaluations in Health Care." *Journal of the American Medical Association* 287 (21): 2809–12.

Jha, P., O. Bangoura, and K. Ranson. 1998. "The Cost-Effectiveness of Forty Health Interventions in Guinea." *Health Policy and Planning* 13 (3): 249–62.

Kandel, R. P., S. R. Rajashekaran, M. Gautam, and K. L. Bassett. 2010. "Evaluation of Alternate Outreach Models for Cataract Services in Rural Nepal." *BMC Ophthalmology* 10: 9.

Khan, A., and S. Zaman. 2010. "Costs of Vaginal Delivery and Caesarean Section at a Tertiary Level Public Hospital in Islamabad, Pakistan." *BMC Pregnancy and Childbirth* 10: 2.

Kong, V., C. Aldous, J. Handley, and D. Clarke. 2013. "The Cost Effectiveness of Early Management of Acute Appendicitis Underlies the Importance of Curative Surgical Services to a Primary Healthcare Programme."*Annals of the Royal College of Surgery England* 95 (4): 280–84.

Koontz, S. L., O. Molina de Perez, K. Leon, and A. Foster-Rosales. 2003. "Treating Incomplete Abortion in El Salvador: Cost Savings with Manual Vacuum Aspiration." *Contraception* 68 (5): 345–51.

Krishna, A., M. C. Misra, V. K. Bansal, S. Kumar, S. Rajeshwari, and others. 2012. "Laparoscopic Inguinal Hernia Repair: Transabdominal Preperitoneal (TAPP) versus Totally Extraperitoneal (TEP) Approach: A Prospective Randomized Controlled Trial." *Surgical Endoscopy* 26 (3): 639–49.

Kruk, M. E., E. Goldmann, and S. Galea. 2009. "Borrowing and Selling to Pay for Health Care in Low- and Middle-Income Countries." *Health Affairs (Millwood)* 28 (4): 1056–66.

Kruk, M. E., C. Pereira, F. Vaz, S. Bergstrom, and S. Galea. 2007. "Economic Evaluation of Surgically Trained Assistant Medical Officers in Performing Major Obstetric Surgery in Mozambique." *British Journal of Obstetrics and Gynaecology* 114 (10): 1253–60.

Kruk, M. E., A. Wladis, N. Mbembati, S. K. Ndao-Brumblay, R. Y. Hsia, and others. 2010. "Human Resource and Funding Constraints for Essential Surgery in District Hospitals in Africa: A Retrospective Cross-Sectional Survey." *PLoS Medicine* 7(3): e1000242.

Kruper, L., J. E. Kurichi, and S. S. Sonnad. 2007. "Methodologic Quality of Cost-Effectiveness Analyses of Surgical Procedures." *Annals of Surgery* 245 (1): 147–51.

Kuper, H., S. Polack, W. Mathenge, C. Eusebio, Z. Wadud, and others. 2010. "Does Cataract Surgery Alleviate Poverty? Evidence from a Multi-centre Intervention Study Conducted in Kenya, the Philippines and Bangladesh." *PLoS One* 5 (11): e15431.

Lansingh, V. C., M. J. Carter, and M. Martens. 2007. "Global Cost-Effectiveness of Cataract Surgery." *Ophthalmology* 114 (9): 1670–78.

Lavernia, C. J., J. F. Guzman, and A. Gachupin-Garcia. 1997. "Cost Effectiveness and Quality of Life in Knee Arthroplasty." *Clinical Orthopaedics and Related Research* Dec (345): 134–9.

Leive, A., and K. Xu. 2008. "Coping with Out-of-Pocket Health Payments: Empirical Evidence from 15 African Countries." *Bulletin of the World Health Organization* 86 (11): 849–56.

Levin, A., T. Dmytraczenko, M. McEuen, F. Ssengooba, R. Mangani, and others. 2003. "Costs of Maternal Health Care Services in Three Anglophone African Countries." *International Journal of Health Planning and Management* 18 (1): 3–22.

Levin, C., D. Grossman, K. Berdichesvsky, C. Diaz, B. Aracena, and others. 2009. "Exploring the Costs and Economic Consequences of Unsafe Abortion in Mexico City before Legislation." *Reproductive Health Matters* 17 (33): 120–32.

Lundström, M., and E. Wendel. 2005. "Duration of Self Assessed Benefit of Cataract Extraction: A Long Term Study." *British Journal of Ophthalmology* 89 (8): 1017–20.

MacKenzie, E. J., S. Weir, F. P. Rivara, G. J. Jurkovich, A. B. Nathens, and others. 2010. "The Value of Trauma Center Care." *Journal of Trauma* 69 (1): 1–10.

Magee, W. P. Jr., R. Vander Burg, and K. W. Hatcher. 2010. "Cleft Lip and Palate as a Cost-Effective Health Care Treatment in the Developing World." *World Journal of Surgery* 34 (3): 420–27.

Malhotra, R., Y. Uppal, A. Misra, D. K. Taneja, V. K. Gupta, and others. 2005. "Increasing Access to Cataract Surgery in a Rural Area: A Support Strategy." *Indian Journal of Public Health* 49 (2): 63–67.

Manuel, M. R., L. M. Chen, A. B. Caughey, and L. L. Subak. 2004. "Cost-Effectiveness Analyses in Gynecologic Oncology: Methodological Quality and Trends." *Gynecologic Oncology* 93 (1): 1–8.

Marseille, E. 1996. "Cost-Effectiveness of Cataract Surgery in a Public Health Eye Care Programme in Nepal." *Bulletin of the World Health Organization* 74 (3): 319–24.

Maru, D. S., R. Schwarz, D. Schwarz, J. Andrews, M. T. Panizales, and others. 2011. "Implementing Surgical Services in a Rural, Resource-Limited Setting: A Study Protocol." *British Medical Journal Open* 1 (1): e000166.

McCord, C., and Q. Chowdhury. 2003. "A Cost-Effective Small Hospital in Bangladesh: What It Can Mean for Emergency Obstetric Care." *International Journal of Gynecology and Obstetrics* 81 (1): 83–92.

Mock, C. N., P. Donkor, A. Gawande, D. T. Jamison, M. E. Kruk, and H. T. Debas. 2015. "Essential Surgery: Key Messages of This Volume." In *Disease Control Priorities* (third edition): Volume 1, *Essential Surgery*, edited by H. T. Debas, P. Donkor, A. Gawande, D. T. Jamison, M. E. Kruk, and C. N. Mock. Washington, DC: World Bank.

Moon, W., H. Perry, and R. M. Baek. 2012. "Is International Volunteer Surgery for Cleft Lip and Cleft Palate a Cost-Effective and Justifiable Intervention? A Case Study from East Asia." *World Journal of Surgery* 36 (12): 2819–30.

Muralikrishnan, R., R. Venkatesh, N. V. Prajna, and K. D. Frick. 2004. "Economic Cost of Cataract Surgery Procedures in an Established Eye Care Centre in Southern India." *Ophthalmic Epidemiology* 11 (5): 369–80.

Murray, C., T. Vos, R. Lozano, M. Naghavi, A. D. Flaxman, C. Michaud, and others. 2012. "Disability-Adjusted Life Years (DALYs) for 291 Diseases and Injuries in 21 Regions, 1990–2010: A Systematic Analysis for the Global Burden of Disease Study 2010." *The Lancet* 380 (9859): 2197–223.

Nathens, A. B., G. J. Jurkovich, P. Cummings, F. P. Rivara, and R. V. Maier. 2000. "The Effect of Organized Systems of Trauma Care on Motor Vehicle Crash Mortality." *Journal of the American Medical Association* 283 (15): 1990–94.

NICE (National Institute for Health and Clinical Excellence). 2008. "Guide to the Methods of Technology Appraisal." NICE, London. http://www.nice.org.uk/media/b52/a7/tamethodsguideupdatedjune2008.pdf.

PATH and M. O. H. Reproductive Health Department, Vietnam (Program for Appropriate Technology in Health and Reproductive Health Department of the Ministry of Health, Vietnam). 2006. *Examining the Cost of Providing Medical Abortion in Vietnam*. Hanoi.

Pizzarello, L., A. Abiose, T. Ffytche, R. Duerksen, R. Thulasiraj, and others. 2004. "VISION 2020: The Right to Sight: A Global Initiative to Eliminate Avoidable Blindness." *Archives of Ophthalmology* 122 (4): 615–20.

Quayyum, Z., M. Nadjib, T. Ensor, and P. K. Suchahya. 2010. "Expenditure on Obstetric Care and the Protective Effect of Insurance on the Poor: Lessons from Two Indonesian Districts." *Health Policy and Planning* 25 (3): 237–47.

Rausch, M., S. Lorch, K. Chung, M. Frederick, J. Zhang, and others. 2012. "A Cost-Effectiveness Analysis of Surgical versus Medical Management of Early Pregnancy Loss." *Fertility and Sterility* 97 (2): 355–60.

Rehan, N. 2011. "Cost of the Treatment of Complications of Unsafe Abortion in Public Hospitals." *Journal of Pakistan Medical Association* 61 (2): 169–72.

Resnikoff, S., D. Pascolini, D. Etya'ale, I. Kocur, R. Pararajasegaram, and others. 2004. "Global Data on Visual Impairment in the Year 2002." *Bulletin of the World Health Organization* 82 (11): 844–51.

Richard, F., C. Ouedraogo, J. Compaore, D. Dubourg, and V. De Brouwere. 2007. "Reducing Financial Barriers to Emergency Obstetric Care: Experience of Cost-Sharing Mechanism in a District Hospital in Burkina Faso." *Tropical Medicine and International Health* 12 (8): 972–81.

Rocconi, R. P., S. Chiang, H. E. Richter, and J. M. Straughn, Jr. 2005. "Management Strategies for Abnormal Early Pregnancy: A Cost-Effectiveness Analysis." *Journal of Reproductive Medicine* 50 (7): 486–90.

Sarowar, M. G., E. Medin, R. Gazi, T. P. Koehlmoos, C. Rehnberg, and others. 2010. "Calculation of Costs of Pregnancy- and Puerperium-Related Care: Experience from a Hospital in a Low-Income Country." *Journal of Health, Population, and Nutrition* 28 (3): 264–72.

Shillcutt, S. D., M. G. Clarke, and A. N. Kingsnorth. 2010. "Cost-Effectiveness of Groin Hernia Surgery in the Western Region of Ghana." *Archives of Surgery* 145 (10): 954–61.

Shillcutt, S., D. Sanders, M. Teresa Butrón-Vila, and A. Kingsnorth. 2013. "Cost-Effectiveness of Inguinal Hernia Surgery in Northwestern Ecuador." *World Journal of Surgery* 37 (1): 32–41.

Singh, A. J., P. Garner, and K. Floyd. 2000. "Cost-Effectiveness of Public-Funded Options for Cataract Surgery in Mysore, India." *The Lancet* 355 (9199): 180–99.

Stroupe, K. T., L. M. Manheim, P. Luo, A. Giobbie-Hurder, D. M. Hynes, and others. 2006. "Tension-Free Repair versus Watchful Waiting for Men with Asymptomatic or Minimally Symptomatic Inguinal Hernias: A Cost-Effectiveness Analysis." *Journal of the American College of Surgeons* 203 (4): 458–68.

Stylopoulos, N., G. S. Gazelle, and D. W. Rattner. 2003. "A Cost-Utility Analysis of Treatment Options for Inguinal Hernia in 1,513,008 Adult Patients." *Surgical Endoscopy* 17 (2): 180–89.

Tengs, T. O., M. E. Adams, J. S. Pliskin, D. G. Safran, J. E. Siegel, and others. 1995. "Five-Hundred Life-Saving Interventions and Their Cost-Effectiveness." *Risk Analysis* 15 (3): 369–90.

Thylefors, B., A. D. Negrel, R. Pararajasegaram, and K. Y. Dadzie. 1995. "Global Data on Blindness." *Bulletin of the World Health Organization* 73 (1): 115–21.

Ungar, W. J., and M. T. Santos. 2005. "Quality Appraisal of Pediatric Health Economic Evaluations." *International Journal of Technology Assessment in Health Care* 21 (2): 203–10.

van Doorslaer, E., O. O'Donnell, R. P. Rannan-Eliya, A. Somanathan, S. R. Adhikari, and others. 2007. "Catastrophic Payments for Health Care in Asia." *Health Economics* 16 (11): 1159–84.

Vlassoff, M., T. Fetter, S. Kumbi, and S. Singh. 2012. "The Health System Cost of Postabortion Care in Ethiopia." *International Journal of Gynecology and Obstetrics* 118: S127–33.

Vlassoff, M., F. Mugisha, A. Sundaram, A. Bankole, S. Singh, and others. 2014. "The Health System Cost of Post-abortion Care in Uganda." *Health Policy and Planning* 29 (1): 56–66.

Vos, T., R. Carter, J. Barendregt, C. Mihalopoulos, L. Veerman, and others. 2010. *Assessing Cost-Effectiveness in Prevention (ACE–Prevention): Final Report*. Brisbane, Australia: University of Queensland; Melbourne, Australia: Deakin University. http://www.sph.uq.edu.au/bodce-ace-prevention.

Warburton, D., and F. Fraser. 1964. "Spontaneous Abortion Risks in Man: Data from Reproductive Histories Collected in a Medical Genetics Unit." *American Journal of Human Genetics* 16 (1): 1–25.

Warf, B. C., B. C. Alkire, S. Bhai, C. Hughes, S. J. Schiff, and others. 2011. "Costs and Benefits of Neurosurgical Intervention for Infant Hydrocephalus in Sub-Saharan Africa." *Journal of Neurosurgery: Pediatrics* 8 (5): 509–21.

Weiser, T. G., S. E. Regenbogen, K. D. Thompson, A. B. Haynes, S. R. Lipsitz, and others. 2008. "An Estimation of the Global Volume of Surgery: A Modelling Strategy Based on Available Data." *The Lancet* 372 (9633): 139–44.

WHO (World Health Organization). 2001. *Macroeconomics and Health: Investing in Health for Economic Development.* Geneva: WHO. http://whqlibdoc.who.int /publications/2001/924154550x.pdf.

———. 2003a. *Safe Abortion: Technical and Policy Guidance for Health Systems.* Geneva: WHO.

———. 2003b. *Surgical Care at the District Hospital.* Geneva: WHO.

———. 2005. *The World Health Report 2005: Make Every Mother and Child Count.* Geneva: WHO.

———. 2006. *Integrated Management for Emergency and Essential Surgical Care Tool Kit.* Geneva: WHO.

———. 2008. *World Health Report: Primary Health Care (Now More Than Ever).* Geneva: WHO.

Wilcox, A., C. Weinberg, J. O'Connor, D. Baird, J. Schlatterer, and others. 1988. "Incidence of Early Loss of Pregnancy." *New England Journal of Medicine* 319 (4): 189–94.

Wittenborn, J. S., and D. B. Rein. 2011. "Cost-Effectiveness of Glaucoma Interventions in Barbados and Ghana." *Optometry and Vision Science* 88 (1): 155–63.

Xia, W., S. She, and T. H. Lam. 2011. "Medical versus Surgical Abortion Methods for Pregnancy in China: A Cost-Minimization Analysis." *Gynecologic and Obstetric Investigation* 72 (4): 257–63.

Xu, K., D. B. Evans, G. Carrin, A. M. Aguilar-Rivera, P. Musgrove, and others. 2007. "Protecting Households from Catastrophic Health Spending." *Health Affairs (Millwood)* 26 (4): 972–83.

Zimmer, Z. 2008. "Poverty, Wealth Inequality and Health among Older Adults in Rural Cambodia." *Social Science and Medicine* 66 (1): 57–71.

Chapter **19**

Task-Sharing or Public Finance for Expanding Surgical Access in Rural Ethiopia: An Extended Cost-Effectiveness Analysis

Mark G. Shrime, Stéphane Verguet, Kjell Arne Johansson,
Dawit Desalegn, Dean T. Jamison, and Margaret E. Kruk

INTRODUCTION

A large fraction of the disease burden is attributable to conditions potentially amenable to surgical treatment (Bickler and others 2015; Mock and others 2015; Shrime, Sleemi, and Thulasiraj 2014). In low- and middle-income countries (LMICs), however, the utilization of surgical services is low, often because of a lack of surgical capacity, sociocultural factors, and cost (Chao and others 2012; Hsia and others 2012; Ilbawi, Einterz, and Nkusu 2013; Knowlton and others 2013; Linden and others 2012). Numerous policies have been proposed to improve access, including making surgery free at the point of care and task-sharing (Bucagu and others 2012; Jadidfard, Yazdani, and Khoshnevisan 2012; Kruk and others 2007).

In Ethiopia, more than 80 percent of the population of 92 million people lives in rural areas (WHO 2012; World Bank 2012), while surgeons are primarily located in urban centers (Berhan 2008; Surgical Society of Ethiopia 2013). As a consequence, access to surgery is particularly low. For example, in 2010, 3.3 percent of women delivered their most recent child by cesarean section—20 percent of the women in Addis Ababa, but as few as 0.5 percent of the poorest women in rural Ethiopia (Central Statistical Agency [Ethiopia] and ICF International 2012). Although traditional preferences

for home delivery play a role, rural women also point to the high cost of care and a lack of providers as reasons for low utilization (Central Statistical Agency [Ethiopia] and ICF International 2012; Shiferaw and others 2013). A patient undergoing surgery in Ethiopia would face, on average, 1,125 Ethiopian birr (Br; I$204) in direct medical costs, as well as Br 1,633 to Br 3,358 (I$297 to I$611) in direct nonmedical costs (Kifle and Nigatu 2010; UN 2014). Even if surgery were publicly financed, the patient would still face direct nonmedical costs, which, in some settings, may be large enough to cause impoverishment.

The World Health Organization (WHO) has stated that health systems have three objectives: to improve health, to provide financial protection, and to advance the equitable distribution of the two (WHO 2007). While health policies typically focus on the first objective, improving health may be in tension with an improvement in either of the other two objectives. In addition, standard health economic evaluations of policies sometimes ignore their expected impact on the private economy of households. Methods for extended cost-effectiveness analyses (ECEAs) have recently been developed to examine all three objectives simultaneously (Verguet, Laxminarayan, and Jamison 2014).

This chapter studies the health and financial risk protection benefits of policies for improving access to

Corresponding author: Mark G. Shrime, MD, MPH, FACS, Harvard University, shrime@mail.harvard.edu surgical care in rural Ethiopia. Using the ECEA framework (Verguet, Gavreau, and others 2015; Verguet, Laxminarayan, and Jamison 2014; Verguet, Murphy, and others 2013), we compare the following:

- A policy of universal public financing (UPF) that makes surgery free at the point of care but does not pay for nonmedical costs
- A policy of task-sharing of surgery with nonsurgeon providers
- A combination of UPF and task-sharing

In addition, because direct nonmedical costs to patients—for transportation, food, and lodging—can be significant drivers of both catastrophic expenditures and decisions to avoid care (Kowalewski, Mujinja, and Jahn 2002), we examine two additional policies:

- UPF with the addition of travel vouchers
- A combination of UPF, task-sharing, and travel vouchers

Finally, we quantify the distribution of these benefits across wealth groups.

METHODS

Selection of Interventions

We defined a basic package of surgery to study in rural Ethiopia, comprising nine surgical procedures treating 13 conditions (table 19.1). This package was chosen because the associated conditions have large, immediate risks of death, and, as a result, the interventions have potentially large individual benefits. For this surgical package, we looked at six scenarios:

- Keeping surgical delivery at the status quo
- Implementing UPF, in which direct medical costs for included procedures are fully paid by the government
- Task-sharing, in which nonsurgeon providers are trained to provide these surgeries, but the cost of accessing care is unchanged from the status quo
- A combination of UPF and task-sharing, in which surgery can be provided by nonsurgeon providers and in which medical costs are fully funded by the public sector
- A policy that implements UPF and provides vouchers to patients for nonmedical costs
- A policy combining UPF, task-sharing, and vouchers, such that surgery can be provided by nonsurgeon providers with no out-of-pocket (OOP) costs for patients

Table 19.1 Surgical Procedures and Treated Conditions Included in the Model

Procedure	Conditions
Appendectomy	Acute appendicitis, complicated or uncomplicated
Exploratory laparotomy	Abdominal trauma
Cesarean section	Obstructed labor
	Other fetal indications
Salpingectomy	Ectopic pregnancy
Hysterectomy	Postpartum hemorrhage
	Uterine rupture
Vacuum aspiration	Spontaneous abortion
	Postpartum sepsis
Chest tube placement	Thoracic trauma
Amputation	Gangrene
Traction	Uncomplicated long-bone fracture

Model Structure, Outcomes, and Data Sources

Model Structure and Outcomes of Interest. We applied ECEA methodology, which is described in annex 19A (Verguet, Murphy, and others 2013; Verguet, Laxminaryan, and Jamison 2014).

We followed a synthetic population of 1 million individuals similar to that in rural Ethiopia and normalized to identically sized wealth quintiles. The structure of the model is given in figure 19.1, which shows one of the 13 surgical conditions. A patient with obstructed labor will seek care conditional on utilization barriers. If she seeks care, she experiences perioperative morbidity or mortality, with probabilities as shown in table 19.2. Total costs, patient-borne costs, direct nonmedical costs, and overall effectiveness are calculated. This structure is essentially identical for the other surgical conditions. The model assumes a single-event analytic horizon and, as such, assumes no discounting of costs or benefits.

Our outcomes of interest were deaths averted, cases of impoverishment averted, cases of catastrophic expenditure averted, average household cost savings (or "private expenditure crowded out" for medical treatment), and governmental costs needed to sustain the program. Note that ECEA methodology does not explicitly calculate the economic benefits of better health, as would be done in a benefit-cost analysis. These benefits are addressed in sensitivity analyses that follow.

Figure 19.1 Basic Chance Tree Structure for Each Surgical Intervention in the Model

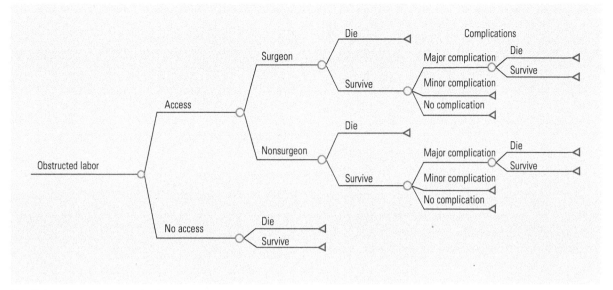

Note: Circles represent chance nodes; triangles represent outcome nodes.

Table 19.2 Condition- and Procedure-Specific Model Inputs
Probability

	Procedure cost (I$)	Perioperative mortality	Mortality, untreated	Major complication rate	Minor complication rate	Prevalence
Cesarean section for obstructed labor	251.81	0.003	0.300	0.109	0.074	Obstetric conditions: 0.020354
Vacuum aspiration for postpartum sepsis	103.07	0.022	0.300	0.154	0.220	
Hysterectomy for uterine rupture	441.02	0.214	0.300	0.140	0.270	
Hysterectomy for postpartum hemorrhage	441.02	0.020	0.300	0.140	0.270	
Salpingectomy	251.81	0.030	0.750[a]	0.046	0.046	
Vacuum aspiration for spontaneous abortion	103.07	0.022	0.300	0.154	0.220	
Cesarean section for other fetal conditions	251.81	0.003	0.300	0.109	0.074	
Appendectomy	301.29	0.012	0.700	0.035	0.140	Appendicitis: 0.0003
Exploratory laparotomy	393.81	0.133	0.923	0.500	0.242	Traumatic conditions: 0.06285
Traction	352.43	0[a]	0.060	0.200	0.067	
Chest tube placement	393.81	0.160	1.000[a]	0.105	0.263	
Amputation	352.43	0.290	0.750	0.086	0.248	

Sources: Procedure cost: Alkire and others 2012; Hu and others 2009; Kifle and Nigatu 2010; Vlassoff and others 2008, 2012. Perioperative mortality: Admasu 2004; Admasu, Haile-Mariam, and Bailey 2011; Alemayehu, Ballard, and Wright 2013; Demissie 2001; Deneke and Tadesse 2001; Gessessew and others 2011; Goyaux and others 2003; Gulam-Abbas and others 2002; Hailu 2000. Mortality, untreated: Abbas and Archibald 2005a, 2005b; Anderson and others 2007; Cobben, Otterloo, and Puylaert 2000; Gulam-Abbas and others 2002; Neilson and others 2003; Thomas and Meggitt 1981. Major complication rate: Ali 1995; Gaym 2002; Hailu 2000; Harris and others 2009; Igberase and Ebeigbe 2008; Mawalla and others 2011; Okeny, Hwang, and Ogwang 2011; Thomas and Meggitt 1981; Thonneau and others 2002. Minor complication rate: Adinma and others 2011; Ali 1995; Gaym 2002; Hailu 2000; Harris and others 2009; Hu and others 2009; Okeny, Hwang, and Ogwang 2011; Razavi and others 2005; Sohn and others 2002; Thomas and Meggitt 1981; Thonneau and others 2002. Obstetric conditions: Admasu, Haile-Mariam, and Bailey 2011; Fantu, Segni, and Alemseged 2010; Gessessew and others 2011; Singh and others 2010; Singh, Remez, and Tartaglione 2010; Thonneau and others 2002; Worku and Fantahun 2006. Appendicitis: Andersson 2007; Groen and others 2012; WHO 2008. Traumatic conditions: Groen and others 2012; Hailu 2000.
a. Assumption.

Data Sources. Parameter estimates (table 19.2) draw on national surveys and published studies. When possible, estimates were derived from rural Ethiopia. If this was impossible, estimates were taken from studies performed—in order—in urban Ethiopia, other Sub-Saharan African countries, and other developing countries. Finally, if no other data were available, estimates from high-income countries and upper-middle-income countries were used.

Costs and Assumptions. All costs, including those from outside the Ethiopian context, are adjusted to and reported in international dollars, using purchasing power parity conversions and GDP deflator estimates published by the United Nations and the World Bank (United Nations 2014; World Bank 2013). Methodology for this conversion has been described previously (Schreyer and Koechlin 2002).

Before the introduction of each program, individuals pay 34 percent of medical costs out-of-pocket, ranging from 19 percent to 78 percent (Vlassoff and others 2012; WHO 2012). Direct nonmedical costs to the patient (for example, for transportation) are paid out-of-pocket under the UPF, task-sharing, and UPF + task-sharing scenarios, and shift to the public sector in the UPF + vouchers and UPF + task-sharing + vouchers scenarios.

To remain conservative, complication and mortality rates for nonsurgeons were assumed to be 1.125 times those of surgeons (Gessessew and others 2011). Similarly, the costs of procedures performed by surgeons were assumed to be 1.47 times higher than those performed by nonsurgeons (Alkire and others 2012; Vlassoff and others 2008). In the base-case analysis, the cost of complications was set at I$25.50 (Vlassoff and others 2008) and varied in sensitivity analyses.

Direct medical costs included the inpatient costs of surgical delivery. Provider salaries are not explicitly added because this analysis is an incremental analysis and, as such, provider salaries would not change with the implementation of UPF or vouchers. Provider salaries in the setting of task-sharing are addressed in a sensitivity analysis below.

Direct nonmedical costs included the costs of transportation, food, and lodging; they did not include the costs of lost productivity due to disease. Because of likely increases in travel costs to centralized providers, nonmedical costs were assumed to be more expensive when care was sought from surgeons than when sought from nonsurgeons (I$611.66 and I$297.45, respectively) (Kifle and Nigatu 2010). Indirect costs were not considered in the base-case analysis, but they were considered in sensitivity analyses.

Catastrophic expenditure was assumed if patients' expenditures brought their incomes to either less than zero or less than 40 percent of their initial nonhealth expenditure, following methods described previously (Habicht and others 2006; Reddy and others 2013). More details are provided in annex 19A. Analyses were conducted using the R statistical software[1] and TreeAge 2013 (TreeAge Software, Williamstown, Massachusetts). Funders had no role in study design, data collection, writing, or submission for publication.

SENSITIVITY ANALYSIS

The base-case analysis did not include the start-up costs for a task-sharing program. These costs, based on estimates from Mozambique (Kruk and others 2007), were included in the sensitivity analysis. These costs included the costs of salaries, training, library buildings, books, computers, and travel. We scaled these estimates linearly for differences in population size and distributed the costs evenly across the population. The linear scale-up results were lower than unpublished estimates from Ethiopia itself; therefore, these unpublished estimates were also used in a separate sensitivity analysis.

Sensitivity analyses of assumptions around baseline utilization, price elasticity of demand for care, the magnitude of direct nonmedical costs, the risk of mortality from untreated disease, the cost of complications, the inclusion of indirect costs, and the effects of taxation were all performed (annex 19A). Finally, heterogeneity in our estimates was modeled using first-order Monte Carlo simulation.

RESULTS

Model Contextualization and Validation

From the 2011 Ethiopia Demographic and Health Survey (Central Statistical Agency [Ethiopia] and ICF International 2012), we calculated an overall rate of obstetric delivery in a medical facility of 16.5 percent, which is nearly identical to published estimates (Shiferaw and others 2013).

The model was then validated against published mortality results from WHO, UNICEF, UNFPA, and World Bank (2012). Because these estimates are for the country as a whole, and, in some cases, for low-income countries as a group, and because the model focuses solely on rural Ethiopia, we allowed the model to predict slightly higher mortality than published estimates. Our model estimated 9,112 maternal deaths per year in Ethiopia, consistent with estimates of 9,000 (WHO 2012); this translates to a predicted maternal mortality ratio of 368 deaths per 100,000 live births, which is also consistent with World Bank estimates of 350 (World Bank 2012). Our model predicted 0.62 deaths per 1,000 population from traumatic conditions and 0.012 deaths per 1,000 population from appendicitis, consistent with World Bank estimates (0.61 and 0.012, respectively) (WHO 2013a).

Base-Case Analysis, without Travel Vouchers

Health Impacts. Nominal health benefits measured in deaths averted are shown in annex table 19A.4,

and health benefits per I$100,000 spent are shown in table 19.3. Per 1 million people per year in rural Ethiopia, UPF averted 21 deaths, at a cost of I$895,000 (2.4 averted deaths per I$100,000 spent, or I$42,600 per death averted). Health gains from UPF varied across disease conditions: per I$100,000 spent, UPF was predicted to avert 40 deaths from obstetric conditions (I$2,500 per death averted), 24 deaths from appendicitis (I$4,200 per death averted), and two deaths from trauma (I$50,000 per death averted).

Task-sharing was predicted to avert 250 deaths per 1 million population per year in rural Ethiopia, at a cost of I$377,200 (65 averted deaths per I$100,000; or I$1,500 per death averted). As with UPF, this

Table 19.3 Summary of Health Gains, Financial Risk Protection, and Costs per 1 Million Population, by Model Scenario

			Wealth quintile					
			Poorest	Poor	Middle	Rich	Richest	Overall
Deaths averted per I$100,00 spent	UPF (no vouchers)	Obstetric	79	47	29	18	4	40
		Appendicitis	45	25	16	11	3	24
		Trauma	5	3	2	1	0	2
		Total	6	3	2	1	0	3
	UPF with vouchers	Obstetric	27	17	11	8	2	15
		Appendicitis	17	10	6	4	1	9
		Trauma	2	1	1	1	0	1
		Total	3	1	1	1	0	1
	Task-sharing	Obstetric	249	249	249	249	249	249
		Appendicitis	495	495	495	495	495	495
		Trauma	57	57	57	57	57	57
		Total	62	64	66	68	72	65
	UPF + task-sharing	Obstetric	137	131	127	124	121	129
		Appendicitis	128	106	90	77	64	99
		Trauma	15	13	11	10	8	12
		Total	17	15	13	12	11	14
	UPF + task-sharing + vouchers	Obstetric	42	39	37	36	35	38
		Appendicitis	33	25	20	17	13	23
		Trauma	4	3	3	2	2	3
		Total	5	4	3	3	2	4
Cases of poverty averted per I$100,000 spent	UPF (no vouchers)	Obstetric	0	−72	−91	216	0	21
		Appendicitis	0	−7	−24	182	0	37
		Trauma	0	−24	−20	221	0	44
		Total	0	−24	−21	221	0	44

table continues next page

Table 19.3 Summary of Health Gains, Financial Risk Protection, and Costs per 1 Million Population, by Model Scenario (continued)

			Wealth quintile					
			Poorest	Poor	Middle	Rich	Richest	Overall
	UPF with vouchers	Obstetric	0	53	96	29	0	35
		Appendicitis	0	91	127	30	0	52
		Trauma	0	88	124	38	0	52
		Total	0	88	124	38	0	52
	Task-sharing	Obstetric	0	−587	−314	0	0	−178
		Appendicitis	0	−531	−307	0	0	−175
		Trauma	0	−454	−287	0	0	−154
		Total	0	−458	−288	0	0	−155
	UPF + task-sharing	Obstetric	0	−307	−166	32	0	−84
		Appendicitis	0	−110	−72	76	0	−20
		Trauma	0	−98	−57	92	0	−10
		Total	0	−101	−59	91	0	−11
	UPF + task-sharing + vouchers	Obstetric	0	20	34	10	0	13
		Appendicitis	0	52	73	18	0	30
		Trauma	0	50	71	22	0	30
		Total	0	50	70	22	0	30
System cost (I$)	UPF (no vouchers)	Obstetric	837	866	1,025	1,213	1,581	5,522
		Appendicitis	345	378	426	478	521	2,147
		Trauma	142,375	155,964	175,976	197,415	215,286	887,016
		Total	143,557	157,208	177,427	199,106	217,388	894,686
	UPF with vouchers	Obstetric	8,005	7,561	8,473	9,687	12,039	45,765
		Appendicitis	2,463	2,654	2,973	3,321	3,597	15,009
		Trauma	889,577	955,658	1,068,886	1,192,590	1,290,102	5,396,812
		Total	900,044	965,874	1,080,332	1,205,597	1,305,738	5,457,585
	Task-sharing	Obstetric	1,896	2,576	3,255	3,934	5,293	16,955
		Appendicitis	193	183	173	163	153	867
		Trauma	80,143	76,009	71,875	67,740	63,606	359,373
		Total	82,233	78,768	75,303	71,838	69,053	377,195
	UPF + task-sharing	Obstetric	4,047	5,296	6,696	8,131	10,990	35,160
		Appendicitis	902	971	1,057	1,148	1,229	5,307
		Trauma	372,217	400,402	435,985	473,213	506,330	2,188,147
		Total	377,166	406,668	443,739	482,492	518,549	2,228,614
	UPF + task-sharing + vouchers	Obstetric	16,464	19,720	24,333	29,247	38,999	128,762
		Appendicitis	4,258	4,648	5,166	5,712	6,188	25,972
		Trauma	1,550,875	1,688,750	1,873,770	2,069,266	2,238,571	9,421,232
		Total	1,571,597	1,713,118	1,903,268	2,104,225	2,283,758	9,575,967

Note: Health and financial risk protection benefits are measured per I$100,000 spent in the indicated quintile (or overall). Hence, the overall column is close to the average, not the total, of the quintile-specific columns. Negative numbers of cases of poverty averted represent cases of impoverishment created by the policy. Note that rows and columns do not sum directly because these reported results are ratios of benefit per dollar spent.

prediction varies by disease condition: per I$100,000 spent, task-sharing averted 249 deaths from obstetric conditions (I$400 per death averted), 495 deaths from appendicitis (I$200 per death averted), and 57 deaths from trauma (I$1,750 per death averted).

Finally, combining task-sharing with UPF was predicted to cost the system I$2,230,000 per million people per year, and to avert 291 deaths, for a total of 14 deaths averted per I$100,000 spent (I$2,222 per death averted). Obstetric conditions accounted for 129 deaths per I$100,000 (I$775 per death averted), appendicitis for 99 deaths per I$100,000 (I$1,000 per death averted), and traumatic conditions for 12 deaths per I$100,000 (I$8,300 per death averted).

Health benefits were not equal across wealth quintiles. The primary beneficiaries of the health benefits of UPF were the poorest quintiles. Under task-sharing, health benefits overall were similar across wealth quintiles, with a slightly higher benefit per dollar spent in the richest. The combination of the two policies maintained a gradient similar to that seen in UPF, with additional health benefits accruing to the richest quintile.

Financial Risk Protection. *Poverty Cases Averted.* Without vouchers, only UPF had financial risk protection effects. Task-sharing alone and task-sharing + UPF both induced impoverishment on average (table 19.3 and annex table 19A.4). UPF averted 366 cases of poverty per million population, amounting to approximately 44 cases of poverty averted for every I$100,000 spent. Poverty was, however, created among the poor. Only the rich saw a financial benefit from UPF.

Task-sharing created 578 cases of poverty per million in the population, or approximately 155 cases created for every I$100,000 spent. No impoverishment was averted, and most of the impoverishment accrued to the poor.

Finally, a policy that combined task-sharing with UPF created 229 cases of poverty, or 11 cases per I$100,000 spent. The distribution of financial risk protection, or lack thereof, was similar to that seen in UPF.

Other measures of financial risk protection—cases of catastrophic expenditure, as well as the crowding out of private expenditure—by policy can be found in annex 19A.

Health and Financial Benefits with Vouchers

When direct nonmedical costs of care-seeking were transferred from patients, overall health benefits increased because of increased demand. However, as a result of the more expensive nature of these interventions, the amount of health benefit bought per dollar (of public money) decreased.

In contrast, financial risk protection benefits increased significantly with this transfer. UPF + vouchers averted only 1 death per I$100,000 spent but averted 52 cases of poverty (I$1,900 per case of poverty averted). Combining UPF, task-sharing, and vouchers averted 4 deaths and 30 cases of poverty per I$100,000 spent (I$25,000 per death averted and I$3,333 per case of poverty averted). Distributionally, financial risk protection continued to accrue primarily to the rich, while health benefits accrued to the poorest.

A comparison of the health benefits and the financial risk protection benefits for each policy, on average, is provided in figure 19.2. These summary statements, however, mask significant variability in outcomes across wealth quintiles, as shown in figure 19.3.

Sensitivity Analysis

Adding the costs for the scaling up of task-sharing—either published from Mozambique or unpublished from Ethiopia—decreased, by a small amount, the health benefit per dollar of any policy that included task-sharing; it had a similarly marginal effect on the distributional equity of health and financial risk protection outcomes. The addition of heterogeneity to the model is shown in figure 19.4. Other sensitivity analyses—on baseline utilization, the price elasticity of demand, the magnitude of direct nonmedical costs, the risk of mortality from untreated disease, the cost of complications, the inclusion of indirect costs, and the impact of taxation to pay for these policies—are in annex 19A.

DISCUSSION

Using an ECEA framework (Verguet, Laxminarayan, and Jamison 2014), this chapter examines the health and financial risk protection benefits of five policies for improving access to surgical services in rural Ethiopia: making surgery free at the point of care (UPF); task-sharing; a combination of UPF and task-sharing; UPF with the addition of travel vouchers; and a combination of UPF, task-sharing, and travel vouchers.

Although surgical services in Addis Ababa approximate those offered in many higher-income countries (Cadotte and others 2010), care in rural Ethiopia is sparse (WHO and GHWA 2008). Because of a lack

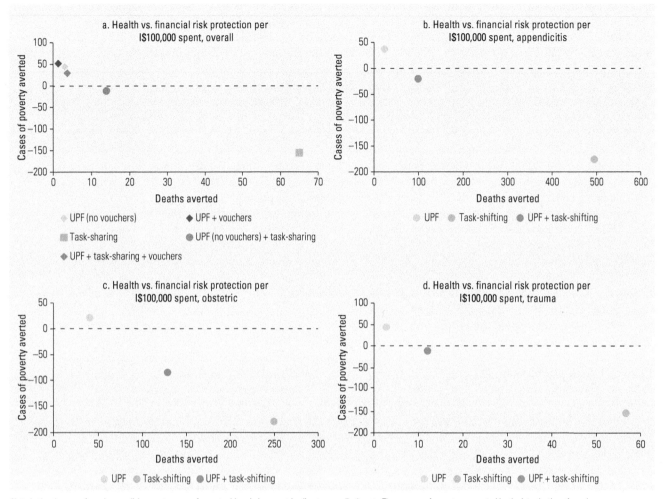

Note: In the absence of vouchers, policies create cases of poverty, driven in large part by direct nonmedical costs. These cases of poverty are averted by the introduction of vouchers.
UPF = universal public finance.

of providers—most of the few surgeons in the country live and work in urban centers (Berhan 2008; Surgical Society of Ethiopia 2013)—as well as high costs, many surgical conditions go untreated, contributing to a large burden of surgical disease in this country. Accordingly, evaluations of policy strategies to improve access to surgical care in this setting are needed.

The provision of universal health care is a focus of the WHO (WHO 2013b). Thus, UPF has been proposed for interventions ranging from rotavirus vaccination (Verguet, Murphy, and others 2013) to dental services (Jadidfard, Yazdani, and Khoshnevisan 2012) to emergency obstetric care (Bucagu and others 2012). Task-sharing has also been promoted, with nonspecialist doctors and nonphysicians increasingly filling a deficit in medical services (Scott and

Campbell 2011) and emergency obstetric care (Ejembi and others 2013; Kruk and others 2007; Sitrin and others 2013). We examined both policies in the setting of surgery.

Unlike many global health interventions, surgery is a relatively nebulous service with indistinct borders. As a result, it is often provided by disparate, poorly organized platforms (Shrime, Sleemi, and Thulasiraj 2014). To facilitate analysis, a bundle of nine surgical procedures for 13 conditions was defined and a model built based on data from nationwide surveys and the published literature (Central Statistical Agency [Ethiopia] and ICF International 2012). This model proved to be well calibrated to current health outcomes in Ethiopia (Shiferaw and others 2013).

The results of this analysis explicitly illustrate tradeoffs between health and financial risk protection. We found,

Figure 19.3 Distribution of Health Benefits and Cases of Poverty Averted, per I$100,000 Spent, across Wealth Quintiles

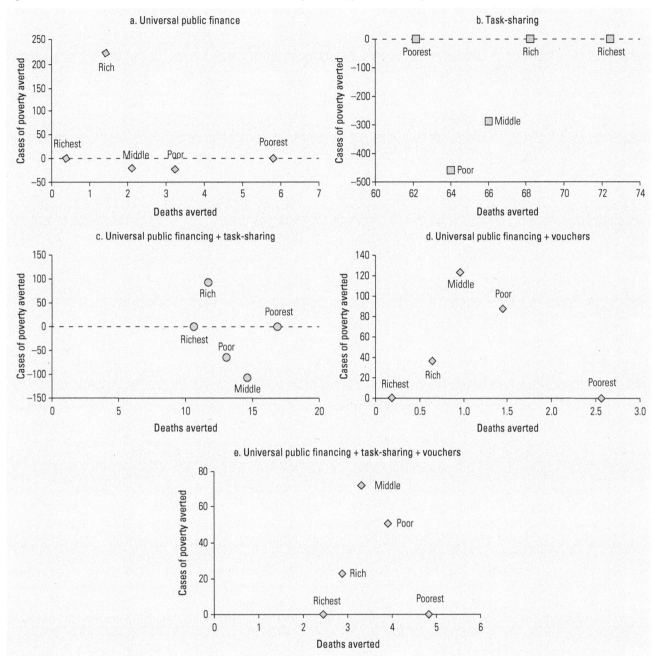

for example, that per I$100,000 spent, task-sharing averts approximately 65 deaths while simultaneously impoverishing 155 individuals. The health benefits accrue preferentially to the wealthiest, whereas the financial burden falls on the poor, in part because the rich, in this model, tended to be more sensitive to a lack of provider than to price.

However, UPF averts only 3 deaths per I$100,000 spent but prevents impoverishment in 44 individuals;

the decreased magnitude of this effect when compared with task-sharing is due to a demand function that is relatively inelastic to price, as well as to the fact that UPF is a more expensive policy. Unlike with task-sharing, the health benefits of UPF accrue to the poor because they are the most price sensitive; they also, however, face the greatest risk of impoverishment. Combining task-sharing with UPF buys more health benefit for all quintiles than does UPF alone, but it does

Figure 19.4 Heterogeneity in Results for Each of the Five Policies

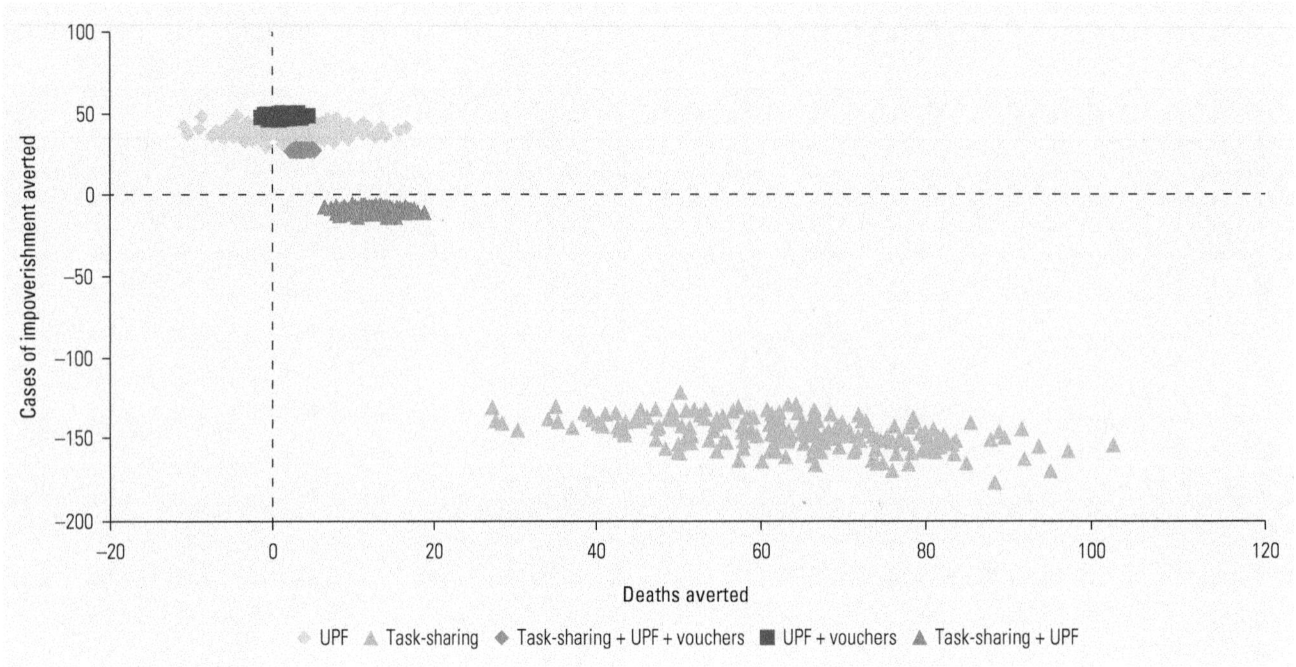

Note: UPF = universal public financing.

so more markedly for the rich. Impoverishment continues to weigh on the poor.

Much of the impoverishment created occurs because, although demand for surgical services is induced by their new availability, these services are not always free, and patients still have to pay for the nonmedical costs of obtaining care. For many patients, these costs prove catastrophic (Kowalewski, Mujinja, and Jahn 2002). This effect is made explicit when travel vouchers are included in the model. Poverty is no longer created, but because these policies are significantly more expensive, the amount of health benefit achieved per dollar spent drops drastically. How such tradeoffs are to be handled is less clear and necessitates further substantial ethical and patient-preference analyses.

Although the cost per quality-adjusted life year cannot be calculated using the methodology employed here, a rough approximation using the median age in Ethiopia of 16.8 and average life expectancy, conditional on attaining that age, of 52.1 additional years (WHO 2012) predicts that task-sharing will cost I$7,200 per life year gained; UPF + task-sharing + vouchers, the most expensive policy, will cost I$184,000 per life year gained.

Although the base-case analysis did not include the start-up costs of a task-sharing program, adding these

costs (Kruk and others 2007) decreased the amount of any benefit bought per dollar by task-sharing policies but had a minimal impact on the distributional pattern for health and financial benefits.

This analysis has limitations. We used an often-employed head-count approach to measuring impoverishment (Garg and Karan 2009; Habicht and others 2006; Honda, Randaoharison, and Matsui 2011; Niens and others 2012). Some authors, however, suggest that a movable threshold (Ataguba 2012) or measures of depth of poverty (Garg and Karan 2009) are more appropriate. We model the former in annex 19A, and the distributional patterns of health and financial risk protection benefits remain essentially unchanged. It should be noted, however, that the latter measure of poverty makes impoverishment in the poorest quintile much more explicit. In the method presented above, individuals in the poorest quintile all fall below the national poverty line. No poverty can be created or averted in these individuals because of that—an artifact which explains the fact that no cases of impoverishment occur in the poorest in table 19.3. The impoverishing impact of each policy on the poorest quintile is, therefore, best seen in annex 19A.

This method is also limited in that it does not measure counterfactual impoverishment well. Were a breadwinner to suffer a catastrophic health event, that death may throw an entire household into poverty. This is not explicitly addressed in our current analysis and is left to future inquiry.

The strength of this analysis is in what it can show: it highlights the significant tradeoffs inherent in policies for increasing access to care in LMICs, which are not dissimilar from those tradeoffs seen in high-income countries and upper-middle-income countries (Baicker and others 2013). In addition, the distribution of these benefits depends on the policy chosen: on the one hand, making surgery free at the point of care appears primarily to improve financial risk protection among the richer segments of the rural Ethiopian population. On the other hand, the small benefits it has on health accrue to the poorest. Conversely, task-sharing without vouchers creates cases of poverty while averting deaths across the entire population; the latter benefit primarily accrues to the richest, while the former harm accrues to the poorest.

Because these are initially counterintuitive findings, the model was tested with multiple sensitivity analyses, including the following: allowing the demand function to be more price elastic, including the costs of start-up for a task-sharing program; increasing the probability of dying from untreated disease; decreasing the direct nonmedical cost; increasing the cost of complications, including indirect costs in three separate ways; and modeling the effect of taxation to pay for the proposed policies. Although the magnitude of the benefits bought per dollar changes with these sensitivity analyses, the changes are often small. More important, except in the case of taxation, the distribution of the benefits across wealth quintiles is robust to these sensitivity analyses.

How to decide among the modeled policies remains a matter of further research, political debate, and ethical analysis. Normative statements about how these choices should be made and their potential unintended consequences on income inequality are not the goal of this chapter. Instead, we believe that this type of analysis can facilitate open, fair, and well-informed deliberative processes for making these decisions.

CONCLUSION

This chapter is the first to examine, simultaneously, the health and financial benefits of policies for improving access to surgical services in LMICs. It highlights tensions between the two sources of benefit and makes explicit their distributional patterns across wealth quintiles. Task-sharing without vouchers appears to improve the health of rural Ethiopia but to simultaneously put the poorest at

risk of impoverishment. Making surgery free protects against impoverishment in the rich; health benefits and impoverishment both accrue to the poor. Perhaps our most important finding is that impoverishment is not fully averted until patients no longer face nonmedical costs of accessing care. Further research is warranted to refine how to choose among these disparate policy benefits.

ANNEX

The annex to this chapter is as follows. It is available at http://www.dcp-3.org/surgery:
- Annex 19A. Extended Cost-Effectiveness Analysis Methodology and Additional Results

NOTES

The World Bank classifies countries according to four income groupings. Income is measured using gross national income (GNI) per capita, in U.S. dollars, converted from local currency using the *World Bank Atlas* method. Classifications as of July 2014 are as follows:

- Low-income countries (LICs) = US$1,045 or less in 2013
- Middle-income countries (MICs) are subdivided:
  - Lower-middle-income = US$1,046 to US$4,125
  - Upper-middle-income (UMICs) = US$4,126 to US$12,745
- High-income countries (HICs)= US$12,746 or more

1. http://www.r-project.org.

REFERENCES

Abbas, Z. G., and L. K. Archibald. 2005a. "Epidemiology of Diabetic Foot in Africa." *Medical Science Monitor: International Medical Journal of Experimental and Clinical Research* 11 (8): 262–70.

———. 2005b. "Tropical Diabetic Hand Syndrome. Epidemiology, Pathogenesis, and Management." *American Journal of Clinical Dermatology* 6 (1): 21–28.

Adinma, J. I. B., E. D. Adinma, L. Ikeako, and C. Ezeama. 2011. "Abortion Treatment by Health Professionals in South-Eastern Nigeria." *Journal of Obstetrics and Gynaecology* 31 (6): 529–32.

Admasu, A. 2004. "Analysis of Ruptured Uterus in Debre Markos Hospital, Ethiopia." *East African Medical Journal* 81 (1): 52–55.

Admasu, K., A. Haile-Mariam, and P. Bailey. 2011. "Indicators for Availability, Utilization, and Quality of Emergency Obstetric Care in Ethiopia, 2008." *International Journal of Gynecology and Obstetrics* 115 (1): 101–05.

Alemayehu, W., K. Ballard, and J. Wright. 2013. "Primary Repair of Obstetric Uterine Rupture Can Be Safely

Undertaken by Non-specialist Clinicians in Rural Ethiopia: A Case Series of 386 Women." *BJOG: An International Journal of Obstetrics and Gynaecology* 120 (4): 505–08.

Ali, Y. 1995. "Analysis of Caesarean Delivery in Jimma Hospital, South-Western Ethiopia." *East African Medical Journal* 72 (1): 60–63.

Alkire, B., J. Vincent, C. Burns, I. Metzler, P. Farmer, and others. 2012. "Obstructed Labor and Caesarean Delivery: The Cost and Benefit of Surgical Intervention." *PLoS One* 7 (4): e34595.

Anderson, D. W., P. A. Goldberg, U. Algar, R. Felix, and R. S. Ramesar. 2007. "Mobile Colonoscopic Surveillance Provides Quality Care for Hereditary Nonpolyposis Colorectal Carcinoma Families in South Africa." *Colorectal Disease* 9 (6): 509–14.

Andersson, R. 2007. "The Natural History and Traditional Management of Appendicitis Revisited: Spontaneous Resolution and Predominance of Prehospital Perforations Imply That a Correct Diagnosis Is More Important Than an Early Diagnosis." *World Journal of Surgery* 31 (1): 86–92.

Ataguba, J. E.-O. 2012. "Reassessing Catastrophic Health-Care Payments with a Nigerian Case Study." *Health, Economics, Policy and Law* 7: 309–26.

Baicker, K., S. L. Taubman, H. L. Allen, M. Bernstein, J. H. Gruber, and others. 2013. "The Oregon Experiment: Effects of Medicaid on Clinical Outcomes." *New England Journal of Medicine* 368: 1713–22.

Berhan, Y. 2008. "Medical Doctors Profile in Ethiopia: Production, Attrition, and Retention." *Ethiopian Medical Journal* 46 (S1): 1–77.

Bickler, S. W., T. G. Weiser, N. Kassebaum, H. Higashi, D. C. Chang, and others. 2015. "Global Burden of Surgical Conditions." In *Disease Control Priorities* (third edition): Volume 1, *Essential Surgery,* edited by D. T. Jamison, R. Nugent, H. Gelband, S. Horton, P. Jha, and R. Laxminarayan. Washington, DC: World Bank.

Bucagu, M., J. M. Kagubare, P. Basinga, F. Ngabo, B. K. Timmons, and others. 2012. "Impact of Health Systems Strengthening on Coverage of Maternal Health Services in Rwanda, 2000–10: A Systematic Review." *Reproductive Health Matters* 20 (39): 50–61.

Cadotte, D. W., K. Viswanath, A. Cadotte, M. Bernstein, T. Munie, and others. 2010. "The Consequence of Delayed Neurosurgical Care at Tikur Anbessa Hospital, Addis Ababa, Ethiopia." *World Neurosurgery* 73 (4): 270–75.

Central Statistical Agency [Ethiopia] and ICF International (2012). *Ethiopia Demographic and Health Survey, 2011.* Addis Ababa, Ethiopia, and Calverton, MD: Central Statistical Agency and ICF International.

Chao, T. E., M. Burdic, K. Ganjawalla, M. Derbew, C. Keshian, and others. 2012. "Survey of Surgery and Anesthesia Infrastructure in Ethiopia." *World Journal of Surgery* 36 (11): 2545–53.

Cobben, L., A. Otterloo, and J. Puylaert. 2000. "Spontaneously Resolving Appendicitis: Frequency and Natural History in 60 Patients." *Radiology* 215 (2): 349–52.

Demissie, M. 2001. "Small Intestinal Volvulus in Southern Ethiopia." *East African Medical Journal* 78 (4): 208–11.

Deneke, A., and B. Tadesse. 2001. "Incidence, Patterns, and Clinical Presentation of Acute Appendicitis in Adults at Zewditu Memorial Hospital (ZMH)." *East and Central African Journal of Surgery* 6 (2): 47–50.

Ejembi, C. L., P. Norick, A. Starrs, and K. Thapa. 2013. "New Global Guidance Supports Community and Lay Health Workers in Postpartum Hemorrhage Prevention." *International Journal of Gynaecology and Obstetrics* 122 (3): 187–89.

Fantu, S., H. Segni, and F. Alemseged. 2010. "Incidence, Causes, and Outcome of Obstructed Labor in Jimma University Specialized Hospital." *Ethiopian Journal of Health Sciences* 20 (3): 145–51.

Garg, C. C., and A. K. Karan. 2009. "Reducing Out-of-Pocket Expenditures to Reduce Poverty: A Disaggregated Analysis at Rural-Urban and State Level in India." *Health Policy and Planning* 24 (2): 116–28.

Gaym, A. 2002. "Elective Hysterectomy at Tikur Anbessa Teaching Hospital, Addis Ababa." *Ethiopian Medical Journal* 40 (3): 217–26.

Gessessew, A., G. A. Barnabas, N. Prata, and K. Weidert. 2011. "Task Shifting and Sharing in Tigray, Ethiopia, to Achieve Comprehensive Emergency Obstetric Care." *International Journal of Gynecology and Obstetrics* 113 (1): 28–31.

Goyaux, N., R. Leke, N. Keita, and P. Thonneau. 2003. "Ectopic Pregnancy in African Developing Countries." *Acta Obstetrica et Gynecologica Scandinavica* 82: 305–12.

Groen, R., M. Samai, K.-A. Stewart, L. D. Cassidy, T. Kamara, and others. 2012. "Untreated Surgical Conditions in Sierra Leone: A Cluster Randomised, Cross-Sectional, Countrywide Survey." *The Lancet* 380 (9847): 1082–87.

Gulam-Abbas, Z., J. Lutale, S. Morbach, and L. Archibald. 2002. "Clincal Outcome of Diabetes Patients Hospitalized with Foot Ulcers, Dar es Salaam, Tanzania." *Diabetic Medicine* 19: 575–79.

Habicht, J., K. Xu, A. Couffinhal, and J. Kutzin. 2006. "Detecting Changes in Financial Protection: Creating Evidence for Policy in Estonia." *Health Policy and Planning* 21 (6): 421–31.

Hailu, S. 2000. "Paediatric Thoracic Empyema in an Ethiopian Referral Hospital." *East African Medical Journal* 77 (11): 618–21.

Harris, A. M., P. L. Althausen, J. Kellam, M. Bosse, and R. Castillo. 2009. "Complications Following Limb-Threatening Lower Extremity Trauma." *Journal of Orthopedic Trauma* 23 (1): 1–6.

Honda, A., P. G. Randaoharison, and M. Matsui. 2011. "Affordability of Emergency Obstetric and Neonatal Care at Public Hospitals in Madagascar." *Reproductive Health Matters* 19 (37): 10–20.

Hsia, R. Y., N. A. Mbembati, S. MacFarlane, and M. E. Kruk. 2012. "Access to Emergency and Surgical Care in Sub-Saharan Africa: The Infrastructure Gap." *Health Policy and Planning* 27 (3): 234–44.

Hu, D., D. Grossman, C. Levin, K. Blanchard, and S. J. Goldie. 2009. "Cost-Effectiveness Analysis of Alternative First-Trimester Pregnancy Termination Strategies in Mexico

City." *BJOG: An International Journal of Obstetrics and Gynaecology* 116 (6): 768–79.

Igberase, G. O., and P. N. Ebeigbe. 2008. "Exploring the Pattern of Complications of Induced Abortion in a Rural Mission Tertiary Hospital in the Niger Delta, Nigeria." *Tropical Doctor* 38 (3): 146–48.

Ilbawi, A. M., E. M. Einterz, and D. Nkusu. 2013. "Obstacles to Surgical Services in a Rural Cameroonian District Hospital." *World Journal of Surgery* 37 (6): 1208–15.

Jadidfard, M. P., S. Yazdani, and M. H. Khoshnevisan. 2012. "Social Insurance for Dental Care in Iran: A Developing Scheme for a Developing Country." *Oral Health and Dental Management* 11 (4): 189–98.

Kifle, Y. A., and T. H. Nigatu. 2010. "Cost-Effectiveness Analysis of Clinical Specialist Outreach as Compared to Referral System in Ethiopia: An Economic Evaluation." *Cost Effectiveness and Resource Allocation* 8 (1): 13.

Knowlton, L. M., S. Chackungal, B. Dahn, D. LeBrun, J. Nickerson, and others. 2013. "Liberian Surgical and Anesthesia Infrastructure: A Survey of County Hospitals." *World Journal of Surgery* 37 (4): 721–29.

Kowalewski, M., P. Mujinja, and A. Jahn. 2002. "Can Mothers Afford Maternal Health Care Costs? User Costs of Maternity Services in Rural Tanzania." *African Journal of Reproductive Health* 6 (1): 65–73.

Kruk, M. E., C. Pereira, F. Vaz, S. Bergstrom, and S. Galea. 2007. "Economic Evaluation of Surgically Trained Assistant Medical Officers in Performing Major Obstetric Surgery in Mozambique." *BJOG: An International Journal of Obstetrics and Gynaecology* 114 (10): 1253–60.

Linden, A. F., F. S. Sekidde, M. Galukande, L. M. Knowlton, S. Chackungal, and others. 2012. "Challenges of Surgery in Developing Countries: A Survey of Surgical and Anesthesia Capacity in Uganda's Public Hospitals." *World Journal of Surgery* 36 (5): 1056–65.

Mawalla, B., S. E. Mshana, P. L. Chalya, C. Imirzalioglu, and W. Mahalu. 2011. "Predictors of Surgical Site Infections among Patients Undergoing Major Surgery at Bugando Medical Centre in Northwestern Tanzania." *BMC Surgery* 11 (1): 21.

Mock, C.N., P. Donkor, A. Gawande, D. T. Jamison, M. E. Kruk, and H. T. Debas. 2015. "Essential Surgery: Key Messages of This Volume." In *Disease Control Priorities* (third edition): Volume 1, *Essential Surgery,* edited by D. T. Jamison, R. Nugent, H. Gelband, S. Horton, P. Jha, and R. Laxminarayan. Washington, DC: World Bank.

Neilson, J., T. Lavender, S. Quenby, and S. Wray. 2003. "Obstructed Labour." *British Medical Bulletin* 67 (1): 191–204.

Niens, L. M., E. Van de Poel, A. Cameron, M. Ewen, R. Laing, and others. 2012. "Practical Measurement of Affordability: An Application to Medicines." *Bulletin of the World Health Organization* 90 (3): 219–27.

Okeny, P. K., T. G. Hwang, and D. M. Ogwang. 2011. "Acute Bowel Obstruction in a Rural Hospital in Northern Uganda." *East and Central African Journal of Surgery* 16 (1): 65–70.

Razavi, S. M., M. Ibrahimpoor, A. S. Kashani, and A. Jafarian. 2005. "Abdominal Surgical Site Infections: Incidence and Risk Factors at an Iranian Teaching Hospital." *BMC Surgery* 5: 2.

Reddy, S. R., D. Ross-Degnan, A. M. Zaslavsky, S. B. Soumerai, and A. K. Wagner. 2013. "Health Care Payments in the Asia Pacific: Validation of Five Survey Measures of Economic Burden." *International Journal for Equity in Health* 12: 49.

Schreyer, P., and F. Koechlin. 2002. "Purchasing Power Parity— Measurement and Uses." OECD Statistics Brief 3. http:// www.oecd.org/std/prices-ppp/2078177.pdf.

Scott, K., and C. Campbell. 2011. "Retreat from Alma Ata? The WHO's Report on Task Shifting to Community Health Workers for AIDS Care in Poor Countries." *Global Public Health* 6 (2): 125–38.

Shiferaw, S., M. Spigt, M. Godefrooij, Y. Melkamu, and M. Tekie. 2013. "Why Do Women Prefer Home Births in Ethiopia?" *BMC Pregnancy and Childbirth* 13: 5.

Shrime, M. G., A. Sleemi, and R. D. Thulasiraj. 2014. "Charitable Platforms in Global Surgery: A Systematic Review of Their Effectiveness, Cost-Effectiveness, Sustainability, and Role in Training." *World Journal of Surgery.* doi:10.1007 /s00268-014-2516-0.

Singh, S., T. Fetters, H. Gebreselassie, A. Abdella, Y. Gebrehiwot, and others. 2010. "The Estimated Incidence of Induced Abortion in Ethiopia, 2008." *International Perspectives on Sexual and Reproductive Health* 36 (1): 16–25.

Singh, S., L. Remez, and A. Tartaglione 2010. Methodologies for Estimating Abortion Incidence and Abortion-Related Morbidity: A Review. New York: Guttmacher Institute.

Sitrin, D., T. Guenther, J. Murray, N. Pilgrim, S. Rubayet, and others. 2013. "Reaching Mothers and Babies with Early Postnatal Home Visits: The Implementation Realities of Achieving High Coverage in Large-Scale Programs." *PLoS One* 8 (7): e68930.

Sohn, A. H., F. M. Parvez, T. Vu, H. H. Hai, N. N. Bich, and others. 2002. "Prevalence of Surgical-Site Infections and Patterns of Antimicrobial Use in a Large Tertiary Care Hospital in Ho Chi Minh City, Vietnam." *Infection Control and Hospital Epidemiology* 23 (7): 382–87.

Surgical Society of Ethiopia. 2013. "List of SSE Members." Addis Ababa: Surgical Society of Ethiopia.

Thomas, T., and B. Meggitt. 1981. "A Comparative Study of Methods for Treating Fractures of the Distal Half of the Femur." *Journal of Bone and Joint Surgery* 63B (1): 3–6.

Thonneau, P., Y. Hijazi, N. Goyaux, T. Calvez, and N. Keita. 2002. "Ectopic Pregnancy in Conakry, Guinea." *Bulletin of the World Health Organization* 80: 365–70.

UN (United Nations). 2014. "Purchasing Power Parities Conversion Factor, Local Currency Unit to International Dollar." United Nations Statistics Division, New York, New York.

Verguet, S., C. Gauvreau, S. Mishra, M. MacLennan, S. Murphy, and others. Forthcoming. "The Consequences of Raising Tobacco Taxes on Household Health and Finances among Richer and Poorer Smokers in China: An Extended Cost-effectiveness Analysis." *The Lancet* Global Health.

Verguet, S., R. Laxminarayan, and D. T. Jamison. 2014. "Universal Public Finance of Tuberculosis Treatment in India: An Extended Cost-Effectiveness Analysis." *Health Economics* 24: 318–32. doi:10.1002/hec.3019.

Verguet, S., S. Murphy, B. Anderson, K. A. Johansson, R. Glass, and others. 2013. "Public Finance of Rotavirus Vaccination in India and Ethiopia: An Extended Cost-Effectiveness Analysis." *Vaccine* 31 (42): 4902–10.

Vlassoff, M., T. Fetters, S. Kumbi, and S. Singh. 2012. "The Health System Cost of Postabortion Care in Ethiopia." *International Journal of Gynaecology and Obstetrics* 118 (S2): S127–33.

Vlassoff, M., J. Shearer, D. Walker, and H. Lucas. 2008. *Economic Impact of Unsafe Abortion-Related Morbidity and Mortality: Evidence and Estimation Challenges.* Research Report 59, Institute of Development Studies, Brighton, U.K.

WHO (World Health Organization). 2007. *Everybody's Business: Strengthening Health Systems to Improve Health Outcomes.* Geneva: WHO.

———. 2008. "Global Burden of Disease 2004 Update: Disability Weights for Diseases and Conditions." WHO, Geneva.

———. 2012. "World Health Statistics: Ethiopia." http://apps.who.int/gho/data/view.country.8500.

———. 2013a. "Global Health Estimates Summary Tables." http://www.who.int/healthinfo/global_burden_disease/en/.

———. 2013b. *World Health Report 2013: Research for Universal Health Coverage.* Geneva: WHO.

WHO and GHWA (Global Health Workforce Alliance). 2008. "Ethiopia's Human Resources for Health Programme." Country Case Study. WHO and GHWA, Geneva.

WHO, UNICEF, UNFPA, and World Bank. 2012. *Trends in Maternal Mortality: 1990–2010.* Geneva: WHO.

Worku, S., and M. Fantahun. 2006. "Unintended Pregnancy and Induced Abortion in a Town with Accessible Family Planning Services: The Case of Harar in Eastern Ethiopia." *Ethiopian Journal of Health Development* 20 (2): 79–83.

World Bank. 2012. "Country Indicators: Ethiopia." World Bank, Washington, DC.

———. 2013. "World Development Indicators, GDP Deflators." World Bank, Washington, DC. http://data.worldbank.org/indicator/NY.GDP.DEFL.ZS.

———. 2014. "Maternal Mortality Ratio (modeled estimate, per 100,000 live births)." http://data.worldbank.org/indicator/SH.STA.MMRT.

Chapter **20**

Global Surgery and Poverty

William P. Schecter and Sweta Adhikari

INTRODUCTION

Surgically treated disorders represent a significant proportion of the burden of the diseases associated with poverty. Furthermore, surgery is a cost-effective method of reducing suffering, prolonging life, and restoring sick and injured people to health and economic productivity.

Some 2 billion people worldwide lack access to surgical care (Funk and others 2010). The maldistribution of surgical resources between high-income countries (HICs) and low- and middle-income countries (LMICs) is striking. HICs have an average of 14 operating rooms and 45 trained surgeons per 100,000 population; LMICs have fewer than 2 operating rooms and 1 trained surgeon per 100,000 population (MacGowan 1987). Only 3.5 percent of the estimated 234 million operations performed annually occur in the poorest countries that spend less than US$100 per capita annually on health care, although these countries account for 34.8 percent of the global population (Weiser and others 2008).

The barriers to surgical access, including lack of awareness, fear, distance, and cultural beliefs, are many. However, the principal barrier appears to be the cost of care (Malhotra and others 2005). For example, 91 percent of the respondents to a survey of cataract patients in Ghana cited cost as a significant barrier to treatment (Gyasi, Amoaku, and Asamany 2007). Similar barriers have been cited for hospital delivery and access to obstetric services in rural Kenya (Myangome and others 2012).

Many hospitals serving poor people charge a fee for care. Sometimes the charge is based on the belief that uncompensated services are not valued by those who receive them, although no literature confirms or refutes this hypothesis. More often, the costs of admission, medications, and food are based on the harsh economic realities of impoverished countries. However, even a nominal fee may serve as a major barrier to destitute patients who need care.

DISPARITIES BETWEEN LOW- AND HIGH-INCOME COUNTRIES

Surgery can have a profound impact on the lives and livelihood of millions of low-income patients worldwide. This section reviews the differential burden of disease and access to surgical care between HICs and LMICs, highlighting conditions with the highest burden and weakest services in LMICs.

Obstetric Conditions

In 2011, approximately 279,000 maternal deaths occurred globally (WHO 2013b). The deaths were primarily due to obstructed labor and peripartum hemorrhage. The burden of these deaths is born primarily by poor women in LMICs; for example, 99 percent of hemorrhage-related peripartum deaths occur in LMICs (Haeri and Dildy 2012). The key to reducing the maternal mortality ratio

Corresponding author: William P. Schecter, MD, FACS, FCCM, University of California, San Francisco, bschect@sfghsurg.ucsf.edu.

is the presence of a trained attendant at every birth and urgent access to obstetric care (Wise and Clark 2010).

Although vesico-vaginal fistula due to obstructed labor is rare in HICs, as many as 3.5 million women may suffer from this condition in LMICs (Wall and others 2008). In a recent study of 278 women with genitourinary fistula in Pakistan, all of the vesico-vaginal fistula were repaired transvaginally, with success rates of 85 percent, 91 percent, and 96 percent, on the first, second, and third attempts, respectively (Sachdev and others 2009). These procedures require advanced training and experience, and the demand greatly exceeds the supply of surgeons and institutions. The ultimate solution is prevention of the initial damage by providing obstetric services to all pregnant women. In the interim, an organized international effort is necessary to help these women who are socially isolated and stigmatized by incontinence and offensive odor.

Trauma

In 2011, nearly 5 million people died of injuries; of these deaths, 88 percent occurred in LMICs (WHO 2013b). Road traffic accidents were the major cause of morbidity and mortality (Hazen and Ehiri 2006).

The vast majority of deaths in LMICs occurs in the field because of the lack of organized prehospital medical care and transport systems (WHO 2004). Patients with lower socioeconomic status have a greater risk of prehospital death (Mock and others 1998). Table 20.1 illustrates this preponderance of prehospital trauma deaths in LMICs compared with HICs.

For every trauma death, many more injured patients sustain temporary or permanent disabilities (Mock and Cherian 2008). Musculoskeletal injuries account for the majority of the disability burden (Peden and others 2004). In most LMICs, musculoskeletal injuries are treated by general surgeons, general practitioners, and nonphysician clinicians (Curci 2012; Mock and

Cherian 2008). Access to trained orthopedists, image intensification, internal fixation, and myocutaneous flap coverage of exposed bone is extremely limited.

Suboptimal quality of trauma and orthopedic care in LMICs leads to an excessive number of amputations, with consequent detrimental effects on mobility and quality of life. A Nigerian study concludes that most of the amputations were preventable and were caused by post-fracture splintage gangrene (Yakubu, Muhammad, and Mabogunje 1996).

Burns

Although few data document the epidemiology of burn injuries, little doubt exists that the global burden of burns is significant, with the majority of cases occurring in Asia and Sub-Saharan Africa (Burd and Yuen 2005). The reasons for the unequal global distribution of burns are unknown, but they probably include the widespread use of open fires for cooking and heating, the absence of fire codes governing building construction, and inadequate burn prevention knowledge in adults (Olabanji and others 2007). The problem is so significant that the World Health Organization (WHO) included burn care education as part of its course on essential emergency surgical procedures in resource-limited facilities (Cherian and others 2004). Burn care has been suggested as an essential part of a context-appropriate curriculum for surgical residents training in Sub-Saharan Africa (Mutabdzic and others 2013).

Cancer

Among the many clinical and sociodemographic factors contributing to disparities in cancer rates, the association between poverty and cancer is so strong that the former director of the National Cancer Institute, Samuel Broder, likened poverty to a carcinogen (Broder 1991; Greenlee and Howe 2009). Each year, 12.4 million cancer cases are newly diagnosed, and nearly 8 million patients with cancer died in 2011; more than half of these cases occurred in LMICs.

The number of new cancer cases diagnosed annually is expected to increase 70 percent by 2030; the largest increases are projected to be in LMICs (Franceschi and Wild 2013). A devastating and largely preventable malignancy in women living in LMICs is carcinoma of the cervix. The annual global burden is 530,000 new cases and 275,000 deaths (Sahasrabuddhe and others 2012). The human papilloma virus (HPV) causes cervical cancer, and the development of an HPV vaccine offers the hope of preventing this malignancy, which almost always presents as advanced disease in poor women (Woo and

Table 20.1 Proportion of Road Deaths by Setting in Three Cities
Percent

Setting	Kumasi, Ghana	Monterrey, Mexico	Seattle, Washington, United States
Prehospital	81	72	59
Emergency room	5	21	18
Hospital ward	14	7	23

Source: Mock and others 1998.

Omar 2011). However, the cultural, religious, educational, and economic barriers to implementation of a worldwide vaccination program are major challenges, particularly in LMICs.

Visual Impairment

Approximately 285 million people are visually impaired; of this number, 39 million are blind, and 246 million have severe or moderate visual impairment. According to the WHO (2013a), 80 percent of the global burden of visual impairment is preventable. Some 90 percent of visually impaired people live in LMICs (VISION 2020, WHO 2013a), and blindness and poverty are closely correlated. In a survey of blind people in Maiduguri, Nigeria, only 8.2 percent were employed, 75.3 percent were engaged in begging, and 69 percent lived on less than US$1 dollar a day (Ribadu and Mahmoud 2010).

Eye surgery is a cost-effective method of treating many common forms of visual impairment and blindness. Providing extracapsular cataract surgery to 95 percent of those who need it would avert more than 3.5 million disability-adjusted life years (DALYs) per year globally. The integrated WHO SAFE (surgery, antibiotics, facial cleanliness, and environmental improvement) program for the treatment of trachoma would avert 11 million DALYs per year globally; cost-effectiveness ranges from I$13 to I$78 per DALY averted across regions (Baltussen and others 2005).[1] Outreach programs to correct refractive errors with inexpensive eyeglasses would greatly reduce the burden of visual impairment.

INEQUITIES IN SURGICAL ACCESS WITHIN COUNTRIES

Substantial inequities exist in access to surgical services within countries based on residence, income, and age among other social stratifiers. For example, access to obstetric surgeries is inadequate in LMICs compared with HICs. Facility-based health services are less equitable than community-delivered services in the area of maternal, newborn, and child health interventions (Barros and others 2012). Skilled birth attendant coverage, an indicator of facility-based care, was found to be the most inequitable service among maternal, newborn, and child health interventions in 54 countries with high maternal and child mortality—the Millennium Development Goals Countdown Countries. Barros and others (2012) report that households in the richest wealth quintile had 52 percent higher utilization of skilled birth attendants than those in the poorest quintile.

Substantial wealth-based differences in access to life-saving obstetric services occur between, across, and within countries. An analysis of cesarean delivery rates over a period of 20 years in 26 countries in South Asia and Sub-Saharan Africa found that the cesarean section rate was less than 2 percent among the poorest quintile in 21 out of the 25 countries, a figure well below the 5 percent to 15 percent threshold suggested by the WHO rate in the richest quintile across countries (figure 20.1) (Cavallaro and others 2013). In the Sub-Saharan African countries included in the study, coverage was less than 1 percent in the poorest quintile. Coverage was also higher for women living in urban areas, with the urban rich faring best, followed by those from rural rich households; the rate was still higher for rural rich women compared with urban poor women (figure 20.2) (Cavallaro and others 2013).

To promote access to care, countries have increasingly implemented user fee exemptions for obstetric surgery. These exemptions have increased utilization of cesarean sections in countries such as Mali and Senegal (Witter and others 2010). However, despite the fee exemptions, women frequently have additional costs for transportation or medical supplies. In Mali, five years after the abolition of user fees for cesarean section, its utilization remained higher among women from richer households; women in the top two quintiles received 58 percent of those surgeries, compared with 27 percent for the bottom two quintiles (El-Khoury, Hatt, and Gandaho 2012). The lack of hospitals in rural areas and high transportation costs continue to be significant barriers to accessing obstetric care in Mali.

FINANCIAL BURDEN OF SURGICAL CONDITIONS

Few poor households are able to save sufficient funds for surgery, particularly emergency surgery, which by definition is unpredictable. The cost of emergency obstetric care is frequently a large economic shock for families and can lead to catastrophic health spending—defined as spending more than 40 percent of annual nonfood income on health care—and impoverishment. Studies from LMICs demonstrate that a major portion of expenditures for obstetric care is for drugs and medical supplies, transportation to the facility, and food and hospital stay. Patients in some LMICs seek private service providers when third-level hospitals lack quality of care and have inadequate supplies; this practice significantly increases patient costs (Kruk 2013).

In Burkina Faso, emergency obstetric surgery imposes a major financial burden on families; 30.5 percent of

Figure 20.1 Rate of Cesarean Sections for 25 Millennium Development Goals Countdown Countries

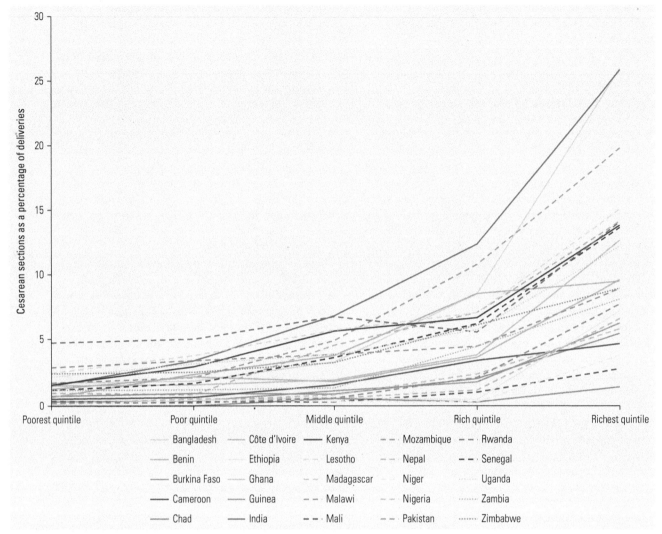

Source: Data from Cavallaro and others 2013.
Note: 2002–06 data for Cameroon, Chad, Côte d'Ivoire, India, Mali, Niger, Mozambique, and Pakistan; 2007–11 data for Bangladesh, Benin, Burkina Faso, Ethiopia, Ghana, Guinea, Kenya, Lesotho, Madagascar, Malawi, Nepal, Nigeria, Rwanda, Senegal, Uganda, Zambia, and Zimbabwe.

women with severe pregnancy complications reported having to borrow money to pay hospital bills, compared with 8 percent of women with normal deliveries. Nearly 33 percent of women in the poorest quintile who experienced severe complications sold assets to pay hospital bills, whereas none of the women in the top two quintiles reported selling assets to cover such costs (Storeng and others 2008).

In Ghana, the cost of a delivery with severe complications, including hemorrhage, was 5 percent to 8 percent of annual cash expenditure of a household, and up to 19 percent of annual household expenditure for the poorest quintile. In Benin, the total cost of

obstetric emergency complicated by dystocia accounted for 34 percent of annual household cash expenditure. About 8 percent of women who received care for severe obstetric complication left the hospital before the discharge date to reduce costs, and 13 percent left the hospital without making any payments (Borghi 2003).

Evidence from Madagascar shows that out-of-pocket costs for cesarean section equate to catastrophic expenses for poorer households (Honda, Randaoharison, and Matsui 2011). Women from the higher socioeconomic group spent 33 percent of their annual nonfood household expenditures on cesarean section, compared with 105 percent for women in the medium socioeconomic group and 109 percent for women in the lower socioeconomic group. Overall, 62 percent of the total cost of cesarean section was for drugs and medical supplies. In an Indonesian study, households reported spending 23 percent to 32 percent of subsistence-level income on complicated obstetric care. Without insurance, 68 percent of the households in the poorest quintile, compared with 8.8 percent in the richest quintile, had catastrophic expenditures for obstetric care (Quayyum and others 2010).

These figures demonstrate the dual burden of poverty in obtaining surgical care. Poor women and men frequently cannot afford the costs of surgery, including transportation to surgical facilities. When they are able to obtain emergency surgery, they suffer financially from high levels of catastrophic spending and impoverishment.

Similar issues pertain to other conditions. For example, injuries can have a devastating effect on low-income households through both the actual treatment costs and the lost wages of the injured persons and family members who must take time off from work or other activities to care for them. One study from Ghana looked at the effect of a serious injury with a disability time of one month or more on families. The majority (64 percent) reported a decline in family income as a result of the injury; a substantial proportion (41 percent) of families had gone into debt. A majority of rural households (54 percent) reported a decline in farm food production due to the loss of labor of the injured persons and others who had to take time off to care for them. A large number (41 percent) of all families, rural and urban combined, reported that family food consumption declined as a result of the injuries. This finding is especially notable given that many of these families already had children who suffered from or were on the brink of malnutrition (Mock and others 2003).

CONCLUSIONS

Poverty and infirmity are closely related. Significant improvement in global health is dependent on the economic development of LMICs, a more equitable distribution of economic resources, and improved education. Emerging data now indicate that surgery is an essential and cost-effective method of treating a significant portion of the global burden of disease engendered by poverty. The international surgical community has a professional responsibility to address the growing disparity in surgical access and standards through an integrated approach of economic, educational, and professional development.

Figure 20.2 Distribution of Cesarean Deliveries by Urban and Rural Households, 2002–11

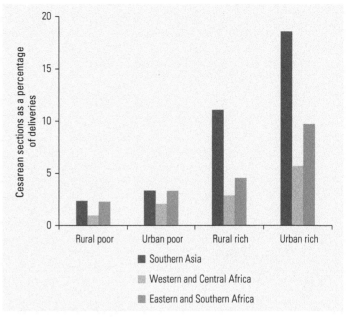

Source: Data from Cavallaro and others 2013.
Note: Figure groups data from 25 Millennium Development Goal Countdown Countries into three categories by geographic region. *Southern Asia* includes Bangladesh, India, Nepal, and Pakistan. *Western and Central Africa* includes Benin, Burkina Faso, Cameroon, Chad, Côte d'Ivoire, Ghana, Guinea, Mali, Niger, Nigeria, and Senegal. *Eastern and Southern Africa* includes Ethiopia, Kenya, Lesotho, Madagascar, Malawi, Mozambique, Rwanda, Uganda, Zambia, and Zimbabwe.

NOTES

The World Bank classifies countries according to four income groupings. Income is measured using gross national income (GNI) per capita, in U.S. dollars, converted from local currency using the *World Bank Atlas* method. Classifications as of July 2014 are as follows:

- Low-income countries (LICs) = US$1,045 or less in 2013
- Middle-income countries (MICs) are subdivided:
  - Lower-middle-income = US$1,046 to US$4,125
  - Upper-middle-income (UMICs) = US$4,126 to US$12,745
- High-income countries (HICs) = US$12,746 or more

1. One I$ was the equivalent of one U.S. dollar in 2000.

REFERENCES

Baltussen, R. M., M. Sylla, K. D. Frick, and S. P. Mariotti. 2005. "Cost-Effectiveness of Trachoma Control in Seven World Regions." *Ophthalmic Epidemiology* 12 (2): 91–101.

Barros, A. J., C. Ronsmans, H. Axelson, E. Loaiza, A. D. Bertoldi, and others. 2012. "Equity in Maternal, Newborn, and Child Health Interventions in Countdown to 2015: A Retrospective Review of Survey Data from 54 Countries." *The Lancet* (9822): 1225–33.

Borghi, J. 2003. "Costs of Near-Miss Obstetric Complications for Women and Their Families in Benin and Ghana." *Health Policy and Planning* 18 (4): 383–90.

Broder, S. 1991. "Progress and Challenges in the National Cancer Program." In *Origins of Human Cancer: A Comprehensive Review*, edited by J. Brugge, T. Curran, E. Harlow, and F. McCormick, 27–33. Plainview, NY: Cold Spring Harbor Laboratory Press.

Burd, A., and C. Yuen. 2005. "A Global Study of Hospitalized Paediatric Burn Patients." *Burns* 31 (4): 432–38.

Cavallaro, F. L., J. A. Cresswell, G. V. A. Franca, C. G. Vitora, A. J. D. Barros, and others. 2013. "Trends in Caesarean Delivery by Country and Wealth Quintile: Cross-Sectional Surveys in Southern Asia and Sub-Saharan Africa." *Bulletin of the World Health Organization* 91 (12): 914–22D. doi:10.2471/BLT.13.117598.

Cherian, M. N., L. Noel, Y. Buyanjargal, and G. Salik. 2004. "Essential Emergency Surgical Procedures in Resource-Limited Facilities: A WHO Workshop in Mongolia." *World Hospitals and Health Services* 40 (4): 24–29.

Curci, M. 2012. "Task Shifting Overcomes the Limitations of Volunteerism in Developing Nations." *Bulletin of the American College of Surgeons* 97 (10): 9–14.

El-Khoury, M., L. Hatt, and T. Gandaho. 2012. "User Fee Exemptions and Equity in Access to Caesarean Sections: An Analysis of Patient Survey Data in Mali." *International Journal for Equity in Health* 11: 49.

Franceschi, S., and C. P. Wild. 2013. "Meeting the Global Demands of Epidemiologic Transition: The Indispensable Role of Cancer Prevention." *Molecular Oncology* 7 (1): 1–13.

Funk, L. M., T. G. Weiser, W. R. Berry, S. R. Lipsitz, A. F. Merry, and others. 2010. "Global Operating Theatre Distribution and Pulse Oximetry Supply: An Estimation from Reported Data." *The Lancet* 376 (9746): 1055–61.

Greenlee, R. T., and H. L. Howe. 2009. "County-Level Poverty and Distant Stage Cancer in the United States." *Cancer Causes Control* 20 (6): 989–1000.

Gyasi, M., W. Amoaku, and D. Asamany. 2007. "Barriers to Cataract Surgical Uptake in the Upper East Region of Ghana." *Ghana Medical Journal* 41 (4): 167–70.

Haeri, S., and G. A. Dildy, 3rd. 2012. "Maternal Mortality from Hemorrhage." *Seminars in Perinatology* 36 (1): 48–55.

Hazen, A., and J. E. Ehiri. 2006. "Road Traffic Injuries: Hidden Epidemic in Less Developed Countries." *Journal of the National Medical Association* 98 (1): 73–82.

Honda, A., P. G. Randaoharison, and M. Matsui. 2011. "Affordability of Emergency Obstetric and Neonatal Care at Public Hospitals in Madagascar." *Reproductive Health Matters* 19 (37): 10–20.

Kruk, M. E. 2013. "Universal Health Coverage: A Policy Whose Time Has Come." *BMJ* 347: f6360.

MacGowan, W. A. 1987. "Surgical Manpower Worldwide." *Bulletin of the American College of Surgeons* 72 (6): 5–7, 9.

Malhotra, R., Y. Uppal, A. Misra, D. K. Taneja, V. K. Gupta, and others. 2005. "Increasing Access to Cataract Surgery in a Rural Area: A Support Strategy." *Indian Journal of Public Health* 49 (2): 63–67.

Mock, C. N., and M. N. Cherian. 2008. "The Global Burden of Musculoskeletal Injuries: Challenges and Solutions." *Clinical Orthopaedics and Related Research* 466 (10): 2306–16.

Mock, C. N., S. Gloyd, S. Adjei, F. Acheampong, and O. Gish. 2003. "Economic Consequences of Injury and Resulting Family Coping Strategies in Ghana." *Accident Analysis and Prevention* 35 (1): 81–90.

Mock, C. N., G. J. Jurkovich, D. nii-Amon-Kotei, C. Arreola-Risa, and R. V. Maier. 1998. "Trauma Mortality Patterns in Three Nations at Different Economic Levels: Implications for Global Trauma System Development." *Journal of Trauma* 44 (5): 804–12; discussion 812–14.

Mutabdzic, D., A. G. Bedada, B. Bakanisi, J. Motsumi, and G. Azzie. 2013. "Designing a Contextually Appropriate Surgical Training Program in Low-Resource Settings: The Botswana Experience." *World Journal of Surgery* 37 (7): 1486–91. doi:10.1007/s00268-012-1731-9.

Myangome, F. K., P. A. Holding, K. M. Songola, and G. K. Bomu. 2012. "Barriers to Hospital Delivery in a Rural Setting in Coast Province, Kenya: Community Attitude and Behaviours." *Rural and Remote Health* 12 (2): 1852.

Olabanji, J. K., A. O. Oladele, F. O. Oginni, and O. G. Oseni. 2007. "Burn Safety Knowledge in Adult Nigerians." *Annals of Burns and Fire Disasters* 20 (3): 115–20.

Peden, M., R. Scurfield, D. Sleet, D. Mohan, A. A. Hyder, and others. 2004. *World Report on Road Traffic Injury Prevention.* Geneva: World Health Organization.

Quayyum, Z., M. Nadjib, T. Ensor, and P. K. Sucahya. 2010. "Expenditure on Obstetric Care and the Protective Effect of Insurance on the Poor: Lessons from Two Indonesian Districts." *Health Policy Plan* 25 (3): 237–47.

Ribadu, D. Y., and A. O. Mahmoud. 2010. "Assessment of Interrelationship between Poverty and Blindness in Maiduguri, Nigeria." *Nigerian Postgraduate Medical Journal* 17 (4): 308–12.

Sachdev, P. S., N. Hassan, R. M. Abbasi, and C. M. Das. 2009. "Genito-Urinary Fistula: A Major Morbidity in Developing Countries." *Journal of Ayub Medical College Abbottabad* 21 (2): 8–11.

Sahasrabuddhe, V. V., G. P. Parham, M. H. Mwanahamuntu, and S. H. Vermund. 2012. "Cervical Cancer Prevention in Low- and Middle-Income Countries: Feasible, Affordable, Essential." *Cancer Prevention Research (Phila)* 5 (1): 11–17.

Storeng, K. T., R. F. Baggaley, R. Ganaba, F. Ouattara, M. S. Akoum, and others. 2008. "Paying the Price: The Cost and Consequences of Emergency Obstetric Care in Burkina Faso." *Social Science and Medicine* 66 (3): 545–57.

Wall, L. L., J. Wilkinson, S. D. Arrowsmith, O. Ojengbedee, and H. Mabeya. 2008. "A Code of Ethics for the Fistula Surgeon." *International Journal of Gynecology and Obstetrics* 101 (1): 84–87.

Weiser, T. G., S. E. Regenbogen, K. D. Thompson, A. B. Haynes, S. R. Lipsitz, and others. 2008. "An Estimation of the Global Volume of Surgery: A Modelling Strategy Based on Available Data." *The Lancet* 372 (9633): 139–44.

WHO (World Health Organization). 2004. *World Report on Road Traffic Injury Prevention: Summary.* Geneva:

WHO. http://www.who.int/violence_injury_prevention/publications/road_traffic/world_report/summary_en_rev.pdf.

———. 2013a. "Blindness: Vision 2020—The Global Initiative for the Elimination of Avoidable Blindness." Factsheet No. 213, World Health Organization, Geneva. http://www.who.int/mediacentre/factsheets/fs213/en/.

———. 2013b. "Global Health Estimates for Deaths by Cause, Age, and Sex for Years 2000–2011." WHO, Geneva.

Wise, A., and V. Clark. 2010. "Challenges of Major Obstetric Haemorrhage." *Best Practice and Research: Clinical Obstetrics and Gynaecology* 24 (3): 353–65.

Witter, S., T. Dieng, D. Mbengue, I. Moreira, and V. De Brouwere. 2010. "The National Free Delivery and Caesarean Policy in Senegal: Evaluating Process and Outcomes." *Health Policy and Planning* 25 (5): 384–92.

Woo, Y. L., and S. Z. Omar. 2011. "Human Papillomavirus Vaccination in the Resourced and Resource-Constrained World." *Best Practice and Research Clinical Obstetrics and Gynaecology* 25 (5): 597–603.

Yakubu, A., I. Muhammad, and O. A. Mabogunje. 1996. "Major Limb Amputation in Adults, Zaria, Nigeria." *Journal of the Royal College of Surgeons of Edinburgh* 41 (2): 102–04.

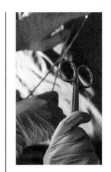

21

Benefit-Cost Analysis for Selected Surgical Interventions in Low- and Middle-Income Countries

Blake C. Alkire, Jeffrey R. Vincent, and John G. Meara

INTRODUCTION

Since surgery was first included in the second edition of *Disease Control Priorities* (DCP2, 2006), research examining the cost-effectiveness of surgical interventions in low- and middle-income countries (LMICs) has expanded substantially (see chapter 18). A growing body of evidence suggests that surgical platforms can be cost-effective in these countries, according to the criteria established by the World Health Organization (WHO) (Grimes and others 2013).

In parallel, a nascent field of study within global health economics has attempted to expand the application of benefit-cost analysis (BCA) to global health interventions in these countries. In contrast with cost-effectiveness analysis, BCA seeks to estimate the net economic benefit of an intervention in monetary terms. The nature of BCA allows researchers to investigate the potential economic return of an investment in global health; it also allows ministries of health and finance to meaningfully compare health care projects to investments in other governmental sectors, such as education and transportation, which are routinely valued with BCA. The use of BCA in global health has

recently become more visible; for example, Jamison, Jha, and Bloom (2008) and Jamison and others (2012) prominently feature BCA in their challenge papers for the 2008 and 2012 Copenhagen Consensus (CC).

Within the surgical cost-effectiveness literature, cleft lip and palate (CLP) has been the subject of at least three cost-effectiveness studies in LMICs; all suggest that CLP can be repaired in LMICs in a cost-effective manner (Corlew 2010; Magee, Vander Burg, and Hatcher 2010; Poenaru 2013). A more thorough review of CLP can be found in chapters 8 and 13 of this volume. The role of cesarean delivery in the context of obstructed labor, and its associated cost and benefit, has been previously studied by the authors (Alkire and others 2012a) and is presented here with updated results. This chapter presents two distinct BCAs:

- An approach for performing BCA using CLP repair as a model surgical intervention using primary data from a subspecialty hospital dedicated to CLP in India
- A BCA based on secondary data that model the benefit and cost of cesarean delivery for treatment of obstructed labor in 47 LMICs.

Corresponding author: Blake C. Alkire, MD, MPH, Harvard University, blake.alkire@post.harvard.edu

BENEFIT-COST ANALYSIS AND GLOBAL HEALTH

The use of BCA to assess global health interventions builds on the economic concept of full income, which reframes how a country's economic performance is measured (Becker, Philipson, and Soares 2003). This approach assumes that gross domestic product (GDP) per capita does not completely capture a country's economic welfare. In addition to the value of goods and services provided during a year, the full income of a country accounts for changes in life expectancy (LE) by valuing additional years of life in monetary terms (Becker, Philipson, and Soares 2003). Changes in LE are valued using the value of a statistical life (VSL) concept, which attempts to measure individuals' willingness to pay for small risk reductions in mortality, and from that it extrapolates what society would be willing to pay to prevent one statistical death; this latter number is termed the value of a statistical life (Hammitt 2007). As an example, if an individual would be willing to pay US$7 to decrease the risk of mortality by 1 in 1 million, then this individual's VSL would be US$7,000,000.

Broadly, economists rely on two different methods to measure VSL: revealed preference studies and stated preference studies. Revealed preference studies rely on behavioral data, such as wage differentials of professions with different mortality risk profiles, to estimate the additional income that workers are willing to accept to be exposed to increased on-the-job mortality risk; stated preference studies use surveys to ask what one is willing to pay for small mortality or morbidity risk reductions. It is striking that among the various approaches to estimating VSL, studies in the United States—where the majority of VSL estimates in the literature have taken place—consistently find VSLs within the same order of magnitude (Viscusi and Aldy 2003). Nomenclature has unfortunately plagued VSL studies because critics tend to argue that, especially when used in LMICs, the notion of differing *values* of life is unethical and morally suspect. The key to resolving this dilemma is to emphasize that VSL does not claim that the value of one's life is equivalent to his or her VSL. VSL studies do, however, suggest that individuals may value reductions in mortality risk differently based on age, income, and other demographic variables (Aldy and Viscusi 2008).

Returning to the concept of full income, Jamison and others argue that when economic performance is measured in full-income terms, a more complete assessment of economic welfare is obtained. Looking to the AIDS epidemic in Sub-Saharan Africa in the 1990s, the Commission on Macroeconomics and Health noted that although GDP per capita remained relatively constant during this period, full income fell and is likely to more closely approximate the economic performance of these countries during this devastating era (WHO 2001). Further discussion of full income and its potential to portray a more complete economic picture than GDP per capita alone can be found in Jamison and others (2012) and in Jamison and others (2013).

If full income can provide a more complete picture of economic performance, then valuing changes in morbidity and mortality according to economic welfare is a valuable exercise in itself. The analysis becomes more powerful, however, if we pair potential economic benefits with economic cost. BCA has long been used by the World Bank to assess development projects (World Bank 2010) and is commonplace in governmental assessments of transportation or environmental projects (Robinson 2007). Applying BCA specifically to global health interventions can allow analysts to demonstrate the potential economic return on investment to governments, nongovernmental organizations (NGOs), and donors; it can also allow stakeholders to compare health care projects with projects in other sectors, such as transportation or education. With these concepts in mind, Jamison and others (2012) perform a BCA for scaling up a number of interventions in LMICs and find benefit-cost (BC) ratios that range from 10:1 for essential surgical services to 35:1 for malaria treatment.

The BCA in this chapter builds on the CC analysis, but it differs in a number of important ways. As in the CC, we also value disability-adjusted life years (DALYs) averted using the VSL methodology. This process involves converting the VSL into its annualized equivalent, the value of a statistical life year (VSLY). The economic benefit of an intervention, then, is as follows:

$$\text{Economic Benefit} = \text{DALYs Averted} \times \text{VSLY}.$$

An important distinction between our analysis and the CC is that the CC chose to value the VSLY equally across LMICs (at US$1,000 or US$5,000). The approach used in this chapter differs because the seminal review of VSL concludes that VSLY strongly correlates with income (Viscusi and Aldy 2003). To be more useful to the governments and NGOs in countries where the studied disease process occurs, our estimates of VSLY are country specific. We also adjust the VSLY for age because economic data suggest that it peaks at roughly two-thirds of LE (Aldy and Viscusi 2008). To maintain consistency, our procedure for adjusting VSLY for age uses the same functional form for age weighting as in the DALY literature.

BENEFIT-COST ANALYSIS OF A CLEFT LIP AND PALATE SURGICAL SUBSPECIALTY HOSPITAL IN INDIA

Cleft Lip and Palate Overview

The incidence of CLP varies by ethnicity and geography. Current estimates range from one in 300 live births to one in 1,500 live births, placing CLP among the most common congenital anomalies (Canfield and others 2006; Poenaru 2013; Vanderas 1987).

Although the pathogenesis of CLP is complex and the subject of ongoing study, current data suggest a complex interplay of environment and genetics (Flint and Cummings 2010). Untreated CLP results in a number of potentially life-altering sequelae, including feeding difficulties, social stigmatization, and speech and hearing developmental delays (Corlew 2010). The primary treatment modality is surgery of the lip, palate, or both within a broader multidisciplinary approach that includes nutrition counseling, speech therapy, audiology, otolaryngology, dentistry, orthodontics, maxillofacial surgery, and possibly nasal surgery. Given that surgery can prevent the majority of the burden of disability, CLP has lent itself well to concentrated efforts such as mission trips and surgical specialty hospitals and is the focus of multiple prominent NGOs (Hughes and others 2012).

CLP has been included in estimates of the global burden of disease (GBD) since its inception. Although earlier GBD studies only considered CLP's contribution to morbidity, the most current iteration by the WHO, the Global Health Estimates (GHE), assumes a mortality risk associated with the burden, with an estimated 4,992 deaths in 2011 (WHO 2013). The most current GHE data for CLP, including the DALY mortality rate by World Bank region, are shown in table 21.1. It is important to note that the estimates for CLP are heavily skewed to LMICs. For example, although South Asia and Sub-Saharan Africa make up roughly 36 percent of the global population in 2011, 62 percent of total CLP DALYs and close to 75 percent of CLP mortality occurred in these two regions (WHO 2013). Of particular relevance to LMICs is the surgical backlog of CLP cases, defined as the total number of patients eligible for CLP repair who have not received it. Poenaru (2013) places the global estimate of the CLP surgical backlog between 420,000 and 2,100,000 cases, with the majority of the backlog in Southeast Asia and Sub-Saharan Africa.

Table 21.1 Disability-Adjusted Life Years per 100,000 and Deaths per 10,000,000, Secondary to Cleft Lip and Palate, by World Bank Region, 2011

World Bank region	DALYs per 100,000	Deaths per 10,000,000
High-income countries	1.90	0.30
East Asia and Pacific	7.99	4.2
Europe and Central Asia	6.73	3.2
Latin America and the Caribbean	6.23	3.1
Middle East and North Africa	8.20	2.2
South Asia	17.85	15.0
Sub-Saharan Africa	16.37	14.3

Source: WHO 2013.

Clearly, LMICs continue to have substantial unmet need for CLP repair.

A number of studies have examined the cost-effectiveness of CLP repair in LMICs. Magee, Vander Burg, and Hatcher (2010) estimate the cost per DALY for nine one-week mission trips to LMICs, which included Kenya and Vietnam, to range from US$7 to US$96 per nondiscounted, non–age-weighted DALY averted. Poenaru (2013) examines the cost-effectiveness of the extensive Smile Train network; using the organization's reimbursement to hospitals as a proxy for cost, he estimates a cost per discounted, age-weighted DALY averted of US$134. Finally, Corlew (2010) finds a cost per discounted, age-weighted DALY of US$70 at a Nepalese hospital staffed primarily by local physicians. Although each study uses a different methodology to estimate cost, and DALYs were not calculated under uniform assumptions (namely, discounting and age-weighting), these estimates fall well within the WHO guidelines for what can be considered a cost-effective intervention (WHO 2002).

Finally, CLP has been the subject of at least two studies that attempt to capture the potential economic benefit of surgical repair. Both Corlew (2010) and Alkire and others (2011) value DALYs averted with a VSLY approach. Each study also values DALYs using the human capital approach, which assumes that people are analogous to machines and that lost years of life are equivalent to lost years of productivity. With this method, gross national income (GNI) per capita is used as a proxy for productivity, and DALYs are valued at a country's GNI per capita. Corlew values the DALYs averted in treated patients in Nepal and finds that with a human capital approach, cleft lip and cleft palate repair result in an economic benefit per patient of US$2,500 and US$7,000, respectively. Using a VSLY approach, the value of cleft lip and cleft palate repair is US$57,000 and US$150,000, respectively (Corlew 2010). Alkire and others (2011) ask what the potential economic benefit to Sub-Saharan Africa would be if all new cases of CLP in one year were surgically repaired. With the human capital approach, the potential ranges from US$252 million to US$441 million; with VSL, the potential economic benefit of the same CLP repair ranges from US$5.4 billion to US$9.7 billion (Alkire and others 2011). Although these figures are significant, it is difficult to draw meaningful conclusions without the context of cost.

Benefit-Cost Analysis of Cleft Lip and Palate Repair

Using cost and patient data supplied by Operation Smile and a model that converts DALYs averted to economic benefit, we estimated the cost and benefit of delivering cleft care in a surgical specialty hospital in Guwahati, India, for one year. Operation Smile is a not-for-profit NGO that focuses on CLP in LMICs; from its inception in 1982 through 2010, it has cared for more than 120,000 children (Magee, Vander Burg, and Hatcher 2010). Although Operation Smile's delivery platform has historically been short-term international missions, recent efforts have focused on establishing subspecialty hospitals within LMICs.

The Operation Smile Guwahati Comprehensive Cleft Care Center (GCCCC) was founded in 2011 with the goal of providing sustainable, high-quality subspecialized surgical care to the Indian state of Assam. Operation Smile chose Guwahati after performing a needs-based assessment and noting a substantial backlog of untreated cleft patients; GCCCC estimates that Assam has up to 1,000 new cleft cases a year and a backlog of 20,000 to 30,000 untreated cases. Furthermore, the vast majority of Assam's 31 million citizens live in rural settings without access to cleft care for reasons both geographic and financial; the average income is roughly US$2 per day.

GCCCC is funded by a combination of government, private business, and NGO resources. In addition to providing primary surgical CLP repair using a full-time staff composed of more than 90 percent local medical professionals, it offers patients additional services such as dentistry, otolaryngology, speech pathology, and nutrition (Campbell 2014). These services are typically offered at cleft centers in high-income countries (HICs), but they are often missing from cleft care delivered in LMICs, especially when the mission model is employed. GCCCC has a team that educates and recruits patients; it has already visited every district within the state (Campbell 2014).

Methods

The basic approach for modeling the economic impact of an intervention is discussed in depth by Corlew

(2013), and the model for valuing DALYs used in this chapter is discussed in more detail in the appendix in Alkire and others (2012b). Given that BCA attempts to measure economic costs and benefits, it is necessary to make adjustments to the financial cost of caring for patients that was provided by Operation Smile. This final cost includes accounting for the opportunity cost to patients' families. To derive economic benefit, we did not use a human capital approach; VSL is the approach favored by economists because it is more firmly rooted in actual human behavior and more accurately approximates the value associated with health risk reduction (Belli and others 2001).

The cost data for surgical care at GCCCC for fiscal year 2012 (April 2012–March 2013) submitted by Operation Smile included the following:

- Operating overhead, including administrative costs such as printing, housekeeping and maintenance, and medical record keeping
- Depreciation of hospital building and equipment, which were costed using standard accounting methodology
- Training, including American Heart Association costs and continuing medical education expenses
- Staff expenses (salary, travel, and food)
- Patient food and travel
- Medicine
- Laboratory testing.

Water and electricity are supplied at no cost to GCCCC by the government of Assam. To capture these costs, we used publicly available data on the average tariff for electricity and water and WHO-CHOICE assumptions to estimate the cost of these resources to society (Indian Power Market 2012; Ministry of Urban Development of India and Asian Development Bank 2008; WHO-CHOICE 2014). In addition to the cost of the center, we attempted to account for opportunity cost to the families of patients using GNI per capita to value days lost secondary to preoperative, perioperative, and postoperative care. Finally, a cost per patient was obtained by dividing the total cost by the total surgical cases for fiscal year 2012; to obtain the cost of primary CLP repair, the total number of primary CLP repairs was multiplied by the cost per patient.

To maintain consistency and facilitate comparison with economic benefits, we converted cost to U.S. dollar estimates using the purchasing-power-parity (PPP) conversion factor for India in 2012 (World Bank 2013).[1] The PPP method compares the relative price levels of a fixed basket of goods between countries to establish a currency conversion rate, such that the price of the basket of goods is the same in both countries when stated in the reference currency. Market exchange rates are dependent upon the supply of and demand for a currency and reflect the price of money. The PPP approach results in a better, and typically more stable, cross-country comparator of the cost of goods. It is worth noting that this approach results in cost estimates that are roughly twice those obtained by using market exchange rates.

Calculating DALYs. The DALY is a health metric that attempts to quantitatively capture the morbidity and mortality secondary to a disease process in a population. One DALY is equivalent to the loss of one healthy year of life from either early death or disability. Disability weights (with 0 = perfect health and 1.0 = death) are used to calculate years lost to disability (YLD). A number of disability weights are available for accounting for CLP morbidity. The original GBD study provided disability weights for treated and untreated CLP (Murray and Lopez 1996), which implies residual morbidity and is most consistent with the reality of CLP; surgery can address a substantial portion of morbidity, but ongoing challenges remain with middle ear disease, speech, and other morbidities. Although there are disability weights for isolated CL and isolated CP, there are no disability weights for combined CLP. We therefore assigned the CP disability weight to patients who underwent repair of combined CLP.

DALYs averted for a surgical intervention rely on estimates of (1) the likelihood (0.0 to 1.0) of disability or mortality without surgery and (2) the likelihood (0.0 to 1.0) of disability or mortality to be averted by surgery (Bickler and others 2010; Gosselin, Maldonado, and Elder 2010; McCord 2003). For the purposes of this analysis, we assumed that CL and CP carry a value of 1.0 for likelihood of disability without surgery, and that CL on its own has a value of 0.9 for disability to be averted by surgery. For CP, we assumed the likelihood of disability to be averted by surgery to be 0.7. These numbers imply that surgery is successful at averting disability in 90 percent of CL cases and 70 percent of CP cases. These rates are largely consistent with the approach taken by Poenaru (2013) and acknowledge that secondary surgery is necessary in some cases of CLP. Our study attempts to estimate the number of DALYs averted secondary to surgical intervention for primary CLP. Although the newest iteration of the GBD study does consider mortality secondary to CLP (Vos and others 2012), we chose not to consider reduction in mortality because the evidence base for mortality rates secondary to

CLP is still being established. Furthermore, we did not include DALYs averted from revision cleft surgery. These assumptions allow us to equate a broader concept (the left-hand side of the following expression) to the quantity we calculated (the right-hand side):

DALYs averted (Primary CLP repair) =
YLD averted (Primary CLP repair).

Discounting and Age Weighting. DALYs can be calculated under different assumptions; the two most important ones pertain to discounting and age weights. The most current iteration of the GBD study has abandoned these assumptions; however, to perform BCA that aligns with empirical economic evidence, we include these assumptions in this chapter. Discounting the value of future DALYs to their present value is common practice and improves the economic comparability of DALYs that occur at different times. All of our DALY estimates are therefore discounted. We used a 3 percent discount rate, which has been used both in studies by the architects of the DALY concept (Murray and Acharya 1997) and in studies by experts on valuing mortality risk reductions (Aldy and Viscusi 2008). The stated justification for age weighting in the DALY literature is that the social value of a year of healthy life is greater for young adults than for children or older adults. An age-weighting parameter, β, determines the age at which the DALY function peaks, with the peak occurring at $1/\beta$. The most common value of β in the DALY literature is 0.04, which implies a peak at age 25. However, we used an alternative, country-specific age-weighting parameter, denoted by $\tilde{\beta}$, which is more consistent with empirical evidence on valuation of health risks (see further discussion of $\tilde{\beta}$ below).

The inclusion of discounting and age weighting results in a complex DALY formula (Murray and Acharya 1997):

$$\text{DALYs} = \int_a^L \{[K \times DW \times Cxe^{-\beta x}e^{-r(x-a)}]$$
$$+ [DW \times (1-K)e^{-r(x-a)}]\}dx \qquad (21.1)$$

in which a = age of onset of disease, L = country-specific life-expectancy if calculating years of life lost (YLL) or the age at onset of a disease plus the duration of disease if calculating YLDs, K = an age-weighting modulation constant (0 = no age weights, 1 = full age weights), DW = disability weight (1 for death), C = age-weighting correction constant, x = age integrated over the duration of disease (YLD) or years of life lost (YLL), r = discount rate (3 percent in this study), and β = age-weighting constant (Lopez and others 2006).

To specify which type of DALY is being considered, we rely on the notation DALYs [r, K, β]. To facilitate comparison with previous studies with regard to cost-utility analysis, we estimated DALYs averted with no age weighting or discounting (DALYs [0,0,0]) and DALYs averted with standard GBD age weighting and discounting (DALYs [3, 1, 0.04]).

For the special case of calculating DALYs to be valued using a VSLY approach, the formula is as follows:

$$\text{DALYs }[3,1,\tilde{\beta}] = \int_a^L \{[DW \times \tilde{C}xe^{-\tilde{\beta}x}e^{-r(x-a)}]\}dx \quad (21.2)$$

Compared with equation (21.1), the integral includes just one term because $K = 1$ (age weighting is turned on because VSLY varies with age [Aldy and Viscusi 2008]), which causes the second term to equal zero. The other key differences are the presence of $\tilde{\beta}$ and $\tilde{C}$, where the tilde indicates that country-specific age-weighting parameters and correction constants were used. Evidence indicates that VSLY peaks at about two-thirds of LE (Aldy and Viscusi 2008), so we modified the age-weighting factor in the DALY formula such that it peaks at two-thirds the LE. Therefore, DALYs [3,1,$\tilde{\beta}$] are discounted at 3 percent and are age weighted such that the maximum weight occurs at two-thirds of LE. Because $(1/\beta)$ = age at which the age-weighting factor peaks, to calculate a country-specific β, we used the following expression to determine $\tilde{\beta}$:

$$\tilde{\beta} = 1/[(2/3) \times LE]. \quad (21.3)$$

The value of C is also country-specific because it varies with β according to table 5.2 in the GBD study (Lopez and others 2006). We fit a cubic polynomial to the values in that table and used it to predict $\tilde{C}$ for a given value of $\tilde{\beta}$.

Converting DALYs Averted to Economic Benefit. To value DALYs using the VSLY approach, we first estimated the VSL using the following formula (Viscusi and Aldy 2003):

VSL (Unknown) = VSL (U.S.)

$$\times \left[\frac{\text{GNIp.c.(Unknown)}}{\text{GNIp.c.(U.S.)}}\right]^{\text{IE-VSL}} \quad (21.4)$$

in which VSL (Unknown) = VSL in a country where VSL studies have not been performed, VSL (U.S.) = VSL in the United States (US$7.4 million in 2006 dollars, updated to reference year),[2] GNI p.c. (Unknown) = GNI

per capita in the desired study year, GNI p.c. (U.S.) = GNI per capita in the United States in the desired study year, and IE-VSL = the income elasticity of VSL.

The key variable in this transfer method is the income elasticity of VSL (IE-VSL), which determines the sensitivity of VSL to income. As IE-VSL increases, the estimated VSL in the lower-income country decreases. Although values of 0.55 to 1.0 are most often used in transferring estimates of VSL, recent evidence suggests that higher values are more appropriate for transfers to low-income countries (Hammitt and Robinson 2011). We used GNI per capita estimates based on the PPP method (Viscusi and Aldy 2003), and an IE-VSL of 1.0 and 1.5. It is worth noting that formal analyses of VSL have been performed in India (Shanmugam 1996) with a minimum VSL estimate of US$1.2 million in 2000 U.S. dollars (Viscusi and Aldy 2003). Other studies have found similar values (Madheswaran 2007; Shanmugam and Madheswaran 2011). These studies, however, have been largely performed in urban settings, and it is difficult to compare these VSL data with a poor region such as Assam.

To calculate the potential economic benefit of an intervention that averts a given number of DALYs [3,1,$\tilde{\beta}$], we multiplied DALYs [3,1,$\tilde{\beta}$] by the value of a statistical life year. VSLY$_x$, the value of a statistical life year at age x, is given by the following expression:

$$\text{VSLY}_x = V \times \tilde{C}xe^{-\tilde{\beta}x} \quad (21.5)$$

in which V = age-neutral (constant) value of a statistical life year (literally, a parameter that converts a single DALY unweighted for age to a monetary value), and $\tilde{C}xe^{-\tilde{\beta}x}$ is the age-weighting factor found in the original DALY formula modified to peak at 2/3 of LE. We discuss the calculation of V in the following section. Using the DALY age-weighting factor creates internal consistency with the age weighting of DALYs and the VSLY.

The formula for estimating the economic benefit of an intervention to the individual receiving it can therefore be written as

$$\text{Economic Benefit} = \int_a^L \{[DW \times \text{VSLY}_x \times e^{-r(x-a)}]\}dx. \quad (21.6)$$

Substituting the equation for VSLY$_x$ into this results in the following:

$$\text{Economic Benefit} = \int_a^L \{[DW \times V \times \tilde{C}xe^{-\tilde{\beta}x} \times e^{-r(x-a)}]\}dx. \quad (21.7)$$

If the constant V is moved out of the integral, the formula can be rewritten as follows:

$$\text{Economic Benefit} = V \int_a^L \{[DW \times \tilde{C}xe^{-\tilde{\beta}x} \times e^{-r(x-a)}]\} \, dx, \tag{21.8}$$

which by equation (21.2) reduces to

$$\text{Economic Benefit} = V \times \text{DALYs}(3,1,\tilde{\beta}) \tag{21.9}$$

The DALY formula already contains the age-weighting factor $(\tilde{C}xe^{-\tilde{\beta}x})$, so we need only multiply DALYs $[3,1,\tilde{\beta}]$ by V, not VSLY_x, which would result in double age weighting. Assuming one has already calculated DALYs $[3,1,\tilde{\beta}]$, the only variable left to define is V, the age-neutral value of a statistical life year. To solve for V, set $DW = 1$ and $a = 0$, which indicates that the disability is equivalent to death at birth. By definition, the economic benefit in this case is the VSL, and L = life expectancy (LE). Therefore, V is defined by the following expression:

$$\text{VSL} = \int_0^{LE} V \times \tilde{C}xe^{-\tilde{\beta}x}e^{-r(x-a)} \, dx. \tag{21.10}$$

We move the constants outside of the integral:

$$\text{VSL} = V \times \tilde{C} \int_0^{LE} xe^{-\tilde{\beta}x}e^{-r(x-a)} \, dx. \tag{21.11}$$

We solve for V and integrate:

$$V = \frac{\text{VSL}}{\tilde{C}} \times \frac{(\tilde{\beta}+r)^2}{1 - e^{-(\tilde{\beta}+r)LE}[1 + LE(\tilde{\beta}+r)]}. \tag{21.12}$$

As described, multiplying V by DALYs $(3,1,\tilde{\beta})$ yields the economic value of averting these DALYs.

Results

During the 2012 fiscal year (April 2012 through March 2013), GCCCC treated 1,498 patients with primary surgical repair for cleft lip, cleft palate, or CLP, resulting in an estimated 9,600 DALYs [0,0,0] averted. The present value of the total economic benefit is sensitive to the assumed income elasticity of demand; using the most conservative (lower bound of VSL) parameters, the estimated economic benefit was US$32 million (in 2012 U.S. dollars). Assuming a total economic cost of US$2.75 million, this resulted in a cost per DALY [0,0,0]

Table 21.2 Economic Cost, Benefit, and DALYs Averted at the Guwahati Comprehensive Cleft Care Center for Fiscal Year 2012

	Outcome
Total cost[a]	US$2,745,000
DALYs averted[b]	
DALYs [0,0,0]	9,600
DALYs [3,1,0.04]	5,400
Cost per DALY averted	
DALYs [0,0,0]	$285
DALYs [3,1,0.04]	$508
Estimated economic benefit[c]	
IE-VSL = 1.5	US$32,000,000
IE-VSL = 1.0	US$116,000,000
Benefit-cost ratio[c]	
IE-VSL = 1.5	12
IE-VSL = 1.0	42

Note: Where dollar figures are used, they are 2012 U.S. dollars. DALY = disability-adjusted life year. IE-VSL = income elasticity of value of a statistical life.

a. Cost includes fixed and variable costs, along with opportunity cost to the families of patients; includes only primary cleft lip, cleft palate, and cleft lip and palate repair.

b. Non–age weighted, nondiscounted disability-adjusted life years (DALYs) are represented with the notation DALY [0,0,0], while discounted, age-weighted DALYs are represented with the notation DALYs [3,1,0.04].

c. Estimates of economic benefit and consequently benefit-cost ratio rely on valuing DALYs in monetary terms. A special form of the DALY was devised to account for the fact that the VSL varies with age.

averted of US$285 and a benefit-cost ratio (BCR) of 12. Estimates using a range of DALY and IE-VSL assumptions are presented in table 21.2.

Discussion and Recommendations

This chapter derives a BCR for CLP repair in a subspecialty surgical hospital in Guwahati, India, and finds a BCR of between 12 and 42, using the more conservative estimates of economic benefit. These findings suggest that investment in CLP repair in a referral center similar to GCCCC is a good economic proposition, with a net positive return on investment. Our cost per DALY averted depends on assumptions regarding age weighting and discounting and ranges from US$285 to US$508. The WHO has provided guidelines for determining an intervention's cost-effectiveness by comparing the cost per DALY averted to GDP per capita, with a cost per DALY averted of less than GDP per capita considered to be highly cost-effective. Although our estimates fall well within that range (WHO 2002), they are greater than previous estimates for CLP repair in the literature. The initial investment in infrastructure and equipment required at GCCCC, the broad range of services offered to CLP patients compared with short-term international missions, and inclusion of the opportunity cost of lost productivity likely explain the observed difference in estimates of cost per DALY averted.

A Model for Delivery of Surgical Care. By performing almost 1,500 primary CLP surgeries in fiscal year 2012, GCCCC has demonstrated that it can begin to address the substantial backlog of 20,000 to 30,000 cases while also addressing the 1,000 new cases each year. Moreover, GCCCC demonstrates a number of important principles for developing sustainable surgical care. In contrast to many short-term missions, GCCCC provides additional services to cleft patients, including otolaryngology, speech therapy, dentistry, and nutrition counseling. Furthermore, the large majority of medical care staff consists of local providers, which facilitates ongoing onsite training and enhances the sustainability of the center. The unique public-private partnership established among NGOs, private business, and the local government—the major funder of GCCCC—has been essential to developing and sustaining this model (Campbell 2014).

In addition to providing care, it is essential that medical organizations track and report their health-related outcomes. Operation Smile has an established track record of publishing outcome data (McQueen and others 2009), and GCCCC has made it clear that reporting and acting on outcome data are important to the center. A review of the more than 8,000 surgical procedures performed revealed no deaths; furthermore, no surgical procedures have required a blood transfusion (two units of blood are always available). Regarding cleft palate–specific outcomes, GCCCC reports a 3.9 percent palatal fistula rate for more than 700 primary repairs, which compares favorably with published data from HICs (Campbell 2014; Cohen and others 1991; Deshpande and others forthcoming). Cleft lip–specific outcomes data for more than 1,800 cases seen in follow-up suggest a total complication rate of 4 percent, largely made up of dehiscence and infection, and a revision rate of only 0.4 percent. In sum, GCCCC demonstrates that high-quality, sustainable, locally supported surgical care can be provided to an underserved population in an LMIC such as India. It further indicates that this care can be provided in a highly cost-effective and economically favorable fashion.

Advantages of Benefit-Cost Analysis. BCA facilitates comparison with investments not only in other medical procedures but also in government programs and development projects. For the 2012 CC, BCRs were calculated for a number of development projects, including investments in global health, education, and agriculture.

- Our BCR of between 12 and 42 is similar to the BCR of 10 for essential surgical services, as estimated by Jamison and others (2012).
- BCRs have also been estimated for reducing the prevalence of stunting through a package of interventions that targeted malnutrition in India, and they range between 44 and 138.6 (Hoddinott, Rosegrant, and Torero 2012).
- Estimate of BCRs for retrofitting schools in India to better withstand earthquakes range from 0.04 to 5.6 (Kunreuther and Michel-Kerjan 2012).

It is difficult to directly compare a project that is aimed at a single disease process, such as cleft repair, to projects that have broader goals, such as investing in nutrition; we present these data, however, as an example of how BCA can be used to compare investment across health sectors. A BCA for essential surgical services in LMICs would lend itself better to these broader comparisons.

The economic valuation of benefits in BCA also allows for a more intuitive discussion with stakeholders who are less academically oriented. For example, the cost per DALY averted of an intervention carries meaning to global health academicians and is necessary for cost-effectiveness analysis, but donors and other stakeholders are not always well-versed in the theory of DALYs. The ability to say that an intervention will return $X for every $1 dollar spent has meaning to all potential audiences, especially those who are making decisions about allocation of funds.

The Bellagio Essential Surgery Group, which comprised physicians, economists, and policy makers and sought to improve access to surgical care in Sub-Saharan Africa, made a number of recommendations regarding essential research questions. Among these recommendations were estimating the burden of surgical disease at the country level, assessing the ability to access surgical care in terms of surgical capacity and patient financial resources, and addressing the quality and effectiveness of surgery at first-level hospitals (Luboga and others 2009). In addition to these necessary efforts, estimates of the economic cost and benefit of surgical intervention are essential to developing the evidence base. Kruk and others (2010) estimate current surgical expenditure at first-level hospitals in three Sub-Saharan hospitals and find that only 7 percent to 14 percent of the total operating cost was allocated to surgery; in addition, they find that the majority of surgical care was delivered by midlevel providers. Quantifying current levels of expenditure on surgical care allows policy makers to make crucial funding decisions; as the burden of surgical disease is further delineated, these types of data will prove essential as decisions are made about how to scale up surgical care delivery. By exploring estimates of economic benefit in addition to cost, policy makers can better understand both current and potential returns on investments in global surgery.

Study Limitations

BCA as performed in this chapter has a number of limitations. One is that we have assumed that the counterfactual in our scenario is the absence of CLP services. This assumption may be an oversimplification of the issue and would drive up our BC ratios if patients receiving CLP care at GCCCC could have received comprehensive cleft care elsewhere. It is a reasonable assumption to make, however, given that the estimated surgical backlog of CLP in India ranges from 233,000 to 544,000 cases (Poenaru 2013) and that GCCCC on its own will require 40 years to 60 years to address the backlog in Assam at the current rate of CLP repair. Furthermore, our results are generalizable only to cleft referral centers with similar characteristics to GCCCC; we are unable to draw conclusions for mission-based models based on these data.

The current analysis focuses on an admittedly narrow subspecialty of surgical care, and estimating the benefits and costs of increasing surgical capacity in LMICs would undoubtedly be a useful contribution to the global surgical evidence base. We recognize that there is uncertainty when deriving economic benefit with a VSL methodology, but we have used the most conservative estimate of VSL. At the recommendation of Hammitt and Robinson (2011), we use an IE-VSL of 1.5 to transfer estimates of VSL from the United States to poor states in LMICs such as Assam, India. If the more commonly used IE-VSL value of 1.0 were used, then our estimates of benefit would increase dramatically. It could be argued that our approach to costing the price per surgery is less rigorous than a micro-costing approach. We are reassured, however, that our cost per surgery falls within the range found by a recent review of surgical cost in India (Chatterjee and Laxminarayan 2013). Our estimate suggests a price of roughly 40,000 rupees per surgery, which compares well with Chatterjee and Laxminarayan's study (2013), which found a range of cost for cesarean delivery (2,500 rupees to 41,000 rupees), hernia repair (5,200 rupees), endoscopic sinus surgery (53,000 rupees), and coronary artery bypass grafting (177,000 rupees).

The DALY age-weighting formula, although adjusted in this study to be more consistent with the VSL literature with regard to age when VSLY peaks, implies VSL curves that peak too early when compared with studies in the VSL literature (Aldy and Viscusi 2008). Consequently, our study may overestimate the VSL of children. The VSL of children is the subject of research; however, the available evidence suggests that the VSL is at least that of an adult, if not higher (Hammitt and Haninger 2010; Roman and others 2012).

Finally, a number of assumptions were used to estimate DALYs averted from cleft surgery. Although we attempted to be consistent with previous methods outlined in the surgical literature (Bickler and others 2010; McCord 2003), the nature of assumptions employed imparts a degree of uncertainty in our results that must be acknowledged.

Future Research

This study examines a specific platform for delivery of surgical care—the surgical specialty hospital. As the global surgery community continues to consider the pros and cons of the various platforms, further economic analyses should be geared toward understanding the benefit and cost of the mission-based model of surgical care. An extensive debate regarding the pros, cons, and possibilities for improvement has taken place in the literature (Dupuis 2004; Farmer and Kim 2008; Meier 2010), yet a robust evidence base with objective outcome and economic data is lacking. A recently published study directly compares the mission-based model to the referral-center model (Rossell-Perry and others 2013). Using outcomes data from CLP operations performed by a single cleft surgeon in Peru in different settings (referral versus mission based), Rossell-Perry and others found a statistically significant difference in palatal fistula, postoperative hemorrhage, and wound dehiscence, with all occurring more frequently in the mission-based model. Although one cannot draw significant conclusions from one study based in one setting, this study should compel further comparative research that includes economic analyses in addition to outcome data.

Conclusions on Cleft Lip and Palate Repair

In summary, we find that investment in a surgical subspecialty center dedicated to CLP repair can be a good economic proposition, and that it is possible to deliver high-quality, sustainable surgical care to underserved populations in LMICs. More broadly, we emphasize that BCA serves as a useful tool for evaluating the potential economic return on investments in global health, allows for the evaluation and discussion of projects both within and outside of global health academia, and facilitates comparisons of investment in health with projects in other governmental sectors. For these reasons, BCA should be applied more broadly in global health analysis, and this chapter demonstrates one manner in which this could be accomplished.

BENEFIT-COST ANALYSIS OF CESAREAN DELIVERY FOR OBSTRUCTED LABOR

Overview

Our second analysis illustrates a higher level (that is, a cross-country) application of the methods presented in the section on cleft lip and palate. Obstructed labor, defined by the WHO as labor in which "the presenting part of the fetus cannot progress into the birth canal, despite strong uterine contractions" (Dolea and AbouZahr 2003, 1), is among the most common causes of maternal death in LMICs (Khan and others 2006). Obstructed labor also results in significant morbidity, including obstetric fistula (Dolea and AbouZahr 2003), which is an abnormal communication between the rectum and vagina (rectovaginal fistula) or the bladder and vagina (vesicovaginal fistula). Beyond the substantial risks to physical health, victims of obstetric fistula are known to suffer from poor mental and social health because they are often banned from their homes and turned away from their communities (Wall 2006; WHO 2005).

The current morbidity and mortality posed by obstructed labor need not be so high, as evidenced by the fact that maternal death and fistula secondary to obstructed labor are rarely seen in HICs (Adler and others 2013; Lozano and others 2012). The sequelae of obstructed labor can be prevented by operative delivery of the fetus, which is most commonly via cesarean delivery (Dolea and AbouZahr 2003; Hofmeyr 2004; Neilson 2003). Timely diagnosis and treatment of obstructed labor with cesarean delivery requires access to emergency obstetric systems, which is unfortunately unavailable to most mothers in LMICs (Paxton and others 2006; Pearson and Shoo 2005). Good evidence suggests that access to emergency obstetric services correlates strongly with decreased maternal mortality (Islam, Hossain, and Haque 2005; Jamisse 2004; Kayongo and others 2006).

The past two decades have seen increased investments in global maternal health, with a consequent 34 percent reduction in maternal mortality rates since 1990 (Lozano and others 2011; WHO and others 2010). Although funding for maternal health in LMICs has increased, the distribution of the funding may not be appropriately aligned. Countries with the highest maternal mortality ratios do not receive a commensurate level of funding, and international aid organizations and governments continue to confront insufficient resources to address maternal health adequately (Pitt and others 2010).

Although the decision-making process behind allocation of financial resources by governments and NGOs is complex, economic evaluations, including BCA, can play an important role. This section evaluates the impact of treating obstructed labor with cesarean delivery across multiple regions, specifically examining countries that the WHO identifies as providing an insufficient number of cesarean deliveries to meet current demand (Gibbons and others 2010). We determine country-specific estimates of both the cost per DALY averted and the BCR for providing cesarean delivery in the context of obstructed labor. The DALYs averted refer only to the mother's experience from neglected obstructed labor, not that of her child.

A more comprehensive discussion of the epidemiology and treatment of obstructed labor and obstetric fistula is provided in chapters 5 and 6 in this volume, respectively, and in *Reproductive, Maternal, Newborn, and Child Health* in this series.

Methods

For the estimations and calculations in this section, *obstructed labor* refers to cases that are neglected or left untreated. The section of this chapter on cleft lip and palate provides a complete discussion of DALYs, VSL, and how DALYs are valued using the VSL approach.

Estimating the Incidence and Sequelae of Obstructed Labor and Obstetric Fistula. The relevant population for this chapter is the estimated number of women who incurred obstructed labor in 2010 in 47 countries noted by the WHO as providing an insufficient number of cesarean deliveries (Gibbons and others 2010).

• To estimate the number of cases of obstructed labor, we used a modeling approach based on a recently performed review of the literature that estimates the global incidence of all cases of obstructed labor, including neglected and treated cases (Adler, Ronsmans, and Filippi forthcoming). Based on these data, we then estimated the incidence of neglected obstructed labor in a country using the estimated proportion of births in a health facility as a proxy for timely treatment of obstructed labor (UNICEF 2013); this modeling approach is based on methodology previously used by the GBD study (Dolea and AbouZahr 2003).

- To estimate the incidence of obstetric fistula and mortality secondary to obstructed labor, we relied on a recent meta-analysis that estimates the incidence of fistula in South Asia and Sub-Saharan Africa (Adler and others 2013). It is worth noting that the prevalence and incidence reported in Adler and others (2013) is lower than previous estimates (Wall 2006), likely because of a more rigorous selection criteria for study inclusion. For mortality estimates, we relied on estimates of mortality rates for South Asia and Sub-Saharan Africa from the GBD 2010 study (Lozano and others 2012). For these two regions, the total number of cases of neglected obstructed labor was estimated, and then cases of maternal death and obstetric fistula secondary to obstructed labor in these regions were divided by all cases of neglected obstructed labor to produce two ratios: maternal deaths per 1,000 cases of neglected obstructed labor and obstetric fistula per 1,000 cases of neglected obstructed labor. Given that maternal death and obstetric fistula should not occur if obstructed labor is treated appropriately—these sequelae are almost never seen in HICs—we calculated the country-specific incidence of these sequelae based on the estimated rate of neglected obstructed labor in a country.

We assume that if left untreated, obstetric fistula is a permanent sequela once present in survivors of obstructed labor. Probabilistic sensitivity analysis was employed for the following variables using Monte Carlo simulation: incidence of all cases of obstructed labor and fistula based on Adler's reviews (Adler and others 2013), and incidence of maternal mortality secondary to neglected obstructed labor based on GBD 2010 (Lozano and others 2012).

We apportioned the incidence of obstructed labor and its sequelae of maternal death and obstetric fistula according to seven maternal age groups: 15–19, 20–24, 25–29, 30–34, 35–39, 40–44, and 45–49. This was accomplished by (1) calculating the total number of births in each of these age groups for every included country in 2010; (2) dividing the number of births in each age group by total births to calculate the relative proportion each age group contributes to total births; (3) calculating the total number of cases of obstructed labor and its sequelae for all women ages 15–49 years; and (4) multiplying the age-specific proportions from (2) by the total number of cases of obstructed labor or its sequelae from (3). An important limitation of this approach is that it does not account for the relationship between parity and obstructed labor: younger women are thought to have increased rates of obstructed labor because they are more likely to be nulliparous.

Establishing the Cost of a Cesarean Delivery. As part of a background report for the 2010 *World Health Report*, the WHO estimated the unit cost of a cesarean delivery for countries that were identified as providing an insufficient quantity to meet demand (Gibbons and others 2010). The inputs for estimating cost included "initiation of labor at referral level, diagnosis of obstructed labor and referral, Caesarean delivery associated devices and medicines, operative facility time, medical human resources time, management of shock including hysterectomy and blood transfusion (assumed for 1% of CS performed), postoperative hospital stay for stabilization…program administration, training, and the corresponding office space, electricity and other services, as well as a variety of standard consumables and equipment" (Gibbons and others 2010, 6).

It is important to note that that study did not include cost associated with vaginal birth, such as clean cord practices and the presence of a birth attendant. To account for this omission, we identified studies that estimated the cost of a vaginal delivery in a health facility in countries in South Asia and Sub-Saharan Africa (Bhat and others 2009; Iyengar and others 2009; Levin and others 2003; Newlands and others 2008; Orach, Dubourg, and De Brouwere 2007; Quayyum and others 2010; Sarowar and others 2010). We established a range of values for the proportion of vaginal delivery cost to the WHO cesarean delivery cost, and we used this to adjust the WHO country-specific estimated cost of cesarean section to more appropriate values. We employed probabilistic sensitivity analysis over a range of vaginal delivery to cesarean delivery cost proportions using Monte Carlo simulation.

Estimating Disability-Adjusted Life Years. Not all cesarean deliveries are meant to address obstructed labor, and not all cases of obstructed labor are treated with cesarean delivery. We estimated that 80 percent of obstructed labor cases require cesarean delivery; the remaining 20 percent can be addressed with instrumental vaginal delivery. These latter cases are excluded from our analysis.

We estimated the number of DALYs that could be averted in the 47 countries included in the WHO cost study if 80 percent of the obstructed labor cases were prevented in a timely fashion with a cesarean delivery. Because cesarean delivery is assigned a disability weight by the GBD study and carries a risk of mortality (Souza and others 2010), we first calculated the gross number of DALYs that would be averted by preventing 80 percent of obstructed labor cases, and then subtracted the number of DALYs that would be incurred secondary to cesarean deliveries to arrive at the net DALYs averted.

This study used disability weights from the GBD study (Lopez and others 2006) to estimate DALYs secondary to cesarean delivery and obstetric fistula.

Estimating the Cost per Disability-Adjusted Life Year Averted and the Benefit-Cost Ratio. To estimate the total cost of providing the necessary number of cesarean deliveries to prevent the sequelae of obstructed labor, we multiplied the country-specific unit cost of a cesarean delivery by the number of cesarean deliveries required to treat 80 percent of the cases in that country. Once the total country-specific cost was calculated, we divided this cost by the total number of DALYs [0,0,0] that cesarean delivery for obstructed

labor was estimated to avert. To calculate the BCA, we divided the country-specific economic benefit of treating obstructed labor by the total cost of providing the cesarean deliveries required to do so; the estimated benefit was based on valuing DALYs $[3,1,\tilde{\beta}]$ averted with the VSL approach. This section uses an IE-VSL of 1.5 to transfer VSL estimates.

Results

Table 21.3 presents the estimated number of cesarean deliveries necessary to treat 80 percent of obstructed labor in each country, along with the number of cases of obstetric fistula and maternal death that would be

Table 21.3 Estimated Number of Cesarean Deliveries Required to Prevent 80 Percent of Obstructed Labor, with the Total Number of Preventable Obstetric Fistulas and Maternal Mortality, 2010

Country	Caesarean deliveries[a]	Preventable obstetric fistulas	Preventable maternal mortality[b]
Algeria	812 (441–1,400)	6 (2–12)	9 (8–11)
Bangladesh	46,429 (25,247–80,086)	362 (100–671)	533 (460–609)
Benin	958 (521–1,653)	7 (2–14)	11 (9–13)
Burkina Faso	4,492 (2,443–7,748)	35 (10–65)	52 (44–59)
Cambodia	3,524 (1,916–6,078)	27 (8–51)	40 (35–46)
Cameroon	6,274 (3,412–10,823)	49 (13–91)	72 (62–82)
Central African Republic	1,466 (797–2,528)	11 (3–21)	17 (15–19)
Chad	9,479 (5,154–16,351)	74 (20–137)	109 (94–124)
Comoros	270 (147–466)	2 (1–4)	3 (3–4)
Congo, Dem. Rep.	13,855 (7,534–23,900)	108 (30–200)	159 (137–182)
Côte d'Ivoire	5,728 (3,115–9,880)	45 (12–83)	66 (57–75)
Eritrea	3,306 (1,798–5,702)	26 (7–48)	38 (33–43)
Ethiopia	56,534 (3,0742–97,518)	441 (121–817)	649 (560–742)
Gabon	154 (84–265)	1 (0–2)	2 (2–2)
Ghana	5,195 (2,825–8,961)	41 (11–75)	60 (51–68)
Guinea	5,093 (2,769–8,785)	40 (11–74)	58 (50–67)
Haiti	4,109 (2,234–7,087)	32 (9–59)	47 (41–54)
India	276,385 (150,291–476,747)	2,157 (592–3,993)	3173 (2,737–36,28)
Indonesia	43,246 (23,516–74,597)	337 (93–625)	496 (428–568)
Kenya	17,442 (9,485–30,087)	136 (37–252)	200 (173–229)
Lesotho	471 (256–812)	4 (1–7)	5 (5–6)
Liberia	1,877 (1,021–3,237)	15 (4–27)	22 (19–25)
Madagascar	9,754 (5,304–16,824)	76 (21–141)	112 (97–128)
Malawi	33,04 (1,797–5,699)	26 (7–48)	38 (33–43)
Mali	7,165 (3,896–12,359)	56 (15–104)	82 (71–94)
Mauritania	1,315 (715–2,268)	10 (3–19)	15 (13–17)

table continues next page

Country	Caesarean deliveries[a]	Preventable obstetric fistulas	Preventable maternal mortality[b]
Mongolia	18 (10–31)	0.1 (0–0.3)	0.2 (0.2–0.3)
Morocco	3,426 (1,863–5,910)	27 (7–49)	39 (34–45)
Mozambique	8,194 (4,455–14,134)	64 (18–118)	94 (81–108)
Nepal	8,879 (4,828–15,315)	69 (19–128)	102 (88–117)
Niger	12,832 (6,978–22,134)	100 (28–185)	147 (127–168)
Nigeria	85,159 (46,307–146,894)	665 (183–1,230)	978 (843–1,118)
Oman	17 (9–30)	0.1 (0–0.25)	0.2 (0.2–0.2)
Pakistan	57,141 (31,072–98,565)	446 (122–825)	656 (566–750)
Philippines	26,402 (14,357–45,542)	206 (57–381)	303 (261–347)
Rwanda	2,557 (1,391–4,411)	20 (5–37)	29 (25–34)
Senegal	2,685 (1,460–4,632)	21 (6–39)	31 (27–35)
Sierra Leone	2,233 (1,214–3,852)	17 (5–32)	26 (22–29)
Sudan	20,044 (10,900–34,575)	156 (43–290)	230 (199–263)
Swaziland	148 (81–256)	1 (0–2)	2 (1–2)
Tanzania	18,198 (9,896–31,391)	142 (39–263)	209 (180–239)
Togo	1,574 (856–2,715)	12 (3–23)	18 (16–21)
Tunisia	394 (214–680)	3 (1–6)	5 (4–5)
Uganda	13,035 (7,088–22,485)	102 (28–188)	150 (129–171)
Vietnam	2,255 (1,226–3,889)	18 (5–33)	26 (22–30)
Yemen, Rep.	11,957 (6,502–20,624)	93 (26–173)	137 (118–157)
Zambia	5,844 (3,178–10,080)	46 (13–84)	67 (58–77)
Total	**811,629**	**6,334**	**9,318**

Note: Table reports mean, with 95 percent uncertainty interval in parentheses.
a. Necessary to prevent 80 percent of obstructed labor.
b. Adjusted for mortality secondary to cesarean delivery.

prevented by providing cesarean delivery for obstructed labor. Maternal mortality is adjusted to account for mortality secondary to cesarean delivery. For the 47 countries, an estimated 815,000 cesarean deliveries would have prevented 6,300 cases of obstetric fistula and 9,400 maternal deaths. Table 21.4 presents the total cost of providing the necessary number of cesarean deliveries to prevent all cases of obstructed labor for the included countries in 2010. For each country, the total cost of providing cesarean deliveries for obstructed labor was then divided by the potential nondiscounted, non-age-weighted DALYs (notated as [0,0,0]) averted if all cases of obstructed labor were treated to create a cost per DALY averted. The average cost per DALY averted varied by country, ranging from US$243 to US$1,192 per DALY averted. The median cost per DALY averted was US$416.

Table 21.4 also presents the country-specific gross economic benefit of preventing obstructed labor.

The mean total benefit across countries was estimated to be US$1.4 billion in 2010 dollars. The last column of table 21.4 shows BCRs for providing cesarean deliveries in each country, calculated by dividing the estimated economic benefit by the total cost of providing cesarean deliveries. The BCR ranges from 0.3 for the Democratic Republic of Congo to 75.5 for Gabon, with a median value of 4.0.

Discussion and Recommendations

Valuing Maternal Health Care. The analysis in this section elucidates the cost and benefit of treating neglected obstructed labor with cesarean delivery across a number of disparate regions. We estimate that cesarean delivery for obstructed labor, depending on the country, costs US$243–US$1192 per DALY [0,0,0], with a median cost of US$416 per DALY for the 47 countries included in

Table 21.4 Total Cost of Treating Obstructed Labor with Cesarean Delivery, Cost per DALY Averted, Gross Economic Benefit, and Benefit-Cost Ratio, US$, 2010

Country	Total cost (thousands)[a]	Cost/DALY averted[b]	Gross economic benefit (thousands)[c]	Benefit-cost ratio[d]
Algeria	245 (130–440)	463 (214–924)	7293 (5,400–9,300)	33.6 (14.2–64)
Bangladesh	7,590 (3,890–13,620)	243 (112–484)	45,702 (34,100–58,300)	6.8 (2.9–13)
Benin	207 (110–370)	349 (161–696)	677 (500–900)	3.7 (1.6–7)
Burkina Faso	1,012 (520–1,820)	386 (178–770)	2,752 (2,100–3,500)	3.1 (1.3–5.9)
Cambodia	812 (420–1460)	364 (168–726)	4,221 (3,100–5,400)	5.9 (2.5–11.2)
Cameroon	1,325 (680–2,380)	363 (167–724)	7,759 (5,800–9,900)	6.6 (2.8–12.6)
Central African Republic	356 (180–640)	551 (253–1103)	361 (300–500)	1.1 (0.5–2.2)
Chad	1,967 (1,010–3,530)	350 (161–698)	5,647 (4,200–7,200)	3.2 (1.4–6.2)
Comoros	61 (30–110)	407 (188–813)	118 (100–200)	2.5 (1–4.7)
Congo, Dem. Rep.	4,415 (2,260–7,920)	581 (267–1159)	1,106 (800–1400)	0.3 (0.1–0.5)
Côte d'Ivoire	1,314 (670–2,360)	395 (182–789)	5,773 (43,00–7,400)	5 (2.1–9.5)
Eritrea	978 (500–1,760)	547 (252–1092)	435 (300–600)	0.5 (0.2–1)
Ethiopia	14,214 (7,290–25,510)	452 (208–902)	21,257 (15,800–27,200)	1.7 (0.7–3.2)
Gabon	80 (40–140)	901 (415–1798)	2,665 (2,000–3,400)	37.4 (15.8–71.4)
Ghana	1,410 (720–2,530)	454 (209–905)	4,322 (3,200–5,500)	3.5 (1.5–6.6)
Guinea	1,249 (640–2,240)	416 (192–830)	1,749 (1,300–2,200)	1.6 (0.7–3)
Haiti	1,009 (520–1,810)	667 (305–1338)	1,570 (1,200–2,000)	1.8 (0.7–3.4)
India	49,033 (25,150–88,000)	279 (129–557)	716,631 (534,700–914,300)	16.5 (7–31.5)
Indonesia	10,777 (5,530–19,340)	395 (182–787)	150,723 (112,400–192,300)	15.8 (6.7–30.1)
Kenya	3,973 (2,040–7,130)	371 (171–741)	14,498 (10,800–18,500)	4.1 (1.7–7.9)
Lesotho	150 (80–270)	685 (314–1,369)	527 (400–700)	4 (1.7–7.6)
Liberia	509 (260–910)	482 (222–962)	232 (200–300)	0.5 (0.2–1)
Madagascar	2,198 (1,130–3,950)	381 (175–760)	3,464 (2,600–4,400)	1.8 (0.8–3.4)
Malawi	752 (390–1,350)	452 (208–903)	949 (700–1,200)	1.4 (0.6–2.7)
Mali	1,528 (780–2,740)	378 (174–754)	3,484 (2,600–4,500)	2.6 (1.1–4.9)
Mauritania	337 (170–600)	439 (202–875)	1,814 (1,400–2,300)	6.1 (2.6–11.6)
Mongolia	6 (0–10)	552 (254–1,101)	58 (0–100)	9.7 (4.1–18.5)
Morocco	867 (440–1,560)	391 (180–780)	13,974 (10,400–17,800)	18.2 (7.7–34.7)
Mozambique	1,900 (970–3,410)	452 (208–902)	2,587 (1,900–3,300)	1.5 (0.6–2.9)
Nepal	1,684 (860–3,020)	283 (130–563)	5,765 (4,300–7,400)	3.9 (1.6–7.4)
Niger	2,923 (1,500–5,250)	386 (178–770)	2,359 (1,800–3,000)	0.9 (0.4–1.7)
Nigeria	20,988 (10,770–37,670)	422 (194–842)	106,203 (79,100–135,600)	5.7 (2.4–10.9)
Oman	14 (10–30)	1,192 (550–2,376)	941 (700–1200)	75.7 (32–144.4)
Pakistan	17,413 (8,930–31,250)	489 (225–976)	107,143 (79,900–136,700)	7 (2.9–13.3)
Philippines	6,315 (3,240–11,330)	365 (168–728)	85,589 (63,900–109,200)	15.3 (6.5–29.2)
Rwanda	577 (300–1040)	379 (175–756)	1,278 (1,000–1,600)	2.5 (1.1–4.8)
Senegal	557 (290–1,000)	343 (158–684)	2,664 (2,000–3,400)	5.4 (2.3–10.3)
Sierra Leone	525 (270–940)	416 (191–829)	978 (700–1,200)	2.1 (0.9–4)

table continues next page

Table 21.4 Total Cost of Treating Obstructed Labor with Cesarean Delivery, Cost per DALY Averted, Gross Economic Benefit, and Benefit-Cost Ratio, US$, 2010 (continued)

Country	Total cost (thousands)[a]	Cost/DALY averted[b]	Gross economic benefit (thousands)[c]	Benefit-cost ratio[d]
Sudan	5,750 (2,950–10,320)	437 (202–872)	20,130 (15,000–25,700)	4 (1.7–7.5)
Swaziland	52 (30–90)	796 (365–1,592)	571 (400–700)	12.5 (5.2–23.9)
Tanzania	4,281 (2,200–7,680)	406 (187–810)	12,029 (9,000–15,400)	3.2 (1.3–6.1)
Togo	316 (160–570)	340 (157–679)	473 (400–600)	1.7 (0.7–3.2)
Tunisia	220 (110–400)	831 (383–1,657)	4,457 (3,300–5,700)	22.8 (9.6–43.6)
Uganda	3,381 (1,730–6,070)	455 (209–907)	6,301 (4,700–8,000)	2.1 (0.9–4)
Vietnam	587 (300–1,050)	357 (165–710)	5,172 (3,900–6,600)	9.9 (4.2–19)
Yemen, Rep.	3,105 (1,590–5,570)	446 (206–891)	19,918 (14,800–25,400)	7.2 (3.1–13.8)
Zambia	1,583 (810–2,840)	518 (238–1,034)	3,627 (2,700–4,600)	2.6 (1.1–4.9)
Median	n.a.	416	n.a.	4.0

Note: n.a = not applicable. Table reports mean, with 95 percent uncertainty interval in parentheses.
a. Total cost to treat 80 percent of cases of neglected obstructed labor with cesarean delivery.
b. The cost per DALY averted using [0,0,0] assumptions. See text for explanation.
c. Estimated by valuing DALYs [3,1,$\tilde{\beta}$] with value of a statistical life year.
d. Benefit-cost ratio calculated by dividing gross economic benefit by total cost.

this study. These estimates compare favorably with the costs reported in chapter 18 of this volume, which summarizes the global surgery cost-effectiveness literature. Using WHO guidelines (WHO 2002), cesarean delivery for obstructed labor is highly cost-effective in the vast majority of countries, and cost-effective in all included countries.

The BCRs in table 21.4, however, convey the main message of this section: the BCR is greater than 1 for nearly every country examined. The exceptions are the Democratic Republic of Congo, Eritrea, Liberia, and Niger, most of which have relatively high costs per DALY averted. These results suggest that devoting appropriate financial resources to cesarean delivery can combat the catastrophic health consequences to mothers in an economically favorable fashion. Indeed, the median BCR for the 47 countries included in our study is 4:1, which represents an excellent return on investment. Our headline results are also our most conservative; we used the largest IE-VSL value (1.5) reported in the literature, which significantly reduces the estimated benefits (see the section of this chapter on cleft lip and palate for more detail regarding the IE-VSL). Even the four countries mentioned above would have BCRs greater than 1 if the more commonly used assumption of IE-VSL = 1 were used.

Implications of Results. Our results have potentially meaningful implications for all involved stakeholders within the continuum of maternal and newborn care. We first emphasize for potential donors and NGOs

the relative cost-effectiveness of cesarean delivery for obstructed labor in comparison with the WHO's per capita income thresholds. We are not the first to suggest that surgical care can be cost-effective, but our results add to the burgeoning evidence base.

Our data further suggest that when prioritizing budgeting of different sectors, governments should recognize that investment in health care can achieve net-positive economic benefits, as indicated by BCRs greater than 1. Specifically, allocating appropriate levels of funding for providing the suggested minimum of emergency obstetric care, considered within the broader context of maternal health care, is a good economic proposition in the vast majority of countries investigated.

It is crucial to note that cesarean delivery is not a panacea. Indeed, the overuse of the procedure in many HICs, along with the associated cost, has been well documented (Gibbons and others 2010). This chapter assesses cesarean delivery in the context of obstructed labor, in which there is a well-defined role for operative delivery. The results of this chapter do not imply that cesarean delivery is always cost-effective; they do suggest, however, that when used appropriately, the economic benefits of the procedure can outweigh the cost.

We also emphasize that we are not advocating vertical programming aimed at providing cesarean delivery or emergency obstetric care in isolation; experience tells us that properly functioning health systems must be in place for mothers to receive appropriate, high-quality care (Maine 2007). The current focus on packages of interventions that are integrated into a functioning health system are envisioned such that women in need of an emergent cesarean delivery are aware of facilities available, are properly diagnosed, are transported to a referral hospital within a reasonable amount of time, and undergo safe cesarean delivery in a capable facility (Fournier 2009; Nyamtema, Urassa, and van Roosmalen 2011). In this broader context, our argument is that cesarean delivery—as part of a larger strategy—can address maternal mortality in an economically favorable fashion.

Study Limitations

The analysis in this section has a number of important limitations. Our methodology rests on the overly simplified assumption that a lack of surgical capacity is the major driver of preventable morbidity and mortality. We may have overestimated the potential benefit of cesarean delivery given other barriers, such as a lack of timely diagnosis and poor transportation infrastructure, that are known to play a role in neglected obstructed labor (Chhabra, Gandhi, and Jaiswal 2000; WHO 2005). However, our calculated BCRs suggest that surgical intervention would still be beneficial even if the number of cesarean deliveries successfully performed were far fewer than the perfect rate we have assumed. At our median estimate of the BCR, surgical intervention would still break even if only 25 percent of the potentially preventable DALYs were actually averted.

A critique of the methods used for placing a dollar value on DALYs is presented elsewhere (Alkire and others 2011; Warf and others 2011). There is uncertainty regarding transfers of VSL estimates to low-income countries for which formal studies are lacking (Hammitt and Robinson 2011), but we have minimized the risk of overvaluing a DALY by using an IE-VSL of 1.5. In fact, our estimates of BCRs are possibly too conservative as a result of using the lower-bound estimate of IE-VSL for valuing DALYs. Most important, our analysis does not account for the benefit of reducing perinatal mortality and morbidity with improved access to cesarean delivery. The perinatal mortality rate as a result of neglected obstructed labor depends on the case series, but ranges from 38 percent to 92 percent (Hofmeyr 2004; Melah and others 2003; Neilson 2003). Finally, there is uncertainty regarding the true number of maternal deaths and fistula worldwide and the contribution that obstructed labor makes to that number; we have attempted to account for this uncertainty with probabilistic sensitivity analysis.

CONCLUSIONS

A case could easily be made for addressing obstructed labor from a strictly humanitarian perspective, yet some continue to suggest that surgery is a luxury. This section demonstrates that investment in cesarean delivery is not only cost-effective; it can yield a net positive economic return within the context of a horizontally functioning health system. More broadly, the analyses used in this chapter can be applied to other interventions and are crucial for better-informed investments in global health care delivery.

ACKNOWLEDGMENTS

The authors acknowledge the support of the government of Assam, the National Rural Health Mission, the Sir Dorabji Tata Trust and Allied Trusts, Operation Smile International, and Operation Smile India for providing infrastructure and funding for the GCCCC, Assam, India. All patients at this center are treated free of cost, with no commercial or financial gain to any member of the team. The authors wish to specifically acknowledge Alex Campbell and William Magee for providing the data used in this analysis.

The section in this chapter on cesarean delivery is based on a paper previously published by the authors, entitled "Obstructed Labor and Caesarean Delivery: The Cost and Benefit of Surgical Intervention" in *PLoS One* (Alkire and others 2012a). The methods and results have been completely revised to reflect the most recent data available. We wish to acknowledge the additional original authors for their efforts in producing the above study: Paul Farmer, Ian Metzler, and Christy Turlington Burns. We also wish to thank Christopher Hughes and Toni Golen for their assistance with the obstructed labor analysis.

NOTES

The World Bank classifies countries according to four income groupings. Income is measured using gross national income (GNI) per capita, in U.S. dollars, converted from local currency using the *World Bank Atlas* method. Classifications as of July 2014 are as follows:

- Low-income countries (LICs) = US$1,045 or less in 2013
- Middle-income countries (MICs) are subdivided:
  - Lower-middle-income = US$1,046 to US$4,125
  - Upper-middle-income (UMICs) = US$4,126 to US$12,745
- High-income countries (HICs) = US$12,746 or more

1. The World Bank: Open Data. http://data.worldbank.org/.
2. United States Environmental Protection Agency. "Frequently Asked Questions on Mortality Risk Valuation." http://yosemite.epa.gov/ee/epa/eed.nsf/webpages/mortalityrisk valuation.html.

REFERENCES

Adler, A., C. Ronsmans, C. Calvert, and V. Filippi. 2013. "Estimating the Prevalence of Obstetric Fistula: A Systematic Review and Meta-Analysis." *Biomed Central Pregnancy and Childbirth* 13 (246): 1–14.

Adler, A., C. Ronsmans, and V. Filippi. Forthcoming. "Prevalence of Obstructed and Prolonged Labour: A Systematic Review."

Aldy, J. E., and W. K. Viscusi. 2008. "Adjusting the Value of a Statistical Life for Age and Cohort Effects." *Review of Economics and Statistics* 90 (3): 573–81.

Alkire, B., C. D. Hughes, K. Nash, J. R. Vincent, and J. G. Meara. 2011. "Potential Economic Benefit of Cleft Lip and Palate Repair in Sub-Saharan Africa." *World Journal of Surgery* 35 (6): 1194–201.

Alkire, B. C., J. R. Vincent, C. T. Burns, I. S. Metzler, P. E. Farmer, and others. 2012a. "Obstructed Labor and Caesarean Delivery: The Cost and Benefit of Surgical Intervention." *PLoS One* 7 (4): e34595.

———. 2012b. "Obstructed Labor and Caesarean Delivery: The Cost and Benefit of Surgical Intervention," Appendix S1 . *PLoS One* 7 (4): e34595. doi:10 .1371/journal.pone.0034595 .s001.

Becker, G. S., T. J. Philipson, and R. R. Soares. 2003. "The Quantity and Quality of Life and the Evolution of World Inequality." Working Paper No. 9765, National Burea of Economic Research, Cambridge, MA. http://www.nber.org /papers/w9765.

Belli, P., J. Anderson, H. Barnum, J. Dixon, and J. P. Tan, eds. 2001. *Economic Analysis of Investment Operations: Analytical Tools and Practical Applications.* Washington, DC: World Bank.

Bhat, R., D. V. Mavalankar, P. V. Singh, and N. Singh. 2009. "Maternal Healthcare Financing: Gujarat's Chiranjeevi Scheme and Its Beneficiaries." *Journal of Health, Population and Nutrition* 27 (2): 249–58.

Bickler, S., D. Ozgediz, R. Gosselin, T. Weiser, D. Spiegel, and others. 2010. "Key Concepts for Estimating the Burden of Surgical Conditions and the Unmet Need for Surgical Care." *World Journal of Surgery* 34 (3): 374–80.

Campbell, A. 2014. "Scalable, Sustainable Cost-Effective Surgical Care: A Model for Safety and Quality in the Developing World." *Journal of Craniofacial Surgery* 25 (5): 1685–89.

Canfield, M. A., M. A. Honein, N. Yuskiv, J. Xing, C. T. Mai, and others. 2006. "National Estimates and Race/Ethnic-Specific Variation of Selected Birth Defects in the United States,

1999–2001." *Birth Defects Research Part A: Clinical and Molecular Teratology* 76 (11): 747–56.

Chatterjee, S., and R. Laxminarayan. 2013. "Costs of Surgical Procedures in Indian Hospitals." *British Medical Journal Open* 3 (6): e002844.

Chhabra, S., D. Gandhi, and M. Jaiswal. 2000. "Obstructed Labour: A Preventable Entity." *Journal of Obstetrics and Gynaecology* 20 (2): 151–53.

Cohen, S. R., J. Kalinowski, D. LaRossa, and P. Randall. 1991. "Cleft Palate Fistulas: A Multivariate Statistical Analysis of Prevalence, Etiology, and Surgical Management." *Plastic and Reconstructive Surgery* 87 (6): 1041–47.

Corlew, D. S. 2010. "Estimation of Impact of Surgical Disease through Economic Modeling of Cleft Lip and Palate Care." *World Journal of Surgery* 34 (3): 391–96.

———. 2013. "Economic Modeling of Surgical Disease: A Measure of Public Health Interventions." *World Journal of Surgery* 37 (7): 1478–85.

Deshpande, G., A. Campbell, C. Restrepo, R. Jagtap, H. Dobie, and others. Forthcoming. "Early Complications after Cleft Palate Repair: A Multivariate Statistical Analysis of 709 Consecutive Patients." *Journal of Craniofacial Surgery*.

Dolea, C., and C. AbouZahr. 2003. "Global Burden of Obstructed Labor in the Year 2000: Version 2." In *Evidence and Information for Policy.* Geneva: WHO.

Dupuis, C. C. 2004. "Humanitarian Missions in the Third World: A Polite Dissent." *Plastic and Reconstructive Surgery* 113 (1): 433–35.

Farmer, P. E., and J. Y. Kim. 2008. "Surgery and Global Health: A View from beyond the OR." *World Journal of Surgery* 32 (4): 533–36.

Flint, P. W., and C. W. Cummings. 2010. *Cummings Otolaryngology: Head and Neck Surgery.* 5th edition, 3 vols. London: Mosby.

Fournier, P. 2009. "Improved Access to Comprehensive Emergency Obstetric Care and Its Effect on Institutional Marternal Mortality in Rural Mali." *Bulletin of the World Health Organization* 87 (1): 30–38.

Gibbons, L., J. M. Belizan, J. A. Lauer, A. P. Betran, M. Merialdi, and others. 2010. "The Global Numbers and Costs of Additionally Needed and Unnecessary Caesarean Sections Performed per Year: Overuse as a Barrier to Universal Coverage." World Health Report 2010, Background Paper 30 for *Health Systems Financing: The Path to Universal Coverage.* Geneva: WHO.

Gosselin, R. A., A. Maldonado, and G. Elder. 2010. "Comparative Cost-Effectiveness Analysis of Two MSF Surgical Trauma Centers." *World Journal of Surgery* 34 (3): 415–19.

Grimes, C. E., J. A. Henry, J. Maraka, N. C. Mkandawire, and M. Cotton. 2013. "Cost-Effectiveness of Surgery in Low and Middle-Income Countries: A Systematic Review." *World Journal of Surgery* 38 (1): 252–63.

Hammitt, J. K. 2007. "Valuing Changes in Mortality Risk: Lives Saved versus Life Years Saved." *Review of Environmental Economics and Policy* 1 (2): 228–40.

Hammitt, J. K., and K. Haninger. 2010. "Valuing Fatal Risks to Children and Adults: Effects of Disease, Latency, and Risk Aversion." *Journal of Risk Uncertainty* 40 (1): 57–83.

Hammitt, J. K., and L. A. Robinson. 2011. "The Income Elasticity of the Value per Statistical Life: Transferring Estimates between High and Low Income Populations." *Journal of Benefit-Cost Analysis* 2 (1): Article 1.

Hoddinott, J., M. Rosegrant, and M. Torero. 2012. "Challenge Paper: Hunger and Malnutrition." Copenhagen Consensus 2012, Copenhagen Consensus Center, Copenhagen.

Hofmeyr, G. 2004. "Obstructed Labor: Using Better Technologies to Reduce Mortality." *International Journal of Gynaecology and Obstetrics* 85: S62–72.

Hughes, C. D., B. Alkire, C. Martin, N. Semer, and J. G. Meara. 2012. "American Plastic Surgery and Global Health: A Brief History." *Annals of Plastic Surgery* 68 (2): 222–25.

Indian Power Market. 2012. "Electricity Prices in Different States of India." http://www.indianpowermarket.com/2012/09/electricity-prices-in-different-states.html.

Islam, M., M. Hossain, and Y. Haque. 2005. "Improvement of Coverage and Utilization of EmOC Services in Southwestern Bangladesh." *International Journal of Gynaecology and Obstetrics* 91 (3): 298–305.

Iyengar, S. D., K. Iyengar, V. Suhalka, and K. Agarwal. 2009. "Comparison of Domiciliary and Institutional Delivery-Care Practices in Rural Rajasthan, India." *Journal of Health, Population and Nutrition* 27 (2): 303–12.

Jamison, D. T., J. G. Breman, A. R. Measham, G. Alleyne, M. Claeson, D. B. Evans, P. Jha, A. Mills, and P. Musgrove, eds. 2006. *Disease Control Priorities in Developing Countries*, 2nd ed. Washington, DC: World Bank and Oxford University Press.

Jamison, D. T., P. Jha, and D. Bloom. 2008. "The Challenge of Disease." Copenhagen Consensus 2008, Copenhagen Consensus Center, Copenhagen.

Jamison, D. T., P. Jha, R. Laxminarayan, and T. Ord. 2012. "Infectious Disease, Injury, and Reproductive Health." Copenhagan Consensus 2012, Copenhagen Consensus Center, Copenhagen.

Jamison, D. T., L. H. Summers, G. Alleyne, K. J. Arrow, S. Berkley, and others. 2013. "Global Health 2035: A World Converging within a Generation." *The Lancet* 382 (9908): 1898–955.

Jamisse, L. 2004. "Reducing Maternal Mortality in Mozambique: Challenges, Failures, Successes and Lessons Learned." *International Journal of Gynaecology and Obstetrics* 85 (2): 203–12.

Kayongo, M., M. Rubardt, J. Butera, M. Abdullah, D. Mboninyibuka, and others. 2006. "Making EmOC a Reality: CARE's Experiences in Areas of High Maternal Mortality in Africa." *International Journal of Gynaecology and Obstetrics* 92 (3): 308–19.

Khan, K. S., D. Wojdyla, L. Say, A. M. Gulmezoglu, and P. F. Van Look. 2006. "WHO Analysis of Causes of Maternal Death: A Systematic Review." *The Lancet* 367 (9516): 1066–74.

Kruk, M. E., A. Wladis, N. Mbembati, S. K. Ndao-Brumblay, R. Y. Hsia, and others. 2010. "Human Resource and Funding Constraints for Essential Surgery in District Hospitals in Africa: A Retrospective Cross-Sectional Survey." *PLoS Medicine* 7 (3): e1000242.

Kunreuther, H., and E. Michel-Kerjan. 2012. "Challenge Paper: Natural Disasters." Copenhagen Consensus 2012, Copenhagen Consensus Center, Copenhagen.

Levin, A., T. Dmytraczenko, M. McEuen, F. Ssengooba, R. Mangani, and others. 2003. "Costs of Maternal Health Care Services in Three Anglophone African Countries." *International Journal of Health Planning and Management* 18 (1): 3–22.

Lopez, A. D., C. D. Mathers, M. Ezzati, D. T. Jamison, C. J. L. Murray, and others. 2006. *Global Burden of Disease and Risk Factors*. Washington, DC: Oxford University Press and World Bank.

Lozano, R., M. Naghavi, K. Foreman, S. Lim, K. Shibuya, and others. 2012. "Global and Regional Mortality from 235 Causes of Death for 20 Age Groups in 1990 and 2010: A Systematic Analysis for the Global Burden of Disease Study 2010." *The Lancet* 380 (9859): 2095–128.

Lozano, R., H. Wang, K. J. Foreman, J. K. Rajaratnam, M. Naghavi, and others. 2011. "Progress towards Millennium Development Goals 4 and 5 on Maternal and Child Mortality: An Updated Systematic Analysis." *The Lancet* 378 (9797): 1139–65.

Luboga, S., S. B. Macfarlane, J. von Schreeb, M. E. Kruk, M. N. Cherian, and others. 2009. "Increasing Access to Surgical Services in Sub-Saharan Africa: Priorities for National and International Agencies Recommended by the Bellagio Essential Surgery Group." *PLoS Medicine* 6 (12): e1000200.

Madheswaran, S. 2007. "Measuring the Value of Statistical Life: Estimating Compensating Wage Differentials among Workers in India." *Social Indicators Research* 84 (1): 83–96.

Magee, W. P., Jr., R. Vander Burg, and K. W. Hatcher. 2010. "Cleft Lip and Palate as a Cost-Effective Health Care Treatment in the Developing World." *World Journal of Surgery* 34 (3): 420–27.

Maine, D. 2007. "Detours and Shortcuts on the Road to Maternal Mortality Reduction." *Lancet* 370 (9595): 1380–82.

McCord, C. 2003. "A Cost Effective Small Hospital in Bangladesh: What It Can Mean for Emergency Obstetric Care." *International Journal of Gynaecology and Obstetrics* 81 (1): 83–92.

McQueen, K. A., W. Magee, T. Crabtree, C. Romano, and F. M. Burkle, Jr. 2009. "Application of Outcome Measures in International Humanitarian Aid: Comparing Indices through Retrospective Analysis of Corrective Surgical Care Cases." *Prehospital and Disaster Medicine* 24 (1): 39–46.

Meier, D. 2010. "Opportunities and Improvisations: A Pediatric Surgeon's Suggestions for Successful Short-Term Surgical Volunteer Work in Resource-Poor Areas." *World Journal of Surgery* 34 (5): 941–46.

Melah, G. S., A. U. El-Nafaty, A. A. Massa, and B. M. Audu. 2003. "Obstructed Labour: A Public Health Problem in Gombe, Gombe State, Nigeria." *Journal of Obstetrics and Gynaecology* 23 (4): 369–73.

Ministry of Urban Development of India and Asian Development Bank. 2008. *2007 Benchmarking and Data Book of Water Utilities in India*. Mandaluyong City, Philippines: Asian Development Bank.

Murray, C. J., and A. K. Acharya. 1997. "Understanding DALYs (Disability-Adjusted Life Years)." *Journal of Health Economics* 16 (6): 703–30.

Murray, C. J., and A. D. Lopez. 1996. The Global Burden of Disease: A Comprehensive Assessment of Mortality and Disability from Diseases, Injuries, and Risk Factors in 1990 and Projected to 2020. Global Burden of Disease and Injury Series. Cambridge, MA: Harvard School of Public Health on behalf of the World Health Organization and the World Bank.

Neilson, J. 2003. "Obstructed Labour." *British Medical Bulletin* 67 (1): 191–204.

Newlands, D., D. Yugbare-Belemsaga, L. Ternent, S. Hounton, and G. Chapman. 2008. "Assessing the Costs and Cost-Effectiveness of a Skilled Care Initiative in Rural Burkina Faso." *Tropical Medicine and International Health* 13 (Suppl 1): 61–67.

Nyamtema, A. S., D. P. Urassa, and J. van Roosmalen. 2011. "Maternal Health Interventions in Resource Limited Countries: A Systematic Review of Packages, Impacts and Factors for Change." *Biomed Central Pregnancy and Childbirth* 11: 30.

Orach, C. G., D. Dubourg, and V. De Brouwere. 2007. "Costs and Coverage of Reproductive Health Interventions in Three Rural Refugee-Affected Districts, Uganda." *Tropical Medicine and International Health* 12 (3): 459–69.

Paxton, A., P. Bailey, S. Lobis, and D. Fry. 2006. "Global Patterns in Availability of Emergency Obstetric Care." *International Journal of Gynaecology and Obstetrics* 93 (3): 300–07.

Pearson, L., and R. Shoo. 2005. "Availability and Use of Emergency Obstetric Services: Kenya, Rwanda, Southern Sudan, and Uganda." *International Journal of Gynaecology and Obstetrics* 88 (2): 208–15.

Pitt, C., G. Greco, T. Powell-Jackson, and A. Mills. 2010. "Countdown to 2015: Assessment of Official Development Assistance to Maternal, Newborn, and Child Health, 2003–08." *The Lancet* 376 (9751): 1485–96.

Poenaru, D. 2013. "Getting the Job Done: Analysis of the Impact and Effectiveness of the Smiletrain Program in Alleviating the Global Burden of Cleft Disease." *World Journal of Surgery* 37 (7): 1562–70.

Quayyum, Z., M. Nadjib, T. Ensor, and P. K. Sucahya. 2010. "Expenditure on Obstetric Care and the Protective Effect of Insurance on the Poor: Lessons from Two Indonesian Districts." *Health Policy and Planning* 25 (3): 237–47.

Robinson, L. A. 2007. "Policy Monitor: How US Government Agencies Value Mortality Risk Reductions." *Review of Environmental Economics and Policy* 1 (2): 283–99.

Roman, H. A., J. K. Hammitt, T. L. Walsh, and D. M. Stieb. 2012. "Expert Elicitation of the Value per Statistical Life in an Air Pollution Context." *Risk Analysis* 32 (12): 2133–51.

Rossell-Perry, P., E. Segura, L. Salas-Bustinza, and O. Cotrina-Rabanal. 2013. "Comparison of Two Models of Surgical Care for Patients with Cleft Lip and Palate in Resource-Challenged Settings." *World Journal of Surgery*. Online in advance of print.

Sarowar, M. G., E. Medin, R. Gazi, T. P. Koehlmoos, C. Rehnberg, and others. 2010. "Calculation of Costs of Pregnancy- and Puerperium-Related Care: Experience from a Hospital in a Low-Income Country." *Journal of Health, Population and Nutrition* 28 (3): 264–72.

Shanmugam, K. 1996. "The Value of Life: Estimates from Indian Labour Market." *Indian Economic Journal* 44 (4): 105–14.

Shanmugam, K., and S. Madheswaran. 2011. "The Value of Statistical Life." In *Environmental Valuation in South Asia*, edited by A. K. Haque, M. N. Murty, and P. Shyamsundar, 412–43. New Delhi: Cambridge University Press.

Souza, J. P., A. Gulmezoglu, P. Lumbiganon, M. Laopaiboon, G. Carroli, and others. 2010. "Caesarean Section without Medical Indications Is Associated with an Increased Risk of Adverse Short-Term Maternal Outcomes: The 2004–2008 WHO Global Survey on Maternal and Perinatal Health." *Biomed Central Medicine* 8: 71.

UNICEF (United Nations Children's Fund). 2013. *The State of the World's Children 2013: Children with Disabilities*. New York: UNICEF. http://www.unicef.org/sowc2013/.

Vanderas, A. P. 1987. "Incidence of Cleft Lip, Cleft Palate, and Cleft Lip and Palate among Races: A Review." *Cleft Palate Journal* 24 (3): 216–25.

Viscusi, W. K., and J. E. Aldy. 2003. "The Value of a Statistical Life: A Critical Review of Market Estimates throughout the World." *Journal of Risk Uncertainty* 27 (1): 5–76.

Vos, T., A. D. Flaxman, M. Naghavi, R. Lozano, C. Michaud, and others. 2012. "Years Lived with Disability (YLDs) for 1160 Sequelae of 289 Diseases and Injuries 1990–2010: A Systematic Analysis for the Global Burden of Disease Study 2010." *The Lancet* 380 (9859): 2163–96.

Wall, L. L. 2006. "Obstetric Vesicovaginal Fistula as an International Public-Health Problem." *The Lancet* 368 (9542): 1201–09.

Warf, B., B. C. Alkire, S. Bhai, C. D. Hughes, S. J. Schiff, and others. 2011. "Costs and Benefits of Neurosurgical Intervention for Infant Hydrocephalus in Sub-Saharan Africa." *Journal of Neurosurgery Pediatrics* 8 (5): 509–21.

WHO (World Health Organization). 2001. *Macroeconomics and Health: Investing in Health for Economic Development*. Report of the Commission on Macroeconomics and Health. Geneva: WHO.

———. 2002. The World Health Report 2002: Reducing Risks, Promoting Healthy Life. Geneva: WHO.

———. 2005. The World Health Report 2005: Make Every Mother and Child Count. Edited by W. V. Lerberghe. Geneva: WHO.

———. 2013. "Global Health Estimates for Deaths by Cause, Age, and Sex for Years 2000–2011." Geneva: WHO. http://www.who.int/healthinfo/global_burden_disease /en/.

WHO-CHOICE. 2014. "Assumptions on Quantities of Resources Use." http://www.who.int/choice/cost-effectiveness/inputs /assumptions/en/.

WHO, UNICEF, UNFPA, and World Bank. 2010. Trends in Maternal Mortality: 1990 to 2008: Estimates Developed by WHO, UNICEF, UNFPA, and the World Bank. Geneva: WHO.

World Bank. 2010. *Cost-Benefit Analysis in World Bank Projects.* Independent Evaluation Group Report. Washington, DC: World Bank.

DCP3 Series Acknowledgments

Disease Control Priorities, third edition *(DCP3)* compiles the global health knowledge of institutions and experts from around the world, a task that required the efforts of over 500 individuals, including volume editors, chapter authors, peer reviewers, advisory committee members, and research and staff assistants. For each of these contributions we convey our acknowledgement and appreciation. First and foremost, we would like to thank our 31 volume editors who provided the intellectual vision for their volumes based on years of professional work in their respective fields, and then dedicated long hours to reviewing each chapter, providing leadership and guidance to authors, and framing and writing the summary chapters. We also thank our chapter authors who collectively volunteered their time and expertise to writing over 160 comprehensive, evidence-based chapters.

We owe immense gratitude to the institutional sponsor of this effort: The Bill & Melinda Gates Foundation. The Foundation provided sole financial support of the Disease Control Priorities Network. Many thanks to Program Officers Kathy Cahill, Philip Setel, Carol Medlin, and (currently) Damian Walker for their thoughtful interactions, guidance, and encouragement over the life of the project. We also wish to thank Jaime Sepulveda for his longstanding support, including chairing the Advisory Committee for the second edition and, more recently, demonstrating his vision for *DCP3* while he was a special advisor to the Gates Foundation. We are also grateful to the University of Washington's Department of Global Health and successive chairs King Holmes and Judy Wasserheit for providing a home-base for the *DCP3* Secretariat, which included intellectual collaboration, logistical coordination, and administrative support.

We thank the many contractors and consultants who provided support to specific volumes in the form of economic analytical work, volume coordination, chapter drafting, and meeting organization: the Center for Disease Dynamics, Economics, and Policy; Center for Chronic Disease Control; Center for Global Health Research; Emory University; Evidence to Policy Initiative; Public Health Foundation of India; QURE Healthcare; University of California, San Francisco; University of Waterloo; University of Queensland; and the World Health Organization.

We are tremendously grateful for the wisdom and guidance provided by our advisory committee to the editors. Steered by Chair Anne Mills, the advisory committee assures quality and intellectual rigor of the highest order for *DCP3*.

The U.S. Institute of Medicine, in collaboration with the Inter-Academy Medical Panel, coordinated the peer-review process for all *DCP3* chapters. Patrick Kelley, Gillian Buckley, Megan Ginivan, and Rachel Pittluck managed this effort and provided critical and substantive input.

The Office of the Publisher at the World Bank provided exceptional guidance and support throughout the demanding production and design process. We would particularly like to thank Carlos Rossel, the publisher; Mary Fisk, Nancy Lammers, Devlan O'Connor, Rumit Pancholi, and Deborah Naylor for their diligence and expertise. Additionally, we thank Jose de Buerba, Mario Trubiano, Yulia Ivanova, and Chiamaka Osuagwu of the World Bank for providing professional counsel on communications and marketing strategies.

Several U.S. and international institutions contributed to the organization and execution of meetings that supported the preparation and dissemination of *DCP3*.

We would like to express our appreciation to the following institutions:

- University of Bergen, consultation on equity (June 2011)
- University of California, San Francisco, surgery volume consultations (April 2012, October 2013, February 2014)
- Institute of Medicine, first meeting of the Advisory Committee to the Editors ACE (March 2013)
- Harvard Global Health Institute, consultation on policy measures to reduce incidence of noncommunicable diseases (July 2013)
- Institute of Medicine, systems strengthening meeting (September 2013)
- Center for Disease Dynamics, Economics, and Policy (Quality and Uptake meeting Sept 2013, Reproductive and maternal health volume consultation Nov 2013)
- National Cancer Institute and Union for International Cancer Control (Cancer consultation Nov. 2013)

Carol Levin provided outstanding governance for cost and cost-effectiveness analysis. Stéphane Verguet added invaluable guidance in applying and improving the extended cost-effectiveness analysis method. Shane Murphy, Zachary Olson, Elizabeth Brouwer, and Kristen Danforth provided exceptional research assistance and analytic assistance. Brianne Adderley ably managed the budget and project processes. The efforts of these individuals were absolutely critical to producing this series and we are thankful for their commitment.

Series and Volume Editors

SERIES EDITORS

Dean T. Jamison

Dean Jamison is a Senior Fellow in Global Health Sciences at the University of California, San Francisco, and an Emeritus Professor of Global Health at the University of Washington. He previously held academic appointments at Harvard University and the University of California, Los Angeles; he was an economist on the staff of the World Bank, where he was lead author of the World Bank's *World Development Report 1993: Investing in Health*. He was lead editor of *DCP2*. He holds a PhD in economics from Harvard University and is an elected member of the Institute of Medicine of the U.S. National Academy of Sciences. He recently served as Co-Chair and Study Director of *The Lancet's* Commission on Investing in Health.

Rachel Nugent

Rachel Nugent is a Research Associate Professor in the Department of Global Health at the University of Washington. She was formerly Deputy Director of Global Health at the Center for Global Development, Director of Health and Economics at the Population Reference Bureau, Program Director of Health and Economics Programs at the Fogarty International Center of the National institutes of Health, and senior economist at the Food and Agriculture Organization of the United Nations. From 1991–97, she was associate professor and department chair in economics at Pacific Lutheran University. She has advised the World Health Organization, the U.S. government, and nonprofit organizations on the economics and policy environment of noncommunicable diseases.

Hellen Gelband

Hellen Gelband is Associate Director for Policy at the Center for Disease Dynamics, Economics & Policy (CDDEP). Her work spans infectious disease, particularly malaria and antibiotic resistance, and noncommunicable disease policy, mainly in low- and middle-income countries. Before joining CDDEP, then Resources for the Future, she conducted policy studies at the (former) Congressional Office of Technology Assessment, the Institute of Medicine of the U.S. National Academies, and a number of international organizations.

Susan Horton

Susan Horton is the CIGI chair in global health economics in the Balsillie School of International Affairs at the University of Waterloo. She has worked in over 20 low- and middle-income countries and has consulted for the World Bank, the Asian Development Bank, several United Nations agencies, and the International Development Research Centre, among others. She led the paper on nutrition for the Copenhagen Consensus in 2008, when micronutrients were ranked as the top development priority. She has served as associate provost of graduate studies at the University of Waterloo, vice-president academic at Wilfrid Laurier University in Waterloo, and interim dean at the University of Toronto at Scarborough.

Prabhat Jha

Prabhat Jha is the founding director of University of Toronto's Centre for Global Health Research and University of Toronto Endowed Professor in Disease Control, Canada Research Chair at the Dalla Lana School of Public Health. He is lead investigator of the Million Death Study in India, which quantifies the causes of death and key risk factors in over two million homes over a 14-year period. He is also Scientific Director of the Statistical Alliance for Vital Events, which aims to expand reliable measurement of causes of death worldwide. He also conducts studies on epidemiology and economics of tobacco control worldwide.

Ramanan Laxminarayan

Ramanan Laxminarayan is Vice President for Research and Policy at the Public Health Foundation of India, and he directs the Center for Disease Dynamics, Economics & Policy in Washington, D.C., and New Delhi. His research deals with the integration of epidemiological models of infectious diseases and drug resistance into the economic analysis of public health problems. He was one of the key architects of the Affordable Medicines Facility for malaria, a novel financing mechanism to improve access and delay resistance to antimalarial drugs. In 2012, he created the Immunization Technical Support Unit in India, which has been credited with improving immunization coverage in the country. He teaches at Princeton University.

VOLUME EDITORS

Haile T. Debas, MD, is Director of the University of California Global Health Institute based at the University of California, San Francisco (UCSF). His career as a physician, researcher, professor, and academic leader spans more than four decades and includes positions at hospitals, medical centers, and universities in Canada and the United States. At UCSF, he served as Chair of the Department of Surgery, Dean of the School of Medicine, Vice Chancellor, Chancellor, and Founding Executive Director of Global Health Sciences. A gastrointestinal surgeon by training, he is the Maurice Galante Distinguished Professor of Surgery, Emeritus at UCSF. Dr. Debas served as the Founding Chair of the Board of Directors of the Consortium of Universities for Global Health. He is a member of the Institute of Medicine and fellow of the American Academy of Arts and Sciences.

Peter Donkor is a Professor of Oral and Maxillofacial Surgery at the Kwame Nkrumah University of Science and Technology (KNUST), Ghana. He studied at the University of Sydney, Australia, and the University of London. He has been a leader in the development of surgical training and provision of services in the West African subregion as Provost, College of Health Sciences, Pro-Vice Chancellor, and former Head, Department of Surgery at KNUST; President, Ghana Surgical Research

Society; Faculty Chief Examiner, Ghana College of Physicians and Surgeons; Council Member, West African College of Surgeons; and Chairman, Ghana Health Workforce Observatory.

Through the Ghana Cleft Foundation, a nonprofit organization that he cofounded, he provides outreach cleft surgery for remote communities throughout Ghana.

He was the Founding President of the Pan African Association for Cleft Lip and Palate and served for a number of years on the International Outreach Committee of the American Cleft Palate–Craniofacial Association and the Advisory Board of the Center for Global Health, University of Michigan.

His research collaborations include head and neck cancer, cleft lip and palate, injury, emergency care, medical education, research training, and global health. He is the Principal Investigator of the President's Emergency Plan for AIDS Relief/National Institutes of Health–funded Medical Education Partnership Initiative project on Emergency Medicine at KNUST.

Atul Gawande is a general and endocrine surgeon at Brigham and Women's Hospital in Boston, Professor in the Department of Health Policy and Management at Harvard T.H. Chan School of Public Health, and Samuel O. Thier Professor in the Department of Surgery at Harvard Medical School. He is Executive Director of Ariadne Labs, a joint center for health systems innovation, and cofounder and chairman of Lifebox, an international not-for-profit that implements systems and technologies to reduce surgical deaths globally. He is also a bestselling author and staff writer for the *New Yorker* magazine.

Dean T. Jamison. See the list of Series Editors.

Margaret E. Kruk, MD, MPH, is Associate Professor of Global Health at Harvard T.H. Chan School of Public Health. Her research focuses on health care utilization and quality, maternal health, and population preferences for health services in low-income countries. Dr. Kruk is interested in the development of novel evaluation methods for assessing the effectiveness of complex interventions and health system reforms. She collaborates with governments and academics in several African countries, most recently Ethiopia, Ghana, Liberia, Mozambique, and Tanzania. She has published more than 60 papers in peer-reviewed journals, was a Commissioner on the Global Health 2035 Lancet Commission on Investing in Health, and serves on the Institute of Medicine

Committee on Health System Strengthening. Before joining Harvard, she was Associate Professor of Health Management and Policy at the Columbia University Mailman School of Public Health and Director of the Better Health Systems Initiative. She was previously Policy Advisor for Health at the Millennium Project, an advisory body to the UN Secretary-General on the Millennium Development Goals. She holds an MD degree from McMaster University and an MPH from Harvard University.

Charles N. Mock, MD, PhD, FACS, has training as both a trauma surgeon and an epidemiologist. He worked as a surgeon in Ghana for four years, including at a rural hospital (Berekum) and at the Kwame Nkrumah University of Science and Technology (Kumasi). In 2005–07, he served as Director of the University of Washington's Harborview Injury Prevention and Research Center. In 2007–10, he worked at the World Health Organization (WHO) headquarters in Geneva, where he was responsible for developing the WHO's trauma care activities. In 2010, he returned to his position as Professor of Surgery (with joint appointments as Professor of Epidemiology and Professor of Global Health) at the University of Washington. His main interests include the spectrum of injury control, especially as it pertains to low- and middle-income countries: surveillance, injury prevention, prehospital care, and hospital-based trauma care. He is President (2013–15) of the International Association for Trauma Surgery and Intensive Care.

Contributors

Richard M. K. Adanu
School of Public Health, University of Ghana, Accra, Ghana

Sweta Adhikari
Mailman School of Public Health, Columbia University, New York, United States

Asa Ahimbisibwe
Department of Obstetrics and Gynecology, University of Western Ontario, London, Canada

Blake C. Alkire
Department of Otology and Laryngology and Department of Global Health and Social Medicine, Harvard Medical School, Cambridge, Massachusetts, United States

Joseph B. Babigumira
Department of Global Health, School of Public Health, University of Washington, Seattle, Washington, United States

Jan J. Barendregt
School of Population Health, University of Queensland, Brisbane, Australia

Jessica H. Beard
Department of Surgery, University of California, San Francisco, California, United States

Staffan Bergström
Department of Public Health Sciences, Karolinska Institute, Stockholm, Sweden

Stephen W. Bickler
Department of Surgery and Rady Children's Hospital, University of California, San Diego, California, United States

David C. Chang
Massachusetts General Hospital and Harvard Medical School, Cambridge, Massachusetts, United States

Anthony Charles
Gillings School of Global Public Health and School of Medicine, University of North Carolina at Chapel Hill, North Carolina, United States

Meena Cherian
World Health Organization, Geneva, Switzerland

Thomas Coonan
Department of Anesthesia, Pain Management, and Perioperative Medicine, Dalhousie University, Halifax, Canada

Dawit Desalegn
School of Medicine, College of Health Sciences, Addis Ababa University, Addis Ababa, Ethiopia

Catherine R. deVries
Department of Surgery and Department of Family and Preventive Medicine, School of Medicine, University of Utah, Salt Lake City, Utah

Delanyo Dovlo
Rwanda Country Office, World Health Organization, Kigali, Rwanda

Richard P. Dutton
Anesthesia Quality Institute and University of Chicago, Chicago, Illinois, United States

Mike English
KEMRI-Wellcome Trust Research Programme, Nairobi, Kenya and University of Oxford, Oxford, United Kingdom

Diana Farmer
UC Davis Children's Hospital and Department of
Surgery, University of California, Davis, California,
United States

Magda Feres
Dental Research Division, Department of
Periodontology, Guarulhos University, Sao Paulo, Brazil

Zipporah Gathuya
Department of Anaesthesia, Gertrude's Children's
Hospital, Nairobi, Kenya

Richard A. Gosselin
Department of Orthopedic Surgery, University of
California, San Francisco, California, United States

Hideki Higashi
Institute for Health Metrics and Evaluation, University
of Washington, Seattle, Washington, United States

Susan Horton
School of Public Health and Health Systems, University
of Waterloo, Waterloo, Canada

Renee Hsia
San Francisco General Hospital and
Department of Emergency Medicine, University of
California, San Francisco, California, United States

Kjell Arne Johansson
Department of Global Public Health and Primary Care,
University of Bergen, Bergen, Norway

Clark T. Johnson
Johns Hopkins University School of Medicine,
Baltimore, Maryland, United States

Timothy R. B. Johnson
Department of Obstetrics and Gynecology, University
of Michigan, Ann Arbor, Michigan, United States

Manjul Joshipura
Academy of Traumatology, Ahmedabad, India

Nicholas J. Kassebaum
Seattle Children's Hospital and
Institute for Health Metrics and Evaluation, University
of Washington, Seattle, Washington, United States

Ramanan Laxminarayan
Center for Disease Dynamics, Economics & Policy and
Public Health Foundation of India, Washington, DC,
United States and New Delhi, India

Carol Levin
Department of Global Health, School of Public
Health, University of Washington, Seattle, Washington,
United States

Katrine Lofberg
Department of Surgery, Oregon Health Sciences
University, Portland, Oregon, United States

Svjetlana Lozo
Division of Global Health and Human Rights,
Massachusetts General Hospital, Boston, Massachusetts,
United States

Jackie Mabweijano
Mulago National Referral Hospital, Kampala, Uganda

Colin McCord
Columbia University (retired)

Barbara McPake
School of Population and Global Health, University
of Melbourne, Melbourne, Australia

Kelly McQueen
Department of Anesthesiology, Vanderbilt
University Medical Center, Nashville, Tennessee,
United States

John G. Meara
Harvard Medical School and
Department of Plastic and Oral Surgery, Boston
Children's Hospital, Boston, Massachusetts, United States

Nyengo Mkandawire
Department of Surgery, College of Medicine,
University of Malawi, Blantyre, Malawi and
School of Medicine, Flinders University, Adelaide,
Australia

Mark A. Morgan
Department of Obstetrics and Gynecology, University
of Pennsylvania Health System, Philadelphia,
Pennsylvania, United States

Mulu Muleta Bedane
Women and Health Alliance International and
University of Gondar, Gondar, Ethiopia

Arindam Nandi
Center for Disease Dynamics, Economics & Policy,
Washington, DC, United States

Richard Niederman
College of Dentistry, New York University, New York,
United States

Emilia V. Noormahomed
Department of Microbiology, Eduardo Mondlane
University, Maputo, Mozambique

Florian R. Nuevo
Department of Anesthesiology, University of Santo
Tomas Hospital and Philippine Heart Center, Manila
and Quezon City, the Philippines

Eyitope Ogunbodede
Faculty of Dentistry, Obafemi Awolowo University,
Ile-Ife, Nigeria

Michael Ohene-Yeboah
Komfo Anokye Teaching Hospital and
Department of Surgery, Kwame Nkrumah University
of Science and Technology, Kumasi, Ghana

Andrew Ottaway
Hobart Anaesthetic Group, Hobart, Australia

Doruk Ozgediz
Department of Surgery, Yale University School of
Medicine, New Haven, Connecticut, United States

Caetano Pereira
Ministry of Health, Mozambique and
Department of Obstetrics and Gynecology,
Central Hospital, Maputo, Mozambique

Mary Lake Polan
Department of Obstetrics, Gynecology, and
Reproductive Medicine, Yale University School of
Medicine, New Haven, Connecticut, United States

N. Venkatesh Prajna
Aravind Eye Hospital, Madurai, India

Raymond R. Price
Intermountain Healthcare and
Department of Surgery and Department of Family and
Preventive Medicine, University of Utah, Salt Lake City,
Utah, United States

Shankar Prinja
Post Graduate Institute of Medical Education and
Research, Chandigarh, India

Thulasiraj D. Ravilla
Lions Aravind Institute of Community Ophthalmology,
Madurai, India

Eduardo Romero Hicks
Ministry of Health of Guanajuato, Guanajuato, Mexico

Sarah Russell
Mailman School of Public Health, Columbia University,
New York, United States

William P. Schecter
San Francisco General Hospital and
Department of Surgery, University of California,
San Francisco, California, United States

Mark G. Shrime
Interfaculty Initiative in Health Policy, Harvard
University, Cambridge, Massachusetts, United States

Nicole Sitkin
Department of Surgery, University of California, Davis,
California, United States

Ambereen Sleemi
Mailman School of Public Health, Columbia
University, New York, United States and
Eritrean Women's Project, Mendefera, Eritrea

David Spiegel
Children's Hospital of Philadelphia and
University of Pennsylvania School of Medicine,
Philadelphia, Pennsylvania, United States

Sathish Srinivasan
University Hospital Ayr and
Ayrshire Eye Clinic and Laser Centre, Ayr, Scotland

Andy Stergachis
School of Public Health, University of Washington,
Seattle, Washington, United States

Amardeep Thind
Schulich School of Medicine and Dentistry, University
of Western Ontario, London, Canada

Stéphane Verguet
T.H. Chan School of Public Health, Harvard University,
Cambridge, Massachusetts, United States

Jeffrey R. Vincent
Nicholas School of the Environment, Sanford
School of Public Policy, Duke University, Durham,
North Carolina, United States

Michael Vlassoff
Guttmacher Institute, New York, United States

Johan von Schreeb
Department of Public Health Sciences, Karolinska
Institute, Stockholm, Sweden

Theo Vos
Institute for Health Metrics and Evaluation, University
of Washington, Seattle, Washington, United States

Thomas G. Weiser
Department of Surgery, Stanford University School of
Medicine, Stanford, California, United States

Iain H. Wilson
Royal Devon and Exeter Hospital, Exeter, United
Kingdom

Ahmed Zakariah
National Ambulance Service, Accra, Ghana

Advisory Committee to the Editors

Reviewers

Wame Baravilala
United Nations Population Fund, Pacific Sub-Regional Office, Suva, Fiji Islands

Chibuike Ogwuegbu Chigbu
University of Nigeria Teaching Hospital, Enugu, Nigeria

Usuf M. E. Chikte
Stellenbosch University, Stellenbosch, South Africa

Kathryn Chu
Harvard Medical School, Cambridge, Massachusetts, United States

Michael Cotton
University Hospital of Lausanne (CHUV), Lausanne, Switzerland

Blami Dao
Jhpiego, an affiliate of Johns Hopkins University, Baltimore, Maryland, United States

Moses Galukande
Makerere University College of Health Sciences, Kampala, Uganda

Raul Garcia
Boston University, Boston, Massachusetts, United States

Sarah Greenberg
Harvard Medical School, Cambridge, Massachusetts, United States

John S. Greenspan
University of California, San Francisco, California, United States

Caris Grimes
King's College London Centre for Global Health, London, United Kingdom

Russell Gruen
Monash University and
The Alfred Hospital, Melbourne, Australia

Jaymie Henry
Global Alliance for Surgical, Obstetric, Trauma, and Anaesthesia Care (G4 Alliance), San Francisco, California, United States

Dhruv S. Kazi
University of California, San Francisco, California, United States

Robert Lane
International Federation of Surgical Colleges, Southampton, United Kingdom

Andrew Leather
King's College London Centre for Global Health, London, United Kingdom

Jenny Löfgren
Umeå University, Umeå, Sweden

Jane Maraka
East of England Deanery, Cambridge, United Kingdom

Kelly McQueen
Vanderbilt University Medical Center, Nashville, Tennessee, United States

Mahesh C. Misra
All India Institute of Medical Sciences, New Delhi, India

Sam W. Moore
Stellenbosch University, Stellenbosch, South Africa

Pär Nordin
Umeå University, Umeå, Sweden

Ebenezer Anno Nyako
University of Ghana Dental School, Accra, Ghana

Akinyinka O. Omigbodun
University of Ibadan, Ibadan, Nigeria

Chris Oppong
Derriford Hospital, Plymouth, United Kingdom

Doruk Ozgediz
Yale University School of Medicine, New Haven,
Connecticut, United States

Norgrove Penny
The University of British Columbia, Vancouver, Canada

Dan Poenaru
Queens University, Kingston, Canada

Teri Reynolds
University of California, San Francisco, California,
United States

Matthias Richter-Turtur
Isar Klinikum, Munich, Germany

Percy Eduardo Rossell-Perry
San Martin de Porres University, Lima, Peru

Andrés Rubiano
South Colombian University, Neiva, Colombia

Iskender Sayek
Hacettepe University Faculty of Medicine, Ankara,
Turkey

Lawrence Sherman
University of Liberia, Monrovia, Liberia

Samuel D. Shillcutt
Johns Hopkins Bloomberg School of Public Health,
Baltimore, Maryland, United States

K. M. Shyamprasad
Martin Luther Christian University, Shillong, India

Hugh R. Taylor
University of Melbourne, Melbourne, Australia

Nitin Verma
University of Tasmania School of Medicine, Hobart,
Australia

L. Lewis Wall
Washington University in St. Louis, St. Louis, Missouri,
United States

Lee Wallis
African Federation of Emergency Medicine, Bellville,
South Africa

Benjamin C. Warf
Harvard Medical School, Cambridge, Massachusetts,
United States

David Watters
Deakin University and Barwon Health, Geelong,
Australia

Andreas Wladis
Karolinska Institute, Stockholm, Sweden

Gavin Yamey
University of California, San Francisco, California,
United States

Index

Boxes, figures, maps, notes, and tables are denoted by b, f, m, n, and t respectively.

Agency for Healthcare Research and Quality (AHRQ), 21, 22
age weighting for benefit-cost analysis, 365
aging population
    blindness and, 197, 199
    cataracts and, 202
    changing demographics, 206
    oral health maladies and, 173
    orthopedics and, 52, 53
    specialty surgical hospitals and, 237
agricultural livelihood, obstetric fistula's effect on women and, 99, 100, 103
Ahimbisibwe, A., 109
AHRQ (Agency for Healthcare Research and Quality), 21, 22
AIDS. *See* HIV/AIDS
airway management during anesthesia, 266
Akoko, L., 154
alcoholic cirrhosis of liver, 64
Alkire, B. C., 361, 363–64
ambulances. *See* prehospital and emergency care; transport of patients
American Board of Surgery, 61
American College of Obstetrics and Gynecology, 90
American Osteopathic Association, Division of State Government Affairs, 309
American Society of Anesthesiologists, 268, 273b, 280
AMOs (assistant medical officers). *See* nonphysician clinicians; Tanzania
amputation, 46, 54, 219–20t, 291–92t, 340t, 354
anesthesia services, 263–78
    accredited professionals, 295t
    airway management, 266
    anesthetist physician assistant programs, 310
    barriers to safe, 265–67
    burden of disease averted by, 263–66
    cardiac perturbations, 266
    cost-effectiveness of techniques, 268–70
    costs of, 268, 269t, 270–72
    data collection related to, 274
    definitions of terms related to technology and patient care, 265
    emergency surgery, 70
    first-level hospitals, 220, 225
    future directions of treatment, 272–74
    hernia repair, 157
    Ketamine, 225, 228n1
    medicines essential for, 268–70, 269t
    mortality rate associated with, 13, 265, 267–68, 267f, 268t, 273–74, 288, 289f
    nurse anesthetists, 310
    overview, 263
    pain management, 266–67
    patient safety, 266–68, 272–74, 291–92

perioperative period, 265, 266–67
pulse oximetry, use of, 13, 292
quality improvement, 73, 273–74, 273b, 291–92
research needs, 274
safety of, 2, 13, 265, 266–68, 269t, 272, 288
shortage of anesthesiologists, 8
standards of practice, 291–92
task-sharing, 272–73, 272t
training of providers, 270–73, 271t
unmet need for, 263, 264m, 265
vigilance, defined, 265
aneurysm repair, 291t
Annan, Kofi, 91
anorectal malformations (ARMs)
    case study, 135–36
    prevalence and mortality rates, 131t, 136
antibiotic use
    burn care, 52
    cataract surgery, 202
    eye infections, 201
    oral disease, 179–81
Apollo Hospital (India), 253b
appendicitis/appendectomy, 23, 63, 72, 219–20t, 340t
    mortality rate following, 283, 284–85t, 285
Apridec Medical Outreach Group, 158–59b
Aravind Eye Hospital (India), 201, 203, 233, 238
ARMs. *See* anorectal malformations
arteriosclerosis, 66, 225
arthritis, 53, 54t
Asia. *See also specific countries and regions*
    abortion complications in, 120
    blindness in, 197
    burn injuries and care in, 354
    contraception, unmet need in, 112
assistant medical officers (AMOs). *See* nonphysician clinicians; Tanzania
associate clinicians. *See* nonphysician clinicians
Association of Anaesthetists of Great Britain and Ireland, 73
asthma, 246
astigmatism, 202
Australia
    anesthesia-related mortality in, 267
    cataract-related blindness in, 198
    cataract surgery in, 199, 204
    cost-effectiveness studies in, 320
    trauma care systems in, 43, 46
autoimmune diseases, 53

B

Babbar Ruga Fistula Teaching Hospital (Nigeria), 232, 237, 238
Babigumira, J. B., 109
Babu, B. V., 164

Baek, R. M., 324
Bainbridge, D., 288
Baltussen, R., 327
banana leaves as burn treatment, 51
Banerjee, A. V., 184
Bangladesh
    burn care in, 50
    cataract surgery in, 328
    DALYs averted by emergency surgery in, 68–69b
    district (first-level) hospitals in, 215, 217,
        217–18t, 219
        costs of care, 222
    obstetric care costs in, 20
    obstetric fistula in, 99
    trauma care system in, 45
Barendregt, J. J., 19
barriers to service delivery. See also access to care
    abortion and postabortion care, 120
    anesthesia, 265–66
    cataract surgery, 202–3, 353
    emergency surgeries, 73
    family planning, 113
    first-level hospitals, 226–27
    obstetric services, 353
    oral health care, 183b, 188
    poverty, 353–57
    surgical care, 8–9, 287–90, 287f
Bayalpata Hospital (Nepal), financial sustainability
        of, 330b
BCA. See benefit-cost analysis
Beard, J. H., 61, 151, 153, 154, 155, 160
Bedane, M. M., 95
Bellagio Essential Surgery Group, 368
benefit-cost analysis (BCA), 7, 361–80
    advantages of, 368–69
    age weighting, 365–66
    cesarean delivery, 83–84, 84t, 87, 370–76, 372–73t
    cleft lip and palate repair, 7, 329, 363–70, 367t
    discounting, 365–66
    future directions for research, 369
    global health interventions, 362–63
    limitations of study, 369, 376
    methods for modeling, 364, 370
    overview, 361
    recommendations for, 367–68
    results, 367
    value of a statistical life (VSL), 362–63
Berger, P., 152
Bergström, S., 307
BethanyKids, 140
Bickler, S. W., 19, 318
biopsies, 21
Birkmeyer, J. D., 290
birth defects. See congenital anomalies

bleeding
    during childbirth, 77, 80, 81, 83
    from esophageal varices, 64
    traumatic injuries and, 49
    ulcers and, 64, 225
blindness. See also cataracts
    costs of, 197–98, 328
    disparities between LMICs and HICs, 355
    expenditures to prevent, 206, 206f
    global challenge of, 197–98
    prevalence of, 197, 206
    risk factors for, 197
    trends in reduction of, 206–7
    visual acuity scale, 197, 198t
blood transfusion, 82
Bloom, D., 361
Bloom, N., 294
Bolivia, first-level hospitals in, 217, 217–18t, 218
bone fractures. See traumatic injuries
bone infections. See infections
Bradley, S., 309
brain drain. See shortage of skilled surgeons
Brazil
    blindness in, 197
    filarial hydrocelectomy in, 165, 166
    hospital management practices in, 294
    lymphatic filariasis in, 164
    tooth paste fluoridation in, 179
    water fluoridation in, 177–78
breech birth. See cesarean delivery; obstetric conditions
Bretlau, P., 234
Broder, S., 354
Brown, M. M., 206
Browning, A., 100, 237, 238
burden of disease, 20–35. See also disability-adjusted
        life years (DALYs); mortality rate
    acute abdominal conditions, 61
    anesthesia services, 263–66
    avertable burden, 6, 6–7t, 7f
        calculation of, 24–25
        research and development on, 35–36
        by scaling up subspecialty surgical care, 28–32, 33t
    burn injuries, 49–50
    cataract, 28, 30, 198–99, 198f, 355
    congenital anomalies, 129, 133–35, 134t, 143, 363
    definition of, 124n12
    emergency surgery, 61–62, 66–67, 221
    family planning and reduction of, 110
    first-level hospitals and surgically treatable disease,
        23, 221
    "global burden of disease," use of term, xi
    hernia, 153–55, 155t
    hydrocele, 162–64
    lymphatic filariasis, 162–64, 163m

obstetric procedures, 87–88, 331*t*, 355–56
oral health care, 187
patient bearing, 12. *See also* catastrophic health spending
prehospital and emergency care, 252–54
sterilization, 116, 117*t*
surgical interventions, 329–31, 331*t*
surgical unit costs, 329–31
transport of patients, 8, 214–15, 285, 288
Council on Health Research for Development, 259
cultural beliefs
abortions and, 120
contraception use and, 111, 113
delay in seeking surgical care due to, 287
filarial hydroceles and, 164
lymphatic filariasis and, 164
obstetric fistula and, 97, 98, 99–100
obstetric procedures and, 88
CURE network, 140

D
DALYs. *See* disability-adjusted life years
Das, J., 290
data collection challenges
anesthesia services, 274
congenital anomalies, 130, 143
cost-effectiveness, 331–32
Debas, H. T., xvi, 1, 20, 61, 67, 215, 222
de Buys Roessingh, A. S., 234
delays in treatment
burn treatment, 50–52
cataracts, 199
congenital anomalies, 130–33, 135–36, 138, 143
emergency care, 259
infant mortality due to, 64, 80
infections as result of, 54
obstetric care, 81, 83, 88
obstetric fistula, 102
surgical care, 285, 287–88
"demographic dividend," 110, 123*n*4
dentistry. *See* oral health maladies
dermatological conditions. *See* skin
Desalegn, D., 339
deVries, C. R., 151
deworming, 184, 185*b*
diabetes
amputation and, 46
cataracts and, 199, 202
cost-effectiveness of treatment, 225
obstetric complications and, 80
oral health and, 179, 180
treatable in prehospital and emergency care, 246
diaphragmatic hernia, congenital, 133*t*

digestive diseases
burden avertable by surgery for, 23, 28, 28*f*
DALYs averted by, 25, 27*t*
deaths prevented by, 25, 26*t*
burden nonavertable by surgical care for, 28, 29*t*
surgery for, 26–27*t*. *See also* appendicitis/appendectomy
dilation and curettage (D&C), 121. *See also* abortion
Dimick, J. B., 290
disability-adjusted life years (DALYs). *See also* burden of disease
assignment to surgical procedures, 22–23
burn injuries, 49, 52
calculating for benefit-cost analysis, 9*b*, 365
averted to economic benefit, 366–67
cataracts, 204, 355
by cause (global), 67, 67*t*
cesarean delivery for obstructed labor, 370, 371–72
congenital anomalies, 129–30
contraceptive surgeries and abortions, 116
converting VSL methodology into, 362
definition of, 20
emergency surgery, 66–67, 67*t*, 68–69*b*
GBD 2010 use of, 20
hernias, 154–55
hydrocele, 163
lymphatic filariasis, 163, 163*m*
obstetric complications, 78–79, 78*t*
obstetric fistula, 101
oral disease, 174–75, 175–76*t*
prehospital and emergency care, conditions treatable in, 246–47, 247*f*
short-term surgical missions, treatment by, 235, 239
surgical interventions, effect on, 7–8, 8*f*, 20, 24–25, 27*t*, 28*f*, 221, 222–24, 281, 319
disabled persons, rehabilitation for, 46
disease burden. *See* burden of disease
Disease Control Priorities in Developing Countries, second edition (*DCP2*), xi–xii, 3*b*, 41, 62, 213, 245
disparities between LMICs and HICs
anesthesia, mortality rate associated with, 13
anesthesiologists, 8–9
anorectal malformations (ARMs), 136
blindness, 355
burden of disease, 353–55
burn injuries, 50, 354
cancer, 354–55
cataract surgery, 200, 355
cesarean delivery, 285, 355
mortality rates, 13
cleft lip and palate repair, 364
congenital anomalies, 130, 134

obstetric procedures in, 87, 89–90
  costs, 101, 356
prehospital and emergency care in, 252
short-term surgical missions in, 233
surgical costs in, 329
trauma care system in, 45, 250*b*
  prehospital mortality, 8
vehicle accident victims, deaths of, 221
Ghana College of Physicians and Surgeons, 12
Ghana Hernia Society (GHS), 158–59*b*
GIEESC. *See* Global Initiative for Emergency and
  Essential Surgical Care
Gilbert, M., 249
gingivitis. *See* oral health maladies
Glasgow Coma Score, 48
Global Burden of Diseases, Injuries, and Risk Factors
  Study 2010 (GBD 2010), 20
  on abortion-related deaths, 120
  burden estimates based on, 23–24
    limitations of methodology, 32
  distinguishing between surgical and nonsurgical
    conditions in, 21, 22*f*
  epidemiological regions and superregions, 24, 24*t*
  on hernia-related DALYs, 154
  on maternal mortality and morbidity, 110
  subspecialty surgical care, types of, 28–29
  on tooth decay, 174
*Global Competency-Based Fistula Surgery Training
  Manual* (International Federation of Gynecology
  and Obstetrics et al.), 103
Global Forum for Health Research, 259
Global Fund to Fight AIDS, Tuberculosis and Malaria,
  33, 34*f*
Global Health 2035 targets, 37
Global Initiative for Emergency and Essential Surgical
  Care (GIEESC), 23, 45, 333
Global Programme to Eliminate Lymphatic Filariasis
  (GPELF), 151, 164
Gogate, P., 201, 202
Goh, J., 99, 100
Goldacre, M. J., 157
Goldmann, E., 328
Gosselin, R. A., 35, 41, 51, 321, 328
gout, 53
GPELF (Global Programme to Eliminate Lymphatic
  Filariasis), 151, 164
Greenland, 234
Grimes, C. E., 155
groin hernia, 151–61. *See also* inguinal hernia
  access to care for, 155–56
  burden of disease due to, 154–55
  clinical features of, 152–53
  cost-effectiveness of repair, 161

definition of, 151
future directions of treatment, 166
mortality rate, 159–60
overview, 151
reducible, 152
repair complications, 157
risk factors for, 152
strangulated, 152
types of, 151–52
gum disease. *See* oral health maladies
Gundre, N. P., 326
Guwahati Comprehensive Cleft Care Center (GCCCC,
  India), 364, 367–68, 367*t*, 369
GVK Emergency Management and Research Institute
  (India), 253*b*
gynecology. *See* obstetric conditions; obstetric fistula

H
Haiti
  cesarean delivery rate in, 280
  costs of surgical care in, 329
    first-level hospital care, 222
  filarial hydrocelectomy in, 166
  lymphatic filariasis in, 164
  trauma, young-adult deaths from, xi
  trauma care system in, 46, 328
    cost-effectiveness of, 321
Haiti earthquake (2010), 28
Hamlin, E. C., 237
Hammitt, J. K., 369
Hanoi Health Department, 12
Hatcher, K. W., 324, 363
head injuries, 47–48, 220*t*
Healing Hands for Haiti, 46
health centers
  availability of, 287
  childbirth care at, 323
  prehospital and emergency care provided by, 252
  primary care, 215
  surgical services provided by, 4–5*t*, 220–21,
    226–27
health insurance. *See* national health plans; universal
  health coverage
health workforce. *See also* nonphysician clinicians;
  shortage of skilled surgeons
  distribution of skilled personnel, 71
  obstetric fistula care, 105
heart disease and heart attacks. *See also* cardiac
  surgery
  prehospital and emergency care, 246, 254
Heitto, M., 321
hemorrhage. *See* bleeding
hemothorax, 65

mortality rate, 279–85, 280f. *See also* burden of disease
   acute abdominal conditions as cause, 61
   anesthesia related, 13, 265, 267–68, 267f, 268t,
      273–74, 288, 289f
   barriers to care as factor for, 287–88
   cesarean delivery, 13, 283, 283–84t
   challenges to reducing, 285–87
   conditions treatable in prehospital and emergency
      care to lower, 246, 247f
   congenital anomalies, 129–33, 131–33t
   disparities between LMICs and HICs in, 283–85
   emergency surgery, 67
   hernia and, 157, 159–60, 283, 285, 286t
   hip fractures and, 53
   improvements in health care practices, effect on,
      291–97
   increased surgical access and, 283
   maternal. *See* maternal morbidity and mortality
   methodology of study, 281–82
   noma, 181
   postoperative care and safety, 290–91, 296t
   rates of, 279–85
   results of study, 282–85
   short-term surgical missions, 234
   strategies for reducing, 291–97
   surgically treatable conditions and, 6, 19,
      25–28, 317
   traumatic injuries, 43
      prehospital, 8
      young-adult deaths, xi
   vehicle accident victims, 221
mosquito-borne parasites, 162, 164
mosquito netting for hernia repair, 157
mouth. *See* oral health maladies
Mozambique
   costs of emergency surgical care in, 68
   first-level hospitals in, 214b
   hernia repair in, 160
   medical training in, 218
   Ministry of Health human resources plan, 313
   obstetric procedures in, 86, 87
   shortage of skilled surgeons in, 307, 308
   técnicos de cirurgia (TCs–nonphysician clinicians)
      in, 12, 309, 310
      acceptability of, 311
      cost-effectiveness, 312–13
      enabling environment, 313
      job satisfaction, 312
      procedures performed by, 310
      retention incentives, 311
      training, 37, 218
      working and living conditions, 312
MSK. *See* musculoskeletal system

Muleta, M., 237
Mullan, F., 309
multiple gestation, 80
Murad, M. K., 254
Muralikrishnan, R., 203, 204
musculoskeletal (MSK) system
   disparities between LMICs and HICs, 354
   infections, 66
   nontraumatic conditions, 53–54, 54t
   surgical procedures performed on, 2
   traumatic injuries, 49, 52–53. *See also* traumatic
      injuries

N
Nandi, A., 317
National Health and Nutrition Examination Survey
   (NHANES), 152, 153
national health plans, xv, 228
National Institute for Health and Care Excellence of
   British National Health Service, 226
Nayak, A. N., 164
neonatal conditions. *See* maternal-neonatal conditions
Nepal
   blindness in, 197
   cataract surgery in, 204, 327
   cleft lip and palate repair in, 327, 363
   financial sustainability of first-level hospital in, 330b
   fluoridation in, 179
   oral health care in, 183b
Netherlands
   mortality rates in
      cesarean delivery, 283
      surgery, 279
   surgical safety checklist, use in, 293
   trauma care systems in, 43
Neuhauser, D., 152
neural tube defects, 12–14, 28, 133, 134t
neurological disabilities, 98
Nevado del Huila volcano (1985), 258b
NGOs. *See* nongovernmental organizations
NHANES (National Health and Nutrition Examination
   Survey), 152, 153
Nicaragua
   cost-effectiveness of orthopedic procedures in, 326
   first-level hospitals in, 218
Niederman, R., 173
Niger
   cesarean delivery in
      costs of, 375
      rate of, 280
   hernia repair in, 160
   obstetric fistula in, 103
   transport options in, 251

Nigeria
    abortion cost-effectiveness in, 122, 321
    anesthesia-related mortality in, 267
    blindness in, 355
    burn care in, 50
    costs of surgical care in, 329
        first-level hospital care, 222
    head injuries in, 47, 48
    hernia repair in, 156, 160
    noma in, 181
    obstetric fistula in, 97, 98, 99, 103, 327
    orthopedic services in, 354
    prehospital and emergency care personnel training
        in, 252
    trauma care system in, 46, 328
        cost-effectiveness of, 321
noma, 174–76, 181–82
noncommunicable diseases, 3b. *See also specific*
        diseases
    superseding infectious diseases as leading cause of
        mortality, 263
nonemergency surgery. *See also specific conditions*
    cost-effectiveness, 323–27
nongovernmental organizations (NGOs)
    platforms for surgical delivery, 231–32
    return on investment to, 362
    self-contained mobile surgical platforms, 233
    short-term surgical missions, 232–36
nonphysician clinicians, 12, 37, 307–16
    acceptability of, 311
    anesthesia, 271, 271t
    cataracts, 203
    congenital anomalies, 141
    cost-effectiveness of, 12, 312–13
    emergency surgery, 71
    enabling environment, 313
    in Ethiopia, 340, 346
    financial incentives, 311
    hernia repairs, 160–61
    job satisfaction, 312
    nonfinancial incentives, 311–12
    obstetric procedures, 86–87, 89, 219, 313
    oral health maladies, 184, 185–86
    overview, 307–8
    research and development, 37
    retention incentives, 311–12
    supervision, 311–12
    task-shifting and task-sharing, 309–10
    training, 309–10, 311–12. *See also* training
    working and living conditions, 312
Noormahomed, E. V., 19
Nordin, P., 161
North Africa. *See* Middle East and North Africa

North America. *See also specific countries*
    international surgical organizations in, 231
NPCs. *See* nonphysician clinicians
Nuevo, F. R., 263
nurse anesthetists, 310
nutrition
    burn injuries healing and, 52
    oral health and, 174

O
obstetric conditions, 23, 77–94. *See also* obstetric fistula
    abnormal fetal presentation, 80
    access to surgical care for, 88
    breech presentation, 80
    burden of preventable deaths and disability, 77–79,
        221, 222
    cesarean delivery, 82–85, 88, 370–76
    challenges in providing care for, 88
    cost-effectiveness of surgery for, 83–85, 321–22t,
        321–23
    costs of surgery for, 87–88, 331t, 355–56
    disability-adjusted life years (DALYs), 78–79, 78t
    disparities between LMICs and HICs, 353–54, 355
    emergency surgery for, 20, 221, 222, 323
    episiotomy, use of, 80
    in Ethiopian study, 339, 340t
    family planning coupled with emergency services, 85
    financial burden on the poor, 355–56
    first-level hospitals, 219–20t, 221, 222
    free emergency obstetrical care, 226
    future directions of treatment, 89–91
    general practitioners performing surgery, 12
    hospital care for, 88–89, 221, 222
    lacerations, 80, 81
    maternal mortality rate (MMR) due to, xv, 77–78,
        85, 221
    models of treatment for, 89–90
    multiple gestation, 80
    nonphysician clinician training, 86–87, 313
    obstructed labor, 370–76
    overview, 79
    pelvic infections with abscesses, 64
    platform for delivery of procedure, 4t
    postpartum hemorrhage, 80. *See also* bleeding
    quality improvement of care, 89–90
    retained placenta, 81
    shoulder dystocia, 80
    subsidization of care for, 85
    surgical intervention for, 20, 219, 219–20t
    task-shifting to increase services for, 86–87
    technology and, 88
    training needs, 86–87, 88–89, 91
    transport of patients with, 88, 89

Pan-African Academy of Christian Surgeons, 140
Papua New Guinea
    short-term surgical missions in, 233
paralytic ileus, 23, 28, 38n3
paramedical personnel. *See also* nonphysician clinicians
    prehospital and emergency care, 248, 250
Patel, T. L., 237, 238
patient transport. *See* transport of patients
Pearse, R. M., 279
pediatric surgery. *See* congenital anomalies
pelvis
    infections with abscesses, 64
    traumatic injuries, 49
peptic ulcer complications, 64, 72
Pereira, C., 307
periodontitis, 174–76, 179–81. *See also* oral health
        maladies
perioperative care, 263–78. *See also* anesthesia services
    safety of, 288–90
perioperative mortality rate (POMR), 273–74
Perry, H., 324
personnel. *See also* nonphysician clinicians; shortage of
        skilled surgeons
    prehospital and emergency care, 248–50
Peru
    cataract-related blindness in, 198
    salt fluoridation in, 179
Philippines
    cataract surgery in, 328
    Fit for School program in, 184, 185b
    oral health care in, 183b
platforms for surgical delivery, 3–4, 4–5t, 231–44.
        See also self-contained mobile surgical platforms;
        short-term surgical missions; specialty surgical
        hospitals
    classification of, 232
    cost-effectiveness by type of, 235, 238–40, 327–28
    literature review, 232, 233f
    nongovernmental organizations (NGOs) as
        providers of, 231–32
    outcomes by type of, 234, 237–38
    recommendations for, 240
    sustainability, 235–36, 238
    temporary, 232–36, 238–39. *See also* short-term
        surgical missions
    training role of, 235–36, 238
pleural disease surgery, 65
pneumonia, 65
pneumothorax, 65
Poenaru, D., 35, 363
Polan, M. L., 95, 118b
POMR (perioperative mortality rate), 273–74
Ponseti method, 138

population, policy, and implementation research
        (PPIR), 12, 13, 14
population health
    subspecialty surgical care, impact on, 30–32
    surgical care, impact on, 25–28
Portugal, prehospital treatment of trauma patients
        in, 254
postabortion care, 119–21, 123
postoperative care and training, 2
    complications and mortality rate, 290–91, 291–92t,
        291f, 296t
    obstetric fistula and, 102–3
    outcomes at first-level hospitals, 222
postpartum hemorrhage, 80
postpartum tubal ligation, 113–14
poverty, 353–60. *See also* disparities between LMICs
        and HICs; *specific conditions and surgeries*
    access to care restricted by, 226, 355–57
    blindness and, 328–29
    burden of disease associated with, 353–56
    burn injuries and, 50
    contraception use and, 111
    financial burden of disease and, 355–57
    oral disease and, 181
    overview, 353
Prajna, N. V., 197
pregnancy. *See* cesarean delivery; family planning and
        contraception; obstetric conditions
prehospital and emergency care, 245–62. *See also*
        emergency surgery
    burden of disease addressable by, 245–47, 246f, 259t
    community-based care. *See* first responders
    cost-effectiveness of, 256
    costs of, 252–54
    deaths due to shortcomings of, 354
    delivery systems for, 247–50
    disparities between LMICs and HICs, 354, 354t
    effectiveness of, 254–55
    equipment and supplies, 251–52
    financing of, 257
    future directions, 256–57
    health facility-based subsystems, 252
    lay first responders, 249, 249b. *See also* first
        responders
    legislation to address, 257, 258b
    notification time, 251
    overview, 245
    paramedical personnel, 248, 250
    personnel roles in, 248–50
    research and development priorities, 257–59
    response time, 251
    scene time, 251
    systems organization, 256–57

affordability of, xv, 28, 288
availability of, xv, 287–88, 287*f*
barriers to service delivery. *See* barriers to service delivery
basic/essential, xv, 23–28, 38*n*2
best practices for LMICs, 37
burden averted value of, 22–35. *See also* burden of disease
checklists for safety, 1, 13–14, 292–95, 293*f*
definition of, 2, 20–21, 21*b*
delays in seeking, 285, 287–88
economic evaluation of, 7, 9*b*
emergencies, 61–76
in Ethiopia study, 340, 340*t*
future directions of treatment, 35–37, 36*f*
intervention categories, 19–20
low- and-middle-income countries (LMICs), need in, 19
models of treatment, 35–37
mortality rate associated with. *See* mortality rate
number of surgeries worldwide, 279, 317
operation, definition of, 21
platform for delivery of procedure, 4*t*. *See also* platforms for surgical delivery
primary health care to include, 35
research and development on, 36–37
priority as global health initiative, 32–33, 34*f*, 37
public health impact of, xv, 19–20, 23, 33
research and development, 35–37
role in global health, 10–11*m*, 19–20, 35
strategies for improving, 291–97
subspecialty, 28, 30–32
surgical sequelae, definition of, 21*b*
surgical trips, 232–35, 238–39
congenital anomalies, 140
sustainability
cataract surgery delivery systems, 203
first-level hospitals, scaling up of, 330*b*
platforms for surgical delivery and, 238
short-term surgical missions, 235–36
specialty surgical hospitals, 238
Sweden
cataract surgery in, 205
hernia repair in, 159, 161, 283
mortality rate following cesarean delivery in, 13, 283
Swedish Hernia Register, 152

T
Tanzania
assistant medical officers (AMOs), 12, 218, 309
cost-effectiveness, 313
enabling environment, 313
job satisfaction, 312

procedures performed by, 310
research on attitudes toward, 311
retention incentives, 311–12
working and living conditions, 312
cesarean delivery auditing in, 310
congenital anomalies treatment in, 142
costs of emergency surgical care in, 68
employment freezes on health personnel, 307
faith-based hospitals in, 218
first-level hospitals in, 214*b*, 215, 217–18*t*, 218, 219
hernia repair in, 152, 153, 155, 156*t*, 160
infrastructure shortcomings as impediment to emergency and surgical care in, 252
lymphatic filariasis in, 162–63
obstetric fistula in, 95, 101
obstetric procedures in, 86, 87, 89
oral health care in, 183*b*
prehospital and emergency care in, 252
shortage of skilled surgeons in, 307, 308
task-sharing and task-shifting. *See also* nonphysician clinicians
anesthesia services, 272–73, 272*t*
cost-effectiveness of, 323
in Ethiopia study, 339–49
inguinal hernia, 160–61
nonphysician clinicians, 1, 309–10
obstetric conditions, 86–87
public finance vs., 339–52
technology. *See also* telemedicine
emergency surgery, 71–73
first-level hospitals, 224, 225, 227
obstetric procedures, 88
técnicos de cirurgia (TCs). *See* Mozambique; nonphysician clinicians
teeth. *See* oral health maladies
telecommunications services, 250–51
telemedicine
burn injuries, evaluation of, 52
congenital anomalies and, 139–40*t*, 141, 144*n*6
exclusion from platform discussion, 232
obstetric procedures and, 88
Thailand
mobile dental clinics in, 184
short-term surgical missions in, 234
trauma care system in, 46, 47*b*
quality improvement programs, 295
Thind, A., 20, 245
third-level hospitals
congenital anomalies treatment, 143
ideal, requirements for, 216–17*t*
levels of care, 214*b*
properly functioning, 213
surgeries, type performed at, 4–5*t*, 281
thorax injuries, 48

von Schreeb, J., 213
Vos, T., 19

W
Waaldijk, K., 97, 98
Warriner, I. K., 309
water fluoridation, 177–80, 178t, 184
Weiser, T. G., 19, 279, 328
Wendel, E., 327
West African College of Surgeons, 70
West African Filariasis Program, 166
western diet, causing need for more surgery, 66
WFSA. *See* World Federation of Societies of
    Anaesthesiologists
WHA. *See* World Health Assembly
WHO. *See* World Health Organization
Wilhelm, T. J., 160
Wilson, I. H., 263
Wisborg, T., 249
Wittenborn, J. S., 327
women. *See* childbirth; family planning and
    contraception; obstetric conditions; obstetric
    fistula
Women and Health Alliance International, 103
Women's Dignity Project and Engender Health, 95
workforce innovations, 307–16. *See also* nonphysician
    clinicians
workforce shortage. *See* shortage of skilled surgeons
working and living conditions
    nonphysician clinicians, 312
    obstetric fistula and, 99–100
World Bank
    benefit-cost analysis used by, 362
    on cost-effectiveness of cataract surgery, 207
World Development Report (1993), 3b
World Federation of Societies of Anaesthesiologists, 73,
    268, 273, 292
World Health Assembly (WHA)
    on people with disabilities, 46
    Resolution 50.29 on lymphatic filariasis, 164
    Resolution 60.22, 41
    on trauma and emergency care, 47
World Health Organization (WHO)
    on abortion safety, 119, 321
    on annual number of surgical operations performed
        globally, 279
    Basic Package of Oral Health Care, 174, 177, 183–
        84b, 185
    on burn care education, 354
    on cataracts and cataract surgery, 198, 201, 203
    on cesarean delivery rates, 79, 86
    on congenital anomalies, 133
    on cost-effectiveness, 367
    Emergency and Essential Surgical Care (EESC)

Project, 9, 23, 333
    on first responders' role, 249, 249b
    Global Alliance for Care of the Injured, 41
    Global Health Estimates, 6, 66, 133, 204, 245, 263
    Global Initiative for Emergency and Essential
        Surgical Care (GIEESC), 2, 23, 45, 333
    Integrated Management of Childhood Illness, 143
    on maternal mortality, 308
    on minimum standards for emergency and surgical
        care, 12, 252, 281
    Monitoring the Building Blocks of Health Systems
        Monitoring and Evaluation Matrix, 36–37
    on nonphysician clinicians, 309
    objectives of health systems, 339
    on obstetric fistula repair, 103
    on obstructed labor, 370
    Patient Safety Pulse Oximetry project, 73
    on properly functioning hospitals, 213
    on quality improvement programs for trauma
        care, 295
    rheumatic disease, community-oriented program
        for, 53
    on rising health costs, 206
    SAFE program, 355
    on standardized metrics for surgical
        surveillance, 279
    Surgical Safety Checklist, 1, 13–14, 292, 293f
    Tool for Situational Analysis to Assess Emergency
        and Essential Surgical Care, 54, 143
    on tooth decay, 174
    trauma care guidelines, 9, 44
    on universal health coverage, 346
    on vaginal delivery, 79
    VISION 2020 Right to Sight initiative, 206, 326–27
    WHO Model List of Essential Medicines, 266, 268, 270
    World Health Report, 333
worms, 63–64, 162

X
Xu, K., 328

Y
years lived with disability (YLD)
    benefit-cost analysis and, 365
    conditions treatable in prehospital and emergency
        care, effect on, 246, 248f
    DALYs and, 20
    scaling up surgical care, impact of, 24–25, 30
years of life lost (YLL)
    benefit-cost analysis and, 365
    conditions treatable in prehospital and emergency
        care, effect on, 246–47, 248f
    DALYs and, 20
    scaling up surgical care, impact of, 24–25, 30

ECO-AUDIT
Environmental Benefits Statement

The World Bank is committed to preserving endangered forests and natural resources. ***Essential Surgery: Disease Control Priorities,*** **third edition, volume 1** was printed on recycled paper with 100 percent postconsumer fiber in accordance with the recommended standards for paper usage set by the Green Press Initiative, a nonprofit program supporting publishers in using fiber that is not sourced from endangered forests. For more information, visit www .greenpressinitiative.org.

Saved:
- 19 trees
- 9 million British thermal units of total energy
- 1,656 pounds of CO_2 equivalent of greenhouse gases
- 8,980 gallons of waste water
- 601 pounds of solid waste

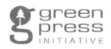